PRACTICAL TRADITIONAL CHINESE MEDICINE

By Prof. Xie Zhufan

FOREIGN LANGUAGES PRESS

First Edition 2000

Home Page:
http://www.flp.com.cn
Email Address:
Info@flp.com.cn
Sales@flp.com.cn

ISBN 7-119-02375-6

Published by Foreign Languages Press
24 Baiwanzhuang Road, Beijing 100037, China
Distributed by China International Book Trading Corporation
35 Chegongzhuang Xilu, Beijing 100044, China
P.O. Box 399, Beijing, China

Printed in the People's Republic of China

CONTENTS

PREFACE

Professor Xie Zhufan is a leading specialist in the area of integrating Chinese and Western medicine. He graduated from the Medical College of Peking University. Since then, he has been working at the First Hospital affiliated to the College as visiting physician, lecturer, associate professor and professor of the Department of Internal (Western) Medicine. In 1955, 1958-59, and 1969-70 he received full-time or part-time in-service training in traditional Chinese medicine (TCM) and engaged in the integration of TCM and Western medicine. In 1970, he was appointed as the chairman of the Department of Traditional Chinese Medicine, and then director of the Institute for Integration of Chinese and Western Medicine. Now, he is the honorary director of the institute. Professor Xie has been invited to teach traditional Chinese medicine in foreign countries on many occasions. He has also worked for the World Health Organization in the field of research and promotion of traditional medicine.

For the purpose of introducing Chinese medicine to Western physicians and foreign friends with medical knowledge but without Chinese language proficiency, he wrote *Practical Traditional Chinese Medicine* in English, based on his decades of clinical and teaching experience and his own understanding of the traditional Chinese medical theories. This book is of very high academic value, and will be of help to people abroad, particularly to medical professionals, who wish to understand Chinese medicine, and facilitate the introduction of Chinese medicine to the rest of the world.

Traditional Chinese medicine is known as the crystallization of the wisdom of the Chinese people achieved in their long-term efforts for treating diseases. For thousands of years, this system of medicine has made indelible contributions to the prosperity of the Chinese nation. Now, it represents the advantage and distinguishing feature of Chinese health care, in coordination with modern medicine. At the same time, traditional Chinese medicine has also had a notable impact on the health of mankind and the culture of the world.

Traditional Chinese medicine was established on the basic concepts of the correspondence between man and nature, the integrity of the human body and mind, and the maintenance of a dynamic balance of life activities under the influences of the internal and external environments. In light of these concepts, traditional Chinese medicine started the study of the human body from the functional aspect. A unique theoretical system, and rich and effective techniques and measures were thus developed for disease prevention and control, and health protection. Tempered and improved by the practice of thousands of years, Chinese medicine has become an important aspect of medical science.

Along with the changes in the human disease spectrum and the concept of health, as well as the aging of the population, traditional Chinese medicine is gaining more and more acceptance, and displaying its special advantages. It is characterized by the preventive viewpoint—"to prevent disease and avoid complications after illness sets in," the "bio-socio-psycho-environmental" medical model, and the unique system of individualized diagnosis and treatment in accordance with climatic and seasonal conditions, geographical localities and the patient's constitution. The curative techniques such as herbal medication, acupuncture, *tuina* (manipulation and massage) and dietotherapy, as well as the theory of maintaining good health—"integration between man and nature, harmonization between body and mind, and combination of action and stability", are attracting attention among medical circles all over the world. To date, academic exchanges in the field of Chinese medicine have been developed between China and over 130 countries and regions, not only among overseas Chinese, but also people without any oriental cultural background. Many occidentals are keen to learn Chinese medicine, but the cultural and language barriers are big obstacles for them. Therefore, there is an urgent need for setting up a bridge of communication, particularly by those who have a deep understanding of both the oriental and occidental culture and also a good command of Chinese medicine to introduce TCM to the outside world.

Taking into account the different cultures of the East and the West, Prof. Xie Zhufan has written *Practical Traditional Chinese Medicine* to meet the needs of Western doctors who do not have a knowledge of Chinese but wish to study TCM. The book explains profound concept in simple terms. The book covers basic theories and major therapeutic measures, i.e., herbal medication and acupuncture. The diseases discussed are limited to those for which Western medical treatment is either hardly effective or likely to produce serious side effects while Chinese medicine may gain better results. The therapeutic methods have been carefully selected; they are quite practical and easy to apply, indicating the characteristic features of traditional Chinese medicine: simplicity and effectiveness. The book not only includes basic knowledge of traditional Chinese medicine, but also Professor Xie's own experience and understanding.

I highly appreciate Professor Xie's unremitting efforts to promote the development of Chinese medicine, and hope that more scholars will pay more attention to studying TCM in order to promote its development.

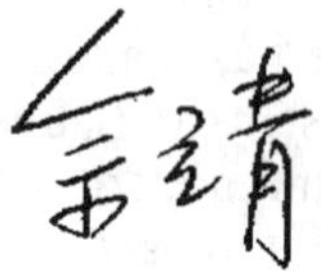

Professor She Jing
Vice Minister of Health and Director-General of the State Administration of Traditional Chinese Medicine, P.R. China
President, China Association of Traditional Chinese Medicine

FOREWORD

Traditional Chinese medicine (TCM) has a history of at least 2,500 years, since *Huangdi's Canon of Medicine* came into being. A century ago, modern Western medicine was introduced to China, and in the first half of the 20th century, official efforts were made to popularize modern Western medicine, particularly in the cities. However, TCM was not brought into this modern system. In rural areas, TCM remained the main means of preventing and treating diseases, and even in urban areas many people would rather consult physicians of traditional medicine. After the founding of the People's Republic of China in 1949, the government formulated a series of policies on traditional medicine, including fostering unity between Chinese and Western-trained doctors, attaching importance to both TCM and Western medicine, calling for the integration of the two systems of medicine, and striving to inherit and develop the tradition of TCM. In this context, TCM hospitals, colleges and institutes have been established, various ways have been devised for Western-trained doctors to learn TCM, and research into the integration of TCM and modern Western medicine has been extensively conducted. Therefore, TCM has not only been preserved, but also greatly developed. In recent years, international medical circles have paid more and more attention to TCM, many patients in other countries have received TCM treatment, and physicians have shown interest in learning this unique system of medicine. In a number of countries, TCM practice has already been formally recognized.

TCM differs from modern Western medicine distinctly. The former is the summarization of careful observation and clinical experience accumulated over thousands of years and approached in the light of traditional Chinese philosophy. The latter is developed on the basis of modern biology, chemistry and physics, and by means of scientific experimentation. The number of TCM books is tremendous, and most of the books, especially the classical works, were written in the ancient Chinese language. This causes great difficulty for the systematic learning of TCM, even for Chinese medical students. Some of the books have been translated into English, but they are still difficult for the medical doctors of the Western world to comprehend, because of the different cultural backgrounds. Therefore, there is an urgent need for the publication of a concise book to introduce essential knowledge of TCM to the people in the West in a way easy for them to understand.

The author of this book, Dr. Xie Zhu-Fan, was originally Western-trained and a professor of the Department of Internal Medicine, Beijing Medical University. Following a systematic study of TCM, he has been engaged in research into the integration of TCM and modern Western medicine for more than three decades. He was appointed chairman of the Department of TCM in the 1970s and has been director of the Institute for the Integration of Chinese and Western Medicine, Beijing Medical University, since the late 1980s. In 1980-1981, he was invited to give lectures on TCM in the United States, at some famous medical schools, such as Harvard Medical

School and UCLA Medical School. Since then, he has been invited to the United States many times to lecture on TCM and its modern research. In addition, he has been a WHO (World Health Organization) short-term consultant or acting medical officer on traditional medicine on four occasions. During two of the appointments, he was asked to assist in holding regional workshops on training in traditional medicine in Manila in 1986 and WHO consultation on training in acupuncture in Milan in 1995. Therefore, he has not only a good command of TCM and its modern research findings, but also has much experience of teaching abroad.

This book has the following distinguishing features: All the TCM concepts are described faithfully to the classical Chinese works, but they are made easily understandable by explaining how they were so formed, and by expounding the rationale of ancient Chinese philosophy. Accounts of the modern achievements of TCM research have been added to the related sections of the book.

The book is divided into four parts: In Part One, the fundamentals and principles of TCM are described precisely and concisely, including the philosophical basis, fundamental concepts, causes and mechanisms of diseases, and the unique methods of TCM diagnosis. In Part Two, discussions on materia medica, herbal formulas and patent drugs as well as their modern pharmacology constitute the main portion of TCM therapeutics. The formulas and patent drugs discussed have been carefully selected for their practical value. Part Three comprises the basic knowledge, techniques and principles of acupuncture treatment. Although TCM covers numerous diseases and the possible prescriptions for treatment are countless, Part Four only covers a limited number of diseases, which can be treated with effective but simple formulas of herbal medication and/or acupuncture. For most of these diseases, there are often difficulties in Western medical treatment, while TCM treatment may give more help to the patients. In summary, the purpose of this book is not to arouse interest in seeking novelty, but rather to provide some effective complementary or alternative measures to Western medical practice.

Of course, the tradition of TCM is extremely rich, and its modern research is just unfolding. Plenty of room remains for studying this traditional system of medicine. However, this book is well worth recommending to medical doctors in the rest of the world as an elementary text for learning TCM.

Rui-cong Peng

Peng Rui-Cong, M.D.
Professor of Public Health
ex-Chancellor of Beijing Medical University

PART ONE

THE FUNDAMENTALS AND PRINCIPLES OF TRADITIONAL CHINESE MEDICINE

CHAPTER 1

PHILOSOPHICAL BASIS OF TRADITIONAL CHINESE MEDICINE —Theories of Essential *Qi*, *Yin-Yang* and the Five Elements

Traditional Chinese medicine is a brilliant component of Chinese culture. Characterized by a unique theoretical system and enriched by thousands of years of practical experience, it still possesses great vitality. This seems to be a miracle in the world history of medicine. How could this happen? There are many reasons; the crucial one is the dialectical viewpoint of ancient Chinese philosophical thought, which provided the theoretical basis for the founding and developing of traditional Chinese medicine. The achievements of traditional Chinese medicine, in turn, further stimulated philosophical thought, thus forming a benign circle. In fact, traditional Chinese medicine is not a collection of piecemeal experiences. Most experiences have been summed up, forming a theoretic system, both medical and philosophical. The philosophical strands that gave the greatest impetus to the development of traditional Chinese medicine are the theories of Essential *Qi*, *Yin-Yang* and the Five Elements.

THE THEORY OF ESSENTIAL *QI*

Originally, *qi* (气) was not a philosophical concept. It meant air, as it is commonly used in the everyday Chinese language. Its meaning was extended to the philosophical field, serving as a symbol for the primordial substance that was thought to constitute the universe. It was believed to be invisible, taking the form of particles, constantly moving and changing, and giving rise to energy and activities. According to ancient Chinese philosophy, the universe originates from *Taiji*, a synonym for original or primitive *qi*. Its essential part, or essential *qi*, was thought to be the basic element out of which the universe is composed, and everything in the world is produced through the movement and changes of *qi*.

It is stated in *The Canon of Medicine (Huangdi's Internal Classic)*: "Human life originates in the *qi* of Heaven and Earth, and develops according to the normal order of the four seasons." That is to say, human life is also endowed with the *qi* of nature. *Qi* is the material basis on which life activities are maintained. Various actions and changes of *qi* accompanied by transformation of energy are the fundamental characteristics of life activities. Without the actions and changes of *qi* there would be no life activities.

It is important to note that, in Chinese medicine, all life activities, including mental activities such as thought, will, and emotions, are based on the actions and changes of *qi*. Since *qi* is material, the theory of *qi* is a kind of materialism which explains mental activities in terms of objective matter. In addition, human beings are derived from the *qi* of nature, so the material world is primary, existing independent of the mind, while human beings are merely a part of nature. Based on this view, Chinese medicine emphasizes that all physiological activities are in conformity with the changes of the natural environment, and so, to preserve health one must keep in harmony with the law of nature.

Since *qi* is invisible and acts as the motive force for all kinds of life activities, the word *qi* in Chinese medicine is often translated into English as "vital energy." This, however, only refers to *qi* in its narrow (physiological) sense, and the word "energy" is comprehended from the viewpoint of modern physics, i.e., matter and energy are regarded as equivalents, mutually convertible.

Actually, *qi* in Chinese medicine can be classified into two main categories: the genuine or normal *qi* and the evil or pathogenic *qi*. The genuine *qi* of human beings comes from three sources: primordial *qi*, *qi* of food essence and air. Primordial *qi* is inborn, inherited from parents, while the *qi* of food essence and air are acquired. Genuine *qi* includes all the materials and energy essential for life activities as well as the body's resistance against disease.

Evil *qi* is harmful to health. It includes various pathogenic agents or factors, for example, abnormal atmospheric changes such as wind, cold, heat, dampness and dryness are all considered evil *qi*, if they happen in an untimely fashion or in excess.

In this context, disease is defined as a process of struggle between the genuine *qi* and evil *qi*. Between these two kinds of *qi*, emphasis is often put on the former, as is stated in *The Canon of Medicine*: "If genuine *qi* prevails, attack of evil *qi* never avails."

Regarding the classification of genuine *qi* and the clinical significance of the various parts of genuine *qi*, a detailed discussion will be found in Chapter II.

THEORY OF *YIN-YANG*

Another philosophical view in traditional Chinese medicine is dialectics. It is expressed as the theory of *yin-yang*. *Yin* and *yang* were and still are two topographical terms designating the shady and sunny sides of a hill, respectively. Since everything under the sun has two sides, the shady and the sunny, by extension, *yin* and *yang* represent two opposites of an object or phenomenon. According to this theory, all things and phenomena in the world contain two opposite aspects: *yin* and *yang*, which are in conflict and at the same time mutually dependent. Therefore, this theory can be taken as a law of unity of opposites.

The theory of *yin-yang* as a dialectical way of thinking can be applied to any field of medicine. There is no conflict between the theory of *qi* and that of *yin-yang*. In fact, *qi,* as the basic element that constitutes the world, can also be divided into two, i.e., *yin qi* and *yang qi*. *Yin qi* chiefly refers to the material aspect of the element, and *yang qi*, the dynamic aspect. *The Canon of Medicine* states, "The clear *yang qi* ascends to form Heaven, while the turbid *yin qi* descends to form Earth."

The quintessence of the theory of *yin-yang* is the law of unity of opposites, which means keeping a dynamic balance. In fact, this law can also be applied to modern physiology at various levels—at the levels of systems, organs, cells, and even molecules. For example, in the nervous system excitation and inhibition, the sympathetic and parasympathetic functions, the actions of acetylcholine and norepinephrine are all in opposition, and between each pair of opposites a dynamic balance should be maintained for normal nervous activities. In the endocrine system there are estrogen and testosterone in opposition; in the kidneys there are diuresis and anti-diuresis, renal tubular secretion and reabsorption; for muscles there are contraction and relaxation; for body temperature there are thermogenesis and thermolysis; for glucose metabolism there are insulin and glucagon; for blood there are coagulation and anticoagulation; in the body fluids there are acid and base; and so on. All these opposites should be kept in dynamic balance. Therefore, it can be concluded that the maintenance of dynamic balance by uniting various opposites is a general law of life activities.

Modern physiology has shown that homeostasis, metabolism and adaptability are the three characteristic features of life activities. In Chinese medicine, these three features are all well discussed, but expressed in different ways: the dynamic balance of *yin-yang* within the body for homeostasis, waxing and waning of *yin-yang* or transformation of *yin-yang* for metabolism, and adaptable conformity between the human being and the external environment for adaptability. If the *yin-yang* theory is compared with modern physiology in this way, it will be easy to find the rationale of this ancient theory from a modern perspective. Of course, there are great differences. The main difference is that the Chinese theory is macrocosmic, while the modern Western theory is microcosmic. The latter has many advantages. The deeper it goes, the more detail and precision attaches to the knowledge. However, it may have the tendency to pay more attention to the local part than to the whole body. The knowledge gained by macrocosmic observation in Chinese medicine is often general and vague, but because of thousands of years of accumulation of experience, there is a wealth of useful knowledge, which is neglected by Western medicine and its microcosmic point of view. That is why integration of the advantages of Chinese medicine with Western medicine may promote the development of world medicine as a whole.

I. The Major Aspects of *Yin-Yang* Theory

1. Opposition of *Yin* and *Yang*

The theory of *yin-yang* holds that everything in the world has two opposite aspects, namely, *yin* and *yang*. The *yin* or *yang* aspect within any phenomenon will restrict the other through opposition. Take the human metabolism as an example. Catabolism (destructive metabolism) and anabolism (constructive metabolism) are the two aspects of metabolism. The former may pertain to *yang*, while the latter to *yin*. They are apparently in opposition, but they should be kept in a dynamic balance so as to guarantee the normal metabolism.

2. Interdependence of *Yin* and *Yang*

Yin and *yang* oppose each other, but at the same time they are mutually dependent. Without anabolism there would be no catabolism, and without catabolism there would be no anabolism. In other words, if no living tissue could be formed through anabolism, the human body would cease to exist, and if no energy could be changed from the living tissue, the human body would die. Therefore, in the theory of *yin-yang* it is said that *yang* exists with *yin* as its prerequisite, and *yin* exists with *yang* as its prerequisite.

3. Inter-Consuming Supporting Relationship of *Yin* and *Yang* (Waxing-Waning of *Yin* and *Yang*)

The balance between *yin* and *yang* is not static, but dynamic. Anabolism and catabolism do not always proceed at the same speed or to the same degree. During daytime activities there is more catabolism than anabolism, while during rest or sleep at night there is more anabolism than catabolism. That is to say, there is an increase of materials at night along with a decrease of activities, and there is an increase of activities in the daytime accompanied by a decrease of its material basis. Of the two opposites of a single entity, increase or excess of the one is usually associated with decrease or deficiency of the other. As stated in *The Canon of Medicine*, "Consumption of *yin* leads to gaining of *yang"* and "consumption of *yang* leads to gaining of *yin*," and the whole process is called "waxing-waning of *yin* and *yang"* for short. In normal conditions, the waxing-waning of *yin* and *yang* is in a state of relative balance. If it goes beyond physiological limits, the *yin-yang* balance will be impaired, resulting in disease.

4. Inter-transformation of *Yin* and *Yang*

During metabolism there is inter-transformation of the living tissue for construction and energy for functional activities. Normally, the inter-transformation takes place within a limited range, forming a dynamic balance. However, in certain circumstances, either *yin* or *yang* may be transformed into its opposite. In an acute febrile disease, there is abnormally increased catabolism to produce a high fever. After persistent high fever, exhaustion may occur, with a sudden drop in body temperature, pallor, cold limbs and profuse sweating. This is a common example to illustrate transformation of *yang* (excess of energy with a heat syndrome) into *yin* (exhaustion of energy with a cold syndrome).

5. Infinite Divisibility of *Yin* and *Yang*

The divisibility of *yin* and *yang* is infinite. As stated in *The Canon of Medicine*, "*Yin* and *yang* can be counted in tens, and can be extended to hundreds, thousands or infinity." For example, day and night can be divided into *yin* and *yang*, in which day is *yang*, while night is *yin*. Each can be further divided into *yin* and *yang*: morning is *yang* in *yang*, while afternoon is *yin* in *yang;* the period from nightfall to midnight is *yin* in *yin*, while the period of the small hours is *yang* in *yin*. If we take metabolism as an example, the divisibility of *yin* and *yang* is more explicit. Either catabolism or anabolism can be divided into opposite processes, and each process can be further divided into opposite aspects. Nutrients (*yin*) and energy (*yang*) are a pair of opposites. A part of energy released in catabolism turns into heat for maintaining the body temperature (*yang* in *yang*), and the rest is stored in adenosine triphosphate (ATP) (*yin* in *yang*). The energy released from ATP is further divided into two parts: one is used for muscular movement as mechanical energy (pertaining to *yang*), and the other is stored in creatine phosphate (pertaining to *yin*).

II. The Applications of *Yin-Yang* Theory in Medicine

The theory of *yin-yang* as a dialectic way of thinking can be applied to any field of medicine. All the life activities, including physiological and pathological processes, can be explained by opposition and transformation of *yin* and *yang*. Dynamic balance of *yin* and *yang* reflects normal physiological activities, while breakdown of the *yin-yang* balance leads to disease. Any treatment is aimed at restoring the normal dynamic balance of *yin* and *yang*. As Zhang Jingyue stated in his well-known *The Complete Works of Jingyue* (1624): "Although medicine is complicated, it can be summed up in one word, namely, *yin-yang*."

1. *Yin-Yang* and Organic Structure

When the theory of *yin-yang* is applied to explain the organic structure of the human body, the underlying premise is that the human body should be viewed as an organic whole. As the whole body is involved, the exterior portion pertains to *yang*, while the interior to *yin*; the back or dorsal aspect pertains to *yang*, while the front or anterior aspect to *yin*; the upper portion pertains to *yang*, while the lower portion to *yin*. Among the *zang-fu* organs, *zang*-organs pertain to *yin*, while *fu*-organs to *yang*. Among the *zang*-organs, the Heart and Lungs, situated in the upper portion of the body (thoracic cavity), pertain to *yang*, while the Liver, Spleen and Kidneys, situated in the lower portion of the body (abdominal cavity), to *yin*. In terms of each organ, it can be further divided into *yin* and *yang*[1], e.g., the Heart can be divided into the Heart *yin* and the Heart *yang*, the Kidneys can be divided into the Kidney *yin* and the Kidney *yang*.

2. *Yin-Yang* and Physiological Functions

All the normal life activities are based on the dynamic balance between *yin* and *yang*, which oppose each other and at the same time unite in coordination. As far as function and matter are concerned, function pertains to *yang*, while matter pertains to *yin*. All physiological activities have their material basis; without material movements, there would be no physiological functions. On the other hand, physiological activities, in turn, promote material metabolism. Therefore, the interrelationship of function and matter is precisely the interdependent and inter-consuming supporting relationship of *yin* and *yang*.

3. *Yin-Yang* and Pathological Changes

The dynamic balance of *yin* and *yang* guarantees health. Once the balance is impaired, disease ensues. Breakdown of the normal balance of *yin* and *yang* is related to both pathogenic and anti-pathogenic factors. There are two types of pathogenic factors: *yin* pathogenic factors and *yang* pathogenic factors. For example, cold and damp are *yin* pathogenic factors, while wind, dryness, heat and fire are *yang* pathogenic factors. Anti-pathogenic factors also include *yin* and *yang*, i.e., the material aspect and the functional aspect. When *yin* pathogenic factors cause disease, this may lead to preponderance of *yin*, which damages *yang* and gives rise to cold syndromes. When *yang* pathogenic factors cause disease, this may lead to an excess of *yang*, which gives rise to heat syndromes and consumes *yin*. (As stated in *The Canon of Medicine*, "*Yin* in excess consumes *yang*, and *yang* in excess consumes *yin*." "*Yin* in excess causes cold syndromes, and *yang* in excess causes heat syndromes.")

If the disease is due to deficiency of the anti-pathogenic factors, there are deficiency syndromes. According to the principle of equilibrium between *yin* and *yang*, deficiency of *yin* leads to relative preponderance of *yang*, giving rise to internal heat, while deficiency of *yang* leads to relative preponderance of *yin*, giving rise to external cold.

In advanced cases, however, deficiency of either *yin* or *yang* may lead to the consumption of the other, known respectively as "impairment of *yin* affecting *yang*" and "impairment of *yang* affecting *yin*."

4. *Yin-Yang* and Diagnosis

Since diseases or syndromes can be classified into *yin* and *yang* according to their nature, and the root cause of the occurrence and development of disease is imbalance between *yin* and *yang*, the key to clinical diagnosis is correct differentiation of the *yin* and *yang* nature of the disease as well as determination of the imbalanced condition of *yin* and *yang*. In this way, complicated clinical conditions can be simplified, and a correct diagnosis can be made.

5. *Yin-Yang* and Treatment

---

[1] *Yin* and *yang* of a *zang-fu* organ denote the material and functional aspects of that organ, respectively. In this context, *yin* refers to the essential materials such as vital essence, nutrients, fluids and blood, and *yang* includes various functional activities as well as heat energy.

Treatment in Chinese medicine is always aimed at restoring the normal balance of *yin-yang*. The following therapeutic principles derived from the theory of *yin-yang* are of the utmost significance.

"Replenish what is in deficiency," "reduce what is in excess," "treat cold with warming measures" and "treat heat with cooling measures" are the general rules of treatment in order to restore the normal balance of *yin-yang*.

An acute disease due to invasion of exogenous pathogenic factors is usually excess in nature, if the patient is normally healthy. In this case, the treatment is to eliminate or reduce the pathogenic factors. For pathogenic factors of a *yin* nature (such as cold), *yang* measures (e.g., warming therapy) should be used, and for pathogenic factors of a *yang* nature (such as heat), *yin* measures (e.g., cooling therapy) are appropriate.

In deficiency syndromes, replenishing or reinforcing measures are indicated. Deficiency of *yin* is usually accompanied by relative preponderance of *yang*, and deficiency of *yang* by relative preponderance of *yin*, and the treatment should be to replenish *yin* and reinforce *yang*, respectively. When the deficiency is put right, the relative preponderance will naturally disappear. In complicated cases, however, the treatment may also be complex. Sometimes it is necessary to "treat the *yang* aspect for diseases of a *yin* nature," and "treat the *yin* aspect for diseases of a *yang* nature," for example, by reducing *yang* to relieve dizziness and headaches in hypertensive patients suffering from *yin* deficiency with relative exuberance of *yang*, and replenish *yin*-fluid in cases of high fever (*yang*-heat) which consumes the body fluids. In acupuncture, it is not unusual to needle the points of the *yang* meridians for disorders of the *yin* meridians, and vice versa.

THE THEORY OF THE FIVE ELEMENTS

The theory of the five elements also belongs to philosophical materialism. It holds that the natural world is made up by five elements, namely, wood, fire, earth, metal and water. The ancient Chinese recognized that each element had its own properties: wood (trees) tends to spread out freely; metal is the material for manufacturing weapons; fire tends to flare upwards; earth produces myriads of things; and water tends to flow downward. By extension of the doctrine, all things can also be classified into five categories according to their properties and actions, each category pertaining to one of the five elements. In addition, there are various interrelationships among the five elements, so that they are all linked together, making the world a unified entity. Applied to medicine, a theoretic system of physiology and pathology was thus formed with the five *zang*-organs, namely, the Liver, Heart, Spleen, Lungs and Kidneys, as the core. The correlation among the *zang*-organs and between *zang*-organs and other organs and tissues as well as various physiological and pathological phenomena could all be explained with reference to the interrelationships of the five elements.

I. Classification of Things According to the Five Elements

In order to categorize physiological phenomena in a systematic way, by using analogy and deduction the ancient Chinese put them into five categories, each having properties or actions similar to one of the five elements. For example, the Liver corresponds to wood because it promotes the spreading of *qi* and blood like a tree spreading out freely. Trees produce green leaves, so green corresponds to wood. Immature fruit, green in color, is usually sour, and so sourness is related to wood. Trees germinate in spring, and the weather in spring is neither too hot nor too cold, but is often windy. So, spring is the season pertaining to wood, and wind is also related to wood. The eyes and tendons all pertain to wood, because the condition of the Liver can be reflected in the eyes, and the Liver controls the tendons. Anger is apt to impair the Liver, and patients with liver troubles are usually irascible. Therefore, among the various emotions, anger is classified into the category of wood. Such classifications are listed in the following table.

Nature					Human Body				
Taste	**Color**	**Atmos. Factor**	**Season**	**Element**	**Zang-organs**	**Fu-organs**	**Sense organs**	**Tissue**	**Emotion**
Sour	Green (Blue)	Wind	Spring	Wood	Liver	Gallbladder	Eye	Tendon	Anger
Bitter	Red	Heat	Summer	Fire	Heart	Small Intestine	Tongue	Vessel	Joy
Sweet	Yellow	Damp	Late Summer	Earth	Spleen	Stomach	Mouth	Flesh	Worry
Pun-gent	White	Dry-ness	Autumn	Metal	Lung	Large Intestine	Nose	Skin & Hair	Sadness
Salty	Black	Cold	Winter	Water	Kidney	Bladder	Ear	Bone	Fear

It is believed that there must be close relationships among the things and phenomena classified in the same category. Sour taste, green color, windy weather, and the season of spring, and the Liver, Gallbladder, eyes and tendons of the human body all correspond to wood, so they should be closely related to each other. The same applies to the other four categories. Therefore, the classification of things and phenomena provides a basis for the conformity of man with nature.

II. Correlation of the Five Elements

According to the five elements theory, correlation is not confined to things and phenomena of the same category of element, it also exists among those of different categories. The interrelationships of the five elements include inter-promoting (producing), interacting (checking), overriding and counteracting. The promoting or producing sequence is: wood → fire → earth → metal → water → wood; the acting upon or checking sequence is: wood → earth → water → fire → metal → wood; the overriding sequence is the same as the acting upon sequence; the counteracting sequence is opposite to the acting upon sequence, i.e., wood → metal → fire → water → earth → wood.

Inter-promoting and interacting are two inseparable aspects of the five elements which both oppose and cooperate with each other, thus forming a relative and dynamic balance and coordination during the development and change of any event or thing. Therefore, each element plays a role of "promoting" (or "producing") and at the same time "being promoted" (or "being produced"), and also role of "checking" and at the same time "being checked." For example, wood promotes fire, and is promoted by water; it checks earth, but is checked by metal. The inter-promoting relationship of the five elements is also known as the "mother-child" relationship, with each element being the "child" of the element that produces it, and the "mother" of the one it produces. For example, wood is the "mother" of fire, and is the "child" of water.

III. The Application of the Five Elements Theory to Medicine

Applied to Chinese medicine, the interrelationships of the five elements further explain the correlation between the various parts of the human body as well as the correlation between the human body and the natural environment. They are particularly useful for explaining the pathogenesis of complicated physiological and pathological conditions. Following are some examples:

Water nourishes wood. This figuratively denotes that a sound Liver needs adequate nourishment of Kidney *yin*. If Kidney *yin* is insufficient, usually there is a deficiency of Liver *yin* accompanied by exuberant Liver *yang*, manifested by dizziness, tinnitus and blurred vision. In the latter case, the pathogenesis is attributed to "failure of water to nourish wood," and the treatment is "replenishing water to nourish wood," i.e., replenishing Kidney *yin* as the major therapeutic measure.

Wood acts on earth. This explains the physiological relationship between the Liver (wood) and the Spleen and Stomach (earth). However, if the Liver is diseased (e.g., depressed or stagnated), it may act on the Spleen and Stomach excessively, causing dysfunction of the latter. This is called the "overriding by wood of earth."

Earth promotes metal. Physiologically the Spleen (earth) transforms the nutrients from food and transports them to the Lungs (metal). This rule can also be used in the treatment of a chronic consumptive disease of the Lungs. In treating such a disease, reinforcement of the Spleen usually plays an important role. This is called "reinforcing earth to strengthen metal."

So far as the "mother-child" relationship is concerned, if the Liver is the "mother" organ, then the Heart is the "child" organ. Deficiency of Heart blood may involve the Liver, causing blood deficiency of both the Heart and Liver. Hyperactivity of the Heart may induce hyperactivity of the Liver, resulting in hyperactivity of both the Heart and Liver. Both of the above examples illustrate the conditions expressed as "a diseased child organ implicates its mother organ."

Closely related to the "mother-child" relationship is the following principle of treatment, which is particularly useful in acupuncture therapy. "Reinforce the 'mother' in deficiency conditions, and reduce the 'child' in excess conditions." This principle is based on the inter-promoting relationship among the five elements. During acupuncture, if the syndrome is deficient in nature, points of the mother meridian are usually selected for reinforcement. For example, in a patient with deficiency of Liver *yin*, reinforcing manipulation at Yingu (KI 10) is often applied, because Yingu is the sea point of the Kidney Meridian. If the syndrome is excess in nature, points of the child meridian are usually selected for reduction. For example, in a patient with exuberant Liver fire, reducing manipulation at Shaofu (HT 8) is often helpful, because Shaofu is the spring point of the Heart Meridian. Of course, in both examples, the points of the Liver Meridian itself can also be selected.

As Chinese medicine developed and became more sophisticated, the original rules and sequences of interrelationships among the five elements were felt to be no longer adequate to explain all the physiological and pathological changes. Therefore, some modifications were made to the five elements theory. For instance, the descending actions of the Lungs (to send down essence and *qi*, to control the passage of water, etc.) are helpful to the Kidneys, but the latter also assist the Lungs in inspiration. (Insufficiency of the

Kidney function may lead to dyspnea characterized by shortened inspiration and prolonged expiration.) According to the five elements theory, we just say "metal promotes water," but clinically we usually say "metal and water promote each other."

Another problem is terminology. Water and fire are two of the five elements, but they are also used in etiology as pathogenic factors, and in diagnosis as names of syndromes. Particularly, the word "fire" is very misleading. Even in physiological conditions, fire, i.e., heat energy necessary for all life activities, particularly for the function of the Spleen in digestion, absorption and assimilation, is produced by the Kidneys. It is called "vital fire," an equivalent to "Kidney *yang*." Although fire (Heart) promotes earth (Spleen) through blood circulation, but by saying "fire promotes earth," we usually mean that the vital fire warms up the digestive function of the Spleen. In chronic diarrhea accompanied by edema and intolerance of cold, the diagnosis is "fire fails to promote earth," and the treatment is "reinforce fire to promote earth." In these statements the word "fire" refers to vital fire, i.e., Kidney *yang*. In some other instances, however, fire still denotes the Heart. "Coordination of water and fire" explains the physiological interrelationship between the Kidneys and the Heart. If Kidney *yin* (water) is insufficient to check the activity of the Heart (fire), there may occur "incoordination of water and fire," marked by restlessness and insomnia.

The confusion in terminology originated in the convoluted course of development of Chinese medicine. The theory of the five elements was formed thousands of years ago, and its application to medicine was first recorded in *The Canon of Medicine*, a product of the Warring States Period (475-221 B.C.). The theory of vital fire was proposed by leading physicians in the 16th century. Since then, the Kidneys have been taken as the "organ of water and fire," in which "water" refers to its *yin* aspect, and "fire" to its *yang* aspect. This doctrine concerns *yin*, *yang*, water and fire within one internal organ; though related to the five elements theory, it cannot be placed on a par with the latter.

Therefore, there have been controversies concerning the validity of the five elements theory. The main objection is to the classification into five categories. For example, the ordinary divisions of the year according to the weather in the temperate zone are the four seasons (spring, summer, autumn and winter) and in the tropical zone only two seasons (dry and rainy). The reason for adding late summer in order to make up the number of seasons to five is far-fetched. However, the quintessence of this theory is not that the number of five should be held sacrosanct, but that the mutual regulatory relationship between different types of matter should be recognized. The inter-promoting (producing) and inter-acting (checking) relationships among different systems or organs, to a great extent, are comparable with the theory of feedback control in Western medicine, but their application to the explanation of physiological phenomena and pathological changes has a much broader spectrum than the feedback mechanism. They can be taken as the basic rules of self-regulation of the human body at various levels. In fact, in modern physiology the significance of feedback control is no longer limited to research into neuro-humoral regulation, it has also been applied to research into immunology, molecular biology, genetic information and gene regulation. In a word, the five elements theory can be regarded as a general rule of correlation and coordination among the various parts of the human body and their functions, though the detailed description may not be precise.

CHAPTER 2

THE FUNDAMENTAL SUBSTANCES FOR LIFE ACTIVITIES —Vital Essence, *Qi*, Fluids, and Blood

All activities have their material basis. The fundamental substances essential for vital activities in human beings are vital essence, *qi*, fluids and blood.

Jing (Vital Essence)

The Chinese character 精 (*jing*) is a polysemant. When it is used as an adjective it means "refined," and when it is used as a noun it means "essence." In traditional Chinese medicine, it may be used in a narrow sense or in a broad sense. In a broad sense, it refers to the fundamental substance that constructs the body and maintains life activities. In a narrow sense, it refers to the substances that produce the body and life of offspring, i.e., sperm and ova; it is also called reproductive essence. In both cases, it is the material basis of life, and so it can generally be called the essence of life or vital essence.

I. Classification of Vital Essence

According to its source, vital essence can be classified into congenital and acquired. The congenital essence is inborn. It stems from the conjugation of the reproductive essence of the parents, and serves as the basic substance for constructing the human body and initiating life activities. The acquired vital essence comes from food. After digestion, the essence of food (nutrient) is assimilated and transformed into vital essence, which is distributed to all the body organs and tissues.

II. Functions of Vital Essence

1. Reproductive function: The reproductive essence is in charge of reproduction, and turns into the congenital essence of the offspring.
2. Promoting growth and development: Vital essence serves as the motive and constructive substance for growth and development.
3. Resistance to exogenous pathogens: The defensive *qi* is transformed from vital essence. When a person is full of vital essence, the body resistance is usually strong.
4. Replenishing the brain and marrow: Marrow, including bone marrow and spinal marrow, is transformed from vital essence, and the brain is regarded as the "sea of marrow." Both the brain and marrow need replenishment of vital essence.
5. Hemopoietic function: Vital essence can be transformed into blood or promote blood formation by replenishing the bone marrow.

III. Difference between Vital Essence and *Qi*

Both *jing* and *qi* have the meaning of essential substance that constitutes the human body and serves as the material basis for life activities. However, *jing* is visible, purely substantial, and hence pertains to *yin*; *qi* is invisible, can only be perceived by its actions, and hence pertains to *yang*. In this context, it seems appropriate to translate them into English as "vital essence" and "vital energy," respectively.

IV. Correlation between Vital Essence and *Qi*

Jing (vital essence) may be transformed into *qi* (vital energy), and *qi* can generate *jing*. They are mutually dependent and transformable, and hence often referred to as *jing-qi*. Since *jing* is stored in the Kidneys, Kidney *yin* chiefly refers to *jing*, and *jing* and *qi* of the Kidneys imply the *yin* and *yang* of the Kidneys, respectively.

Qi

In this chapter, *qi* is discussed only in its physiological sense. Physiological *qi* provides energy for all kinds of life activities of the human being, and is often translated as "vital energy."

Physiological *qi* of the human body comes from three sources: (1) congenital *qi*, or inborn *qi*, derived from the reproductive essence of the parents, and stored in the Kidneys, serving as the initiative power that forms a new life and playing its role in the whole process of the succeeding life activities; (2) the nutrients derived from food, also called "essential *qi* of food and drink," obtained through digestion and assimilation by the Stomach and the Spleen and distributed by the Spleen; (3) the clean *qi* of nature, i.e., the fresh air (oxygen) inhaled by the Lungs. The latter two pertain to acquired *qi*. The inborn *qi* and the acquired *qi* are mutually dependent and complementary. Without incessant replenishment and nourishment from the acquired *qi*, the inborn *qi* would be exhausted. Without the action of the inborn *qi*, there would be no generation and metabolism of the acquired *qi*. Combination of the inborn and acquired *qi* forms the physiological *qi*, which is traditionally called "genuine *qi*," "normal *qi*," or simply "*qi*."

I. Physiological Functions of *Qi*

The *Lei Jing* (*Classified Canon*) states, "All the human life depends upon *qi*." Physiologically, *qi* has the following functions:

1. Dynamic (Propelling) function

Qi serves as the dynamic force promoting the growth and development of the human body, the physiological activities of the various organs and tissues, formation and circulation of blood, and formation, distribution and excretion of fluids. If *qi* is insufficient, growth and development will be retarded, the functions of the organs and tissues will be diminished, and the formation, circulation and distribution of blood and fluids will be impaired.

2. Warming function

Qi provides heat energy for maintaining the body's temperature and guarantee the normal activities of the organs and tissues. If its warming function is insufficient, as in deficiency of *yang-qi*, there will be aversion to cold and cold limbs in association with various diminished functions of organs and tissues.

3. Protecting function

Qi protects the human body against attacks of exogenous pathogens. As stated in *The Canon of Medicine*, "If an exogenous pathogen invades the body, the *qi* must be insufficient." *Qi* is responsible for closing the pores to prevent the invasion of exogenous pathogens. If the pathogen has already entered, *qi* has the ability to fight against it and drive it out of the human body.

4. Retaining function

Qi holds the internal organs in their proper places, keeps the blood flowing within the blood vessels, and prevents excessive loss of the various body fluids (including sweat, urine, saliva and seminal fluid). Weakening of the retaining function of *qi* may result in abnormal loss of blood and body fluids, such as chronic bleeding, spontaneous perspiration, polyuria or incontinence of urine, salivation, watery diarrhea, spermatorrhea or premature ejaculation.

5. Transforming (metabolizing) function

The action of *qi* is closely related to all kinds of metabolism, including the mutual transformation of *qi*, blood, fluids and essence. The transforming function of *qi* is particularly connected with the water metabolism. Since water metabolism involves the functions of *qi* of the Lungs, Spleen and Kidneys, the organs situated in the Upper, Middle and Lower Energizers (body cavities) respectively, the process of water metabolism is also called the transforming function of the Triple Energizer. Impairment of this function is often manifested by accumulation of water in the body, particularly edema.

II. Classification and Distribution of *Qi*

Qi (genuine *qi*) of the human body can be generally classified into inborn *qi* and acquired *qi*. According to their functions and distribution, they can be further classified as follows:

1. Primordial *qi* (*Yuan-qi*)

Yuan-qi or primordial *qi* is inborn, derived from the reproductive essence of the parents, serving as the most fundamental substance and initiative force of life activities. It is stored in the Kidneys, constantly nourished by the essential essence from food, and distributed to the other *zang-fu* organs to ensure their functions. When one grows up, a part of primordial *qi* in the Kidneys will turn into reproductive *qi* and become the inborn *qi* of the offspring. Deficiency of primordial *qi* usually results in retarded growth and development, and diminished functions of the *zang-fu* organs.

2. Pectoral *qi* (*Zong-qi*)

Zong-qi or pectoral *qi* refers to the *qi* stored in the chest. It is formed in the Lungs by combining the essential *qi* derived from food and fresh air (oxygen) from nature. So the functions of the Stomach and the Spleen in digestion, assimilation and transportation, and the function of the Lungs in respiration directly determine the condition of pectoral *qi*. Pectoral *qi* thus formed accumulates in the chest, and spreads to the throat and the Heart. The main functions of pectoral *qi* are: (1) to supply energy for respiration and the voice; (2) to promote the heartbeat and regulate the heart rate and rhythm for blood circulation. Deficiency of pectoral *qi* is manifested by disorders of the Heart and the Lungs, such as weakened respiration, feeble voice, arrhythmia and sluggish blood circulation.

3. Nutritive *qi* (*Ying-qi*)

Ying-qi or nutritive *qi* is derived from the essential part of food digested and assimilated by the Stomach and the Spleen. The refined particles of food essence are transmitted into the blood vessels, turning into nutritive *qi,* which circulates throughout the body via the Lung vessels and then other vessels. Since nutritive *qi* circulates together with blood, they are often collectively called *ying*-blood. The main functions of nutritive *qi* are: (1) to provide nutrients for all organs and tissues, and (2) to serve as a component part for the formation of blood.

4. Defensive *qi* (*Wei-qi*)

Wei-qi or defensive *qi* is also derived from the essential part of food. Being transported to the Lungs by the Spleen, some effectual part of the food essence turns into defensive *qi* and spreads throughout the body, particularly the exterior part of the body. Unlike nutritive *qi*, defensive *qi* moves outside the vessels. Its main functions are: (1) to protect the exterior part of the body against the attack of exogenous pathogens; (2) to warm and nourish the internal organs, skeletal muscles and body surface; and (3) to control sweating by regulating the secretion of sweat for maintaining the body's temperature stable. In addition, defensive *qi* is related to sleep. When it goes into the interior part of the body, one falls asleep, and when it moves out to the body surface, one wakes up. Deficiency of defensive *qi* often results in constitutional weakness, vulnerability to exogenous affections, abnormal cutaneous sensation, and spontaneous sweating. Abnormal circulation of defensive *qi* may cause sleep disorders, either insomnia if defensive *qi* flows in the exterior part of the body for a long time, or somnolence if it moves in the interior part of the body for a long time.

Both defensive *qi* and nutritive *qi* are derived from the food essence, but there are differences between them. Defensive *qi* flows outside the blood vessels, chiefly protecting the exterior part of the body; nutritive *qi* circulates within the blood vessels, chiefly nourishing the blood and internal organs. Therefore, defensive *qi* pertains to *yang*, while nutritive *qi*, to *yin*. Between them, a *yin-yang* balance should also be kept. Either strong defensive *qi* with weak nutritive *qi* or strong nutritive *qi* with weak defensive *qi* is abnormal. Disharmony between nutritive *qi* and defensive *qi* is manifested by chills and fever with anhidrosis or excessive sweating.

5. *Qi* of the *zang-fu* organs

Genuine *qi* distributed to each *zang-fu* organ becomes the *qi* of that organ, providing energy for corresponding functional activities. For example, Heart *qi* is the dynamic force of blood circulation and mental activities, Lung *qi* provides energy for respiration and voice, Stomach *qi* takes charge of digesting food and sending the gastric contents downwards.

6. *Qi* of the meridian system

This is the genuine *qi* responsible for the functional activities of the meridian system. *Qi* of a certain meridian is closely related to *qi* of the corresponding *zang-fu* organ. For example, *qi* of the Large Intestine Meridian is directly connected with *qi* of the Large Intestine.

Blood

In traditional Chinese medicine, blood is defined as the red liquid that circulates in the vessels throughout the body for nourishing and moistening the organs and tissues. So it has the same meaning as it in Western medicine. However, regarding the production, circulation and functions of blood, traditional Chinese medicine has its own views in certain respects.

I. Production of Blood

The main factors related to the production of blood are food essence and vital essence.

1. Food essence is derived from food by the Stomach and the Spleen. As early as in *The Canon of Medicine,* the relationship between assimilation of food essence and production of blood was known: "The Stomach and the Spleen absorb the nutrients from food, extract the fluid part and transform it into a red liquid which is called blood." So it is often said that the Spleen and the Stomach are the source from which blood is generated.

Blood contains nutritive *qi.* The latter is composed of nutritive essence and the fresh air (oxygen) inhaled by the Lungs. So the Lungs are also involved in the production of blood. "The Stomach and the Spleen assimilate the nutrients and pour them into the vessels of the Lungs for production of blood."

2. Vital essence is also one of the basic substances for the production of blood. Vital essence is stored in the Kidneys and can be transformed into bone marrow. "When the bone marrow is firm, so are *qi* and blood." In addition, the vital essence of the Kidneys transported to the Liver can also be transformed into blood in the Liver. So it is often said that the vital essence and blood have the same source.

From the above discussion, it can be seen that food essence and vital essence are the main factors in the production of blood, and the Stomach, Spleen, Lungs, Kidneys and Liver are all involved in this process.

Compared to the modern theory of hemopoiesis, the traditional Chinese description, though roughly similar, is obviously crude. However, according to the above theoretical consideration, a large amount of experience has been accumulated in the treatment of anemia. Recent studies have shown that herbal formulas to invigorate the Spleen and those to reinforce the Kidneys can have good effects in the treatment of nutritional anemia and aplastic anemia respectively.

II. Circulation of the Blood

The concept of blood circulation is clearly expressed in *The Canon of Medicine*. "Blood constantly flows in the vessels without cessation." "The blood vessels are linked together like an endless ring." Normal blood circulation depends on the propelling and retaining functions of *qi*. The following *zang*-organs are involved:

1. "The Heart rules blood circulation." Heart *qi* drives the blood flow by means of heartbeats.

2. "All blood vessels lead to the Lungs." Not only does the blood get rid of the stale air and help the Lungs absorb fresh air, pectoral *qi* formed by the Lungs also helps the Heart propel the blood flow.

3. "The Liver stores blood." By storing blood, the Liver regulates the circulating blood volume.

4. "The Spleen keeps the blood flowing within the vessels," so that no blood spontaneously escapes from the vessels when the Spleen is functioning normally.

All these factors related to blood circulation are of significance in clinical practice.

For example, insufficiency of Heart *qi* is often accompanied by sluggish blood flow (blood stasis), failure of the Liver to store blood may result in massive hemorrhage such as hematemesis, failure of the Spleen to keep the blood flowing within the vessels often leads to chronic hematochezia or uterine bleeding.

III. Functions of the Blood

1. Nourishing and moistening functions

"One can see while the Liver receives blood; one can walk while the feet receive blood; one can grasp with the hands while the hands receive blood; and one can pinch with the fingers while the fingers receive blood." All parts of the body, including the internal organs, sense organs, trunk and limbs, can only work while adequate blood is supplied. In addition, the nourishing function of blood is manifested by a rosy complexion, thick and robust muscles, and smooth and sleek skin and hair. Inadequate blood supply with reduction in nourishing function may be manifested by dizziness, blurred vision, pallor or sallow complexion, dry and withered hair, dry skin, numbness of the limbs and clumsiness in movement, in addition to diminished functions of the *zang-fu* organs.

2. Serving as material basis of mental activities

"Blood supplies energy for the mental functions." This conclusion is based on clinical observations. Normal mental activities need an adequate blood supply. Blood deficiency or disordered circulation may have mental manifestations, e.g., insomnia and dream-disturbed sleep due to blood deficiency in the Heart and Liver, and restlessness or even loss of consciousness resulting from a massive loss of blood.

IV. Correlation between *Qi* and Blood

Qi and blood are closely related to each other, particularly in their production, circulation and distribution. Their correlation is usually expressed as "*Qi* is the commander of blood, and blood is the mother of *qi*."

1. "*Qi* is the commander of blood" implies the following three points:

Qi is the dynamic force for the production of blood. The processes of blood formation, including assimilation of the essential parts of food, transformation of food essence into nutritive energy and body fluids, and formation of blood from nutritive energy and fluids, are all due to the functions of *qi*. Vigorous *qi* leads to abundant production of blood, while insufficient *qi* results in deficiency of blood. That is why replenishing *qi* is usually necessary for the treatment of blood deficiency.

Qi is also the dynamic force for the circulation of blood. Heart *qi* drives the blood flowing in the vessels. Lung *qi* and Liver *qi* also take part in propelling and regulating blood circulation. So in traditional Chinese medicine there is a saying: "*Qi* in motion keeps the blood circulating."

Qi controls blood circulation, keeping blood flowing within the vessels. Various kinds of chronic bleeding may be attributed to deficiency of *qi*, and in these cases, to replenish *qi* is of great significance in arresting bleeding.

2. "Blood is the mother of *qi*" implies the following two points:

Firstly, blood is the carrier of *qi*. *Qi* can exist in the human body only when it is attached to blood or body fluids. If *qi* loses its carrier, it will scatter and flee. So great loss of blood may lead to shock (prostration of *qi*).

Secondly, blood constantly supplies *qi* with food energy. So blood deficiency may also result in deficiency of *qi*.

Body Fluids

Jin-ye[1] is a general term for all kinds of normal body fluids. It includes fluids existing within various tissues and organs, normal secretions (such as gastric juices, intestinal fluids, saliva, tears, mucus and sweat), and also the metabolite of fluids (urine). All of them come from food and drink.

I. Formation, Distribution and Excretion of Body Fluids

The whole metabolic process of body fluids is briefly described in *The Canon of Medicine* as follows: "After drink enters the Stomach, it is absorbed and transmitted to the Spleen. The Spleen disseminates the essential fluid and sends it to the Lungs, which, in turn, regulates the water passages, sending the fluid downward until it is introduced into the Urinary Bladder. Thus, the essential fluid is distributed throughout the body and flows in all the vessels of the organs and tissues."

In fact, according to the theory of traditional Chinese medicine regarding the *zang-fu* organs, the Stomach, Intestines, Spleen, Lungs, Kidneys, Urinary Bladder and Liver are all related to water metabolism. Having entered the Stomach, food and drink are partially digested and sent to the Small Intestine, and then the Large Intestine. In the intestines the essential fluid is absorbed and then transported by the Spleen to the Heart and the Lungs. The residue of food, which normally contains a small amount of water, is excreted as feces. The essential fluid is dispersed from the Heart and Lungs throughout the body to nourish and moisten various organs and tissues. The fluid that comes to the skin may be excreted as sweat under the control of defensive *qi*. By its descending action, the Lungs regulate the water passages and send a part of the body fluids down to the Kidneys. Controlled by the "sluice-valve" of the Kidneys, the surplus fluid is sent to the Urinary Bladder, and excreted as urine. The smoothing and regulating function of the Liver also helps the body fluid to circulate normally.

Metabolism of body fluids is regulated in accordance with physiological conditions and weather changes. For example, with less fluid intake, there is less urine; with more fluid intake, there is more urine; in the hot season there is more sweating; in the cold season, less sweating. Thus, a dynamic *yin-yang* balance is maintained.

II. Functions of the Body Fluids

Generally speaking, the functions of the body fluids are moistening and nourishing, but different fluids may have different functions. As the basic component of blood, the circulating fluid nourishes the organs and tissues throughout the body. The thin fluid that permeates the skin and muscles is chiefly for moistening; the thick fluid that fills in the joints, sense organs (e.g., mucus and tears), and the craniospinal cavity (cerebrospinal fluid) is not only for moistening but also for protecting the corresponding organs and tissues.

---

[1]In traditional Chinese medicine, both *jin* (津) and *ye* (液) refer to body fluids, but they are some minor differences. *Jin* is thin fluid that permeates the skin and muscles. *Ye* is thick fluid that fills in the joints, sense organs (such as mucus and tears) and the craniospinal cavity (cerebrospinal fluid).

III. Impairment of Fluid Metabolism

The two main types of impaired fluid metabolism are consumption of body fluids and retention of water.

Consumption of body fluids is often caused by high fever, profuse sweating (e.g., due to hot weather or misuse of diaphoretics), severe vomiting or diarrhea (e.g., due to insanitary food), and polyuria (e.g., in diabetes).

In the process of fluid metabolism, the Spleen transports the fluid to the Lungs, the Lungs distribute the fluid and send it downward through the water passages, and the Kidneys regulate the excretion of urine by controlling the "sluice-valve." Dysfunction of any of the above three *zang*-organs may cause retention of water, manifested by edema. In addition, dysfunction of the Liver may play an auxiliary role in the retention of water.

IV. Correlation between *Qi* and the Body Fluids

Qi pertains to *yang*, while fluids pertain to *yin*. Both of them originate from the essential part of food and drink. They are closely related in the process of formation and distribution.

1. *Qi* promotes the formation of body fluids.

Qi provides energy for the functional activities of the Stomach and Spleen, including assimilation of essential substances from food and drink, and transformation of the essential substances into body fluids.

2. *Qi* facilitates the flow of fluid.

Qi provides the dynamic force for the distribution and excretion of body fluids. If the movement of *qi* stagnates, distribution and excretion of fluids will be impeded ("failure of *qi* to move the fluid"). On the other hand, if fluid stagnates and accumulates in a certain part of the body, it can interfere with flow of *qi*, resulting in *qi* stagnation ("retention of fluid with stagnation of *qi*").

3. *Qi* controls the excretion of fluids.

Both excretion of urine and secretion of sweat are controlled by *qi*. Deficiency of *qi* may lead to polyuria and profuse sweating.

4. Fluids serve as the carrier of *qi*.

Qi, particularly defensive *qi*, is attached to body fluids. Along with massive loss of fluids, *qi* may be exhausted (collapse due to dehydration).

CHAPTER 3

STRUCTURE AND FUNCTIONS OF THE HUMAN BODY —Manifestations of the *Zang-Fu* Organs

As early as 2,000 years ago, autopsies were performed in China. A description of a postmortem examination in *The Canon of Medicine* reads, "A well-developed man can be measured from outside on the skin and flesh, and after death the body can be dissected to examine the firmness of the *zang*-organs, the size of the *fu*-organs, the volume of food contents, the length of vessels, the turbidity of blood, the content of *qi*, and whether the meridians are abundant in blood but lack *qi*, lack blood but are abundant in *qi*, abundant in both blood and *qi*, or lack both blood and *qi*: All these changes can be roughly estimated." Many anatomical descriptions recorded in *The Canon of Medicine* are basically correct from the perspective of modern anatomy. For example, it is recorded there that the ratio between the esophagus and intestines in length is 1:35, this figure being very close to 1:37 of modern anatomy. Based on anatomy, blood circulation is described: "The heart governs the blood flowing in the vessels," and "the blood flows around incessantly in a complete circuit." However, owing to the influence of ancient Chinese natural philosophy and dialectics, and also owing to the lack of modern science and technology, the development of traditional Chinese medicine was not based upon progress in anatomy. On the contrary, anatomy was neglected for many generations after China's unique system of medicine was established on the basis of holism. According to the holistic view, traditional Chinese medicine puts emphasis on the complicated internal and external relations and interactions, and studies the rules of physiological activities and pathological processes from the perspective that the human body and its environment are regarded as an organic whole. Although essential *qi* is considered as the fundamental substance that constitutes the human body and maintains life activities, it is not regarded as a kind of substantial particle with definite form or shape; its existence is merely reflected in a series of constant movements and changes in the material formation of the human body and its activities. Therefore, the cognition of essential *qi* did not lead to morphological studies of the human body, but spurred the study of the interrelation and mutual regulation between different organs as well as the interaction and dynamic balance between the human body and its outer environment. The theory of organ manifestations was thus established to expound on the structure and functions of the human body.

It is called the theory of organ manifestations because knowledge of the functions of the various organs was not obtained by experimental studies, as in modern physiology. In traditional Chinese medicine, it is believed that anything that happens in the interior of the body must have some manifestations on the exterior. Thus, by observing the outward manifestations of healthy persons and patients, the normal and abnormal functional states of human beings can be recognized and comprehended. The theory of organ manifestations is the summarization of the observations of physiological functions and pathological changes of various organs and tissues, particularly of the correlation among the organs and tissues in both normal and abnormal states.

The theory of organ manifestations is also called *zang-fu* theory. *Zang-fu* is the collective name for all internal organs. There are five *zang* organs—the Heart, Lungs, Spleen, Liver and Kidneys, and six *fu* organs—the Gallbladder, Stomach, Small Intestine, Large Intestine, Bladder and Triple Energizer. In addition, there are extraordinary organs —the brain, marrow, bones, vessels and uterus (also the Gallbladder). The *zang*-organs are mostly solid organs, characterized functionally by transforming, producing and storing essential substances but not discharging them, and the *fu*-organs are hollow ones, characterized functionally by transporting and digesting food and drink and discharging the metabolites. The extraordinary organs also store essential substances, but are different from the *zang* organs in some other respects. The Gallbladder is considered both a *fu*-organ and an extraordinary organ, because it stores bile (regarded as a kind of refined essence) and also discharges it.

Vital essence, *qi*, fluids and blood, the fundamental substances for the body's construction and life activities, are also included in the theory of organ manifestations. They have already been discussed in Chapter II.

Some of the unique features of the theory of organ manifestations are the following:

1. The five *zang*-organs are regarded as the core of the structure and functions of the human body. Each *zang*-organ is closely related ("interior-exteriorly related"[1]) to a corresponding *fu*-organ by the meridians, and also related to certain sense organs and tissues. The functions of *zang*-organs coordinate with each other by mutually promoting and restraining, and are closely linked with emotional and psychic conditions as well as the conditions of the natural environment, so that a relative balance and stability is maintained in the inner environment and also between the human body and the outer environment.

2. The *zang*-organs, though named on the basis of anatomy, are not confined to anatomical entities. They can be regarded as functional systems. For example, the Kidneys store vital essence, govern growth, development and reproduction, regulate water metabolism, help the Lungs receive air, produce marrow, dominate the bones, replenish the brain, have their health reflected in the hair, have the ears as their "windows," control urination and bowel movements, and are interior-exteriorly related to the Bladder. Therefore, the Kidneys, Bladder, bones, marrow, brain, hair, ears, genitals and anus form the Kidney system. Functionally, the Kidneys in traditional Chinese medicine include the urogenital, skeletal, endocrine systems and part of the nervous systems in modern Western medicine.[2]

3. Knowledge of the functions of the *zang-fu* organs is not only derived from observing healthy persons, but also from sick ones. For example, obstruction of the Stomach, Intestines, Gallbladder and Bladder usually causes serious illness, and removal of the obstruction cures the illness. Thus, it is concluded, "The *fu*-organs function well when they are unobstructed." A disorder of the Stomach is often manifested by nausea, vomiting and acid regurgitation, and Spleen dysfunction is marked by diarrhea with undigested food.

---

[1]All the *zang-fu* organs are situated inside the human body, but the *fu*-organs usually communicate with the outside, while the *zang*-organs have no such connection. Therefore, the *zang*-organs are situated deeper in the interior than the *fu*-organs, and a *zang*-organ and its closely related *fu*-organ, e.g., the Kidneys and the Bladder are said to be interior-exteriorly related.

[2]Since great disparities exist in the concept of the internal organs between the two systems of medicine, the names of the *zang-fu* organs in traditional Chinese medicine are written with an initial capital letter in this book.

Thus, "the Stomach has the function of sending its contents down" and "the Spleen sends the food essence upward." Therefore, the theory of organ manifestations is a combination of anatomy, physiology and pathology, and is very useful for clinical practice.

THE FIVE *ZANG* ORGANS

The Heart

The Heart is the seat of the mind, the ruler of blood circulation and the source of the vascular system. It is covered by the pericardium for protection, and is regarded as the "monarch organ" and the "supreme ruler of all the *zang-fu* organs." The Heart has its outward manifestation in the face, and a direct connection with the Small Intestine via meridians. In addition, the Heart has its "window" in the tongue, denoting that the condition of the Heart is usually reflected in the tongue. Thus, the Heart system consists of the Heart itself, the Small Intestine, the blood vessels, the face and the tongue. According to the theory of the five elements, the Heart corresponds to fire.

Anatomical Description

The Heart is described in *The Canon of Medicine* and the *Classic of Difficulties* (1st or 2nd century B.C.) as an organ "situated in the thorax," with "its apex contacting the diaphragm and the Lungs, and its beat can be seen or felt under the left nipple, serving as the source of the pulse beat." "Inside the Heart there are seven hollow places,"[3] and "surrounding the Heart is the pericardium." "The Heart looks like a lotus in bud, below the Lungs and above the Liver" (*Yi Xue Ru Men* or *The ABC of Medicine*, 1575). From the above description, the Heart in Chinese medicine apparently refers to the same organ as in Western medicine.

Physiology and Pathology

The main physiological functions of the Heart are ruling blood and vessels, and housing the mind.

1. Ruling blood and vessels. The beats of the Heart drive blood to circulate continuously through the vessels to nourish all parts of the body. This concept is similar to that of Western medicine. To accomplish this physiological function, two basic factors are necessary: The blood in the Heart and vessels ("Heart blood") and the dynamic force that drives blood to circulate ("Heart *qi*"). Normal heartbeats depend on adequate Heart *qi*. Only when Heart *qi* is abundant can the heart beat at a normal rate, rhythm and strength, maintaining normal blood circulation. On the other hand, normal blood circulation also depends on a sufficient volume of Heart blood (circulating blood in the Heart and vessels). If Heart *qi* is insufficient, there will be cardiac palpitation, shortness of breath and weak pulse. In severe cases, the blood flow will be impaired, manifested by a dark complexion, cyanotic lips and tongue, precordial pain, and a rapid and irregular or hesitant pulse.

2. Housing the mind. The Heart governs mental activities, including spirit, consciousness, thinking, expressions and behavior. According to these functions, the

---

[3]The seven hollow places refer to the two ventricular and two auricular cavities, the orifices of the aorta, pulmonary artery and vena cava.

"Heart" in Chinese medicine actually refers to a part of the central nervous system, particularly the cerebral cortex. Although this concept seems to be entirely different from that of modern Western medicine, a similar concept did once exist in the Western world. Even at present, similarities can easily be found in the English language, for example, "take heart" means "be confident," "heart-break" means "overwhelming sorrow," "hearten" means "cheer up," and "know by heart" means "know from memory."

In Chinese medicine, not only the Heart, but all the *zang*-organs share in taking charge of mental activities as well as emotions. This is one of the holistic views of Chinese medicine, i.e., all mental activities are reflections of physiological functions of *zang-fu* organs. The mental activities and emotions related to each *zang*-organ are listed in Table III-1.

Table III-1. Attribution of Mental Activities and Emotions to *Zang*-Organs

Zang-organ	Mental activities	Emotions
Heart	*Shen* (spirit, consciousness)	Joy
Liver	*Hun* (soul, courage)	Anger
Lung	*Po* (mengal vigor, liveliness)	Sadness and grief
Spleen	*Yi* (idea, thought with purpose)	Worry
Kidney	*Zhi* (will, remembrance)	Fear and fright

Among all the *zang-fu* organs, the Heart is the "supreme ruler." The *Lei Jing* (*Classified Canon of Medicine*, 1624) states, "As the Heart is the commander of all *zang-fu* organs, the mental activities including *hun* (soul and courage), *po* (mental vigor and liveliness), *yi* (idea and thought with purpose) and *zhi* (will and remembrance), though pertaining to other organs, are all controlled by the Heart. To sadness in the Heart, the Lungs respond; to worry in the Heart, the Spleen responds; to anger in the Heart, the Liver responds; to fear in the Heart, the Kidneys respond." This explains the relation of the Heart to other *zang*-organs in terms of mentality and emotion. Therefore, it can be concluded that the Heart plays the most important role in the higher nervous activities.

Why such important nervous activities are attributed to the Heart cannot be explained by semantics. On the contrary, semantics only reflects medical knowledge in this case. Among all physical functions blood circulation is of utmost importance. Once the blood circulation stops, all other functions will also stop. Among all mental activities, *shen* is of utmost importance. *Shen* means the comprehensive manifestation of life activities, especially the spirit, consciousness and thinking. There is a close relation between blood circulation and *shen*. "Blood gives energy for mental activities." "Only when the blood circulation is normal can *shen* be in good order." Therefore, as the "supreme ruler," the Heart not only rules all the physical activities of other *zang*-organs, but also governs all the mental activities related to other *zang*-organs.

The functions of the Heart and their physiological and pathological significance are summarized in Table III-2.

3. Relations with the sense organs and tissues

(1) The Heart and the vessels

As mentioned above, the Heart rules the vessels. The vascular system is directly connected with the Heart, and the blood circulating within the vessels is driven by Heart *qi*.

(2) The Heart and the face (complexion)

The color and luster of the face chiefly depend upon blood circulation. A normal complexion reflects a normal condition of the Heart. The face turns pale if Heart *qi* or the circulating blood is insufficient, it becomes cyanotic if the blood circulation stagnates, and it flushes if there is exuberant Heart fire.

(3) The Heart and the tongue

"The tongue is the 'window' of the Heart." Normal color of the tongue depends upon normal blood circulation. In addition, the tongue is a movable organ in the mouth used in tasting and talking.

Table III-2. Functions of the Heart

	Physiological significance	Pathological significance
Ruling blood and vessels	Driving blood to circulate in the vessels to transport nutrients	Deficiency of the Heart qi: pallor, weak pulse; Stagnation of the Heart qi and blood: dark complexion, cyanotic lips and tongue, precordial pain, arrhythmia
Housing the mind	Maintaining normal mental activities	Impaired consciousness, chaotic thinking, slow reactions

Inspection of the tongue gives information about the condition of the Heart. When the Heart is functioning normally, the tongue has a normal red color, lustrous, moderately moistened, flexible and nimble, and is sensitive to taste and fluent in talking. Disorders of the Heart are often reflected in the tongue. When Heart *qi* or blood is insufficient, the tongue becomes pale. Excessive fire in the Heart results in a reddened tongue tip with ulceration. Stagnation of Heart blood is manifested by a purple color of the tongue or purple spots on the tongue. Mental derangement may be accompanied by stiffness of the tongue or aphasia.

The relations of the Heart with the sense organs and tissues, and their physiological and pathological significance are summarized in Table III-3.

4. Relations with the emotions

The Heart is particularly related to joy. Generally speaking, joy is an emotional response to a benign stimulus, beneficial to the physiological activities of the Heart. However, excessive joy may be harmful. On the other hand, disorders of the Heart as the "house" of the mind may be manifested by incessant laughing. In addition, as the "supreme ruler of all the *zang-fu* organs," any kind of emotional disturbance not only injures the corresponding *zang-fu* organ, it also impairs the normal mental activities controlled by the Heart.

5. Relations with the fluids

Both sweat and the liquid part of blood originate from the fluid assimilated from food and drink. So it is said that sweat and blood have the same source. Since blood is ruled by the Heart, and sweat comes from the liquid part of blood, it is also said that "sweat is the fluid of the Heart." The close relationship between blood and sweat exists not only in physiological conditions, but also in pathological changes. Excessive sweating may cause loss of fluid and reduction of blood volume, impairing Heart *qi* and blood, manifested by cardiac palpitation or even collapse. On the other hand, deficiency of Heart *qi* often leads to spontaneous sweating (sweating in the daytime, not connected with physical exertion, hot environment or thick clothing), and deficiency of Heart *yin* is manifested by night sweating (sweating during sleep).

[Appendix] The Pericardium

The pericardium is the membranous sac surrounding the Heart. Its function is to protect the Heart. In the theory of *zang-fu* manifestations, the Pericardium is not a *zang*-organ, but merely an attachment of the Heart. It is believed that the Heart, being the site where mental activities take place and serving as the supreme ruler of all the *zang-fu* organs, can hardly be invaded by exogenous pathogens. If the Heart itself were invaded, the mental activities would cease, and life immediately ended. Therefore, in febrile diseases with mental derangement, such as delirium or loss of consciousness, it is thought that the Pericardium is attacked by heat pathogens ("invasion of the Pericardium by heat").

Table III-3. Relations of the Heart with the Sense Organs and Tissues

	Physiological significance	Pathological significance
Blood vessels (ruled by the Heart)	The Heart is directly connected to blood vessels and drives the blood to circulate.	Impairment of blood circulation.
Face (reflecting the Heart's brilliance)	Lustrous complexion reflects normal functions of the Heart in both ruling the blood and housing the mind.	Pallor and lusterless complexion due to deficiency of Heart qi and blood; cyanosis due to blood stasis
Tongue (as the "window" of the Heart)	A normal reddish, moistened tongue with free movement, normal taste and fluent speech indicates abundant qi and Heart blood.	Abnormal color of the tongue in circulatory disorders; abnormal movement of the tongue due to mental (or neurological) disorders

The Lungs

The Lungs in traditional Chinese medicine have a broader connotation than the same term used in Western medicine. The Lungs include the whole respiratory system, and even some functions other than respiration. They dominate *qi*, administer respiration, take charge of superficial body resistance and regulate water passages. The Lungs are closely related to the body's surface, have their specific body opening in the nose and direct connection with the Large Intestine via meridians. Thus, the Lung system consists of the Lungs themselves, the Large Intestine, skin and body hair (the superficial part of the body), and the nose. According to the theory of the five elements, the Lungs correspond to metal.

Anatomical Description

Among the *zang-fu* organs, "only the Lungs and the Heart are situated above the diaphragm" (*The Canon of Difficulties: the 32nd Problem*), "forming a cap on top of the other *zang-fu* organs." (*The Canon of Medicine*) "The Lungs are honeycomb-like organs, but the cells have no opening underneath. They become full during inhalation and shrink during exhalation." (*Yi Zong Bi Du* or *Essentials of Medicine*, 1637) Apparently, the Lungs in Chinese medicine are the same organs as in Western medicine.

Physiology and Pathology

The main functions of the Lungs are dominating *qi* (respiration) and regulating the water passages.

1. Dominating *qi*

The Lungs dominate *qi* in two aspects. One aspect is that the Lungs take charge of respiration; breathing in fresh *qi* (air containing oxygen) and breathing out stale *qi* (air containing carbon dioxide). It is in the Lungs that the gas exchange takes place. Therefore, the movements of *qi* in the Lungs include ascending, descending, coming in and going out. Through these movements of *qi* in different directions, the Lungs regulate the movements of *qi* in general. In the process of respiration, the air passages should be kept clean and unobstructed. If any pathogenic factor impedes the smooth flow of air during respiration, there will be coughing and dyspnea due to "upward perversion of Lung *qi*." It should be noted that the Lungs need the assistance of the Kidneys in respiration. Some chronic respiratory disorders, such as coughing and dyspnea in emphysema and chronic asthma, are often attributed to impaired function of both the Lungs and the Kidneys.

The other aspect is the role of the Lungs in the formation of *qi*, especially pectoral *qi*. Pectoral *qi* is formed by combining essential *qi* derived from food and fresh air (oxygen) inhaled by the Lungs. The *qi* thus formed in the Lungs is collected in the chest. It provides energy for respiration and the voice on the one hand, and assists Heart *qi* to promote blood circulation on the other. With normal functioning of the Lungs in dominating *qi*, abundant *qi* can be supplied to all the *zang-fu* organs. Impairment of this function usually results in insufficient formation of pectoral *qi* and disordered movements of *qi* in general, manifested by shortness of breath, feeble voice, lassitude and lack of energy.

2. Regulating the water passages

This is one of the unique points in traditional Chinese medicine. The Lungs are believed to take part in the regulation of water metabolism. They disseminate fluid to the body's surface, and disperse a part of the body's fluids through the pores as sweat. They also constantly send fluid downwards to the Kidneys for the excretion of urine. The latter function is known as "regulating the water passages." If this function is impaired, fluid will be retained, transformed into phlegm in the Lungs, or accumulated in the tissues, resulting in edema, especially edema of the upper portion of the body.

The Lungs' function in regulating the water passages is a conclusion drawn from clinical observations. Edema manifested in the upper portion of the body (e.g., acute nephritis) is often associated with respiratory symptoms and can be relieved with herbal medicines commonly used for treating respiratory diseases (such as *Herba Ephedrae*).

The functions of the Lungs and their physiological and pathological significance are summarized in Table III-4.

3. Relations with the sense organs and tissues

(1) The Lungs and the body's surface

The body's surface includes the skin, body hair and sweat pores. They protect the body against exogenous affections. Superficial defensive *qi* is derived from pectoral *qi* and disseminated to the body's surface by the Lungs. Sound Lung *qi* strengthens superficial defensive *qi*, strengthening the body resistance against the attack of exogenous pathogens. Superficial defensive *qi* also controls the closing and opening of the sweat pores. If Lung *qi* is insufficient, the body resistance is weakened, accompanied by excessive sweating and vulnerability to colds.

Table III-4. Functions of the Lungs

	Physiological significance	Pathological significance
Dominating qi	Normal respiration and formation of pectoral qi	Impaired respiration: coughing and dyspnea; insufficient pectoral qi: shortness of breath and feeble voice
Regulating water passages	One of the key links in water metabolism	Edema, particularly in the body, when the Lungs fail to regulate the water passages

(2) The Lungs and the nose

"The nose is the specific body opening (or 'window') of the Lungs." Through nose the breath passes. Sense of smell is also one of the functions of the Lungs. If the Lungs function well, the breathing is smooth through the nose, and the sense of smell acute. Stuffed nose, sneezing, running nose or dryness of the nose, and impaired sense of smell indicate that the Lungs are diseased.

(3) The Lungs and the larynx

The larynx is not only the passage for the breath, but also the organ of the voice. If the Lungs are sound, the voice is normal. Feeble voice, hoarseness of voice and aphonia all indicate disorders of the Lungs.

The relations of the Lungs with the sense organs and tissues, and their physiological and pathological significance are summarized in Table III-5.

Table III-5. Relations of the Lungs with the Sense Organs and Tissues

	Physiological significance	Pathological significance
Skin and hair (ruled by the Lungs)	Superficial defensive qi derived from pectoral qi in the Lungs protects the body against exogenous affections.	Weakened Lung qi lowers the body's resistance, causing spontaneous sweating and vulnerability to colds.
Larynx (managed by Lung qi)	One with sound Lungs has a normal voice.	Deficiency of Lung qi: feeble voice or aphonia; Obstruction of Lung qi: hoarseness of voice.
Nose (as the "window" of the Lungs)	Even breathing through the nose and normal sense of smell when the Lungs are healthy.	Disturbance of the Lung function: stuffed and running nose, impaired sense of smell.

4. Relations with the emotions

It is believed that sadness is apt to consume *qi*. Since the Lungs dominate *qi*, they are particularly vulnerable to sadness. Moreover, one with chronic Lung disease (for example, pulmonary tuberculosis) often feels sad and becomes pessimistic.

5. Relations with the fluids

Among the fluids, nasal mucus secreted for moistening the nostrils is specifically related to the Lungs. In wind-cold affection of the Lungs there is excessive secretion of thin nasal mucus, and in wind-heat affection of the Lungs, there is muco-purulent nasal discharge.

The Spleen

The Spleen and the Stomach digest food, and assimilate and distribute the nutrients for life activities. Therefore, it is said that "the Spleen and the Stomach provide the material basis of the acquired constitution," serving as "the source of nutrients for the production of *qi* and blood." The Spleen is closely related to the Stomach, nourishes the flesh, and has its outward manifestation in the lips and its "window" in the mouth. Thus, the Spleen system consists of the Spleen itself, the Stomach, flesh, lips and mouth. According to the theory of the five elements, the Spleen corresponds to earth.

Anatomical Description

The records about the location and morphology of the Spleen in Chinese medical literature can be summarized as follows: "Under the diaphragm there is the Stomach, which receives food and digests it. To the left of the Stomach is the Spleen, which is surrounded by the same membrane as the Stomach." (*Yi Guan* or *Key Link of Medicine*, 1687) "The Spleen has a flattened, oblong shape, with a fatty appendage." (*Canon of Difficulties: the 42nd Problem*) "It looks like a horse's hoof or a sickle." (*Yi Xue Ru Men* or *The ABC of Medicine*, 1575) According to these descriptions, the Spleen in Chinese medicine refers to what Western medicine regards as the spleen together with the pancreas. Its physiology and pathology, however, cannot be covered by the spleen and pancreas in the Western sense.

Physiology and Pathology

The main physiological functions of the Spleen are: (1) ruling transformation and transportation, (2) reinforcing *qi* and regenerating blood, (3) controlling the blood flow (keeping blood flowing within the blood vessels), and (4) sending essence upward.

1. Ruling transformation and transportation

The Spleen plays the most important role in the process of digestion and assimilation. The Stomach partially digests the ingested food and sends its contents to the intestines. The Spleen further digests the food and transforms the food into food essence (nutrients), absorbs it and transports it to the Heart and Lungs for nourishing the whole body. The activities of all organs and tissues need the food essence provided by the Spleen; generation of *qi* and blood also depends on the supply of food essence by the Spleen. Since the Spleen has such a vital function, it is considered the source of essential substances for growth and development, forming the basis of one's acquired constitution.

If the Spleen function in transformation and transportation is impaired, there will be anorexia, abdominal distension, loose stools, and even lassitude, emaciation or other manifestations of *qi* and blood deficiency.

The transforming and transporting function of the Spleen also includes absorption and distribution of fluid. In the process of water metabolism, the Spleen assimilates fluid and transports it throughout the body. The Spleen not only provides fluid for the organs and tissues, but also removes the surplus fluid from them.

If the Spleen function is in disorder, there will be accumulation of water-damp in the body, manifested by profuse expectoration or edema. This is often described as "production of dampness due to insufficient Spleen function," "the Spleen being a source of phlegm formation," or "edema due to insufficiency of the Spleen."

2. Reinforcing *qi* and regenerating blood

Genuine *qi* is the dynamic force of all kinds of life activities. It is composed of inborn *qi* originating from the innate essence stored in the Kidneys, and acquired *qi* derived from the food essence assimilated by the Spleen and the fresh air (oxygen) inhaled by the Lungs. Therefore, a sound Spleen provides materials for the production of *qi*, while a weak Spleen often leads to deficiency of *qi*. If genuine *qi* is abundant, normal functioning of the *zang-fu* organs is guaranteed; if it is insufficient, various functions of the organs may be impaired. Clinically, if a patient with *qi* deficiency has manifestations of insufficient Spleen function, failure of the Spleen to reinforce *qi* is usually considered the cause, and combined use of *qi* tonics and Spleen tonics is the rule of treatment. Since the Spleen has the function to reinforce *qi*, even in *qi* deficiency of other organs, e.g., deficiency of the Lungs, therapy to invigorate the Spleen is also helpful.

The food essence assimilated by the Spleen also provides the material basis for the regeneration of blood. In traditional Chinese medicine, the Spleen is taken as an important organ for hemopoiesis. Tonification of the Spleen is an effective measure for treating anemia.

3. Controlling the blood flow (keeping blood circulating within the blood vessels)

In the process of blood circulation, the Heart, the Liver and the Spleen are the major links. Heart *qi* serves as the dynamic force of blood circulation; the Liver regulates the volume of the circulating blood and makes the blood flow smoothly; Spleen *qi* has the function of keeping the blood flowing within the vessels. If the Spleen fails to prevent the circulating blood from extravasation, chronic bleeding ensues, often occurring as subcutaneous hemorrhage, hematochezia, hematuria or uterine bleeding.

4. Sending essence upward

Qi of the Spleen is characterized by its ascending action. It sends the food essence upward to the Lungs and Heart. This is a part of the Spleen's function in transformation and transportation. In addition, Spleen *qi* also has the action of supporting the visceral organs at the right place. If Spleen *qi* is weakened, downward displacement of the visceral organs will occur, such as gastroptosis, prolapse of the uterus or prolapse of the rectum.

The functions of the Spleen and their physiological and pathological significance are summarized in Table III-6.

3. Relations with the sense organs and tissues

(1) The Spleen and flesh (muscles)

In Chinese medicine, muscles consist of two parts: flesh and tendon. The flesh of the muscles is the somatic element, which gives the body its characteristic shape and physical strength. Since this part of the muscles particularly needs a supply of nutrients, it has a special relationship with the Spleen. The muscle tendon responsible for the movement of the body and limbs, however, is controlled by the Liver. Therefore, weakness, emaciation, lack of strength, and even muscular atrophy are usually attributed to impairment of the Spleen in transforming and transporting food essence, while abnormal muscular movements, such as tremors, twitching or convulsions, are usually attributed to dysfunction of the Liver.

Table III-6. Functions of the Spleen

	Physiological significance	Pathological significance
Ruling transformation and transportation	Normal digestion, assimilation and distribution of nutrients	Disorders in digestion and assimilation: anorexia, abdominal distension, loose stools, sallow complexion, and emaciation
	One of the major links in water metabolism	Disorders in water metabolism: retention of phlegm, edema, diarrhea
	Reinforcing qi and blood	Deficiency of qi and blood, regenerating blood
Controlling blood flow	Keeping blood flowing within the vessels	Failure of the Spleen to control blood: chronic bleeding
Sending essence upward	Transporting food essence to the Lungs and Heart	Lack of source for producing qi and blood: deficiency of qi and blood
	Maintaining the proper position of the visceral organs	Sinking of the Spleen qi: visceroptosis, protracted diarrhea

(2) The Spleen and the lips

The color and luster of the lips reflect the condition of *qi* and blood. Since *qi* and blood are derived from the food essence absorbed by the Spleen, red, moist and lustrous lips signify normal functioning of the Spleen, and pale lips often indicate impaired function of the Spleen. This is expressed as "The Spleen has its brilliance reflected in the lips."

(3) The Spleen and the mouth

"The mouth is the 'window' of the Spleen." Here, by "mouth" is particularly meant the sense of taste. Normal taste with a good appetite reflects a sound Spleen. "Spleen *qi* goes to the mouth. When the Spleen functions in harmony, different tastes of food can be clearly differentiated." When the Spleen is weak, all food becomes insipid and the appetite is lost.

The relations of the Spleen with the sense organs and tissues, and their physiological and pathological significance are summarized in Table III-7.

4. Relations with the emotions

All the emotions may influence the functions of the Spleen, but worry is thought to be the most prominent one. Worry or anxiety usually impairs the flow of Spleen *qi*, dulling the appetite.

5. Relations with the fluids

Among the fluids, the thin saliva running from the mouth is taken as the fluid of the Spleen. It moistens the mouth and protects the mucous membrane. Its secretion increases during the taking of food to help digestion and facilitate swallowing. Normally, it does not run out of the mouth, but salivation occurs when there is disharmony between the Spleen and the Stomach.

Table III-7. Relations of the Spleen with the Sense Organs and Tissues

	Physiological significance	Pathological significance
Flesh and muscles (ruled by the Spleen)	Well-developed muscles with great strength indicate healthy Spleen qi	Weak and flaccid muscles, emaciation, lassitude, lack of strength in Spleen insufficiency
Lips (reflecting the Spleen's brilliance)	Red, moist and lustrous lips reflect a sound Spleen	Pale lips in weakness of the Spleen
Mouth (as the "window" of the Spleen)	Normal taste with good appetite indicates abundant Spleen qi	Anorexia and dysgeusia in weakness of the Spleen

The Liver

The Liver is the seat of the soul and place where blood is stored. Its main function is to smooth and regulate the flow of *qi* and blood. This function also involves the secretion of bile as well as digestion of food and assimilation of nutrients by the Spleen and Stomach. The Liver is directly connected with the Gallbladder, controls the tendons for bodily movement, and has its outward manifestation in the nails, and its "window" in the eyes. Thus, the Liver system consists of the Liver itself, the Gallbladder, tendons, nails and eyes. According to the theory of the five elements, the Liver corresponds to wood.

Anatomical Description

"The Liver as a *zang*-organ is situated in the right upper part of the abdomen in front of the right Kidney." (*Shisi Jing Fahui* or *Exposition of the Fourteen Meridians*, 1341) "The Liver can be generally divided into the right and left lobes, and further divided into lobules." (*Nan Jing Ji Zhu* or *Collection of Annotations on the Classic of Difficulties*) "The Liver is under the diaphragm" and "The gallbladder is attached to the Liver." (*Yi Guan* or *Key Link of Medicine*, 1687) According to the anatomical descriptions, the Liver in Chinese medicine refers to the organ of the same name in Western medicine.

Physiology and Pathology

The main physiological functions of the Liver are storing blood, and smoothing and regulating the flow of *qi*.

1. Storing blood

The Liver stores blood and regulates the volume of circulating blood. "Blood returns to the Liver when one is lying down, and circulates in the vessels when one is moving." "With the blood supply, one is able to see with the eyes, to walk with the feet, to hold things with the hands, and to take things with the fingers." This roughly conforms to the modern Western concept. However, the blood-storing function of the Liver is far beyond the regulation of the circulating blood volume.

Impairment of the Liver in storing blood may give rise to two kinds of disorders: One is inadequate storage of blood in the Liver and the other is discharge of blood from the vessels. When the blood stored in the Liver is inadequate ("deficiency of Liver blood"), sufficient blood cannot be supplied to meet their needs of the organs and tissues. If the eyes are involved, there will be blurred vision or night blindness; if the tendons of the limbs are involved, there will be muscular contraction, numbness of the limbs, or abnormal movements, such as tremors, twitching and even convulsions. If deficiency of Liver blood occurs in women of child-bearing age, there will be oligomenorrhea or even amenorrhea.

Discharge of blood from the vessels due to disturbance of the Liver in storing blood is called "failure of the Liver in storing blood." There may be hematemesis, epistaxis, or menorrhagia. In a typical case, hemorrhaging occurs after a fit of anger.

2. Smoothing and regulating the flow of *qi*

Qi provides energy for various functional activities. First of all, the smooth flow of *qi* is prerequisite for maintaining normal blood circulation. So, this Liver function can also be called smoothing and regulating the flow of *qi* and blood. This function plays important roles in the following fields:

(1) Regulating psychic and emotional activities

Although psychic and emotional activities are ruled by the Heart, they are also closely related to the Liver. It is stated in *The Canon of Medicine*: "The Liver is in charge of planning and consideration." With normal Liver function in smoothing and regulating the flow of *qi*, Liver *qi* is neither excessive nor depressed. Under such a condition, one will be easy in mind, clear in reasoning and quick in thinking. Dysfunction of the Liver with stagnant flow of *qi* often results in depression, while over-exercised function of the Liver usually leads to irritability and irascibility, and in some cases even mania.

(2) Promoting digestion and assimilation

The Liver promotes the digestive and assimilative functions of the Stomach and the Spleen by regulating the movement of their *qi* and secreting bile. Coordination of the descending function of the Stomach and ascending function of the Spleen guarantees normal digestion and assimilation. Dysfunction of the Liver may either impair the descending function of the Stomach, resulting in nausea, vomiting, belching, loss of appetite, epigastric distension and constipation ("disharmony of the Liver and Stomach"), or impair the ascending function of the Spleen, manifested by abdominal distension and loose stools ("disharmony of the Liver and Spleen").

Bile is secreted by the Liver and stored in the Gallbladder. "After a meal, food fills the Small Intestine and stimulates the Gallbladder, so that bile is excreted into the intestine to facilitate digestion and transportation of the intestinal content." (*Yi Yuan* or *Key Link of Medicine*, 1687)

(3) Maintaining normal movement of *qi* and blood

The Liver is directly responsible for the normal movement of *qi*. "*Qi* in motion keeps the blood circulating." Heart *qi* makes blood circulate, Lung *qi* assists the Heart in blood circulation, and Spleen *qi* controls blood flowing within the blood vessels: all these functions require a condition of smooth movement of *qi* regulated by the Liver. If the function of the Liver in maintaining normal movement of *qi* is in disorder, stagnation of *qi* will occur, manifested by distension and pain in the chest, breasts or lower abdomen. Stagnation of *qi* may further lead to blood stasis, manifested by stabbing pains, mass formation, and various blood disorders.

(4) Assisting water metabolism

Water metabolism is accomplished by the Lungs, Spleen and Kidneys, but the Liver also plays an auxiliary role by regulating *qi* of the Triple Energizer[4] and facilitating the

---

[4]"The Triple Energizer can be compared to water communications, controlling the circulation of body

smooth flow of water.

(5) Regulating the Thoroughfare and Conception Vessels

The Thoroughfare and Conception Vessels play special roles in female physiology. Both vessels communicate with the Liver Meridian, and their functions are regulated by the Liver. When the Liver functions well, menstruation, leukorrhea, and the process of pregnancy and delivery will be normal. Dysfunction of the Liver in smoothing and regulating *qi* may cause menstrual disorders, abnormal leukorrhea, disorders during pregnancy and infertility.

The functions of the Liver and their physiological and pathological significance are summarized in Table III-8.

Table III-8. Functions of the Liver

	Physiological significance	Pathological significance
Storing blood	1. To regulate circulating blood volume 2. To prevent hemorrhaging	Deficiency of Liver blood: insufficient blood supply for tendons and eyes Failure of the Liver in storing blood: hematemesis, excessive uterine bleeding
Smoothing and regulating the flow of qi	1. To regulate psychic and emotional activities: ease of mind when the Liver functions normally 2. To promote digestion and assimilation by secreting bile and regulating Stomach and Spleen qi 3. To maintain the normal flow of qi and blood 4. To assist normal water metabolism 5. To regulate the Thoroughfare and Conception Vessels: normal menses, pregnancy and delivery	Psychic and emotional changes: irritability, irascibility or depression Disharmony between the Liver and the Stomach (or Spleen): impaired digestion and assimilation Impaired flow of qi and blood: stagnation of qi and blood stasis Disordered water metabolism: accumulated phlegm, edema Disturbances of the Thoroughfare and Conception Vessels: various gynecological and obstetric disorders

3. Relations with the sense organs and tissues

(1) The Liver and tendons

Tendons are the fibrous cords by which the muscles are attached to bones or other structures. Since the movement induced by muscular contraction and relaxation is through the tendons, it is believed in traditional Chinese medicine that the tendons are in charge of movement, while the muscles give strength. When the Liver blood is abundant, sufficient blood is provided for the tendons, so that the body and limbs can move freely and quickly. Decrease of Liver blood in the aged causes difficulty and slowness in motion. In morbid conditions insufficiency of Liver blood impairs the blood supply to the tendons. This may lead to tremors, numbness and contraction of the extremities, or even twitching and convulsions.

(2) The Liver and the nails

"The brilliance of the Liver is reflected in the nails." In traditional Chinese medicine,

fluids." Since the Lungs are situated in the Upper Energizer, the Spleen in the Middle Energizer and the Kidneys in the Lower Energizer, this function of the Triple Energizer actually refers to the comprehensive functions of the Lungs, Spleen and Kidneys in water metabolism.

the nails are taken as "the odds and ends of tendons," which also need nourishment from Liver blood. Since the condition of the Liver determines the luster of the nails, lustrous nails signify a sound Liver. If Liver blood is insufficient, the nails will be thin, soft, withered, or even deformed and chipped.

(3) The Liver and the eyes

Although the eye is related to all the *zang-fu* organs, there is a special relationship between the Liver and the eyes, because the Liver Meridian connects the Liver and the eye connectors[5], and eyesight depends on the smoothing and regulating function of the Liver and nourishment of Liver blood. It is said that the eye is the "window" of the Liver. When the Liver is normal, the vision is acute, and the eyes are lustrous. Disorders of the Liver often have manifestations in the eyes, e.g., dryness, blurred vision or night blindness when Liver blood is insufficient, conjunctivitis when wind-heat attacks the Liver Meridian, inflammation of the eye or keratitis when Liver fire flames up, deviation of the eyes when Liver wind stirs, and yellow discoloration of the sclera when damp-heat accumulates in the Liver and Gallbladder.

The relations of the Liver to the sense organs and tissues, and their physiological and pathological significance are summarized in Table III-9.

Table III-9. Relations of the Liver with the Sense Organs and Tissues

	Physiological significance	**Pathological significance**
Tendons (ruled by the Liver)	Normal and free movements of body and limbs indicate abundant Liver blood.	Motor disturbances due to deficiency of the Liver yin- blood (tremors, twitching, contraction or even convulsions)
Nails (reflecting the Liver's brilliance)	Smooth and lustrous nails reflect a sound Liver.	Thin, soft, withered, deformed or chipped nails due to deficiency of Liver blood
Eyes (as "windows" of the Liver)	Acute eyesight indicates abundant Liver blood.	Dryness of the eyes with blurred vision due to deficiency of Liver yin-blood; inflammation of the eye when the Liver fire flames up; deviation of the eyes when Liver wind stirs up

4. Relations with emotions

The Liver is particularly related to anger. Anger is a strong feeling that comes when one has been insulted or when one sees injustice. This feeling often makes people want to quarrel or fight, and disturbs the normal movement of *qi*, causing upward perversion of *qi* and blood. An outburst of fury may injure the Liver, and excessive rising of Liver *qi* may sometimes result in hematemesis or even sudden loss of consciousness. Moreover, one with deficiency of Liver *yin* or blood is irritable and irascible. "It is difficult to treat one who is easily made angry. The only way is to soothe the Liver." (*Za Bing Yuan Liu Xi Zhu* or *Analysis of the Sources of Miscellaneous Diseases*, 1773)

5. Relations with fluids

---

[5]The "eye connector" consists of the ophthalmic blood vessels and the optic nerve.

Among body fluids, tears are most closely related to the Liver, as "the eyes are the 'windows' of the Liver." Dryness of the eyes stemming from deficiency of Liver blood is actually due to insufficient secretion of tears. When the Liver Meridian is attacked by wind-heat, tears often become mucopurulent, with excessive lacrimation induced by the irritation of wind.

The Kidneys

The function of the Kidneys in traditional Chinese medicine is by no means confined to secretion of urine. It stores *jing* (vital essence) which serves as the source of life, and is hence regarded as the "congenital foundation" of the human body. It provides vital essence for all organs, and also governs the vital fire, which warms the body, promotes growth and development, and activates the functioning of all other organs. "Kidneys" are probably the most confusing term in Chinese medicine or at least as confusing as "Spleen." Besides the Kidneys themselves, the Kidney system includes the bladder, marrow, brain, head hair, ear, genitals and anus. According to the theory of the five elements, the Kidneys correspond to water.

Anatomical Description

"The lumbar region is the seat of the Kidneys." (*The Canon of Medicine*) "Each has the shape of a cowpea, placed in opposition, lateral to the spine." (*Yi Guan* or *Key Link of Medicine*, 1687) Apparently, the Kidneys in Chinese medicine refer to the same organ in Western medicine, though the former probably includes the suprarenal gland as well.

Physiology and Pathology

The main physiological functions of the Kidneys are storing *jing* (vital essence), producing marrow, governing the vital fire, dominating water metabolism, and helping inspiration of air.

1. Storing *jing* (vital essence)

Jing is a general term for the basic structural substances. The embryo is formed by the conjugation of the parents' *jing* (sperm and ovum, both of which are called reproductive essence) and depends on the nutrients supplied by the mother for its development. The *jing* inherited from parents is stored in the Kidneys. After birth, the basic structural substances should be further acquired from food through the metabolism in the various *zang-fu* organs. They are also stored in the Kidneys and are supplied to all *zang-fu* organs whenever necessary. Thus, the Kidneys store two kinds of vital essence: congenital (or inherited) and acquired.

The vital essence stored in the Kidneys has the following functions:

(1) Reproduction, growth and development

Jing is the source of reproduction. A new human life starts after fusion of the parents' reproductive essence (ovum and sperm). After birth, the congenital essence is stored in the Kidneys and continuously nourished by essence acquired from food, making possible the child's growth and development. The relationship of the Kidney function to growth, development and reproduction is described in *The Canon of Medicine* as follows:

"In the female, at seven years of age her Kidney *qi* becomes full, her permanent teeth appear, and her hair grows long. At the age of fourteen years, the sex-stimulating essence comes in with maturation of reproductive essence, the Conception Vessel is open and the Thoroughfare Vessel is filled with blood, so menstruation begins and pregnancy is possible. At twenty-one years, her Kidney *qi* is in *yin-yang* balance[6], the wisdom teeth emerge, and her body is fully developed. At twenty-eight years, the tendons and bones are firm, the hair grows to its extreme, and the body to the height of development. At thirty-five, the Stomach and Large Intestine Meridians begin to be depleted[7], facial wrinkles appear and the hair begins to thin. At forty-two, all the *yang* meridians related to the face are depleted, the entire face is wrinkled and the hair begins to turn grey. At forty-nine, the Conception Vessel is empty, the Thoroughfare Vessel is depleted, the reproductive essence is exhausted, the menstruation ceases, and the woman is no longer able to conceive.

"In the male, at eight years of age, Kidney *qi* becomes full, his hair grows long, and the permanent teeth appear. At the age of sixteen years, Kidney *qi* is full, the sex-stimulating essence comes in with seminal discharge; intercourse and procreation is possible. At twenty-four years, his Kidney *qi* is in *yin-yang* balance, the wisdom teeth emerge, and his body is fully developed. At thirty-two years, the tendons and bones are firm and muscles full-grown. At forty, Kidney *qi* begins to decline, the hair begins to thin and the teeth become loose. At forty-eight, *yang-qi* to the head begins to deplete, the face becomes wrinkled and the hair grey. At fifty-six, Liver *qi* weakens, and the tendons become stiff; the sex-stimulating essence is exhausted, the sperm becomes less, and with the waning of the Kidneys the body deteriorates. At sixty-four, the hair and teeth are lost. The Kidneys store the excess essence of all the organs. But now, the organs are all weakened with age and their essence has become depleted; the tendons and bones become frail and stiff, and the movements hampered. Since the Kidney reservoir becomes empty, there is no more reproductive essence for conception."

Therefore, the Kidneys rule development, maturation and reproduction as well as aging through its function of storing vital essence (*jing*). Various sexual disturbances and reproductive problems (such as impotence or sterility) are usually attributed to dysfunction or hypofunction of the Kidneys. Premature senility may be prevented by using Kidney tonics.

(2) Producing marrow, dominating the bones and replenishing the brain

These functions are also closely related to the vital essence (*jing*) stored in the Kidneys. Marrow includes the bone marrow and spinal marrow. Both are produced from the Kidney essence. The bone marrow fills and nourishes the bones, so the condition of the bones is determined by the Kidney function of storing vital essence. Deficiency of Kidney essence is a common cause of defective skeletal development in children and other bone disorders involving bone solidity, such as osteomalacia and osteoporosis.

The upper part of the spinal marrow (spinal cord) is connected with the brain. In traditional Chinese medicine, the brain is also called a "sea of marrow" or taken as a part of the marrow. When the Kidneys function well with abundant storage of vital essence (*jing*), the activities of the brain are normal, full of vim and vigor, quick in thinking, nimble in reactions, acute in hearing and vision. If the Kidney essence is insufficient, the patient lacks vigor, and suffers from dizziness, tinnitus, forgetfulness, soreness in the loins and weakness of the legs.

(3) Transforming essence into blood

---

[6]*Qi* can be divided into *yin-qi* and *yang-qi*. In children, *yang-qi* is exuberant and the children are said to have "a pure-*yang* constitution." In adults, *yin-qi* and *yang-qi* should be kept in balance, but in old people, *yang-qi* is usually declining. These are the physiological changes that come about with age.

[7]The Yangming Meridians of the hands and feet (Large Intestine and Stomach Meridians) are connected with the face for supplying nourishment.

"If the bone marrow is sound, both *qi* and blood are produced." The bone marrow is formed from the Kidney essence. So the Kidneys are also related to the regeneration of blood. Clinically, tonifying the Kidneys and replenishing their essence are effective therapies for aplastic anemia and anemia in other blood diseases.

Table III-10. Functions of the Kidney

	Physiological significance	Pathological significance
Storing essence	1. To promote reproduction	Decrease of reproductive function: sterility
	2. To promote development	Retardation of development, premature senility
	3. To produce bone marrow and spinal marrow, and replenish the brain	Defective skeletal development Disorders of brain function: e.g., forgetfulness
	4. To transform essence into blood	Deficiency of blood
Governing vital fire	1. To supply heat energy for warming the body and activating zang-fu organs	Insufficient vital fire: aversion to cold, cold limbs; diarrhea before dawn
	2. To serve as the motive force of sex ("ministerial fire")	Insufficient "ministerial fire": hyposexuality Excessive "ministerial fire": hypersexuality
Dominating water meta-bolism	To maintain normal water	Disordered water metabolism metabolism: oliguria with edema or polyuria
Assisting respiration	To help the Lungs keep normal respiration	Failure of the Kidneys to receive air: dyspnea with prolonged exhalation

2. Governing the vital fire

The vital fire refers to the heat energy distributed throughout the body for activating the functions of organs and tissues, maintaining the body temperature, and promoting development in youngsters. When the vital fire is deficient, the most common manifestation is aversion to cold, with cold limbs. Among all the visceral organs, the Spleen needs a particular supply of vital fire, as the process of digestion is figuratively described as "stewing" the food. Decline of vital fire, therefore, may lead to digestive disorders characterized by diarrhea with undigested food in the stool. Owing to the circadian rhythmic changes of *yin* and *yang,* with the least *yang* in the small hours of the morning, diarrhea due to decline of vital fire usually occurs daily before dawn.

The vital fire is also the motive force of the sexual function. This part of vital fire bears the specific name of "ministerial fire" in order to differentiate it from the vital fire with other actions. If the "ministerial fire" is insufficient, there will be hyposexuality, frigidity or impotence, premature ejaculation and spermatorrhea. On the other hand, the "ministerial fire" may also be in relative excess, usually due to deficiency of Kidney *yin.* In this case, there is hypersexuality and nocturnal emission.

3. Dominating water metabolism

Water metabolism includes two major processes: Distribution of fluids throughout the body for nourishing the organs and tissues, and excretion of turbid (waste) fluids after utilization and metabolism. The Kidneys are involved in both processes. Although the fluids derived from food and drink are assimilated and transported by the Spleen and dispersed by the Lungs, these functions depend upon the warming action of the vital fire governed by the Kidneys, which is called "vaporization" by the Kidneys metaphorically. When fluid is sent down to the Kidneys, it is separated into two parts: the clear (useful) and the turbid (waste). The clear part is retained, while the turbid part flows into the urinary bladder and is excreted as urine. Figuratively, the Kidneys work like a sluice gate, regulating the body fluid volume by appropriately opening and closing the gate. Normally, the opening and closing of the gate is in coordination, maintaining a relatively stable volume of body fluid. If the function of the Kidneys in regulating the water metabolism is impaired, disorders of the water metabolism will occur. Excessive closing with insufficient opening will result in oliguria and edema, while excessive opening with insufficient closing will lead to polyuria.

4. Assisting inhalation

The Kidneys assist the Lungs to inhale to accomplish the normal exchange of gases. This concept is based on the following facts: Dyspnea with prolonged exhalation and shortened inhalation that is considered to be "failure of the Kidneys to receive air" can be treated with Kidney tonics. During *qigong* practice, only when the sensation of *qi* comes down to the lower abdomen can the *qigong* state be achieved.

The functions of the Kidneys and their physiological and pathological significance are summarized in Table III-10.

5. Relations with the sense organs and tissues

(1) The Kidneys and the bones

See above: "Producing marrow, dominating the bones and replenishing the brain."

(2) The Kidneys and the ears

The ears can be taken as the "windows of the Kidneys," for healthy Kidneys ensure acute hearing, while dysfunction of the Kidneys is often accompanied by impaired hearing and tinnitus. Deafness in the aged develops along with the decline of Kidney *qi*.

(3) The Kidneys and the genitals and anus

The genitals (including the urethra) and the anus are also related to the Kidneys. The former are sexual organs and at the same time have the function of discharging urine. The latter is the opening through which the stool passes out of the body. Since dysfunction of the Kidneys may lead to sexual disturbances, abnormal urination and diarrhea, the genitals and the anus are considered to be the specific openings of the Kidneys.

The relations of the Kidneys with the sense organs and tissues, and their physiological and pathological significance are summarized in Table III-11.

6. Relations with the emotions

Fear and fright are thought to be the emotions most closely related to the Kidneys. This is probably because fright may cause incontinence of urine and stools.

7. Relations with the fluids

Among the fluids, saliva has a special relationship with the Kidneys. Here, the saliva refers to the thick natural liquid present in the mouth. The thin fluid running from the mouth is related to the Spleen. In traditional Chinese medicine, saliva is believed not only to moisten and digest food, cleanse and protect the mouth, but also to nourish the Kidney essence as it is transformed from the latter. That is why during *qigong* and many other health-preserving exercises, the saliva should be swallowed.

Table III-11. Relations of the Kidneys with the Sense Organs and Tissues

	Physiological significance	Pathological significance
Bone	Well-developed bones and firm teeth	Defective skeletal development; loosening and loss of teeth
Hair	Thick and lustrous hair	Withering or loss of hair
Ear	Acute hearing	Tinnitus and deafness
Genitalia and anus	Normal sexual ability, micturition and bowel movements	Sexual disturbances, disorders of micturition, diarrhea or constipation

THE SIX *FU*-ORGANS

The six *fu*-organs are the Gallbladder, Stomach, Small Intestine, Large Intestine, Bladder and Triple Energizer. The common feature of their functional activities is to pass the digested food or metabolites. So their functions are characterized by "going downward" and ensured by "opening without obstruction." Except for the Triple Energizer, all the other *fu*-organs have the same anatomical descriptions as in Western medicine. Their functions, though quite similar to those described in modern Western physiology, still have some peculiarities that need discussion.

The Gallbladder

The Gallbladder stores bile and excretes it into the intestines to help digestion. If the excretion of bile by the Gallbladder is impeded, digestion by the Stomach and Spleen would be impaired, manifested by anorexia, abdominal distension and diarrhea. If the passage of bile is obstructed, staining of the skin and sclera by the overflowing bile results in jaundice.

Beside excretion of bile, the Gallbladder also has something to do with mental activities. It is believed that the Gallbladder is particularly related to decisiveness and courage. This concept has had a profound influence on Chinese culture. Even now, a coward is customarily called "one with a small gallbladder" in the Chinese language. Clinically, insomnia with nightmares and susceptibility to fright can be diagnosed as "weakness of Gallbladder *qi*" and treated accordingly.

The Stomach

The Stomach receives and temporarily stores food and drink, so this organ is also called a "sea of food and drink." The food is partially digested in the Stomach, and transformed into chyme, which is sent down to the Small Intestine. Stomach diseases with impairment of the receiving function are usually manifested by anorexia and epigastric distension. If digestion is impaired, the undigested food will be retained in the Stomach, causing epigastric pain with foul belching.

Coordination of the Stomach with the Spleen safeguards the entire process of digestion, assimilation and distribution of the nutrients, and provision of material basis for the acquired constitution. So, "the root of the acquired constitution" is often attributed to the Spleen and the Stomach instead of the Spleen alone.

The function of the Stomach to send its food contents downward into the Intestines is also important. Disturbances of the descending function of the Stomach will result in upward perversion of Stomach *qi*, manifested by nausea and vomiting. In this context, it should be noted that by "Stomach" is sometimes meant the whole gastro-intestinal tract instead of just the Stomach itself, because the downward transmission of the intestinal contents is also attributed to the action of Stomach *qi*. Accumulation of pathogenic heat in the Stomach and Intestines resulting in high fever, severe thirst, profuse sweating, constipation or discharge of hard fecal masses, and abdominal pain is diagnosed as "excess in the Stomach" instead of "excess in the Stomach and Intestines."

Traditional Chinese medicine pays much attention to Stomach *qi*. "Stomach *qi* is the root of human life." If Stomach *qi* is strong, the *zang*-organs can maintain their normal activities. But if Stomach *qi* is weak, all the *zang*-organs will decline. And if Stomach *qi* dissipates, life will stop.

The Small Intestine

The Small Intestine receives partially digested food and drink from the Stomach for further digestion and "separation of the clear (nutrients) from the turbid (waste)." The nutrients are absorbed and then transported and transformed by the Spleen. The waste contains two parts: food dross and surplus water. Food dross is transmitted to the Large Intestine and discharged through the anus as feces. The surplus water is sent to the Kidneys and Bladder, and discharged as urine. This description is different from the concept of modern Western medicine, but it has practical value. In some cases of diarrhea accompanied by oliguria, increased water content of the stool and decreased volume of urine is thought to be due to impaired function of the Small Intestine in sending the surplus water to the Kidneys and Bladder, and the appropriate treatment is the use of diuretics.

The Small Intestine has its meridian connected with the Heart Meridian, and is hence closely related to the Heart physiologically and pathologically. Some Heart disorders, such as excessive fire in the Heart, may involve the Small Intestine, resulting in hematuria and a burning sensation during micturition.

The Large Intestine

The main function of the Large Intestine is to pass food dross and discharge feces. It transmits the waste material sent down from the Small Intestine, absorbs part of the fluids and finally excretes the waste as feces. So it is also called "an organ of transmission."

Dysfunction of the Large Intestine is often manifested by disordered transmission of its contents or impaired absorption of fluid. In the former case there may be constipation or diarrhea. In the latter case, diarrhea with borborygmi often occurs.

The Bladder

The main function of the Bladder is to temporarily store urine and eventually excrete it from the body. The Bladder is exterior-interiorly related to the Kidneys, not only because of their anatomical connection, but also due to the connection through the meridians. The function of the Bladder depends upon the action of Kidney *qi*, and can be taken as a part of the Kidney function. If Kidney *qi* is weakened, there will be difficulty in micturition or even retention of urine. If Kidney *qi* fails to arrest the discharge of urine, there will be dribbling or incontinence of urine. All these disturbances of urination are diagnosed as dysfunction of the Kidneys and should be treated from the Kidneys instead of the Bladder. Only when the Bladder is invaded by exogenous pathogens, such as damp-heat, should the Bladder itself be treated directly.

The Triple Energizer

The Triple Energizer is a unique term used in traditional Chinese medicine. It is composed of the Upper, Middle and Lower Energizers, and is regarded as one of the *fu*-organs. There have been arguments regarding the anatomical descriptions of the Triple Energizer, and it has even been said that the Triple Energizer is not an anatomical entity, but just a functional system. From the present knowledge of Chinese medicine, the Triple Energizer refers to the body cavities, i.e., the Upper, Middle and Lower Energizers refer to the thoracic cavity, upper abdominal cavity and lower abdominal cavity, respectively. As a functional system, it is in charge of water metabolism and *qi* (energy) metabolism.

"The Upper Energizer is like a sprayer," because the Heart and the Lungs housed in it spread *qi* and blood throughout the body and send fluids down to the Kidneys.

"The Middle Energizer resembles a fermentation tank," because the Stomach and the Spleen housed in it decompose and digest food.

"The Lower Energizer works like a sewer," because the Kidneys, Bladder and Large Intestine housed in it drain off waste and surplus water.

Therefore, the Triple Energizer serves as a container or passage by which digestion of food and drink, distribution of the essential substances, and excretion of the waste take place. Since the distribution of *qi* and fluid is the key link in the process of *qi* (energy) and fluid metabolism, the Triple Energizer often implies the passages of *qi* and fluids. The meridians are pathways of *qi*, but they are different from the Triple Energizer. The meridian system only connects the internal organs and the body surface, and the internal organs to each other. The Triple Energizer, however, governs *qi* in general, including the *qi* of all the organs and tissues, and also the *qi* of the meridians.

The distribution of fluids is closely related to the flow of *qi*. Without the movement of *qi*, there would be no movement of fluids. Moreover, *qi* cannot exist independently; blood and fluids are the carriers of *qi*. Therefore, distribution of *qi* and distribution of fluids are the two aspects of the same function of the Triple Energizer. The most common disorder of the Triple Energizer is disturbance of the water metabolism. Various kinds of retention of water and formation of edema due to different mechanisms—failure of the Lungs to send the fluids downwards, insufficiency of the Spleen in transporting fluids and weakness of the Kidneys in secreting urine are collectively called "dysfunction of the Triple Energizer."

THE EXTRAORDINARY ORGANS

The extraordinary organs include the brain, marrow, bones, blood vessels, Gallbladder and uterus. They are so called because they are said to resemble the *fu*-organs in form but the *zang*-organs in function.

The Brain

In ancient China, the function of the brain was not clearly known. Although there are some statements regarding the brain in *The Canon of Medicine*, such as "Intelligence comes from the head," and "If the sea of marrow (the brain) is weakened, there will be dizziness or vertigo, tinnitus, loss of vision and lassitude," the mental activities were attributed to the *zang-fu* organs, particularly the Heart. Later, it was recognized that the brain is in charge of psychic activities as well as thinking, memory and emotions. "The brain is the seat where mental activities take place." (*Ben Cao Gang Mu* or *Compendium of Materia Medica*, 1590) "Intelligence and memory depend on the function of the brain but not the Heart." (*Yi Lin Gai Cuo* or *Errors in Medicine Corrected*, 1830) However, since the theory of traditional Chinese medicine is self-justified, and the *zang-fu* organs actually imply functional systems rather than anatomical entities, it is not of much importance whether the organ in charge of psychic activities is called the brain or Heart. In addition, according to the theory of *zang-fu* manifestations, different brain functions are attributed to different *zang-fu* organs, e.g., consciousness to the Heart, memory to the Kidneys, consideration to the Liver. These conclusions were achieved not by imagination but chiefly by observation of daily life and therapeutic effect. For example, some people are born clever, and some slow-witted. This is apparently related to heredity. As the inborn (genetic) factors are associated with the reproductive essence (germ cells) stored in the Kidneys (uro-genital system), the Kidney essence has thus been taken as "the basis of the inborn constitution." In the aging process along with the decline of reproductive ability, memory starts to fail, and thinking and action slow down. These facts put more weight on the attribution of some brain functions to the Kidneys. Furthermore, Kidney-replenishing treatment does have some effect on preventing and improving the impaired brain functions.

Similar examples can also be listed for demonstrating the relationships of some other brain functions to the *zang-fu* organs. Therefore, if the basic concepts about the psychic, mental and nervous activities were changed from the functions of various *zang-fu* organs into the functions of the brain, the entire theoretic system of traditional Chinese medicine would have to be changed accordingly. Such a big change would cause great confusion among practitioners of Chinese medicine. In addition, most of the effective therapies for neurological and psychic conditions could hardly be applied to clinical practice. Of course, this does not mean that the traditional Chinese medical theories should always be the same, and there should be no change. Re-systematization and promotion of Chinese medical theories can only be accomplished after a thorough study of all their advantages by modern scientific means.

The Marrow

The marrow is the soft, fatty substance that fills the hollow parts of bones, the vertebral canal and the skull. As stated above, marrow in Chinese medicine includes bone marrow, spinal cord (spinal marrow), and even the brain ("sea of marrow"). All of them are believed to be transformed from and nourished by Kidney essence. Deficiency of Kidney essence may lead to retardation of development in children manifested by delayed closure of the fontanel, short stature, feeble-mindedness and slow action, and may also result in asthenia of the brain in adults manifested by dizziness, tinnitus, poor vision, weakness in the loins and legs, and loss of memory.

The bone marrow nourishes the bones. Firm bones need a sufficient supply of the marrow, and so deficiency of the Kidney essence also impairs the firmness of the bones.

"If the bone marrow is sound, *qi* and blood will be produced normally." (*The Canon of Medicine*) Impairment of the bone marrow may cause deficiency of blood, and replenishing Kidney essence is useful in the treatment of certain kinds of anemia.

The Bones

The bones form the body's shape and support it. They are also responsible for the body movements. The condition of the bones is closely related to Kidney essence as mentioned above. A person with deficiency of Kidney essence cannot stand for long or walk with vigorous strides.

The Blood Vessels

Strictly speaking, "the vessels are conduits for blood." (*The Canon of Medicine*) But *qi* and blood cannot be totally separated: Blood is the carrier of *qi*, and the circulation of blood depends upon the movement of *qi*. So, it is usually said that the blood vessels are the tubes through which *qi* and blood circulate.

Now, a question should be raised: Since both the blood vessels and the meridians are taken as the conduits through which *qi* and blood flow, what is the difference between them? In Chinese medicine there are several related terms: *xue-mai* (血脉) blood vessels, *jing-mai* (经脉) cardinal vessels (meridians), *luo-mai* (络脉) branches of cardinal vessels (collaterals), and *sun-mai* (孙脉) subdivided small branches of vessels or capillaries. From the terminology, the vascular system and meridian system can hardly be differentiated. The English word "meridian" (or formerly "channel") is the translation of the Chinese character 经 (*jing*), which actually refers to 经脉 (*jing-mai*) for short and means the cardinal vessels coursing vertically. Similarly, the complete name of "the twelve meridians" should be "the twelve cardinal (or longitudinal) vessels." In fact, even in the English translation, the word "vessel" is also retained in the eight extra meridians, e.g., the Governor Vessel, the Conception Vessel.

It is difficult to identify the anatomical difference between the vascular system and meridian system, for many concepts in Chinese medicine are not based on anatomy. Functionally, there are differences between the two systems. Blood vessels are used for transporting blood (which carries nutrients and vital energy) to the various parts of the body, while the meridians are used for connecting the internal organs with superficial organs and tissues, and also for connecting different internal organs to make the human body an integral whole. The latter function may be partially performed by the vascular system, but it cannot be totally accomplished by it. Therefore, many modern researchers have been searching for the anatomical basis of the meridian system from the known body structure (blood vessels, lymph vessels and nervous system) or even trying to discover some new structure unknown to modern anatomy. However, so far no conclusion can be drawn on this issue.

The Uterus

The uterus is a female organ in which offspring are carried and nourished before birth. It is also in charge of menstruation. Its functions are closely related to the Thoroughfare and Conception Vessels, and to the Liver, Kidneys, Heart and Spleen.

The uterus becomes mature when Kidney *qi* is full, approximately at the age of fourteen years, according to *The Canon of Medicine*. "Both the Thoroughfare and Conception Vessels originate in the uterus." The Conception Vessel, meeting the three *yin* meridians of the foot, regulates all the *yin* meridians of the body and is called "sea of *yin* meridians." The Thoroughfare Vessel, running in parallel to the Governor Vessel, regulates the *qi* and blood of the twelve meridians and is called "sea of blood." When blood is abundant in the twelve meridians, it floods into the Thoroughfare and Conception Vessels and reaches the uterus, forming menstruation, which is regulated by the two vessels. In childhood when Kidney *qi* is not full, the uterus is not mature, the Conception Vessel is not open, the Thoroughfare Vessel is lacking in blood, and so there is no menstruation. By the age of fifty, the Kidney essence-*qi* declines, resulting in insufficient filling of the Thoroughfare and Conception Vessels, and so the menstruation becomes scanty, and finally ceases. Pathologically, disorders of the Thoroughfare and Conception Vessels are manifested by irregular menstruation, abnormal uterine bleeding, amenorrhea, infertility and abortion.

The chief component of menstruation is blood. The Heart rules blood, the Liver stores blood, the Spleen controls blood and the Kidneys transform its essence into blood. The function of any of these *zang*-organs may influence menstruation. Failure of the Liver to store blood or failure of the Spleen to control blood usually results in excessive menstrual flow with shortened cycles and prolonged periods, or even abnormal uterine bleeding out of the period. Diminished function of the Spleen may impair the production of blood, giving rise to insufficiency of Heart blood with oligomenorrhea or even amenorrhea. Injury to the Liver by depression causing stagnant flow of *qi* may also lead to menstrual disorders.

THE RELATIONS BETWEEN THE *ZANG-FU* ORGANS

The human body is regarded as an integral organic whole. All its component parts, including organs and tissues, should function harmoniously. Physiologically, they are mutually connected, dependent and restraining. Pathologically, they are mutually influencing and transmit the diseases according to certain rules.

The Relations between *Zang* and *Zang* Organs

I. The Heart and the Lungs

Both the Heart and the Lungs are situated in the Upper Energizer. The Heart rules blood and the Lungs dominate *qi*. So, the relationship between the Heart and the Lungs is actually the relationship between *qi* and blood. The Heart pumps blood and makes it circulate, but the circulation is also driven and regulated by Lung *qi*. On the other hand, *qi* is distributed throughout the body by attaching to the blood. Without the drive of *qi*, the blood would be stagnant; without blood as the carrier, *qi* would perish. Therefore, the following sayings are very commonly used in Chinese medicine: "*Qi* is the commander of blood" and "blood is the mother of *qi*"; "*Qi* in motion keeps blood circulating," and "stagnation of *qi* causes stasis of blood."

Pathologically, the following conditions are frequently encountered: weakness of Lung *qi* results in stagnation of Heart blood; deficiency of Heart *qi* leads to dysfunction of the Lungs; deficiency of *qi* of the Heart and Lungs gives rise to blood stasis.

II. The Heart and the Spleen

The Heart rules blood, and the Spleen regenerates and controls blood (keeps blood flowing within the blood vessels). So the relationship between the Heart and Spleen is chiefly reflected in the regeneration and flowing of blood. Physiologically, the Spleen functions well with adequate assimilation of food essence which is transformed into blood, and Heart blood is thus abundant. On the other hand, when Heart blood is abundant, the Spleen is well nourished and functions normally. Normal blood flow depends on the drive of Heart *qi*, circulating throughout the whole body, and also on the control of Spleen *qi*, which keeps the blood flowing within the blood vessels.

Pathologically, diseases of the Spleen may involve the Heart: weakness of the Spleen leads to inadequate regeneration of blood, and hence deficiency of Heart blood. Diseases of the Heart, in turn, may involve the Spleen: When Heart blood is consumed, the Spleen will be poorly nourished, leading to deficiency of Spleen *qi*. No matter whether deficiency of Spleen *qi* leads to deficiency of Heart blood, or deficiency of Heart blood results in deficiency of Spleen *qi*, "deficiency of both the Heart and the Spleen" will ensue.

III. The Heart and the Liver

The relationship between the Heart and the Liver is reflected in blood supply and mental activities.

The Liver stores blood. If the Heart blood is abundant, some blood can be stored in the Liver for regulating the circulating blood volume. Blood pertains to *yin*. Adequate blood supply nourishes the Liver and restrains the activity of Liver *yang*. Furthermore, a well-nourished Liver usually has a normal function in smoothing and regulating the flow of *qi* and blood. This, in turn, helps the Heart to promote blood circulation.

As for mental activities, the Heart governs mental activities, and the Liver smoothes the flow of *qi* and blood, regulating psychic and emotional activities. If the functions of both organs are in good coordination, normal mental activities can be maintained.

Pathologically, the mutual influences of the Heart and the Liver are reflected in deficiency of blood and mental disorders. Insufficiency of Liver blood may lead to consumption of Heart blood, and insufficiency of Heart blood may result in consumption of Liver blood. In both cases pallor, insomnia and palpitation may occur, indicating deficiency of Heart blood, and dizziness, numbness in the limbs, withered nails and oligomenorrhea, indicating deficiency of Liver blood. Blood deficiency in the Heart and the Liver may influence mental activities, bringing about depression with insomnia and irritability. In addition, deficiency of *yin*-blood may be accompanied by relative exuberance of *yang*-fire. Exuberance of Heart and Liver fire is one of the pathogenic bases of mania.

IV. The Heart and the Kidneys

1. Coordination between the Heart and the Kidneys

The Heart controls fire (pertaining to *yang*), and the Kidneys regulate water (pertaining to *yin*). Normally, the fire of the Heart comes down to warm the Kidneys and the water of the Kidneys goes up to irrigate the Heart. Thus, a *yin-yang* balance between the Heart and the Kidneys is maintained. This is called "coordination of the Heart and the Kidneys," also "coordination of fire and water."

If this balanced relationship breaks down, there will be a series of fire symptoms of the Heart together with deficiency of Kidney *yin*. This is called "incoordination of the Heart and the Kidneys."

2. Mutual transformation of vital essence and blood

The Heart rules blood, and the Kidneys store vital essence. Both vital essence and blood are essential substances for maintaining life activities. Vital essence regenerates blood, and blood nourishes vital essence. It is believed that vital essence can be transformed into blood, and vice versa.

Pathologically, patients with deficiency of blood often have manifestations of deficiency of both Heart blood and Kidney essence.

3. Mutual dependence of vital essence and mental activities

Jing (vital essence) is the material basis of *shen* (mental activities, especially consciousness, expression and concentration), and the mental activities are the manifestations of vital essence. The Heart governs mental activities and the Kidneys store vital essence. Normal mental activities depend on soundness of the Heart and Kidneys.

Clinically, either consumption of Heart blood or deficiency of Kidney essence may be manifested as mental symptoms such as insomnia, dream-disturbed sleep and forgetfulness.

V. The Lungs and the Spleen

The Spleen is the source generating *qi* and the Lungs, taking charge of respiration, dominate *qi*. The Spleen transports fluid to the Heart and Lungs, and the Lungs disperse fluids throughout the body and send fluids downward to the urinary system. Thus, these two *zang*-organs have a close relationship in the formation of *qi* and distribution of fluids.

Normally, the fresh air (oxygen) inhaled by the Lungs and the essence of food and drink transported upward by the Spleen combine together, forming acquired *qi*. The essence of food and drink assimilated by the Spleen is distributed throughout the body by the dispersing action of the Lungs. On the other hand, the activities of the Lungs need the essence of food and drink provided by the Spleen. So it is said that the Spleen assists the Lungs to replenish *qi*.

In water metabolism, the Spleen sends fluids upwards, and the Lungs disperse fluids throughout the body and send them down through the water passages. So, a harmonious combination of the Spleen and the Lungs is an important link in the process of water metabolism.

Pathologically, deficiency of Lung *qi* in a long run will lead to deficiency of Spleen *qi*, and weakness of the Spleen usually lowers the resistance of the Lungs against pathogens. As a treatment principle, weakness of the Lungs should be treated with Spleen tonics. This is also called "reinforcing earth (the Spleen) to strengthen metal (the Lungs)."

Insufficiency of the Spleen in transformation and transportation may cause retention of fluids, forming damp-phlegm which invades the Lungs and results in chronic cough and expectoration. So, in traditional Chinese medicine, expectoration in chronic respiratory diseases is explained in a peculiar way: "The Spleen is the source from which phlegm is produced, while the Lungs are the organs that store phlegm."

VI. The Lungs and the Liver

The action of the Liver is characterized by ascent, and the action of the Lungs by descent. Harmonious actions of these two organs ensure normal movement of *qi* and blood. Hyperactivity (fire) in the Liver may impair the normal descending function of the Lungs, resulting in paroxysms of coughing, sometimes accompanied by hemoptysis. This is also called "Fire of wood (the Liver) invading metal (the Lungs)."

VII. The Lungs and the Kidneys

The Lungs, regulating the water passages, are "the upper source of water flow," and the Kidneys are the organs in charge of water metabolism. The Lungs dominate respiration and the Kidneys assist the Lungs to receive air. So the two organs cooperate in water metabolism and respiration.

Pathologically, dysfunction of the Lungs in sending down fluids through the water passages will impair the Kidneys' function in regulating water metabolism, causing retention of water and edema. If the Kidneys fail to receive air, respiration will be impaired, manifested by dyspnea with prolonged exhalation and shortened inhalation.

VIII. The Liver and the Spleen

The Liver and the Spleen function harmoniously in digestion and blood circulation. The Liver's smoothing function facilitates secretion of bile and guarantees the normal function of the Spleen in digestion, assimilation and transportation. On the other hand, the Liver needs nourishment from the Spleen. In addition, the Liver stores blood and smoothes the flow of blood, and the Spleen regenerates blood and controls blood circulation to prevent extravasation. So, the two organs also act in coordination in blood circulation.

If the Liver function is depressed, the digestive function of the Stomach and the Spleen will be impaired. This is called "depressed wood (the Liver) encroaching earth (the Spleen)."

When the Spleen is diseased, dampness may be retained. If dampness impairs the Liver function, particularly the secretion of bile, jaundice may occur.

Weakness of the Spleen may impair the regeneration of blood or the normal flow of blood within the blood vessels. Impaired regeneration of blood or excessive loss of blood may lead to insufficiency of Liver blood.

IX. The Liver and the Kidneys

The relation between the Liver and the Kidneys is very close. There is even a saying: "The Liver and the Kidneys have the same source." This is chiefly because the Liver stores blood and the Kidneys store vital essence; and vital essence and blood have the same origin as they can be transformed into each other. In addition, the Liver needs an adequate supply of Kidney *yin* (vital essence) for nourishment, so that a normal *yin-yang* balance can be maintained in the Liver. The Liver and the Kidneys also act in coordination in the sexual and reproductive function. This is not only because they provide the material (vital essence and blood) for menstruation in the female and seminal discharge in the male, but also because both the Liver and the Kidneys govern the "ministerial fire"[8] which is the

---

[8]It is believed that the "ministerial fire" originating from the Kidneys stay in the Liver, the Gallbladder and the Triple Energizer.

motive force of the sexual function.

Pathologically, deficiency of Kidney *yin* (vital essence) is often accompanied by deficiency of Liver *yin*. The latter will lead to relative excess of Liver *yang*, manifested by dizziness, headache, irritability and tinnitus. In a severe case, even twitching or convulsions may occur. On the other hand, fire of the Liver may also involve the Kidneys, resulting in consumption of Kidney *yin* or hyperactivity of the "ministerial fire" manifested by nocturnal emission and sexual hyperesthesia.

X. The Spleen and the Kidneys

The Kidneys are the "root of the congenital constitution," and the Spleen, the "root of the acquired constitution," providing the material basis for regeneration of *qi* and blood. The Kidneys control the excretion of water, and the Spleen controls the transportation of fluid. Therefore, the two organs collaborate in promoting the constitution and accomplishing water metabolism.

Normally, digestion and assimilation of food by the Spleen needs the warming action of Kidney *yang*. Moreover, the congenital essence stored in the Kidneys should be constantly nourished by the acquired essence from the Spleen.

In the process of water metabolism, transportation of fluids by the Spleen also needs the warming and vaporizing action of Kidney *yang*. The Kidneys govern the discharge of water by opening and closing the sluice gate, which, in turn, is influenced by Spleen *qi*. This is called "earth restraining water."

If Kidney *yang* is insufficient, the Spleen function will be impaired. The typical condition is diarrhea occurring daily before dawn. If the Spleen's action in restraining water is insufficient, water will flood from the Kidneys, causing edema or ascites.

The Relations between the *Zang*- and *Fu*-Organs

The *zang*-organs pertain to *yin,* and *fu*-organs to *yang*. The relationship between the *zang*- and *fu*-organs actually refers to the coordination of *yin* and *yang*. Each *zang*-organ has a *fu*-organ as its partner, directly connected by meridians and functioning in coordination. Since the *zang*-organs are situated in the interior of the body without direct connection with the outside, while the *fu*-organs are more exteriorly situated, discharging their contents out of the body, each *zang*- and *fu*-organ in coordination is said to be interior-exteriorly related. The interior-exteriorly related *zang-fu* organs are: the Heart and the Small Intestine; the Lungs and the Large Intestine; the Spleen and the Stomach; the Liver and the Gallbladder; and the Kidneys and the Bladder. Besides the direct connection via meridians, some of them also have anatomical connections. It should be noted that each pair of interior-exteriorly related *zang-fu* organs function in coordination physiologically and influence each other in diseased conditions. But, this does not rule out the relations between other *zang-fu* organs.

I. The Heart and the Small Intestine

The Heart and the Small Intestine have no direct anatomical connection. Their connection is achieved by meridians, as the Heart Meridian originates in the Heart and is connected with the Small Intestine, and the Small Intestine Meridian is connected with the Heart. The clinical significance of the interior-exterior relationship is reflected in some morbid conditions, e.g., Heart fire may move downward to the Small Intestine, causing disturbance of the latter; and heat from the Small Intestine may go upward to the Heart, impairing the Heart function.

II. The Lungs and the Large Intestine

The Lungs and the Large Intestine are also connected by their meridians. They have a close relationship in their functional activities. The Lungs regulate the passages of water and the Large Intestine absorbs fluid. Both take part in controlling water metabolism. If the Lungs function normally, there will be neither retention of water nor consumption of fluid in the Large Intestine, and normal stools will be discharged. Furthermore, the transmission of intestinal contents by the Large Intestine depends on the descending action of Lung *qi*. If Lung *qi* is weak, the transmission function of the Large Intestine will be impaired, resulting in constipation, which can be effectively treated by replenishing Lung *qi*. On the other hand, if the transmission of the intestinal contents is impeded by excess heat in the Large Intestine itself, the descent of Lung *qi* can also be impaired, leading to dyspnea and stuffiness in the chest. In this case, cathartics may relieve the respiratory disorders.

III. The Spleen and the Stomach

The Spleen and the Stomach coordinate in digestion and assimilation. Both organs are regarded as the "root of acquired constitution" and the "source of regenerating *qi* and blood." In fact, the characteristic features of their functions are in opposition: the Stomach "receives" food, while the Spleen "sends out" the food essence; the Stomach "sends downward" the turbid (preliminarily digested food), while the Stomach "sends upward" the clear (nutrients); the Stomach is intolerant of dryness, while the Spleen is intolerant of dampness. Precisely because of their opposite functional properties, the Stomach and Spleen complement and mutually restrain each other, so that their physiological activities can be kept in harmony. This is a general rule of coordination between two organs, and the relation between the Stomach and the Spleen is illustrative of this.

Pathologically, the Stomach and the Spleen influence each other, and in many digestive disorders both organs are involved. In herbal treatment, stomachic and Spleen-invigorating drugs are often used in combination.

IV. The Liver and the Gallbladder

The Liver secretes bile as a part of its smoothing function, and the Gallbladder stores and discharges bile. Coordination of the two organs plays an important role in digestion. In addition, both organs are related to psychic activities, particularly to courage and decisiveness.

Pathologically, the Liver and the Gallbladder influence each other. For example, damp-heat often invades both organs, causing jaundice and bitterness in the mouth (symptoms of the Gallbladder) together with hypochondriac pain and distension (stagnation of Liver *qi*).

V. The Kidneys and the Bladder

The Kidneys secrete urine and the Bladder stores and discharges urine. The function of the Bladder is actually controlled by the Kidneys, and can be taken as a part of the Kidney function. Particularly in diminished function of the Bladder, the treatment is usually to reinforce the Kidneys.

CHAPTER 4

CAUSES OF DISEASE AND PATHOGENIC FACTORS

In traditional Chinese medicine, diseases are defined as the struggling process of genuine or normal *qi* (body resistance) against evil *qi* (pathogenic factors). Between these two opposing aspects, the former is often more emphasized. As stated in *The Canon of Medicine*, "If genuine *qi* prevails, the attack of evil *qi* never avails." "If evil *qi* invades the body, genuine *qi* must be insufficient." Emphasis on genuine *qi* does not mean that evil *qi* can be neglected. On the contrary, in some acute cases, evil *qi* may play a determinant role in the occurrence of a disease. Therefore, there are two general rules of treatment: one is to strengthen genuine *qi* (the body's resistance), and the other is to dispel evil *qi* (the pathogenic factors). The above two rules are often expressed in a more complete way: "Strengthen genuine *qi* so as to eliminate evil *qi*" and "Dispel evil *qi* so as to strengthen genuine *qi*." This indicates that any disease process must involve two opposite aspects: genuine *qi* and evil *qi*.

In this connection, we can now discuss "deficiency syndromes." In Chinese medicine, there are a number of diseases or syndromes characterized by insufficient vital energy, diminished functional activities or deficiency of essential substances. They are called deficiency syndromes. In diagnosing those syndromes, probably no evil *qi* is mentioned, unless they are further complicated by an apparent attack of evil *qi*. However, in an uncomplicated deficiency syndrome, evil *qi* does exist, though only in a relative sense. Chinese medical theory stresses the adaptability of the human body to the environment. If a functional system of the human body is in a insufficiency state, a normal event occurring in the environment may become an evil factor. For example, for a person with decreased function of the Spleen, a normal diet may cause indigestion; for a person with deficiency of Heart *qi*, moderate physical activities will lead to shortness of breath and palpitations; for a person with deficiency of Lung *qi*, a minute weather change may cause flu. Normal diet, moderate physical activities and minute weather changes certainly cause no harm to healthy persons, but they have the effects of improper diet, overwork and stormy weather changes in those with deficiency conditions.

CAUSE OF DISEASE

According to the above discussion, the causes of disease can be generally divided into two categories: invasion of pathogenic factors (evil *qi*) and reduction of the body's resistance (genuine *qi*). Generally, a disease usually results in the following three conditions: (1) The pathogenic factor is so strong that it intrudes into the human body even though genuine *qi* is normal. (2) Genuine *qi* is so weak that any factor negligible for a normal person may become pathogenic and cause disease. (3) Genuine *qi* is weak and the pathogenic factor strong, and so disease is inevitable. In conclusion, the cause of a disease is always the failure of genuine *qi* to prevent the attack of pathogenic factors. This concept is of crucial significance in the treatment and prevention of disease.

Another important issue is the cause of insufficient genuine *qi*. Genuine *qi* has two natures: inborn (prenatal) and acquired (postnatal). First of all, an inherited defect may cause insufficiency of genuine *qi*. But in most cases, genuine *qi* is impaired postnatally by various pathogenic factors. For example, prolonged improper diet impairs the function of the Spleen, leading to deficiency of Spleen *qi*; over-indulgence in sex consumes the vital essence, resulting in deficiency of Kidney *yin*. Therefore, the pathogenic factors stated below may cause deficiency conditions, even though they are no longer present.

Customarily, pathogenic factors are classified into two categories: external or exogenous, and internal or endogenous. The exogenous pathogenic factors refer chiefly to abnormal weather changes and various infectious agents. The diseases caused by these factors are collectively called "exogenous affections." The endogenous pathogenic factors refer chiefly to emotions. The diseases caused by excessive or persistent emotional changes are called "endogenous injuries." There are other pathogenic factors, such as trauma, improper diet, overwork, mental stress and over-indulgence in sex. They are called non-exogenous and non-endogenous factors, but in fact they are also either exogenous or endogenous. Generally speaking, most cases of exogenous affection are acute and infectious, and most endogenous injuries, including those caused by overwork, mental stress and sexual indulgence are chronic and non-infectious. But there are exceptions, for example, some cases of exogenous affection may be chronic, as encountered in a chronic infectious disease, and some endogenous injuries may be acute, as seen in a sudden occurrence of *yin-yang* imbalance during a fit of emotional upset.

PATHOGENIC FACTORS

The Six Evils

The six evils primarily refer to excessive or untimely weather changes. They are wind, cold, summer-heat, damp, dryness and fire. Their occurrence is often seasonal. Since most infectious diseases are marked by seasonal epidemicity, the exogenous upsets caused by the six evils also include many infectious diseases.

The weather always changes from time to time, and man is adapted to them. But if it suddenly becomes too hot or too cold or it changes in an untimely fashion, one may get sick because of inadaptability. However, there is no clear-cut demarcation line between normal and abnormal or non-pathogenic and pathogenic changes of weather. *The Canon of Medicine* states, "A pathogenic factor such as wind, rain, cold or heat is unable to cause damage unless there is insufficient genuine *qi*. That is why people with good resistance, though caught in a heavy rain or strong wind, will not become ill." A sudden violent change of weather may not harm individuals with strong constitutions, while those with weak constitutions may become sick even because of a mild weather change. Therefore, a practitioner cannot determine the cause of an exogenous affection merely by observing weather changes. In addition, owing to the limitations of natural science and technology in ancient times, there was no laboratory means to find out the pathogens that cause exogenous affection, though the latter actually include many viral and bacterial infections.

In this connection, two questions should be answered first: (1) What is the rationale of the six evils hypothesis? (2) In clinical practice, how can the pathogenic factors be determined in patients with exogenous affections?

Deduction from analogy

Deduction from analogy was a common way of reasoning in ancient China. The theory of the five elements in traditional Chinese medicine is actually based on analogy. This is also true for the hypothesis of cause of disease, especially for knowledge about the six evils. Take wind for example. Some patients suffering from attacks of wind really have histories of being caught in draughts, but most patients with wind syndrome have no such history. Wind was taken as one of the pathogenic factors because of the similarities between the symptoms and the natural wind. Since the wind blows the branches of a tree slantwise, Bell's palsy, characterized by the twisting sideways of the face, is usually diagnosed as a wind syndrome and thought to be caused by pathogenic wind. Among the common natural phenomena, the wind is most likely to start suddenly and subside quickly. On this account, many morbid conditions characterized by abrupt onset and disappearance (e.g., urticaria and angioneurotic edema) are considered to be wind syndromes. Since things can be moved by the wind in a gust, pathological changes marked by migratory features (e.g., acute rheumatic arthritis) are also attributed to wind.

Reasoning from analogy may provide brilliant insights, but not a logical trend of thought. A deduction drawn from analogy always needs further evidence to prove it. In traditional Chinese medicine, the strongest argument for the hypothesis of the cause of a disease are the results of clinical treatment, i.e., all the above-mentioned diseases can be effectively treated by "wind-dispelling" medicines. Therefore, it can be concluded that all these morbid conditions must have a common pathogenic or pathogenetic factor. This is more important than arguing about whether the factor should be called "wind" or not.

Clinical determination of the exogenous pathogenic factor

In internal injuries, the causal factor can often be determined by tracing the history of the condition, taking into account such factors as overwork and emotional upset. For exogenous affection, the history may not be much help. For example, most patients with a wind syndrome have no history of being caught in a draught. The usual way of determining the pathogenic factor is to analyze the symptoms and signs. This is actually a part of the diagnostic process known as etiological differentiation of syndromes. In other words, the determination of the pathogenic factor and the etiological differentiation of the syndrome in exogenous affection are practically the same. In modern Western medicine, once the pathogen is found, the etiological diagnosis can be ascertained. But in traditional Chinese medicine, the reverse may be more appropriate in most cases, i.e., once the syndrome differentiation is determined, the pathogenic factor can be determined. Take rheumatoid arthritis for example. Theoretically, it is caused by a combined attack of pathogenic wind, cold and damp, but in an individual case, one of the pathogenic factors may play the major role. In some cases, particularly in those with acute exacerbation, heat may also be the pathogenic factor. If multiple joints are involved, with migratory arthralgia accompanied by aversion to wind and fever, the diagnosis is wind-arthritis. In this case, wind should be considered as the pathogenic factor, and wind-dispelling therapy should be applied. If the joint pain is severe and fixed, aggravated by exposure to cold, alleviated by applying warmth and not accompanied by local hotness and redness, the diagnosis is cold-arthritis; cold is regarded as the major pathogenic factor, and cold-dispelling therapy is the main treatment. If the joint pain is accompanied by local swelling and a sensation of heaviness, and the patient's tongue coating is greasy and white, the diagnosis is damp-arthritis. In this case, damp is considered to be the major pathogenic factor, and damp-eliminating therapy should be applied. If there is acute exacerbation of the arthritis with joint pain, redness and hotness, accompanied by fever, thirst, yellow tongue coating and rapid pulse, the diagnosis is heat-arthritis, and the major pathogenic factor is heat. From the above examples, it can be clearly seen that the pathogenic factor is determined by identifying the syndrome or syndrome pattern. The terms used to designate the pathogenic factors are the same as the names of the syndromes.

The Six Endogenous Evils

Another puzzling issue is that in some endogenous injuries there may also be symptoms and signs similar to above-mentioned natural phenomena, and terms such as wind, cold, heat, damp, dryness and fire are also used for naming both the syndromes and the pathogenic factors. As pathogenic factors, they are not exogenous and have no direct relation to the climate. In most cases, they are the products of other morbid processes, and in turn, they further give rise to pathological changes. For example, long-term stress may consume Liver *yin*, with relatively exuberant *yang* (as in hypertension). When exuberant *yang* reaches a high level, there may be attacks of vertigo. During the attack, the patient feels that his head is spinning and the surroundings are moving or rotating. Since the symptoms possess the characteristic features of wind, they also constitute a morbid condition that is called a "wind syndrome." In this case, the wind by no means originates from outside the human body, but is a product of highly exuberant *yang*, and is hence endogenous. In order to differentiate this from pathogenic wind from outside, it is called "endogenous wind." Besides endogenous wind, there are endogenous cold, endogenous heat, endogenous dampness, endogenous dryness and endogenous fire.

Endogenous wind is apparently different from exogenous wind. Why didn't the ancient Chinese use different terms for these, to avoid confusion? Initially, in some endogenous diseases the pathogenic factors were thought to be exogenous. For example, stroke was believed to be a disease stemming from exogenous wind, and was thus called wind-stroke. Later, strokes were found to be unrelated to exogenous wind, but practitioners of Chinese medicine as well as ordinary Chinese people have persisted in using the same name. This is not merely because they are accustomed to this terminology; clinical findings may also play a certain role. The general principle of treating wind syndrome is to get rid of pathogenic wind. After numerous trials, quite a few herbal drugs were found to have the effect of eliminating both exogenous wind (in treating "catching wind," "wind-rash," "windy arthritis," and "wind-edema") and endogenous wind (in treating convulsions, vertigo and some premonitory symptoms of apoplexy, such as numbness of the limbs). This is true for other evils, too. The herbal drugs that are prescribed to eliminate exogenous damp and endogenous damp and to relieve exogenous dryness and endogenous dryness are almost the same.

In summary, although the six evils originating from weather changes are taken as pathogenic factors of exogenous affections, they actually serve as guidelines for the classification of syndromes, and identification of the corresponding syndromes is of more significance than determination of the pathogenic factors themselves. In addition, many syndromes which are not caused by exogenous pathogenic factors are also classified under the six headings. Therefore, it is appropriate to discuss the pathogenic factors together with their corresponding syndromes, and the differentiation between exogenous and endogenous conditions.

I. Wind and Wind Syndromes

1. The properties of wind and the characteristics of wind syndromes

Wind is air in motion. It usually comes and goes abruptly, makes things move, sways the branches of trees, and blows harder at the tops of mountains than at the bottoms. Symptoms or diseases with features similar to wind are believed to result from wind, and are grouped under the heading of wind syndromes.

(1) Symptoms or diseases with sudden onset and quick disappearance, e.g., mild cases of upper respiratory infection or allergic rhinitis with only sneezing and running nose, which are soon righted ("catching wind"), urticaria ("wind-rash") and angioneurotic edema.

(2) Diseases with lesions that move from one place to another, e.g., rheumatic arthritis with migratory joint pains ("wind-arthritis"), and cutaneous pruritus with no fixed location.

(3) Generalized diseases with marked symptoms in the head and face, e.g., acute nephritis with puffy eyelids ("wind-edema").

(4) Symptoms or diseases characterized by the sudden onset of abnormal involuntary movements or sensation of abnormal movements, e.g., diseases marked by tremors, twitching, convulsions, or vertigo, apoplexy with sudden onset of hemiplegia ("wind-stroke"), and facial paralysis.

2. Differentiation between exogenous and endogenous wind

The above conditions can be classified into two categories: exogenous wind syndromes (such as colds, acute rheumatic arthritis and allergic reactions) and endogenous wind syndromes (such as convulsions, vertigo and stroke). As far as facial paralysis is concerned, it may be caused by exogenous wind as in Bell's palsy, or by endogenous wind as in stroke.

Exogenous wind as a pathogenic factor comes from outside the human body in any season. Usually, it invades the upper respiratory tract (as in allergic rhinitis), the skin (as in cutaneous pruritus) and the meridians (as in migratory arthritis and Bell's palsy).

Endogenous wind originates inside the human body, and is usually due to dysfunction of the Liver. The Liver controls the tendons (the movements of the limbs). Dysfunction of the Liver may lead to disturbances in motion of some part of the body, such as hemiplegia and involuntary movements of the limbs. Exuberance of Liver *yang* may cause vertigo or even fainting. As stated in *The Canon of Medicine*, "Wind syndromes characterized by convulsions and vertigo are mostly due to some dysfunction of the Liver."

Therefore, the differentiation of exogenous and endogenous wind chiefly depends on which organ is involved. Involvement of the Lungs (including the body surface) and meridians indicates exogenous wind, while involvement of other internal organs, particularly the Liver, suggests endogenous wind.

II. Cold and Cold Syndromes

1. Properties of cold and characteristics of cold syndromes

Cold is a common weather change in winter, but it may happen in any season. In Chinese medicine, the following properties of cold are stressed: Cold makes things contract and congeal, and is apt to impair the *yang-qi* (consume heat energy). Symptoms grouped under the heading of cold syndrome are:

(1) Chill with cold limbs. Chill, an unpleasant feeling of cold, is subjective, while cold limbs can be detected by others. The cold feeling may be generalized over the whole body or localized in a certain part of the body, such as in the back, abdomen or a joint.

(2) Stiffness of joint(s) with contracture. It is often associated with pain, as in rheumatoid arthritis and other arthropathies.

(3) Stagnation of *qi* and blood due to the congealing effect of cold, manifested by severe pain aggravated by exposure to cold and alleviated by warmth.

2. Differentiation between exogenous and endogenous cold

The above cold syndromes may result either from exogenous cold or from endogenous cold. The differentiation is usually easy to make, because exogenous cold causes an acute illness involving the superficial part of the body as seen in the common cold or early stage of other infections, while endogenous cold is always due to deficiency of *yang* after a long-standing course of derangement of *zang-fu* organs, particularly the Kidneys. Among the *zang-fu* organs, the Spleen and the Stomach may be directly affected by exogenous cold, resulting in abdominal pain with vomiting and diarrhea, but an acute onset is helpful for the differentiation of exogenous affection from endogenous cold. Chronic arthritis aggravated by cold weather is not infrequently encountered. In this case, exogenous cold should be considered, but if a disease is long-standing, derangement of some *zang-fu* organs, particularly the Kidneys, is inevitable.

The most common symptom of cold syndromes is chill. Chill in an exogenous cold syndrome, particularly occurring at the onset of an infectious disease, cannot be alleviated by heavy clothing and a warm environment, while chill due to decreased heat metabolism in endogenous cold syndromes can be easily alleviated by applying warmth.

III. Damp and Damp Syndromes

1. Properties of damp and characteristics of damp syndromes

A damp atmosphere and wet environment may cause disease, but more often damp syndromes are endogenous, due to dysfunction of *zang-fu* organs, especially the Spleen, which produces damp within the body. In the natural world, damp makes things sticky, heavy, turbid and dirty. As a pathogenic factor, damp may cause symptoms or diseases possessing these features, or it could be said that symptoms or diseases with these features are attributed to damp. The following symptoms or diseases indicate damp syndromes.

(1) Lingering disease with other manifestations indicating the presence of dampness. As damp makes things sticky, in a disease caused by damp, the patient finds it difficult to get rid of the pathogenic factor, and the course of the disease often persists for a long time.

(2) Impairment of the Spleen function. It is believed that the Spleen is intolerant of damp. Damp is apt to impair the transporting and transforming function of the Spleen, resulting in anorexia, diarrhea or edema.

(3) Heaviness in the head (as if it were tightly bound), body and limbs: a pathognostic symptom of damp affection.

(4) Pathological changes characterized by turbid discharge, such as morbid leukorrhea, turbid urine and exudation from skin lesions.

(5) Symptoms due to obstruction of the normal flow of *qi*, such as sensation of fullness in the chest, dyspnea and coughing with expectoration when the Lungs are affected by damp; epigastric or abdominal distension, anorexia, nausea, vomiting and diarrhea when damp is accumulated in the Spleen and the Stomach.

2. Differentiation between exogenous and endogenous damp

The differentiation between exogenous and endogenous damp syndromes is not always easy. It is common sense to diagnose a case of exogenous affection if the syndrome has an acute onset after exposure to damp (e.g., being caught in the rain), with symptoms involving the body's exterior, such as fever and chill, headache as if the head were tightly bound, and pain and swelling with a heavy sensation in the joints. However, if the *zang-fu* organs are involved, the differentiation may be difficult. Generally speaking, exogenous damp syndromes are more or less acute, with damp symptoms occurring before other manifestations of dysfunction of the *zang-fu* organs, while endogenous damp syndromes are usually chronic, with damp symptoms occurring after the presence of other manifestations indicating the dysfunction of the *zang-fu* organs.

IV. Dryness and Dryness Syndromes

1. Properties of dryness and characteristics of dryness syndromes

Attacks of dryness usually occur in the dry season. Such attacks are apt to impair the body fluids, resulting in a series of dry symptoms, particularly dryness of the Lungs, manifested by dry nose, dry throat and dry cough.

Deficiency of body fluids due to other causes, such as insufficient fluid intake, profuse vomiting, severe diarrhea, excessive perspiration, massive hemorrhage, high fever, chronic consumption, and excessive administration of warming and desiccating drugs, also brings about a dryness syndrome, endogenous but not exogenous.

2. Differentiation between exogenous and endogenous dryness

Exogenous dryness syndromes occur in dry weather, marked by dryness of the upper respiratory tract, which is directly exposed to the dry atmosphere.

For an endogenous dryness syndrome, it is not difficult to identify the cause of fluid deficiency, as it is either due to insufficient intake or to excessive loss. The clinical manifestations are not confined to the respiratory tract, but are usually generalized, such as wizened skin and constipation as well as dry mouth, dry lips, and thirst.

V. Summer-Heat and Summer-Heat Syndromes

Summer-heat is purely an exogenous factor that affects the human body. It causes heat stroke or sunstroke manifested by irritability, mental confusion, thirst and high fever. In severe cases, owing to the exhaustion of body fluid and *qi*, there may be loss of consciousness and coldness in the limbs.

In summer, the hot weather is often associated with high humidity. Affection by summer-heat together with damp is not infrequently encountered. The syndrome consists of fever and thirst, accompanied by a heavy feeling in the limbs, stuffiness in the chest, nausea and loose stools.

VI. Fire[1] (or Heat) and Fire (or Heat) Syndromes

Fire and heat belong to the same category of pathogenic factors. They mainly differ in degree. Heat as a pathogenic factor due to weather is called summer-heat, as discussed above. According to the traditional mode of thinking in Chinese medicine, syndromes with manifestations similar to heat or fire in the natural world are called heat or fire syndromes and assumed to be caused by heat or fire. Of course, heat and fire syndromes do not refer to heat-stroke or burns. In fact, they are a number of diseases or pathological changes caused by microbic pathogens. Owing to lack of modern scientific techniques, ancient Chinese doctors could only assume the existence of pathogenic factors which cause infectious or inflammatory diseases, but were not able to identify the individual microbic pathogens, and so the pathogens, are collectively called heat or fire.

1. Properties of fire (or heat) and characteristics of fire (or heat) syndromes

(1) Heat is high temperature, and fire is intense heat. So, the most common feature

---

[1]The word "fire" in traditional Chinese medicine has many connotations. Other pathogenic factors — wind, cold, damp, dryness and heat may have dual meanings: They are the names of pathogenic factors and also the names of the syndromes imitating the corresponding natural phenomena. They are only used in a pathological sense. But the word "fire" has both physiological and pathological senses. Even in its physiological sense, "fire" has a dual meaning: It refers to the Heart in the theory of the five elements, and also to Kidney *yang* as the fire of the vital gate. The latter is probably of more significance than the former. When we say "fire generates earth," we usually mean that the vital fire but not the Heart (fire) promotes the function of the Spleen (earth). In the terminology of pathological conditions, the word "fire" may be used in its pathological sense or physiological sense. In the syndrome "decline of the vital fire," the fire is physiological; but in *liu-huo* (流火) or "flowing fire," a Chinese medical term for erysipelas of the leg, or in the syndromes such as "flaming of the Heart fire" and "fire in the Liver," the fire is pathological. Therefore, the word "fire" has many different meanings besides that of one of the pathogenic factors; its real meaning can only be judged from the context.

of heat or fire is elevated body temperature, either general or local. In the case of fire, the hotness is accompanied by redness.

(2) Fire tends to flare upward. Clinically, fire or intense heat may disturb mental activities, causing insomnia, irritability, delirium or impaired consciousness.

(3) Fire or heat evaporates fluids. Clinically, a fire or heat syndrome is often accompanied by consumption of body fluids manifested by thirst, dryness of the throat and tongue, excretion of scanty and concentrated urine, and constipation.

(4) Extreme heat may give rise to wind. Convulsions may occur during a high fever. In addition, fire and heat may damage the blood vessels, resulting in hemorrhages.

2. Differentiation between exogenous and endogenous fire (or heat)

Exogenous affections due to heat or fire are often characterized by high fever or acute inflammation, accompanied by thirst, flushed face, reddened eyes, parched lips, dry and yellow tongue coating, and full, rapid pulse. Such a condition is called "heat or fire of excess type" (or "excess heat" or "excess fire" for short).

Syndromes of endogenous heat or fire due to disharmony of *qi* and blood or due to consumption of essence usually have a gradual onset and prolonged course. There is only low-grade fever with a hot sensation in the chest, palms and soles, accompanied by malar flush, night sweating, uncoated tongue, and thready, rapid pulse. Such syndromes are called "heat or fire of deficiency type" (or "deficiency heat" or "deficiency fire" for short).

However, excess fire may also occur in endogenous injuries, particularly when the Liver or the Heart is disturbed by emotional influence or mental stress.

Appendix: Toxic Pathogens

The concept of toxic pathogens was developed after the hypothesis of the six evils. In severe cases of heat and fire, and sometimes damp affections, the patients were so badly ill that ordinary treatment to remove those pathogenic factors could not give much help. This suggested the high virulence of the pathogens. The pathogens were thought to contain certain toxic substances, and they were thus named toxic heat, toxic fire and toxic damp. After repeated trial and error, a group of herbal drugs were discovered to be effective for treating those toxic pathogens, and called "detoxifying febrifugals."

It is interesting to note that modern research has found that some detoxifying febrifugals really show counteractions against bacterial toxins (including endotoxins) experimentally and have a therapeutic effect for toxemia in severe bacterial infections clinically.

Pestilential Pathogens

Pestilential pathogens are pathogens that cause epidemic or fulminating infectious diseases such as plague, cholera, diphtheria, epidemic encephalitis, epidemic meningitis, scarlet fever, mumps and fulminating dysentery.

The Seven Emotions

Emotions are feelings or mental reactions to stimuli. Normally they do not cause disease. Only when a sudden, violent or prolonged emotion exceeds the range of normal physiological activities is the *qi* disturbed, the equilibrium between *yin* and *yang* as well as the harmonious coordination of *qi* and blood is impaired, and disease ensues.

In Chinese medicine, emotions are classified into the following seven categories, namely, joy, anger, worry, anxiety, sadness, fear and fright. They can be further merged into five: joy, anger, anxiety, sadness and fear, relating to the Heart, Liver, Spleen, Lungs and Kidneys, respectively. *The Canon of Medicine* states, “Anger injures the Liver;” “Excessive joy injures the Heart;” “Anxiety injures the Spleen;” “Sadness injures the Lungs;” and “Fear injures the Kidneys.” The emotions injure the internal organs by disturbances of *qi*. “Excessive joy makes Heart *qi* sluggish;” “Anger makes Liver *qi* flow adversely upward;” “Anxiety makes Spleen *qi* depressed;” “Sadness consumes Lung *qi*;” and "Fear makes Kidney *qi* sink.” Therefore, different emotions may cause different disturbances of *qi*, resulting in damage to different *zang-fu* organs.

In clinical practice, however, the relationships between emotions and corresponding *zang-fu* organs are not absolute and exclusive. From the holistic viewpoint, any excessive emotional change may exert an impact on multiple internal organs. This is emphasized in *The Canon of Medicine*: “The Heart is the ruler of all the *zang-fu* organs.... Emotions such as sadness, worry and anxiety are feelings aroused in the Heart, but will stir all the *zang-fu* organs.”

Among the five *zang*-organs, the Heart controls blood and houses the mind; the Liver stores blood and regulates the flow of *qi*, and the Spleen, situated in the middle Energizer, serves as the pivot of ascent and descent of *qi*, as well as the source of formation of *qi* and blood. Since emotions cause disease by disturbing the harmonious coordination of *qi* and blood, internal injuries by emotions often involve the Heart, Liver and Spleen. For example, worry and anxiety usually cause a deficiency condition in both the Heart and the Spleen, manifested by insomnia, dream-disturbed sleep, loss of appetite, abdominal distension, loose bowels and lassitude. Anger is apt to injure the Liver, causing stagnation of *qi* along the Liver Meridian, manifested by hypochondriac distension and frequent sighing. If stagnated *qi* further leads to blood stasis, there will be hypochondriac pain and formation of abdominal mass, or dysmenorrhea and other menstrual disorders in women.

Besides the disturbance of *qi* and blood, the pathological changes caused by emotions may be transformed into fire, such as excessive Heart fire, and up-flaming of Liver fire. These syndromes will be discussed in detail in Chapter VI entitled “Differentiation of Syndromes.”

A point worth emphasizing is that in Chinese medicine the emotions are regarded as the pathogenic factors, but not the stimuli that lead to emotional reactions. This is of great significance for the prevention of disease. In order to avoid the harmful emotional effects, one is not advised to escape reality, but is asked to cultivate good character and exercise self-control to distract the mind from unfavorable emotions.

Improper Diet

Irregular food intake with excessive hunger and overeating is a common cause of dysfunction of the Spleen and Stomach. Constantly indulging in a rich, fatty diet may produce internal heat, making one apt to contract pyogenic infections. Contaminated food causes gastro-intestinal disorders.

Partiality for certain foods may also be harmful to the health. For example, partiality for extremely cold food may injure Spleen and Stomach *yang*, resulting in the formation of endogenous cold-damp, manifested by chronic diarrhea and abdominal pain. Partiality for extremely hot and spicy food may cause accumulation of heat in the Stomach and Intestines, giving rise to thirst, epigastric distension, abdominal pain, constipation or hemorrhoids.

Partiality for a certain taste should also be avoided. It is believed that each type of taste has its affinity for a certain *zang*-organ, namely, sour for the Liver, bitter for the Heart, sweet for the Spleen, pungent for the Lungs and salty for the Kidneys. Long-term partiality for a certain taste will cause the corresponding organ to function excessively and result in disorder. For example, partiality for sweets may injure the Spleen and Stomach, causing acid regurgitation.

Fatigue and Lack of Physical Exercise

Excessive stress and strain, particularly over a long period, may give rise to various diseases. For example, mental strain and fussiness may injure the Heart and the Spleen, resulting in forgetfulness, insomnia, dream-disturbed sleep, anorexia, abdominal distension and loose stools.

Lack of physical exercise is also harmful to the health. *The Canon of Medicine* states, "Lying in bed all the day impairs *qi*." It makes one lack strength, with weak Spleen and Stomach function, or results in obesity with palpitation and shortness of breath even during mild exertion.

Overindulgence in Sex

The vital essence is considered to be the most valuable substance for constructing the human body and maintaining life activities. It is stored in the Kidneys, and is hence called Kidney essence. Reproductive essence is an important portion of Kidney essence. Overindulgence in sex may consume Kidney essence, resulting in sexual disorders such as hyposexuality, impotence and premature ejaculation, as well as general weakness, listlessness, dizziness and tinnitus.

Phlegm and Retained Fluid

Both phlegm and retained fluid are pathological products of disordered water metabolism. Their formation is closely related to dysfunction of the Lungs, Spleen and Kidneys. Accumulation of a large amount of excessive water in the subcutaneous tissues, and in the thoracic and abdominal cavities gives rise to edema, hydrothorax and ascites, respectively.

If excessive fluid accumulates in a certain part of the body and condenses, phlegm is formed. Phlegm affecting the Lungs causes coughing, asthma and expectoration of sputum. In addition, phlegm can produce a variety of syndromes or diseases other than respiratory disorders. Retained in the Heart, it disturbs the normal mental function, leading to impaired consciousness or epilepsy, and in combination with fire it causes mania. Retained in the Stomach, it gives rise to nausea, vomiting and fullness in the epigastrium. Retained in the meridians, it blocks the normal flow of *qi* and blood, causing numbness of the limbs in mild cases, and paralysis in serious ones. Retained subcutaneously, it becomes masses or nodules, such as enlarged lymph nodes. The above-mentioned diseases seem to have nothing to do with each other, but they are all attributed to phlegm and grouped together under the category of phlegm syndromes. This had several explanations in the ancient textbooks, such as "Queer diseases are mostly due to phlegm;" "Phlegm is turbid and thick, so it can impede the normal flow of *qi* in various internal organs." However, the most convincing explanation probably lies in the therapeutic effect, namely, various phlegm syndromes can all be treated with "phlegm-dispelling" therapy.

Stagnated Blood

Stagnated blood refers to extravasated blood or blood remaining within a blood vessel when the circulation is impeded. It is a pathological product, but, in turn, it serves as a pathogenic factor causing a variety of pathological changes.

1. Formation of stagnated blood

(1) Trauma. The term "stagnated blood" was initially used in traumatology to indicate extravasation with ecchymosis, as the extravasated blood stops flowing.

(2) Disorders of *qi*. *Qi* is the dynamic force of the blood flow. Either stagnation of *qi* or deficiency of *qi* may cause stagnation of the blood flow (blood stasis).

(3) Pathogenic cold and heat. The congealing action of cold is a common cause of the formation of stagnated blood. Pathogenic heat directly invading the blood may induce blood coagulation.

2. Clinical features of pathological changes caused by stagnated blood

The pathological changes caused by stagnated blood have different manifestations according to the location. For example, if the Heart vessel is involved, there occurs precordial pain with cardiac palpitation and a stuffy sensation in the chest; if the Stomach is involved, there is epigastric pain with vomiting of blood and passage of bloody or tarry stools; and if the uterus is involved, dysmenorrhea and other menstrual disorders are frequently encountered. Generally, the pathological changes caused by stagnated blood have the following common clinical features:

(1) Pain. There is a saying in Chinese medicine: "Wherever there is obstruction, there is pain." Stagnated blood is the result of obstructed blood flow, and can induce further obstruction of the blood flow. So, pain is a very common feature. The pain caused by stagnated blood is usually stabbing or pricking in character, fixed in location and accompanied by tenderness.

(2) Mass formation. Long-standing stagnation of blood may induce mass formation. The mass formed in ectopic pregnancy is a typical example. Hepatomegaly, splenomegaly, and hysteromyoma are all believed to be caused by or associated with blood stasis.

(3) Purple discoloration.

(4) Hemorrhage. Blockage of the blood flow by stagnated blood may induce escape of blood from blood vessels, resulting in hemorrhage. The blood discharged is usually dark in color, mixed with blood clots.

CHAPTER 5

METHODS OF EXAMINATION

The recording of the history of the condition and physical examination are the main methods of collecting data for making diagnosis. In traditional Chinese medicine, the former is called "inquiry," and physical examination includes inspection, auscultation, olfaction and palpation. Usually, inspection comes first in examining a patient, because it starts as soon as the doctor sees the patient. Although the methods of examination used in Chinese medicine are quite similar to those used in Western medicine, there are many differences in choosing the key points and considering their clinical significance. For example, such a question as whether the patient wants to drink if he (she) feels thirsty is seldom asked by a doctor of Western medicine, but it is an important question in Chinese medicine. Pulse taking is used chiefly for examining the cardiovascular system in Western medicine, but it is used for obtaining information about all the *zang-fu* organs in Chinese medicine. In this chapter, only the unique points of diagnostic examination in Chinese medicine will be discussed in detail.

INSPECTION

I. Inspection of *shen* (vitality)

Shen is the general manifestation of the life activities. Here, it is translated as vitality. Clinically the condition of vitality can be determined by comprehensive examination of the complexion, expression, posture, speech and consciousness. The expression in one's eyes usually gives the most important information about the condition of vitality, because it is believed that the vital essence and energy of all the *zang-fu* organs pour into the eyes. Generally speaking, the condition of vitality can be classified on three levels: full of vitality, loss of vitality and false vitality.

1. Full of vitality: If a patient is conscious, with the eyes glowing with radiating vigor and moving freely, speaks clearly with quick response, and behaves naturally and nimbly, he (she) is full of vitality without severe deterioration of the *zang-fu* organs, and the prognosis is usually good.

2. Loss of vitality: A patient with loss of vitality is listless with a dull look in his (her) eyes, slow in reacting, feeble in breathing, or even delirious with floccitation. This indicates that the patient is critically ill, with poor prognosis.

3. False manifestation of vitality: A critically ill patient may have a momentary spurt of activity just before death. It is customarily called "the flash of lucidity of the dying."

II. Inspection of the Complexion

The natural color and luster of the skin, especially of the face, should be carefully ascertained. The luster of the skin reflects the general condition of the internal organs. A withered or haggard face suggests deterioration of the vital essence and energy. Change of the skin color provides information about the pathological process and the organ(s) involved.

1. Pallor. A bloodless face or one with little color is often seen in patients with deficiency of *qi* or loss of blood. Pallor indicates inadequate blood supply. Since *qi* drives the blood flow, deficiency of *qi* leads to insufficient blood supply to the face, and results in pallor in the same way as deficiency of blood does. But, there is some difference between the complexions of the two conditions: In deficiency of blood the face looks pale and wan, while in deficiency of *qi* the face is pale and bright.

2. Sallowness. A sallow appearance of the skin and sclera is a sign of jaundice. It is usually due to impairment of the Spleen or the Liver and Gallbladder by damp. A bright yellow appearance indicates damp-heat, and a dull yellow appearance is a sign of cold-damp. A sallow complexion with no discoloration of the sclera is not a sign of jaundice. It suggests diminished function of the Spleen.

3. Red color. Flushing of the face indicates the presence of heat. It occurs in both excess and deficiency conditions. If the heat is of the excess type, the whole face is flushed; if the heat is of the deficiency type, there is only malar flush in the afternoon. The latter usually appears in patients with a chronic consumptive disease.

4. Blue color. Bluish discoloration of the skin is often seen in cold syndromes, severe pain, blood stasis and convulsions. In all cases the bluish discoloration is due to retardation of the blood flow.

5. Dark color. Dark color of the skin or complexion is seen usually in severe and chronic cases of blood stasis, and deficiency-cold syndrome due to decline of Kidney *yang*. In the former, the skin is not only dark but also scaly dry. In the latter, the dark color may involve the whole body or appear chiefly around the eyes.

III. Inspection of the Physical Build and Gesture

A well-developed and nourished person with strong muscles usually has a good constitution. Poor development with meager physique indicates a weak constitution. But an obese person with soft muscles, shortness of breath and poor strength is "full in shape but lacking in energy," often suffering from deficiency of *qi* or insufficiency of the Spleen. Emaciation with pale, dry and wizened skin is a sign of deficiency of *yin* and blood.

Some disorders can be recognized immediately by observing the patient's posture, gait and motions. If a patient lying in bed moves restlessly and dislikes covers, he (she) is probably suffering from an excess-heat syndrome. If the patient lies still in bed and prefers thick covering, he (she) probably has a deficiency-cold syndrome. In patients with coughing and dyspnea, sitting with the head turned upwards suggests an excess syndrome of the Lungs with accumulation of phlegm; sitting with the head hanging down often indicates a deficiency syndrome of the Lungs or failure of the Kidneys to assist the Lungs in breathing. Hemiplegia due to stroke, shaking of the head due to Liver wind, swelling of joints with difficulty in motion due to arthritis and loss of normal power of motion due to paralysis, all can be discovered by inspection.

IV. Inspection of the Head

1. The hair. Thick and lustrous hair reflects abundance of Kidney *qi*. Sparse and withered hair is a sign of deficiency of vital essence and blood. Premature greying of the hair may be due to deficiency of Kidney *qi* if the greying is accompanied by deficiency symptoms of the Kidneys, or due to mental stress with impairment of the blood if the greying is accompanied by deficiency symptoms of the Heart.

2. The eyes. Although the eyes are regarded as the "windows" of the Liver, they are actually related to all the internal organs. As stated in *The Canon of Medicine*, "The vital essence and *qi* of all the *zang-fu* organs pour into the eyes and become the vital essence of the latter." Therefore, vitality is reflected in the expression of the eyes, and information about the changes of individual internal organs may also be obtained by inspection of the eyes.

According to the hypothesis of the Five Orbiculi, the eye can be divided into five parts: the eyelid, canthus, white of the eye, black of the eye, and pupil, reflecting the condition of the Spleen, Heart, Lungs, Liver and Kidneys, respectively. Reddening of the canthus is attributed to Heart fire, reddening of the white of the eye to Lung fire, reddening, swelling and festering of the eyelid to Spleen fire, swelling and reddening of the whole eyeball to Liver fire, and cataracts with impaired vision to Kidney deficiency.

3. The ears. A thick and well-shaped helix indicates abundance of Kidney *qi*, while a thin and small helix may be due to deficiency of Kidney *qi*. Withering of the helix is a sign of extreme consumption of Kidney yin, and atrophy of the helix, a sign of exhaustion of Kidney *qi* in a critical case. A scaly, dry helix is seen in chronic cases of blood stasis.

4. The nose. Discoloration of the nose may give useful diagnostic clues. Bluish discoloration is often seen in cases of severe abdominal pain; yellow discoloration indicates the presence of damp-heat; pallor of the nose may be due to loss of blood; a reddened nose is a sign of heat in the Spleen and Lungs; and grey color of the nose suggests retention of fluid.

5. The lips, teeth and gums. A normal person has red and lustrous lips, indicating abundance of Stomach *qi* and harmony of *qi* and blood. Pale lips are usually seen in patients with deficiency of blood or deficiency of both *qi* and blood. Deep-red and dry lips are caused by heat, and cracked lips by consumption of body fluids. Cyanotic lips suggest cold or blood stasis.

The teeth are considered odds and ends of bone. Since the Kidneys are in charge of the bones, the teeth may reflect the condition of the Kidneys. Clean, white and lustrous teeth indicate abundance of Kidney *qi* and body fluid. Yellow and dry teeth in a febrile disease suggest exuberant heat with impairment of body fluid. If the teeth are as dry as a dead bone, Kidney *yin* is exhausted. Grinding the teeth during sleep is mostly due to internal heat or retention of undigested food. Swollen and tender gums with or without bleeding indicate excessive heat in the Stomach. But bleeding from painless gums without inflammation is often due to deficiency of *qi* or deficiency of Kidney *yin* with endogenous fire.

V. Inspection of the Tongue

Inspection of the tongue is one of the important diagnostic methods in Chinese medicine. The tongue proper reflects the condition of the internal organs, and the tongue coating gives information about the pathogenic factors as well as Stomach *qi*. In recent years, observation of the sublingual vein has also been included in inspection of the tongue.

Partition of the tongue: The tongue is usually divided into the following portions: the tip, middle, root and borders, revealing pathologic changes of the Heart (and Lungs), Spleen (and Stomach), Liver (and Gallbladder), and Kidneys (and Bladder), respectively. For example, a scarlet tongue tip suggests exuberant fire of the Heart; bright red borders of the tongue indicate heat in the Liver and Gallbladder; retention of undigested food in the Stomach gives rise to a thick greasy coating particularly prominent at the central part of the tongue.

(I) Observation of the Tongue Proper

1. Color

The normal color of the tongue is light-red and moistened. The following changes in color are often seen in pathological conditions.

(1) Pale tongue: A tongue less red than normal is often due to deficiency of blood, *qi* or *yang*. Since the flow of blood is driven by *qi*, in deficiency of *qi* or *yang* the supply of blood to the tongue is inadequate, and so the tongue becomes pale as in deficiency of blood. A pale tongue due to deficiency of blood is usually not accompanied by change in shape or size. In deficiency of *qi*, the tongue is not only pale, but also plump and flabby due to tissue edema. In deficiency of *yang,* which is usually accompanied by cold syndrome, the tongue is pale and more moist than normal.

(2) Reddened tongue: A tongue redder than normal indicates pathogenic heat, either of excess type or of deficiency type. The reddened tongue due to a heat syndrome of excess type is usually accompanied by a yellow coating, while that in a heat syndrome of deficiency type has a thin coating or is furry and fissured. According to modern studies, a reddened tongue is mostly due to increased metabolism with dilation of capillaries and increased blood flow.

(3) Crimson tongue: Deep redness of the tongue indicates intense heat. In an exogenous febrile disease, a crimson tongue accompanied by a yellow coating indicates that the *yin* system is involved. According to modern studies, this is not only due to increased metabolism with dilation of capillaries, but is also related to increase of fungiform papillae which contain more capillary loops with accelerated blood flow caused by toxins in a severe infection.

A crimson tongue is also frequently found in deficiency of *yin* with endogenous heat, but in this case the tongue is dry and shriveled, with a scanty or no coating. This is due to increased metabolism accompanied by atrophy and degeneration of the periglottis and the minor salivary glands.

(4) Purplish tongue: Purple indicates blood stasis, extreme heat or extreme cold. The purple color may cover the whole tongue, or only the borders or the tip. It is not infrequently accompanied by purple spots, ecchymosis, and varicose sublingual veins. Clinically, purple of the tongue is seen in patients with liver or gallbladder diseases, heart

diseases and malignant tumors. According to modern studies, it is chiefly due to venous congestion, sluggish blood flow and hypoxia. Venacaval or portal congestion slows down the blood flow and gas exchange in the tissues, so that oxidized hemoglobin is decreased and reduced hemoglobin increased, making the blood dark and the tongue purple. A purple tongue is usually accompanied by serious microcirculatory disturbances, such as increase of minute vessels with slow blood flow, aggregation of blood cells and even extravasation. In hypoxia the blood is remarkably dark in color. It has been shown by animal experiments that the color of the tongue is generally parallel to the degree of hypoxia. The greater the degree of hypoxia, the more purple the tongue becomes. It has also been revealed that patients with purple tongues usually have elevated capillary fragility, increased blood platelet aggregation, high blood viscosity and other hemorheological changes. In cancer patients, successful chemotherapy usually leads to a marked decrease in purple color, as well as in the hemorheological indices. Therefore, observation of the tongue may serve as an index for assessing the therapeutic effect in the treatment of cancers.

2. The shape of the tongue

(1) Enlarged or plump tongue: A plump and flabby tongue is usually pale and accompanied by tooth prints on its edges, indicating deficiency of Spleen *qi* or Kidney *yang*. This is often caused by low plasma protein with tissue edema. Disturbance of water metabolism with edema may also result in a plump tongue. The enlarged tongue presses against the teeth, forming tooth prints on its borders.

A swollen, reddened and painful tongue is due to inflammation of the tongue itself.

(2) Thin tongue: A thin tongue is smaller and thinner than normal. A thin tongue pale in color indicates deficiency of *qi* and blood. A thin, dry and deep red tongue is a manifestation of deficiency of *yin* with hyperactive fire. Modern research has shown that a thin tongue is related to inadequate blood supply or lack of body fluid.

(3) Shriveled tongue: A dry and shriveled tongue indicates consumption of body fluid. If it is deep red in color, the body fluid is consumed by excessive heat. Modern research has shown that shriveling of the tongue is due to diminished saliva secretion or insufficient water content in the saliva, and can be taken as an early manifestation of dehydration from various causes.

(4) Cracked tongue: Irregular streaks or cracks on the tongue indicate consumption of body fluid by excessive heat if the tongue is deep red in color. In severe cases, the cracks often appear on shriveled tongue. They also indicate deficiency of blood if the tongue is pale. However, a cracked tongue may be present in a normal person. In this case, the cracks are not deep, and remain there all the time without change. The formation of streaks or cracks is related to atrophy of the lingual mucosa or fusion of the lingual papillae.

(5) Thorny tongue: The fungiform papillae over the surface of the tongue swell up like thorns. A thorny and red tongue indicates accumulation of pathogenic heat in the interior of the body. The more severe the pathogenic heat is, the more enlarged and profuse the thorns will be. Thorny tongue is formed by atrophy of the lingual buds and exfoliation of cornified cells; in such cases, the fungiform papillae greatly increase in number.

3. Movement of the tongue

(1) Deviated tongue: The tongue turned to one side while stuck out is often seen in

apoplexy.

(2) Rigid tongue: A rigid tongue lacks flexibility and is difficult to protrude, retract or roll. In exogenous febrile diseases it indicates invasion of the Pericardium by heat, retention of turbid phlegm in the interior, or excessive pathogenic heat consuming body fluid. In non-febrile diseases, it is a sign of apoplexy.

(3) Flaccid tongue: A flaccid tongue is weak in motion, and often indicates extreme deficiency of *qi* and blood if it is pale. A flaccid and deep red tongue may be seen in extreme consumption of *yin* fluid.

(4) Tremulous tongue: Tremor of the tongue is often seen in endogenous wind or alcohol intoxication. If the tongue is pale, the tremor is often due to deficiency of *qi* and blood, with endogenous wind from blood deficiency. If the tongue is dark red, the tremor results from Liver wind or wind produced by extreme heat. If the tongue is purplish red and the tremor only occurs when the tongue is stuck out, this suggests alcohol intoxication.

(II) Observation of the Tongue Coating

On observing the tongue coating, attention should be paid to its thickness and color. A healthy person has a thin layer of whitish coating which is moderately moistened. The thicker the coating, the deeper the pathogenic factors. The color of the tongue coating indicates the nature of pathogenic factors—white for cold and yellow for heat. In addition, the formation of the tongue coating is related to the Stomach function. No coating will be produced if Stomach *qi* and *yin* are exhausted. Therefore, observation of the tongue coating can produce information about the nature and location of the pathogenic factors as well as the condition of Stomach *qi* and *yin*.

According to modern studies, the appearance of the tongue coating depends on the functional and structural changes of filiform and fungiform papillae of the tongue.

1. Quality of the tongue coating

(1) Thick coating vs. thin coating: The tongue coating is considered thin if the tongue proper can be distinctly seen, and considered thick if the tongue proper is not clearly visible. The thickness of the coating usually gives important information on the severity of the pathogenic factors and progression of the pathological conditions. In the case of exogenous affection at the early stage, when the pathogenic factor only invades the superficial portion of the body, the coating is usually thin. Along with the inward transmission of the pathogenic factor, the tongue coating becomes thick. Retention of damp, phlegm or food in the interior also produces a thick tongue coating. Generally speaking, thickening of the coating is a sign of aggravation of the disease; thinning of the coating indicates elimination of the pathogenic factor, and hence alleviation of the pathological condition. (However, sudden and total disappearance of the coating may indicate something different.)

(2) Moist coating vs. dry coating: Moisture of the tongue coating gives information on the condition of the body fluid. A normal tongue coating is moist and lustrous, but not slippery. A dry tongue coating indicates consumption of body fluid. If the tongue surface is excessively moistened, the coating looks slippery. This is usually due to upward surging of water and damp.

(3) Sticky coating and curdy coating: It is a sticky coating if the tongue is covered by a turbid layer of fine greasy substance which is hard to be scraped off. A sticky coating

is often seen in retention of turbid damp-phlegm or retention of food. A curdy coating is coarse, loose and thick, looks like a layer of curds, and is easily scraped off. It reflects retention of undigested food in the Stomach.

(4) Shedding of the tongue coating: The tongue with map-like shedding of its coating is known as a "geographic tongue." It indicates consumption of *qi* and *yin* of the Stomach or intestinal parasitosis. A geographic tongue, however, may be of little clinical significance if it has been there for many years without any change. If the tongue sheds all its coating, leaving a mirror-like surface, it is known as a "glossy tongue." Glossy tongue is a sign of exhaustion of Stomach *yin* and severe damage to Stomach *qi*, particularly when the shedding happens suddenly in the course of a disease.

2. Color of the tongue coating

(1) White coating: A thin white coating is normal. In morbid conditions white coating indicates cold. A thin white coating is seen in exterior cold syndrome, while a thick white coating occurs in interior cold syndrome. If the thick white coating is greasy, it indicates damp-phlegm. Since the coating reflects the existence of pathogenic factors, if the interior cold syndrome is of deficiency type, the tongue coating is white and thin.

(2) Yellow coating: A yellow coating usually indicates heat in the interior of the body. The deeper yellow the coating is, the more severe pathogenic heat it indicates. Intense heat with impairment of body fluid produces a yellow and dry coating. Accumulation of damp-heat is often reflected in a yellow and greasy coating.

(3) Grey coating: A grey coating indicates an interior syndrome involving either heat or cold-damp. If a grey coating is tinged with yellow and dry, it signifies excessive heat with consumption of body fluid. If the coating is whitish and moist, it implies retention of cold damp, phlegm or fluid in the interior of the body.

(4) Black coating: A black coating is often the further development of a grey coating. It is often present at the severe stage of an illness, indicating extreme heat or excessive cold in the interior of the body. If a black coating is yellowish and dry, possibly with thorns, it signifies extreme heat with consumption of body fluid. A pale black and slippery coating implies excessive cold due to *yang* deficiency.

According to modern studies, the formation of a thick white coating is chiefly due to changes in the filiform papillae. In healthy persons the foreign substances between the filiform papillae and exfoliated keratinized epithelium are washed away by saliva, food and drink. The tongue coating is therefore thin and white. In patients, the "self-clearing" of the tongue is impaired due to decreased intake of food and drink, inadequate secretion of saliva, and diminished chewing actions for the mechanical removal of the tongue coating, so that there is prolongation of the filiform papillae with accumulation of dirt, forming a thick white coating.

If the hyperkeratinized filiform papillae are increased, mixed with exfoliated epithelia, leukocytes, bacteria and fungi, and accumulated on a thick white coating, the coating will look greasy.

A yellow coating of the tongue is often seen in inflammation with fever or severe indigestion. In cases of inflammation, there is increased keratinization and ramification of filiform papillae with accumulation of large amount of bacteria and inflammatory exudate.

Manifold pathogenic bacteria may be cultured from the yellow coating. Therefore, the yellow coating is formed by the inflammatory exudate, accumulation of inflammatory cells and growth of certain species of bacteria. In digestive disorders, there is usually generalized and distinct keratinization of papillae, on which a precipitated and adsorbed layer of the regurgitated gastric contents forms the yellow coating. The thickness of the coating is directly proportional to the amount of regurgitated substances and the severity of digestive disturbance.

AUSCULTATION

Auscultation in Chinese medicine chiefly includes listening to the patient's voice, and sounds of breathing, coughing, belching and hiccup.

I. The Voice

By listening to the patient's voice, some clue may be obtained to the diagnosis. A patient with cold deficiency syndrome usually speaks with a feeble voice. Hoarseness may be due to an attack on the Lungs by exogenous pathogens or due to deficiency of body fluids.

II. Breathing

1. Asthenic breathing: Lack of strength in breathing is usually due to deficiency of *qi*.

2. Rough breathing: Forceful respiration with harshness is usually due to the presence of excessive heat.

3. Shortness of breath: The breathing is short and rapid, but not labored due to physical activity. It is often due to deficiency of Lung *qi*; but may also occur in excess cases of retained fluid in the chest or stagnation of *qi* in the epigastrium or abdomen.

4. Dyspnea without wheezing: Difficulty in breathing, may be accompanied by flaring nares and indrawing of the soft tissues of the neck, but no wheezing. This may occur either in deficiency conditions (deficiency of Lung or Kidney *qi*) or in excess conditions (excess heat in the Lungs). In cases of deficiency, the breathing sound is feeble, while in cases of excess, the breathing sound is loud and harsh.

5. Dyspnea with wheezing (asthma): Dyspnea attended by a whistling sound, i.e., during an acute attack of asthma, is mostly due to invasion of exogenous pathogens in people with insidious retention of phlegm.

III. Coughing

A muffled coughing sound is often due to cold-damp. A clear coughing sound suggests dryness-heat, especially when the coughing is not associated with expectoration. Coughing with a feeble sound and shortness of breath is a sign of deficient Lung *qi*. In a paroxysm of whooping cough there is a series of short coughs of increasing intensity, and then a deep inspiration with a gasping sound like the cry of an egret. (Whooping cough is also called "egret cough" in Chinese medicine.)

IV. Belching and hiccuping

Both belching and hiccuping are symptoms indicating reverse flow of Stomach *qi*. Hiccuping associated with a sharp, short and loud sound is usually due to excess heat; hiccuping with a low, prolonged and a feeble sound indicates cold deficiency. Persistent hiccuping occurring in a chronic case may be a sign of deterioration of Stomach *qi*, foreboding a poor prognosis. Belching commonly occurs after a heavy meal, resulting from indigestion, disharmony of the Liver and the Stomach, or diminished function of the Stomach.

V. Sighing

Frequent sighing is a symptom of stagnation of Liver *qi*, caused by emotional disturbance, particularly depression.

OLFACTION

Smelling the odor of the patient, his (her) compartments and his (her) secretions and excretions may be taken as a reference for diagnosis. Sour smell in the patient's mouth is a sign of indigestion. Foul breath indicates presence of heat in the Lungs or the Stomach. Offensive smells are often given off by cancerous discharge.

INQUIRY

Traditionally Chinese physicians have used a standard list of questions for history taking. This list was first recommended by Zhang Jiebin (1563-1640) and revised by Chen Xiuyuan (1753-1823). It is customarily called the "ten questions." In fact, they are questions about ten aspects: (1) chill and fever; (2) perspiration; (3) headache and body pains; (4) urination and defecation; (5) appetite; (6) feeling in the chest and abdomen; (7) hearing; (8) thirst; (9) past diseases; and (10) cause of the present illness. In addition, inquiry should be made into the efficacy of medicine taken, and about menstruation for women patients.

I. Inquiry about Chill and Fever

Both chill and fever refer to subjective symptoms in traditional Chinese medicine. If the patient complains of chill and fever, the following points should be clarified: (1) occurrence of both chill and fever, or chill or fever alone; (2) severity of chill and fever; (3) time of occurrence; (4) length of persistence; and (5) accompanying symptoms.

1. Chill together with fever

At the onset of an exogenous affection, chill and fever are the main manifestation of an exterior syndrome. In the exterior syndrome of wind-cold, chill is more severe than fever, while in the exterior syndrome of wind-heat, heat is more severe than chill. The chill in an exogenous affection is characterized by the patient still feeling cold even when wearing more clothes and warming him(her)self near a source of heat.

2. Chill with no fever

Chill without fever is usually due to deficiency-cold in *yang*-deficiency patients. The sensation of cold is relieved when the patient wears more clothes and warms him(her)self near a source of heat.

3. Fever with no chill

Fever without chill indicates heat in the interior, and can be divided into the following patterns:

(1) High fever: Persistent high fever with desire for cold and aversion to heat indicates a syndrome of excess heat. Usually, the fever is accompanied by perspiration and thirst.

(2) Tidal fever: Fever appears at fixed hours of the day, usually in the afternoon, so that the fever rises and subsides like a tide. Tidal fever can be further divided into three patterns:

Tidal fever due to deficiency of *yin*: It is characterized by a hot sensation in the chest, palms and soles, often accompanied by night sweating, malar flush, a dry throat and reddened tongue with only a thin coating.

Tidal fever due to damp-warm: Fever appears in the afternoon, and is characterized by its recessiveness, namely, the hotness of the patient's skin can only be felt by the physician after lengthy palpation. In this case, the fever is thought to be obscured by pathogenic damp.

Tidal fever in Yangming[1] disease: Fever appears late in the afternoon, accompanied by abdominal pain and tenderness, constipation, deep and forceful pulse, and a prickled tongue with a yellow, dry coating. This kind of fever is caused by accumulation of pathogenic heat in the Stomach and Large Intestine.

(3) Low fever: Prolonged low fever may be due to deficiency of *yin*, deficiency of *qi* or emotional depression. Deficiency of *yin* often leads to relative exuberance of *yang*, resulting in fever and other manifestations as described above. Deficiency of *qi* may also cause persistent low fever when *yang-qi* cannot be normally distributed throughout the body but is retained in the superficial portion. Low fever due to deficiency of *qi* is aggravated by physical labor, and accompanied by spontaneous sweating and lassitude. Occasionally, deficiency of *qi* may also cause high fever.

(4) Alternate spells of chill and fever: If the spells occur at not fixed times and is accompanied by fullness and a choking sensation in the chest and costal region, bitterness in the mouth, dry throat, nausea, loss of appetite, and taut pulse, it indicates a half-exterior-half-interior syndrome, i.e., the exogenous pathogen is going inward but has not reached the interior of the body, so that the normal *qi* fights against the pathogenic *qi* between the exterior and interior. If the spell comes at fixed times daily or every two or three days, it is characteristic of another kind of half-exterior-half-interior syndrome, as seen in malaria.

II. Inquiry about Perspiration

1. Perspiration in an exterior syndrome

In an exterior syndrome inquiry about perspiration can provide information about

---

[1]The Hand Yangming Meridian is the meridian of the Large Intestine, and Foot Yangming Meridian, the meridian of the Stomach. Therefore, Yangming refers to both the Large Intestine and the Stomach. In addition, the Stomach may not be limited to the digestive pouch below the esophagus, it sometimes refers to the entire gastro-intestinal tract.

the property of the pathogen and the condition of defensive *qi*.

(1) Exterior syndrome with no perspiration, accompanied by more chill than fever, headache, and a floating and tense pulse, is a syndrome of an attack of wind-cold.

(2) Exterior syndrome with perspiration: If it is accompanied by aversion to wind and a floating and relaxed pulse, it is an exterior-deficiency syndrome (deficiency of defensive *qi*); if it is accompanied by moderate fever with mild chill, headache, sore throat, and a floating and rapid pulse, it is a syndrome of wind-heat attack.

2. Perspiration in an interior syndrome

(1) Spontaneous perspiration: Sweating in the daytime spontaneously, not caused by physical exertion or thick clothing, often accompanied by lassitude and lack of strength, is a sign of *qi* deficiency. If there are accompanying cold symptoms such as aversion to cold and cold limbs, the spontaneous sweating is due to *yang* deficiency.

(2) Night sweats: Sweating occurring during sleep and stopping immediately after waking up, is often due to *yin* deficiency. It may be accompanied by tidal fever and malar flush. Its mechanism is explained as follows: During sleep, when superficial defensive *qi* goes into the interior so that the pores cannot close firmly, the endogenous heat due to *yin* deficiency "evaporates" the body fluid out and discharges it as sweat. When the patient wakes up, defensive *qi* that controls the pores returns to the superficies, and so the sweating stops.

(3) Profuse sweating: This may occur in cases of excess-heat with high fever, flushed face, dire thirst and a gigantic pulse. In such a case, the fluid is "evaporated" by the intense heat from the interior to the superficies, and excreted as sweat. But if the patient breaks out in a profuse cold sweat together with pallor, cold limbs and scarcely perceivable pulse, collapse or shock will ensue.

3. Localized perspiration

In some patients abnormal perspiration is localized at the head, one side of the body or the palms and soles. Sweating confined to the head is often due to the presence of pathogenic heat in the Upper Energizer or accumulation of damp-heat in the Middle Energizer. If sweating from the head occurs after recovery of a severe disease or in an aged person with shortness of breath, it indicates a deficiency state. If it suddenly occurs at the late stage of a severe disease, it may be a sign of impending collapse. Perspiration on one side of the body, or to put it more accurately, no perspiration on the other side, as seen in hemiplegia, is due to obstruction of the meridians and collaterals, resulting in anhidrosis. Hyperhidrosis in the palms and soles is often related to dysfunction of the Spleen in fluid transportation, with extra fluid reaching the palms and soles and secreted as sweat.

III. Inquiry about Headache and Body Pains

1. Headache

According to the location of the headache, the affected meridian can be ascertained. Frontal headache is related to the Foot Yangming (Stomach) Meridian, temporal headache to the Foot Shaoyang (Gallbladder) Meridian, occipital headache to the Foot Taiyang (Bladder) Meridian, and vertical headache to the Foot Jueyin (Liver) Meridian.

According to the features of the headache, the property of the syndrome can be determined. An acute attack of headache, severe and continuous, with a short course, is usually due to exogenous affection and pertains to an excess syndrome. If the headache involves the nape and the patient is averse to wind, the pathogenic factor is most likely wind-cold. If the patient is averse to heat, and has a flushed face and reddened eyes, he (she) is probably affected by wind-heat. Headache accompanied by such a feeling as if the head were tightly bound is a symptom of wind-damp.

Chronic headache with the attacks on and off is mostly an endogenous injury and pertains to a deficiency syndrome. If the headache has continued for a long period of time and is aggravated by overwork, it is due to deficiency of *qi*. Headache accompanied by dizziness and pallor is a symptom of blood deficiency. Headache with an empty sensation in the head and weakness of the legs is a symptom of Kidney deficiency.

2. Chest pain

Chest pain is often associated with disorders of the Heart and the Lungs, both of which are situated in the chest. The common pathogenic factors are deficient *yang-qi*, stagnated *qi* and blood, turbid phlegm, heat and fire.

Chest pain with fever, cough and dyspnea often results from heat in the Lungs. Chest pain with hectic fever, night sweating or hemoptysis suggests deficiency of Lung *yin* with endogenous heat, as occurs in pulmonary tuberculosis. Chest pain with no definite location, accompanied by distension and alleviated by sighing is usually due to *qi* stagnation. Attacks of precordial pain in the shoulder or arm are often due to cold congealing the Heart vessel or blood stasis, as seen in coronary heart disease with angina pectoris. Severe persistent precordial pain accompanied by cold sweating indicates stagnation of *qi* and blood with decline of *yang-qi*, as occurring in myocardial infarction.

3. Costal and hypochondriac pain

The costal and hypochondriac regions are the sites where the Liver and Gallbladder Meridians cross. Pain in these regions is mostly due to obstruction of either or both of the meridians by stagnated *qi* or blood, damp-heat, or exuberant *yang*.

4. Epigastric pain

The epigastric region is the place where the Stomach is located. Epigastric pain is usually due to dysfunction of the Stomach, such as cold or heat in the Stomach, retention of undigested food, or attack on the Stomach by the Liver *qi*.

5. Abdominal pain

In Chinese medicine the abdomen is customarily divided into three regions: the greater abdomen (the portion above the umbilicus), the lower abdomen (the portion below the umbilicus) and the iliac region. The greater abdomen is related to the Spleen and the Stomach, the lower abdomen to the Kidneys, Bladder, Intestines and Uterus; the iliac region is the site traversed by the Liver Meridian.

Abdominal pain may be seen in many excess syndromes, such as attacks of cold, accumulation of heat, stagnation of *qi*, stasis of blood, retention of undigested food, and parasitosis. It may also be seen in deficiency conditions, such as *qi* deficiency, blood deficiency, and deficiency-cold (*yang* deficiency).

6. Lumbar pain

The lumbar region is the seat of the Kidneys. Lumbar pain of deficiency type is usually due to disorders of the Kidneys. But it may also be seen in excess conditions such as obstruction of the meridians and collaterals by pathogenic wind, cold and damp, or by stagnated blood.

7. Pain in the limbs

Either joint pain or muscle pain in the limbs is the result of impeded flow of *qi* and blood by invasion of pathogenic wind, cold and damp. Pain in the heel (not caused by local lesion), sometimes radiating to the lower back, is a pathognostic symptom of Kidney deficiency.

8. Property of pain

Inquiry about the property of the pain is helpful for differentiating the cause and mechanism of pain. A distending pain is characteristic of *qi* stagnation, a stabbing pain is usually due to blood stasis, and a continuous dull pain is seen in deficiency conditions.

Tenderness should also be examined. Pain with tenderness is usually pain of the excess type, while pain that can be alleviated by pressure is of the deficiency type.

IV. Inquiry about the Appetite and Tastes in the Mouth

1. Appetite

Appetite depends upon the functions of the Spleen and the Stomach. Loss of appetite in a chronic case is usually due to weakness of the Spleen and the Stomach. Diminished food intake accompanied by fullness in the chest, distension in the abdomen and a greasy tongue coating is seen in disturbance of the Spleen by damp. Polyphagia with frequent hunger is a sign of exuberant fire of the Stomach. Hunger but no desire for food indicates deficiency of Stomach *yin*.

2. Tastes in the mouth

Tastelessness in the mouth is mostly due to diminished function of the Spleen and the Stomach.

Sweetness in the mouth suggests accumulation of damp-heat in the Spleen and the Stomach.

Sourness in the mouth is often seen in cases of indigestion.

Bitterness in the mouth indicates the presence of excessive heat, particularly in the Liver and the Gallbladder.

Saltiness in the mouth is usually due to deficiency of the Kidneys.

V. Inquiry about Thirst and Fluid Intake

Thirst indicates impairment of body fluids. Generally, patients with excess heat feel thirsty and like cold drinks. If the patient has no thirst and likes hot drinks, he (she) is probably suffering from a cold syndrome. In cases of interior retention of damp or phlegm, the patient feels thirsty but only drinks small amounts of hot water.

VI. Inquiry about Sleeping

Abnormal changes in sleep include insomnia and somnolence. Insomnia may result from deficiency of *yin* and blood, with exuberance of *yang,* which disturbs the mind, or result from phlegm-fire or retained food, which interferes with sleep. Difficulty in falling asleep accompanied by unease, vivid dreams, night sweating, aching back and weak legs is due to incoordination of the Heart and the Kidneys. Abnormal wakefulness accompanied by cardiac palpitation, impaired appetite, lack of strength, and pale tongue indicates deficiency of both Heart blood and Spleen *qi*. Insomnia associated with epigastric distention, belching, and thick greasy tongue coating is related to retention of undigested food.

Somnolence is often caused by weakness of the Spleen with accumulation of phlegm-damp which stops the essence and energy absorbed from food ascending to the head.

VII. Inquiry about Urination and Defecation

1. Urination

Polyuria often results from weakened Kidney *qi* which is unable to hold fluid. Oliguria may be either due to consumption of body fluid or due to dysfunction of the Kidneys with inadequate formation of urine from the body fluid.

Frequency and urgency in urination, painful urination, and dripping of urine are common manifestations of accumulation of damp-heat in the Bladder at the acute stage.

Incontinence of urine and enuresis are both attributed to deficiency of Kidney *qi*.

2. Defecation

Constipation: Infrequent or difficult evacuation of feces is either due to inadequacy of the intestinal fluid or due to retardation of transmission in the Large Intestine. If it occurs in a patient with high fever, accompanied by abdominal distension, reddened tongue and dry yellow coating, it is a case of excess heat with impairment of the intestinal fluid. If a patient with constipation is pale, likes hot drinks, and has a deep and slow pulse, he (she) is suffering from "cold constipation," i.e., intestinal *qi* stagnates because of accumulated cold. A constipated patient with a reddened tongue, scanty coating, and thready, rapid pulse, is deficient in *yin*-fluid in the Intestines. Constipation after a chronic disease, in aged or postpartum patients, is usually due to deficiency of *qi* and fluid. Deficiency of *qi* makes one incapable of defecating, and lack of fluid makes defecation difficult.

Diarrhea: The causes of diarrhea are multifarious, including exogenous attack by cold-damp or damp-heat, impairment of the Spleen by retention of undigested food, diminished function of the Spleen, deficiency of Kidney *yang* to warm up the Spleen, and attack on the Spleen by stagnant Liver *qi*. A detailed inquiry may give some clue to the diagnosis. Passage of watery stools accompanied by chills and fever often indicates exogenous attack of cold-damp. Diarrhea with offensive odor from the stools and burning sensation in the anus is usually caused by damp-heat. Passage of sour and fetid stools suggests indigestion. Chronic diarrhea accompanied by abdominal distension, impaired appetite and sallow complexion signifies weakness of the Spleen. Diarrhea daily before dawn is a typical symptom of deficiency of Kidney *yang*. Diarrhea immediately after the onset of abdominal pain but without alleviation of abdominal pain after emptying the bowels is seen in attacks on the Spleen by stagnant Liver *qi*. Frequent passage of stools containing blood and mucus occurs as a result of dysentery.

VIII. Inquiry about Menstruation and Leukorrhea

1. Menstruation

(1) Menstrual cycle: If the menstrual cycle is shortened by more than seven days, it is called "advanced menstruation" and usually results from heat which propels the blood flow or from deficiency of *qi* to control the blood flow. If the menstrual cycle is prolonged by more than seven days, it is called "delayed menstruation" and may be seen in deficiency of blood, congealing of blood due to cold, stagnation of *qi*, or stasis of blood. Irregular menstrual cycle with the menstruation sometimes advanced and sometimes delayed is either due to stagnation of Liver *qi* or due to deficiency of the Spleen and the Kidneys.

(2) Amount of menstrual flow: Normally, the amount of menstrual flow varies in different individuals. Abnormally profuse menstruation may be caused either by excess of heat or by deficiency of *qi*. In the former case the blood discharge is thick and red, while in the latter case it is light-colored. Abnormally scanty and light-colored menstruation indicates deficiency of vital essence and blood.

(3) Color of menstrual blood: Thin and light-colored menstruation is seen in deficiency of *qi* and/or blood. Thick and bright-colored menstruation suggests the presence of heat. Dark-colored menstrual discharge mixed with blood clots signifies blood stasis.

2. Leukorrhea

Normally, leukorrhea is a whitish, viscid discharge from the vagina. Profuse leukorrhea, thick, foul and yellow-colored indicates the presence of damp-heat. Whitish, viscid leukorrhagia is usually due to weakness of the Spleen, and whitish, thin leukorrhagia is due to deficiency of the Kidneys.

PALPATION

Palpation includes pulse-taking and examination of the other parts of the body by feeling with the hand or fingers.

Pulse-taking

Pulse-taking is a diagnostic method unique to Chinese medicine. It gives important information about the condition of *qi*, blood and internal organs, and helps differentiate the syndromes of exterior vs. interior, cold vs. heat, and deficiency vs. excessiveness. Wang Xi (also known as Wang Shuhe, 210-285) wrote *The Pulse Classic*, the first comprehensive book on sphygmology now extant. In 1564 Li Shizhen (also known as Li Binhu) wrote *Binhu's Pulse Studies*, in which 27 kinds of pulses and their diagnostic value are given in detail in lucid verses. In ancient Chinese literature, the pulse conditions are classified into 28 types according to depth, rate, strength, volume, tension, shape and rhythm. They are: floating, sinking (deep), slow, rapid, slippery, hesitant, feeble, forceful, long, short, full, faint, tense, relaxed, taut, hollow, tympanic, firm, soft, weak, scattered, fine, hidden, tremulous, running, knotted, intermittent and gigantic. Among these pulse conditions, the following 12 types are the most commonly encountered clinically: floating, sinking, slow, rapid, feeble, forceful, knotted. intermittent, slippery, hesitant, taut and tense.

I. Formation of the Pulse

According to Chinese medical theory, the following factors are involved in the formation of a pulse.

1. The Heart, vessels, *qi* and blood

"The Heart governs the blood which circulates in the vessels." The heart beat drives the circulation of blood, causing pulsation of the arteries, i.e., the pulse. Pectoral *qi* accumulated in the chest is not only responsible for respiration, but is also the motive force of the heart beat and blood circulation. Thus, pectoral *qi* plays an important role in the formation of pulse. The pulse is normal only when pectoral *qi* is adequate; otherwise morbid conditions of the pulse will occur. Therefore, the Heart, vessels, *qi* and blood are the basis on which a pulse is formed.

2. Coordination of the functional activities of *zang-fu* organs

"All blood vessels lead to the Lungs." The Lungs help the Heart to drive the blood flow. "The Spleen has the function of keeping the blood flowing within the blood vessels," and so it guarantees the normal circulation of blood in the vessels. "The Liver stores blood," serving as a reservoir to regulate the circulating blood volume, also relating to the blood flow in the vessels. "The Kidneys store the essence," from which blood is derived for replenishing the circulation. Therefore, coordinated actions of all the *zang*-organs are necessary to form a normal pulse.

II. Method of Pulse Taking

1. Position of Pulse Taking

In ancient times the pulse was taken on three parts of the body: the head, the upper limbs and the lower limbs. In each part pulses of three arteries were examined: the temporal artery at Taiyang (EX-HN 5) for the state of the head; the auricular artery at Ermen (TE 21) for the ears; the arteria buccinatoria at Dicang (ST 4) and Daying (ST 5) for the mouth and teeth; the radial artery at Taiyuan (LU 9) for the Lungs; the ulnar artery at Shenmen (HT 7) for the Heart; pulse at Hegu (LI 4) for the chest, pulse at Wuli (LR 10) and Taichong (LR 3) for the Liver, pulse at Qimen (LR 14) and Chongyang (ST 42) for the Spleen and Stomach; pulse at Taixi (KI 3) for the Kidneys. This is called "three-portion and nine-position pulse taking."

In the first or second century B.C., when the *Classic of Difficulties* appeared, only the pulse of the radial artery on the wrist was taken. This portion of the radial artery is called *cunkou*, in which *cun* is a unit of measure of length, approximately equal to one inch, and *kou* means entrance or exit. It is so called because it is about one inch from Yuji (LU 10, a point on the radial side of the midpoint of the first metacarpal bone, and on the dorso-ventral boundary of the hand), where the pulsation of the radial artery emerges. This part of the radial pulse is divided into three sections, designated as *cun* (the front or distal section), *guan* (the middle section) and *chi* (the proximal or rear section), in which *guan* means the entrance or exit, and *chi* is also a unit of measure of length, approximately equal to a cubit, an old measure of length. The rear section is so called because it is about one *chi* distal to the cubital crease. The styloid process of the radius is taken as a landmark for locating the three sections. The region opposite to this bony eminence is *guan*, that just distal to *guan* is *cun*, and that just proximal to *guan* is *chi*.

2. Division of *cunkou* pulse

Disorders of the *zang-fu* organs can be reflected in the changes of the radial pulse on the wrist. It is generally acknowledged that the three sections—*cun*, *guan* and *chi* of the left hand—reflect, respectively, the conditions of the Heart, the Liver and the Kidneys; and *cun*, *guan* and *chi* of the right hand, reflect, respectively, the conditions of the Lungs, the Spleen and the Kidneys. In addition, according to the correlations between *zang-* and *fu-*organs, disorders of the *fu*-organs can also be reflected in the radial pulse. The reason why the radial pulse on the wrist can reflect the disorders of all the internal organs is that *cunkou* is a segment of artery pertaining to the Lung Meridian. Since the vessels of all internal organs lead to the Lungs, disorder of any internal organ is bound to be reflected on the Lung Meridian. About the correspondence of the three sections of *cunkou* pulse to the five *zang*-organs there have been various descriptions, though they are fundamentally compatible. The explanation of the correspondence is as follows: since *cun* is the front section, it corresponds to the internal organs in the upper portion of the body (i.e., the Heart and the Lungs); since *guan* is the middle section, it corresponds to the middle portion of the body (i.e., the Liver and the Spleen); and since *chi* is the rear section, it corresponds to the lower portion of the body (i.e., the Kidneys). Then, according to the *yin-yang* theory that the left pertains to *yin* and the right to *yang*, the Heart governs blood and the Liver stores blood, both being *yin zang*-organs, while the Lungs dominate *qi* and the Spleen replenishes *qi*, both being *yang zang*-organs. Therefore, the left *cun* corresponds to the Heart and the right *cun* to the Lungs; the left *guan* corresponds to the Liver and the right *guan* to the Spleen; and both the left and right *chi* correspond to the Kidneys (the left *chi* to Kidney *yin* and the right *chi* to Kidney *yang* or the "vital gate"). It is hard to say whether this is a strained explanation, but the relationships between the changes in different sections of the radial pulse and disorders of the internal organs are of pragmatic significance, for they were summarized from clinical observations.

3. How to take the pulse

The patient should adopt a sitting or supine position, with the arm at the level of the heart, the wrist straight and the palm upward. It is advisable to put a small cushion under the wrist.

When taking the pulse, the physician uses the index, middle and ring fingers. He first palpates the process styloid of the radius with the middle finger to locate the *guan* section. Then, he locates the *cun* section distal to *guan* with the index finger, and the *chi* section proximal to *guan* with the ring finger. The distribution of the three sections of the pulse should accord with the patient's height. In other words, the three examining fingers should be set somewhat apart when taking the pulse of a long arm, and closed up when taking the pulse of a short arm. In the case of infants, the pulse is taken with the thumb only.

There are three manipulations used in pulse taking: touching, pressing and searching. By touching is meant resting the fingers on the patient's wrist very lightly; by pressing is meant feeling the pulse with proper force; and by searching is meant varying the force and moving the fingers to get a more distinct pulse reading. Therefore, by using light, moderate and heavy force at each three sections, nine examinations of the pulse can be executed on each side. The manipulations can be performed with the three examining fingers simultaneously, or with one finger first and then another.

III. Normal Pulse

1. Description of a normal pulse

A normal pulse in a healthy individual is neither floating nor sinking, and neither large nor small; it is of moderate tension and force, and even in rhythm—4-5 beats to one cycle of the physician's respiration (i.e., 60-80 beats per minute). It may have some changes in accordance with the climate, environment and the person's physical activities.

2. Characteristics of a normal pulse

The three characteristic features of a normal pulse are: It beats with adequate Stomach *qi*, with vitality and with root. A pulse with adequate Stomach *qi* is a pulse that beats unhurriedly with regular rhythm and normal frequency. A pulse with vitality is a pulse that beats with moderate but enough strength. A pulse with root means that the pulse can be felt at all the three sections (*cun, guan,* and particularly *chi*) with deep palpation.

Stomach *qi* is a very important factor in human life, according to *The Canon of Medicine.* It states that one lives on Stomach *qi* and will die if Stomach *qi* fades away. Therefore, Stomach *qi* is highly emphasized in pulse taking. A pulse with adequate Stomach *qi* is normal, a pulse with insufficient Stomach *qi* is abnormal, and a pulse with no Stomach *qi* is fatal.

The vitality or strength of a pulse is directly related to the condition of the Heart. If Heart *qi* is abundant and the vessels are full of blood, the pulse will beat with vitality.

The Kidneys are the foundation of the inborn constitution, and supply motive power to all the body organs and tissues. Therefore, the Kidneys are regarded as the root of life, and their function is reflected in the pulse. A pulse with root implies the existence of adequate Kidney *qi*. "Even though the *cunkou* pulse is hardly perceptible, pulsation felt at the *chi* position with deep pressure means that the stream of life can be continued." (cited from the *Mai-Jue* or *Key to Pulse-Taking*.)

3. Physiological factors that may influence the pulse condition

Age, sex, constitution, physical activity, mental state and climate may influence the pulse condition. In children, the younger the age, the more rapid the pulse. A young adult with a strong constitution usually has a forceful pulse, while a weak elderly person has a feeble pulse. A woman's pulse is often soft and weak, whereas a man's pulse tends to be more forceful. The pulse is generally somewhat floating in thin persons, and slightly sinking in obese ones. During intense physical exercise or emotional upset the pulse is rapid and forceful. The pulse at night is slower and weaker than in the daytime. In addition, the pulse may be varied in different seasons: in spring it may be slightly taut, in summer somewhat full, in late summer moderately soft, in autumn rather floating and taut, and in winter a little bit sinking.

IV. The Clinical Significance of Abnormal Pulse Conditions

Since the condition of the pulse depends upon the condition of the Heart, vessels, *qi* and blood, as well as coordination of the functions of the various internal organs, changes of any of the factors may be reflected in the pulse. Generally speaking, from the pulse one can judge the exuberance or decline of *qi* and blood, the functional state of the internal organs, and the situation of the *yin-yang* balance.

The following are abnormal pulses commonly found in clinical practice, and their clinical significance.

1. Pulses characterized by abnormal depth in location

1) Floating Pulse vs. Sinking Pulse

The differentiation between floating and sinking pulses is based on the depth of location of the pulse. A floating or superficial pulse can be easily felt with a light touch but fades when heavy pressure is applied. This is attributed to the resistance of the body's defense against attacks of pathogens on the superficial portion of the body. So, it usually indicates an exterior (superficial) syndrome. It often occurs at the initial stage of an exogenous disease.

A sinking or deep pulse can only be felt while pressing hard. This is attributed to confrontation between the genuine *qi* and pathogenic factors in the interior of the body, and hence indicates an interior syndrome. If the sinking pulse is forceful, it indicates an interior excess syndrome, and if it is weak, it indicates an interior deficiency syndrome.

2) Scattered Pulse and Hollow Pulse

Scattered pulse and hollow pulse are pulses similar to floating pulse in depth of location. A scattered pulse feels diffuse and feeble to a light touch and faint when hard pressure is applied. It happens in critical cases, indicating exhaustion of *qi*. A hollow pulse is floating, large, soft and hollow, and feels like a scallion stalk. It may be encountered in massive loss of blood.

3) Hidden Pulse and Firm Pulse

Hidden pulse and firm pulse are pulses similar to sinking pulse in depth of location. A hidden pulse can only be felt by pressing on the bone, and is located even deeper than a deep pulse. It may be found in cases of syncope, shock or excruciating pain. A firm pulse is forceful and taut, felt only upon hard pressure, suggesting accumulation of *yin* cold and mass formation.

2. Pulses characterized by abnormal frequency

1) Slow Pulse vs. Rapid Pulse

The differentiation between slow and rapid pulses is based on the pulse rate. A slow or retarded pulse has less than four beats to one cycle of the physician's respiration (or less than 60 beats per minute). It reflects inhibited activity of *qi* by pathogenic cold, and hence indicates a cold syndrome.

A rapid pulse has more than 5 beats to one cycle of the physician's respiration, or more than 90 beats per minute. It is usually caused by pathogenic heat which accelerates the blood circulation, and hence it indicates a heat syndrome. A forceful rapid pulse is usually found in an excessive heat syndrome, while a weak rapid pulse is found in a deficiency-heat syndrome.

2) Swift Pulse and Tremulous Pulse

A swift pulse has more than 7 beats to one cycle of the physician's respiration, or more than 120 beats per minute. It is not infrequently encountered in severe case of febrile disease or exhaustion of *yin* with extreme hyperactivity of *yang*.

A tremulous pulse is quick and jerky, and feels like a bouncing pea. It may occur in cases of fright or severe pain.

3. Pulses characterized by abnormal strength

1) Depleted (or Feeble) Pulse vs. Replete (or Forceful) Pulse

The differentiation between depleted and replete pulses depends on the strength of the pulse felt by the physician. A depleted pulse feels feeble and void to the physician's finger. This is attributed to deficiency of *qi* and blood. When *qi* is inadequate to drive the circulating blood, the pulse will be feeble, and when the blood circulating in the vessels is insufficient, the pulse will feel void. So, a depleted or feeble pulse is a sign of deficiency. A replete pulse feels vigorous and forceful to both light and heavy pressure. It shows that both the pathogenic factors and genuine *qi* are strong, and there is an intense struggle of genuine *qi* against the pathogenic factors. So, it is a sign of excess.

2) Weak Pulse and Faint Pulse

Weak pulse and faint pulse are also pulses with decreased strength. A weak pulse feels deep and soft. It indicates deficiency of *qi* and blood. A faint pulse feels thready and soft, scarcely perceptible. It is a sign of extreme exhaustion.

4. Pulses characterized by change in smoothness

1) Slippery Pulse vs. Hesitant Pulse

The differentiation between slippery and hesitant pulses depends upon whether the pulse feels smooth. A slippery or smooth pulse is extremely fluid, and feels like beads rolling on a plate. It often occurs in accumulation of phlegm and dampness, stagnation of food, and excess heat when excessive pathogenic factors cause excited activity of *qi* with surging blood flow. It also occurs in pregnancy, when extra blood is needed to nourish the fetus.

A hesitant pulse comes and goes irregularly, with a fine, slow rhythm, like scraping bamboo with a knife. It indicates sluggishness of blood circulation caused by deficiency of blood or stagnation of *qi* and blood.

5. Pulses characterized by change in volume

1) Full Pulse (Surging) vs. Fine (or Thready) Pulse

A full pulse beats like dashing waves. It results from excessive heat in the interior, which causes dilation of the blood vessels and rapid flow of blood. So, it indicates the existence of excessive pathogenic heat.

A fine pulse is as thin as a thread, feeble yet always perceptible. In most instances, it is due to deficiency of *qi* and blood, so that the vessels are not filled with enough blood and the circulation is not adequately motivated. However, it may also result from obstruction of circulation by dampness. So, it indicates deficiency of *qi* and blood and other kinds of deficiency syndromes; sometimes it can be a sign of dampness.

2) Gigantic (or Large) Pulse

A large or gigantic pulse is a pulse with a high wave which lifts the examining finger to a greater height than normal, either forceful (seen in cases of undamaged body resistance and excessive heat in the interior) or weak (seen in general debility).

6. Pulses characterized by change in tension

1) Tense (or Tight) Pulse vs. Relaxed (or Loose) Pulse

A tense pulse feels like a tightly stretched cord. It indicates cold, pain or retention of food.

Relaxed or loose pulse is a pulse with diminished tension and moderate frequency. It is a sign of dampness or weakness of the Spleen.

2) Stringy Pulse and Tympanic Pulse

Stringy pulse and tympanic pulse are also pulses with increased tension.

Stringy pulse is a pulse that feels straight and long, like a violin string. It usually occurs in Liver and Gallbladder troubles, and cases of severe pain. Tympanic pulse feels hard and hollow, as if touching the surface of a drum. It can be encountered in patients after loss of blood or spermatorrhea.

3) Soft Pulse

Soft Pulse is also a pulse with diminished tension. It cannot resist pressure, and is felt only upon a light touch, but fades away upon heavy pressure. In this respect, it has some similarities to a floating pulse, but it feels thinner and softer than the latter. It is a sign of deficiency or dampness.

7. Pulses characterized by change in extent—Long Pulse vs. Short Pulse

Long pulse is a pulse with large extent and prolonged stroke. A long pulse with moderate tension may be found in normal persons, but a long and taut pulse indicates excess of *yang* or heat.

Short pulse is a pulse with short extent, easily felt at the *guan* section, but not obviously felt at the *cun* and *chi* sections. It strikes the finger (namely the middle finger) sharply and leaves it quickly. A forceful short pulse indicates *qi* stagnation, while a feeble short pulse is a sign of *qi* consumption.

8. Pulses characterized by arrhythmia—Intermittent Pulse, Knotted Pulse and Running Pulse

Intermittent pulse is a slow and weak pulse pausing at regular intervals. It may result from feebleness of the internal organs with consumption of *qi* and blood, indicating a severe condition; but it may also occur in one who is seized with terror or pain, which causes interruption of the flow of *qi* to the pulse. In the latter case, an intermittent pulse does not signify a severe disease.

Knotted pulse is characterized by pauses at irregular intervals, resulting from excess of *yin* with disharmonious *yang*. It usually occurs in *qi* stagnation due to excess of *yin* or blood stasis due to cold phlegm.

Running pulse is a rapid pulse with irregular intermittence, usually caused by extreme *yang* heat with disharmonious *yin*. It indicates excessive heat, *qi* stagnation and blood stasis.

9. Combination of pulse conditions

All the pulses listed above are simple patterns of pulse conditions. Many patients have two or more pulse conditions, namely, compound pulses. The following compound pulses are often found in clinical practice.

A floating-tense pulse indicates an exterior-cold syndrome caused by exogenous pathogenic cold attacking the exterior portion of the body.

A floating-relaxed pulse is a sign of exterior-deficiency syndrome, in which defensive *qi* is weak while there is an invasion of exogenous pathogenic wind.

A floating-rapid pulse is a sign of exterior-heat syndrome caused by an attack on the exterior portion of the body by exogenous wind-heat.

A deep-slow pulse indicates interior-cold.

A stringy-rapid pulse is often found in fire syndrome produced by a depressed Liver or attack on the Liver and Gallbladder by pathogenic damp-heat.

A slippery-rapid pulse indicates phlegm-heat, phlegm-fire or food stagnation.

A full-rapid pulse signifies excessive heat at the *qi* level, as occurring in exogenous affection with high fever.

Palpation of the Body

I. The Skin

Palpation of the skin is chiefly for determining temperature, moisture and swelling. Generally, the skin feels hot in the case of heat syndromes and cool in the case of cold syndromes. If the palm feels much hotter than the back of the hand, the heat is endogenous, due to deficiency of *yin*. If the body feels hot at first, and the hotness becomes less after a long palpation, the heat is in the exterior portion of the body. If the heat increases after a long palpation, the heat is in the interior of the body. Dry and shriveled skin suggests deficiency of body fluid. Dry and scaly skin is a sign of blood stasis.

II. Abdomen

If there is abdominal pain, palpation helps to differentiate between excess and deficiency. Pain alleviated by pressure is a pain of the deficiency type, and pain with tenderness is a pain of the excess type.

If the abdomen is distended, palpation together with percussion is useful for differentiation between tympanites and ascites.

If there is an abdominal mass, palpation may give information about its shape, size, consistency and tenderness.

III. Acupoints

Tender points reflecting diseases of the internal organs may be found by pressing on acupoints with the fingers. For instance, tenderness at Weishu (BL 21) or Zusanli (ST 36) usually indicates a stomach disease; tenderness at Lanwei (EX-LE 7) often occurs in patients with appendicitis. Sometimes a small nodule may be felt at certain acupoints. For instance, a nodule may be felt at Feishu (BL 13) in pulmonary diseases.

Appendix: Modern Research into Chinese Sphygmology[2]

Pulse-taking is a unique diagnostic method in Chinese medicine. By taking the pulse a lot of information can be obtained which may help to determine the location of a disease, the condition of *qi* and blood, the functional activities of the various internal organs and the presence of pathogenic factors, as well as the prognosis. All the knowledge about pulse-taking is the result of practical experience accumulated over thousands of years. But this has been felt to be inadequate from the standpoint of modern science, and research has been carried out in an effort to identify objective standards of the various pulse conditions which can stand up to scientific scrutiny.

In order to develop objective standards to substitute for the subjective feeling in pulse-taking, several types of sphygmochronography have been designed. The main component of the sphygmochronograph for Chinese pulse study is a device to transform the pulse beat into electronic information, which can be displayed on a fluorescent screen after amplification and filtration, and recorded as a sphygmogram. The device includes a detector which can exert different levels of pressure on the radial pulse.

The development of sphygmochronographic studies proceeds in three stages. The first stage is the recognition of the pulse condition from the shape of the recorded pulse wave. Success has been achieved in this regard, for the shape of the pulse waves is stable in a long recording. The disadvantage is that it is only a pattern recognition, without quantitative analysis.

The second stage is to perform quantitative analysis according to multiple parameters of the sphygmogram. In order to obtain the normal range of each parameter and its range in various pulse conditions, thousands of sphygmograms have been analyzed. Quantitative analysis of a sphygmogram is now available, but manual measuring of the parameters and calculation are time-consuming. Although computer programming has made it much easier, this device is still not ideal, because a Chinese physician usually takes the pulse with three fingers at the same time. However, a new pattern of sphygmochronograph has been developed with three detectors for simultaneously recording the pulses at *cun*, *guan* and *chi* sections. Experiments are still being carried out.

The third stage is the design of a scheme for the comprehensive recognition of abnormal pulses. Abnormal pulse conditions can be analyzed according to the following eight factors: depth of location, volume (or thickness), strength, rate, rhythm, smoothness, tension and extent (or length). Any pulse condition is a combination of the above eight factors. Such an analysis makes the direct computer recognition of the pulse condition feasible. However, a vast amount of scientific data needs to be collected for assessing its clinical value.

Below is a brief discussion on the sphymographic features of the major abnormal

---

[2]Special References for the Appendix

(1) Huang, Shi-Lin, et al. *Zhongyi Maixiang Yanjiu* (Chinese Sphygmology Studies) (in Chinese), Beijing, People's Medical Publishing House, 1986.

(2) Chen, Jie-Wen: *Maixiang de Shenglixue Jichu* (Physiological Basis of Chinese Sphygmology) in *Xiandai Zhongyi Shenglixue Jichu* (Physiological Basis of Modernized TCM) (in Chinese), Ist ed, Ji, Zhong-Pu (editor-in-chief), Beijing, Xueyuan Press, 1991, pp. 147-164.

pulse conditions described in Chinese medicine.

A pulse wave is composed of two parts: an ascending limb and a descending limb. They form the main wave. On the descending limb there are two minor waves and an incisure, which are called the tidal wave, dicrotic wave and dicrotic notch, respectively.

Normal Pulse (Fig. V-1)

The normal ranges of the sphygmographic parameters in adults are as follows:

1. Pulse rate: 60-100/min.
2. Ascending angle: 80-87°.
3. Ascending time of the ascending limb (t_1): 0.07-0.11 sec.
4. Half-ascending time <0.04 sec.
5. Pattern of the ascending limb: steep without notch.
6. Height of the main wave (h_1): 9-22mm.
7. Angle of the main wave: 19-42°.
8. Height of the dicrotic notch (h_3)/h_1: 30-55%.
9. Amplitude of the dicrotic wave (h_4): 0.5-2mm.
10. The best pressure for pulse taking: 150g.

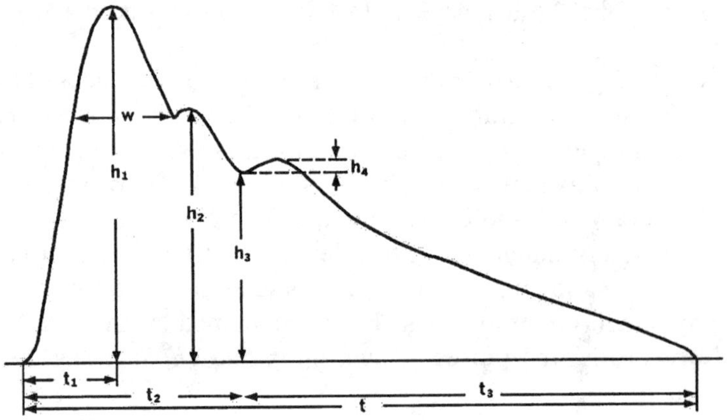

Fig. V-1 Measurements of the pulse wave

Rapid Pulse and Swift Pulse vs. Slow Pulse

The pulse rate is related to the heart rate, which is controlled by neuro-humoral factors, body temperature, acidity of the body fluids and concentration of various ions. Clinically, rapid pulse is most commonly found in cases of fever and sympathetic excitation with more secretion of epinephrine. It is characterized by increased frequency at the range of 100-130/minute and regular rhythm. If it is not combined with other abnormal pulse conditions, the pattern of each pulse wave is basically the same as that of a normal pulse. A swift pulse has an even greater frequency, ranging from 140-170/minute.

Slow pulse is often caused by vagus excitation, low body temperature, increased blood potassium ions, or conduction block of the heart. It is characterized by low frequency at the range of 40-59/minute and basically regular rhythm.

Floating Pulse vs. Sinking Pulse (Fig. V-2 and Fig. V-3)

Adequate blood volume and normal cardiac output are necessary for filling the blood vessels with blood. The elastic fibers of the arterial wall allow the arteries to dilate, and the smooth muscles of the arterial wall limit the dilation. Therefore, the arteries are in a slightly dilated state normally, maintaining a certain volume and pressure. The smooth muscles of the arterial wall are controlled by the sympathetic nerve, excitation of which causes contraction of the smooth muscles and reduction in caliber of the arteries. On the other hand, decreased excitation of the sympathetic nerve causes dilation of the blood vessels. Some humoral factors, such as norepinephrine and angiotensin, cause vascular contraction, while vaso-active substances cause vascular dilation. Cold and heat also cause contraction and dilation of the blood vessels, respectively. The depth of the radial artery felt during pulse-taking chiefly depends upon its location and state of contraction and dilation, but is also related with the cardiac output and vascular filling.

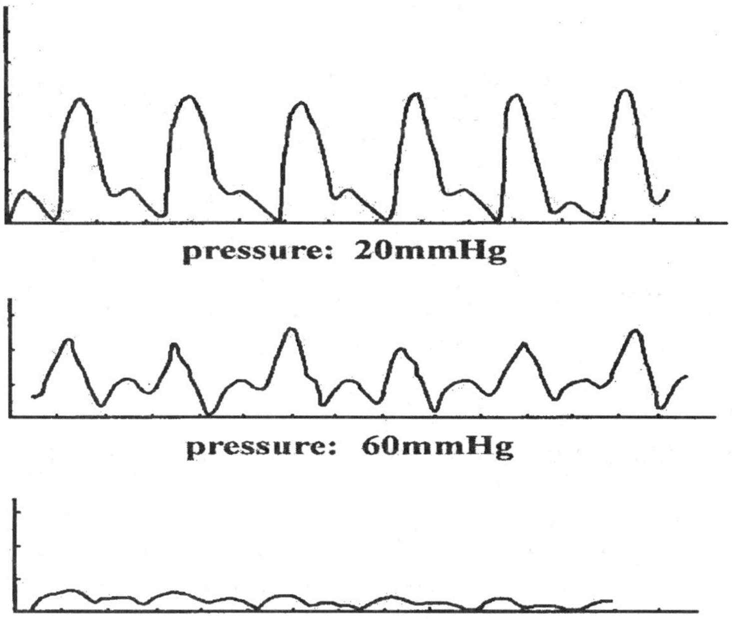

Fig. V-2 Floating pulse

A floating pulse is superficially located, easily felt with a light touch and fading away upon hard pressure. Physiologically, it may be encountered in thin persons, with the radial artery of the wrist located just beneath the skin, or in hot weather, which causes dilation of the peripheral arteries. As a pathological pulse condition, it is often seen in colds and influenza or at the initial stage of an acute infectious disease. In most cases it is due to the action of pyrogen, which causes fever, increased metabolism, and increased cardiac output. In addition, there is reflective dilation of peripheral vessels for heat dissipation, with consequent free circulation of the blood due to lowered vascular resistance. Therefore, the main factors for the formation of a floating pulse are increased cardiac output, dilation of peripheral arteries and free blood circulation. The sphygmographic features of a floating pulse are: (1) With a light touch with a pressure of 20-40mmHg, a higher main wave can be obtained with a steep ascending limb and shortened ascending time. (2) The location of the dicrotic wave is lowered, and h_3/h_1 is less than 30%. (3) The sphygmogram record at moderate pressure (50-80mmHg) or heavy pressure (90-120mmHg) shows marked decrease in amplitude of the main wave and changes of wave pattern.

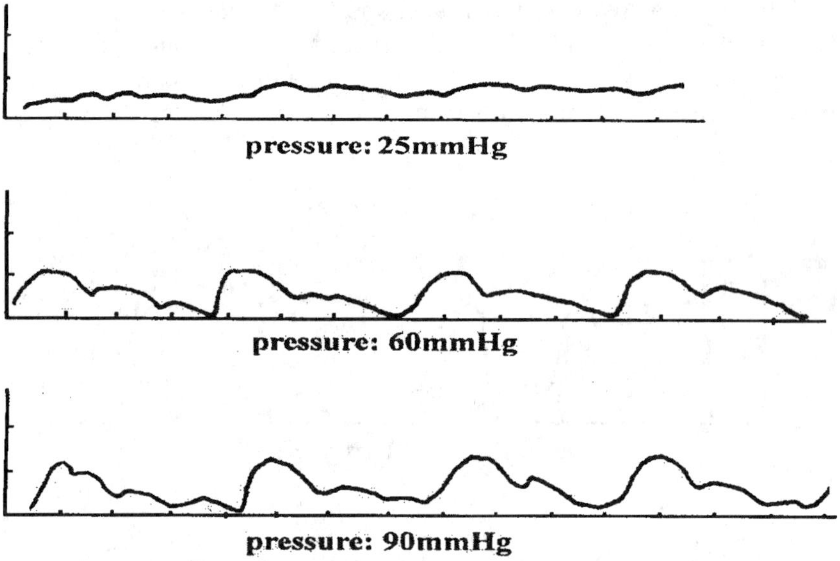

Fig. V-3 Deep (sinking) pulse

Sinking pulse is a pulse deep under the skin, which is not perceptible to a light touch, and can only be felt with hard pressure. In obese persons the pulse is often sinking because of the thick subcutaneous fat. A normal pulse sinks in somewhat cold weather, which causes contraction of the peripheral vessels by a reflex action. A pathological sinking pulse may be due to reduced cardiac output with lowered blood pressure, insufficient filling of blood vessels and slow blood circulation. In this case, the sinking pulse is weak. Arteriolar spasm with increased peripheral resistance may also give rise to a sinking pulse, which is usually thready and forceful. In cases of severe edema when the distance between the radial artery and the skin is increased, the pulse is certainly felt to be sinking. The sphygmographic features of a sinking pulse are: the ascending limb of the main wave has a less steep slope followed by a blunt peak, and the pulse waves can only be distinctly recorded when the pressure is heavy. Lowered and deformed pulse waves are recorded when the pressure is moderate or light.

A hidden pulse is deeper in location and weaker than a sinking pulse. Even with heavy pressure, the pulse waves recorded may not be distinct.

Full Pulse vs. Fine Pulse (Fig. V-4 and Fig. V-5)

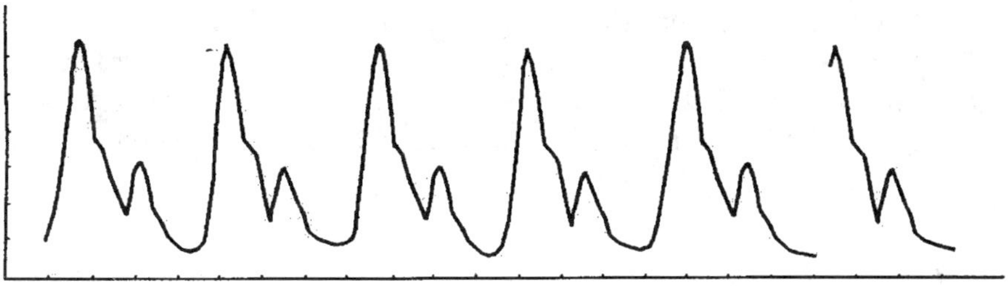

Fig. V-4 Full pulse

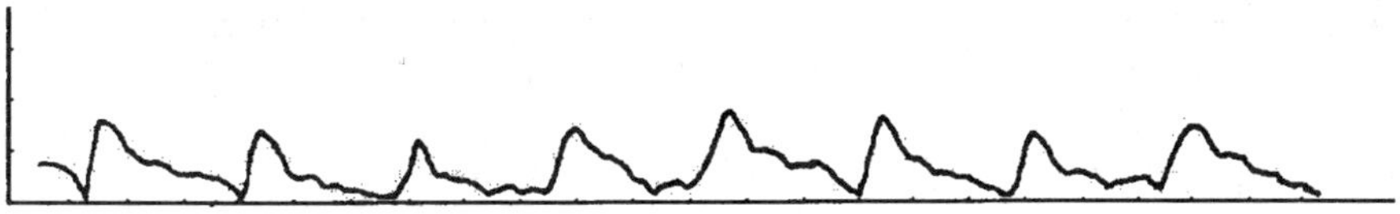

Fig. V-5 Fine (thready) pulse

The difference between the systolic pressure and diastolic pressure is pulse pressure. The systolic pressure chiefly depends on the cardiac output, while the diastolic pressure chiefly depends on the peripheral resistance. Therefore, the pulse pressure is a comprehensive reflection of both the cardiac output and the peripheral resistance. The changes in pulse pressure have a direct impact on the volume of the pulse. A high pulse pressure leads to a full pulse, and a low pulse pressure to a fine pulse.

Full pulse is formed by intensified ventricular systole and dilation of the peripheral blood vessels. Because of the intensified ventricular systole which accelerates the ejection and causes an abrupt rising of intravascular pressure, there is a forceful rising of the pulse. The dilation of the peripheral arteries not only makes a remarkable rising and declining of the pulse wave, but also gives a feeling of increased volume of the pulse. Full pulse usually occurs in cases of excessive heat, such as high fever, which is associated with strengthened cardiac contraction, shortened systolic time, increased cardiac output and accelerated blood flow, as well as dilated peripheral blood vessels for heat dissipation. It is also present in aortic insufficiency and hyperthyroidism. The sphygmographic features of a full pulse are: (1) The main wave has a large amplitude. (2) The ascending limb is steep with a shortened ascending time, followed by rapid descending, so that the angle of the main wave is usually less than 20°. (3) The dicrotic wave is located at the lower portion of the descending limb, and h_3/h_1 is less than 30%. (4) Distinct sphygmograms can be obtained with light, moderate and heavy pressures.

Fine pulse is a pulse felt as fine as a thread, but is distinctly perceptible. It may be due to peripheral vascular contraction with decreased pulse pressure, but it may result from diminished cardiac output in cardiac insufficiency or decreased blood volume. Thus, fine pulse can be further divided into two patterns: forceful fine pulse and weak fine pulse. A fine pulse due to deficiency of both *qi* and blood is usually a weak and fine pulse. A fine and stringy pulse is not infrequently encountered in hypertension. The sphygmographic feature of a fine pulse is small amplitude of the main wave with a small or invisible dicrotic wave.

Slippery Pulse vs. Hesitant Pulse (Fig. V-6 and Fig. V-7)

The velocity of blood flow is related to the dynamic force of the cardiac contraction and the resistance of the blood flow. Besides the length and caliber of the blood vessels, blood viscosity plays an important role in influencing the velocity of blood flow. Normally,

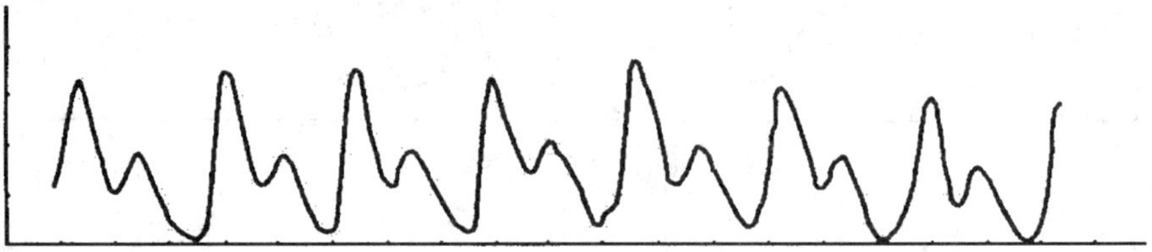

Fig. V-6 Slippery pulse

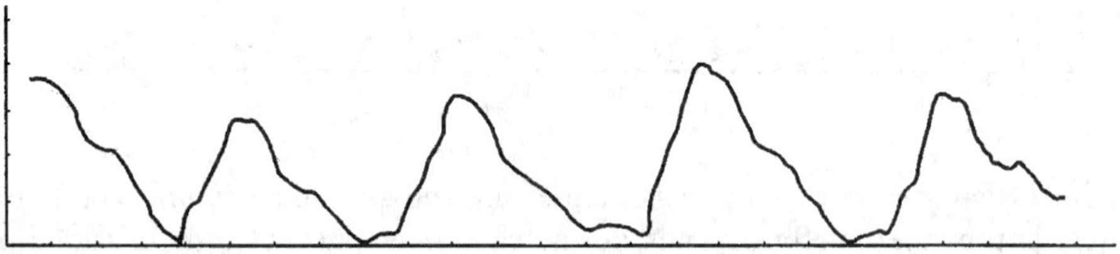

Fig. V-7 Hesitant pulse

the viscosity of blood is about 4.5 times that of water. It is in proportion to the resistance of the blood flow. The more viscous the blood is, the greater the resistance of the blood flow, and hence the more slowly the blood flows. On the other hand, the blood flow will be accelerated if the blood is less viscous. The blood viscosity is chiefly related to the number of red blood cells and the content of plasma protein. High red blood cell count is accompanied by increased blood viscosity, and low red blood cell count by decreased blood viscosity. Elevated plasma protein level also leads to increased blood viscosity, and lowered plasma protein level to decreased blood viscosity. Increased blood viscosity causes sluggish blood flow, and hence a hesitant pulse, whereas decreased blood viscosity makes the blood flow smooth, and hence a slippery pulse.

Slippery pulse is a pulse which comes and goes smoothly. In anemia, liver cirrhosis with ascites and nephrosis with edema, the pulse is usually slippery, either due to a decreased red blood cell count or due to low plasma protein. In pregnancy, owing to the action of estrogen, there is retention of water both intra- and extra-vascularly, and the slippery pulse is physiological, indicating increased circulating blood volume, particularly plasma volume. The sphygmographic features of a slippery pulse are: (1) The ascending limb rises almost vertically with shortened ascending time, followed by a sharp peak. (2) There is an apparent tidal wave or deep dicrotic notch. (3) The dicrotic wave starts at the lower portion of the descending limb and has a large amplitude; h_3/h_1 is less than 30%. Therefore, a slippery pulse often shows a double-waved or triple-waved pattern.

Hesitant pulse is a pulse which comes and goes irregularly, with a small, fine, slow jogging tempo. Its main mechanism is increased blood viscosity. The causes of increased blood viscosity are various. Typical hesitant pulse is seen in dehydration due to severe vomiting and diarrhea, polycythemia, and hyperlipemia. The sphygmographic feature is the slow ascending limb with a prolonged ascending time, followed by a blunt peak, while the tidal wave and dicrotic wave are usually absent.

Stringy Pulse and Tense Pulse (Fig. V-8 and Fig. V-9)

The transmission of the pulse wave is closely related to the elasticity of the arteries. An elastic artery transmits the pulse wave slowly, so the three palpating fingers are slow to feel it. An artery with poor elasticity transmits the pulse faster, and so the pulse is felt by the three fingers almost simultaneously.

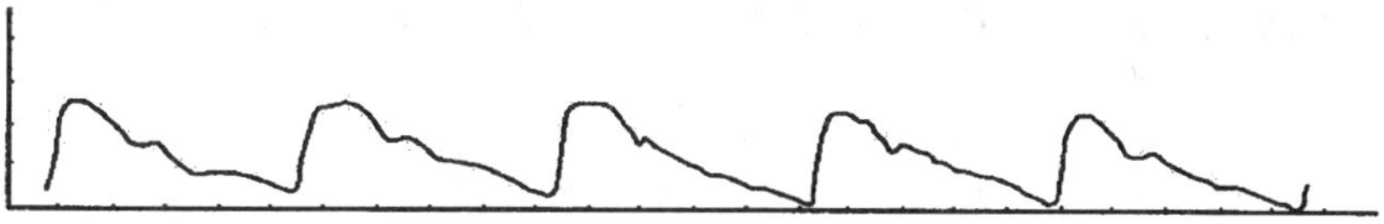

Fig. V-8 Stringy pulse

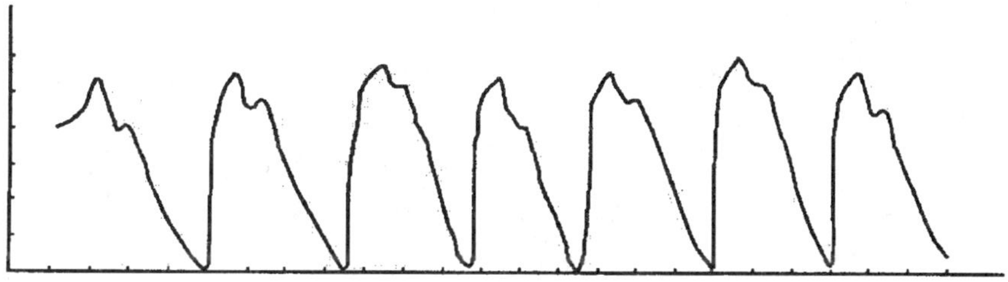

Fig. V-9 Tense pulse

Contraction of the smooth muscle of an artery elevates the tension of the arterial wall, reduces the caliber of the artery and increases the resistance of blood flow. The heart contracts more energetically to overcome the increased resistance, resulting in elevation of the blood pressure. Because of the increased tension of the arterial wall and elevated blood pressure, the pulse is felt to be tense.

Stringy pulse is a pulse that feels straight and long, like a violin string. Its mechanism is multifarious, including: (1) increased tension of the vascular smooth muscle by sympathetic excitation or some humoral factors; (2) reduced elasticity of the arterial wall with increased resistance of peripheral blood flow. Clinically, a stringy pulse is often found in patients with hepatitis, liver cirrhosis, hepatic carcinoma, hypertension, atherosclerosis, severe pains, and emotional upset. In liver diseases, stringy pulse might be caused by some humoral factors as the result of metabolic disturbances. In hypertension, a stringy pulse is probably related to the increased peripheral resistance and elevated arterial blood pressure. In atherosclerosis, the reduced elasticity of the arterial wall makes the pulse stringy. In cases of severe pain and emotional upset, secretion of epinephrine and the like causes increased peripheral resistance, and hence a stringy pulse. In a healthy volunteer, intravenous dripping of norepinephrine can turn the normal pulse into a stringy pulse. The sphygmographic features of a stringy pulse are: (1) The angle of the main wave is increased, and the peak is often vaulted or replaced by a plateau. (2) The tidal and dicrotic waves are located at the upper portion of the descending limb, and h_3/h_1 is over 50%. (3) The dicrotic wave is also located at the upper portion of the descending limb, or even at the same level as the main wave, but with a small amplitude.

Tense pulse is quite similar to stringy pulse. It feels like a tightly stretched cord. Its mechanism is intense contraction of the peripheral vessels with increased cardiac output. It is often seen at the initial stage of an infection, when the heat regulating center is stimulated by pathogens or toxins. Impulses are then sent out through the sympathetic nerve to cause intense contraction of the peripheral blood vessels and muscles, and hence the tense pulse and chills. It also occurs in cases of acute pain, when there is a sympathetic-adrenomedullary response which makes the peripheral blood vessels highly contracted. Its sphygmographic features are similar to those of the stringy pulse, but the height of the main wave is usually increased with an incisure at the peak, while the dicrotic wave disappears.

CHAPTER 6

DIFFERENTIATION OF SYNDROMES

In traditional Chinese medicine, syndrome differentiation is the major part of diagnosis. It is more important than disease diagnosis, for the treatment is usually based upon the syndrome. Both "syndrome" and "disease" in traditional Chinese medicine have different implications from the same terms used in Western medicine. In many instances, "disease," or more precisely "illness," mainly refers to what the patient feels or complains of. For example, diseases in traditional Chinese medicine include coughing, headaches, and diarrhea, which are simply symptoms; and jaundice, ascites and goiter, which are signs, often discovered by the patients themselves. Even in the case of a disease diagnosis more or less equivalent to that of Western medicine, such as *xiao-ke*[1] (diabetes mellitus), it is still insufficient for giving proper treatment, and further determination of the "syndrome" is necessary. In this respect, there are some similarities between Western and Chinese medicine. Diabetes mellitus cannot be properly treated by a Western medical doctor if the doctor does not know whether it is insulin-dependent or non-insulin-dependent. In traditional Chinese medicine, *xiao-ke* is classified into different syndrome patterns such as dryness-heat of the Lungs and the Stomach, dysfunction of the Spleen and the Stomach, and *yin* deficiency of the Liver and the Kidneys, upon which proper treatment can be administered. However, there are disparities. In Western medicine, differentiation of insulin-dependence and non-insulin-dependence is specific for diabetes mellitus but useless for other diseases. In traditional Chinese medicine, on the contrary, any of the above-mentioned syndrome patterns can be found in many other diseases and different diseases, with the same syndrome pattern can be treated with the same (or at least similar) therapy. Therefore, a disease is usually treated differently according to different syndromes, and different diseases may be treated with similar therapy if they show the same syndrome.

In traditional Chinese medicine, a syndrome[2] is not merely a collection of symptoms and signs, but comprises the following components: location of the pathological changes, cause and pathogenesis of the disease, nature of the syndrome and the ability of the body to resist the pathogenic factors. These components are deduced by comprehensive analysis of

---

[1]*Xiao* means consumption and *ke* means thirst. *Xiao-ke* is a disease characterized by polyphagia, polydipsia and polyuria, with thirst. It has also been known since the 8th century that the urine discharged by patients suffering from *xiao-ke* tastes sweet.

[2]The English translation of the Chinese medical term 证 (*zheng*) has given rise to much controversy. The original meaning of this word is "evidence." As a medical term, it refers to the conclusion made after an overall analysis of the symptoms and signs in the light of traditional Chinese medical theory. Syndrome is not an exact English equivalent; it should be comprehended as described in the text. "Pattern," "state" and other translations have been proposed. However, since they do not bear the sense of abnormal or morbid conditions of the body or mind, they are not adopted in this book. Transliteration of this term as *zheng* is somewhat confusing, because at least five terms commonly used in Chinese medicine can be transliterated as *zheng*, and for three of them the English equivalents are difficult to find.

the symptoms and signs from a holistic perspective.

Among these components, location may only refer to the depth of the disease, i.e., whether the disease involves the exterior portion of the body or it has penetrated into the interior of the body; if the disease is in the interior, which organ(s) is(are) involved. Even if an internal organ is involved, it is involved only in a very broad sense. For example, the Kidneys comprise a big system with multiple functions such as urine secretion, reproduction, osteogenesis, hemopoiesis and assisting of respiration, as well as many endocrine functions and some brain activities. In addition, disorders in the correlation between the diseased organ and other organs is more emphasized than the impairment of the diseased organ itself. Deficiency of Kidney *yin* usually leads to deficiency of Liver *yin* and Heart *yin*, and deficiency of Kidney *yang* may impair the function of the Spleen or influence the function of the Heart or the Lungs. Thus, the location of the disease in traditional Chinese medicine can only be considered as a classification of syndromes according to the involved functional systems. Unlike Western medicine, traditional Chinese medicine has no concept of disease entity based on patho-anatomy, except for some superficial pathological changes that can be observed from the outside.

The pathogenic factors in traditional Chinese medicine are usually very general. Emotional influences, improper diet and unhealthy life style are by no means specific to a particular disease. Even atmospheric factors are not comparable with the bacteria and viruses identified by Western medicine. It is preferable to consider them as the responses of the human body to pathogens rather than the pathogens themselves.

Pathogenesis explains how *yin-yang* is imbalanced. Although there are various approaches to explain different patterns of imbalance, most of them are not specific to a given disease. For example, in some diabetic patients with deficiency of Liver and Kidney *yin*, deficiency of Liver *yin* leads to relative hyperactivity of the Liver in promoting the flow of *qi*, which helps excretion of water, and deficiency of Kidney *yin* implies impairment of its capacity of storing essential substances and reserving body fluids. Therefore, there is polyuria with excretion of large amounts of essential substance (glucose). However, deficiency of Liver and Kidney *yin* also occurs in many other diseases, such as hypertension, anxiety disorder, Ménière's syndrome, menstrual disorders and menopausal syndrome. Deficiency of Liver and Kidney *yin* leads to exuberance of Liver *yang*, and hence the elevation of blood pressure with dizziness and irritability in hypertension, vertigo and tinnitus in Ménière's syndrome, and insomnia and irritability in anxiety disorder. The Liver and the Kidneys are closely related to the Thoroughfare and Conception vessels. *Yin* deficiency of these two organs deprives the Thoroughfare and Conception vessels of adequate supplies of blood and essence, and hence produces oligomenorrhea or menopausal syndrome. The crucial point is that all these diseases can be effectively treated with the same therapeutic principle or even with the same formula, if they show an identical syndrome indicating the same pathogenesis or pathological basis.

GENERAL PARAMETERS OF SYNDROME DIFFERENTIATION —THE EIGHT PRINCIPAL SYNDROMES

It is usually said that there are eight general parameters for differentiation of syndromes in traditional Chinese medicine. But it should be noted that they are not at the same level. Two are at the primary level, i.e., *yin* and *yang*, which are most generalized.

Differentiation of *yin* syndromes and *yang* syndromes is of theoretical significance; it gives information about the general character of a syndrome, but no concrete treatment can be determined merely based upon a diagnosis of *yin* or *yang* syndrome. In fact, the exterior syndromes, excess syndromes and heat syndromes are all *yang* syndromes, and the interior syndromes, deficiency syndromes and cold syndromes are *yin* syndromes.

The other six parameters are at the secondary level. They are exterior versus interior, cold versus heat, and deficiency versus excess. They are of more practical significance, and in some cases diagnosis at this level can already make treatment possible, though in the majority of cases further differentiation of syndromes is necessary.

The six parameters or three pairs of parameters can not serve as independent guiding principles for the classification of syndromes. They are concerned with different aspects of a syndrome—exterior and interior indicating the depth or location of the disease, cold and heat indicating the nature of the disease, and deficiency and excess indicating the relative force of the body's resistance (genuine or normal *qi*) and the pathogenic factors (evil *qi*) in their confrontation. Therefore, they should be considered in combination during the differentiation of syndromes. For example, a syndrome may be exterior in location, cold in nature and at the same time have an excess of pathogenic factors.

Only in typical cases can the parameters be distinctly determined; in many other cases both the exterior and interior may be involved, deficiency of normal *qi* and excess of evil *qi* may be present simultaneously, and there may be interlocking of cold and heat. In addition, the parameters may change in the course of a disease. For example, an exterior syndrome may turn into an interior one, a cold syndrome may transform into heat, and an excess syndrome may become a deficient one. The most complicated issue is the appearance of "false" symptoms. A cold syndrome may appear as a heat syndrome, and a heat syndrome as a cold syndrome. A deficiency syndrome may have pseudo-excess symptoms, and an excess syndrome, pseudo-deficiency symptoms.

Exterior versus Interior

Exterior and interior indicate the depth or location of a disease. The exterior refers to the superficial portion of the body, including the subcutaneous tissue, sweat glands, skeletal muscles, and the meridians and collaterals running through this portion. The interior refers to the internal (*zang-fu*) organs.

Exterior syndromes

Invasion of exogenous pathogenic factors (exogenous affection) usually causes an exterior syndrome at the early stage. The common clinical features of exterior syndromes are chills and fever, headache, aching of the body or joints, thin coating on the tongue and floating or superficial pulse. Since the Lungs are closely related to the body's surface, exterior syndromes may also include upper respiratory symptoms, such as stuffy and running nose, sore throat and coughing.

According to the nature of the exogenous pathogenic factor and the response of the human body, exterior syndromes can be classified into those involving exterior cold and exterior heat.

Exterior cold syndrome: marked chills with mild fever, normal tongue with thin white coating, no thirst, floating and tense pulse.

Exterior heat syndrome: marked fever with mild chills, sometimes mild thirst, reddened tip of the tongue and thin white or yellowish coating, floating and rapid pulse.

Both of the above syndromes are of the excess type. They usually occur in previously healthy individuals with no deficiency of normal *qi* after an attack of excessive pathogenic factors. An exterior syndrome occurring in those with weak constitutions (either deficiency of *qi* or deficiency of *yang*) gives different manifestations, and is called an "exterior deficiency syndrome."

Exterior deficiency syndrome: chills and fever, aversion to wind, spontaneous sweating, floating and feeble pulse.

The distinguishing features for differentiating an exterior deficiency syndrome from exterior excess syndromes are spontaneous sweating and feeble pulse.

It should be noted that local diseases of the skin and subcutaneous infections do not pertain to exterior syndromes. They are called "external syndromes."

Interior syndromes

Interior syndromes, associated with diseases of the internal organs, may be caused in any of the following three ways:

1. Transmission of exogenous pathogenic factors from the exterior to the interior. For instance, following an exterior syndrome with chills, fever, headache and floating pulse, the chills disappear and a high fever occurs, accompanied by dyspnea, expectoration of yellow sticky sputum, chest pains, dire thirst, reddened tongue with a thick yellow coating, and forceful and rapid pulse. This is an interior syndrome (heat in the Lungs) due to transmission of the pathogenic factor from the exterior.

2. Direct attack of exogenous pathogenic factors on the internal organs. For instance, catching a cold results in vomiting, abdominal pain and diarrhea, indicating that the Stomach and the Spleen are affected—a syndrome of direct attack on the interior by cold.

3. Dysfunctioning of the internal organs due to internal injuries. For instance, emotional turmoil can result in headache, dizziness, bloodshot eyes and tinnitus, with stringy rapid pulse and reddened tongue with a yellow coating, indicating hyperactivity of the Liver—a syndrome of Liver fire.

The key points for differentiating exterior syndromes from interior syndromes are as follows: Most exterior syndromes are caused by exogenous pathogenic factors (such as the six evils from the natural environment). Exterior syndromes occur at the early stage of exogenous affections and last for a short period of time, then they are either cured or transformed into interior syndromes. The common manifestations of exterior syndromes include chills or aversion to cold (or wind), thin coating of the tongue and floating pulse. Among them, the presence of chills (including aversion to wind) is of crucial importance. As it is commonly said, "So long as chills exist, the exterior syndrome is there." Interior syndromes are characterized by dysfunction of the internal organs. If there is fever, it is not accompanied by chills or aversion to cold (or wind). The other symptoms of interior syndromes are extremely diverse, as different internal organs may be involved.

In addition to those mentioned above, there are two other categories of syndromes which may be related to both the exterior and interior. One is a syndrome due to an affection located between the exterior and the interior, and the other is a syndrome due to affection of both the exterior and the interior.

Half-exterior and half-interior syndrome: This is a syndrome due to an affection located between the exterior and interior, marked by alternate chills and fever, fullness and a choking feeling in the chest and costal region, bitter taste in the mouth, dry throat, nausea, loss of appetite and stringy pulse.

Affection of both the exterior and interior: This is marked by coexistence of exterior and interior syndromes.

Cold vs. Heat

Syndromes cold or heat in nature reflect the deficiency or excess of *yin-yang*. As stated in *The Canon of Medicine*, "Predominance of *yang* gives rise to heat, and predominance of *yin* gives rise to cold." In addition, as the rules of treatment, "cold syndromes should be treated with hot-propertied drugs, and heat syndromes should be treated with cold-propertied drugs." Therefore, the differentiation between the cold and heat nature of a syndrome is of great clinical importance.

Differentiation of cold and heat in exterior syndromes has been discussed in the previous section. Cold and heat syndromes of the interior are much more complicated, for the different causes and different internal organs involved give rise to diversified manifestations. Generally speaking, cold syndrome of an internal organ refers to hypofunction of that organ, and heat syndrome to hyperfunction. The common features of interior cold syndromes and those of interior heat syndromes can be described as follows:

Interior cold syndromes: Pallor, intolerance of cold, absence of thirst, loose stools, clear profuse urine, pale tongue with a white coating and slow or tense pulse. If there is pain, it is aggravated by cold and alleviated by warmth. If there is expectoration, the sputum is thin, frothy and whitish.

Interior heat syndromes: Flushed face, fever or feverishness, thirst, irritability and restlessness, constipation, deep-colored scanty urine, reddened tongue with a yellow coating and rapid pulse. If there is pain, it is aggravated by heat and alleviated by cold. If there is expectoration, the sputum is thick, sticky and yellowish.

These criteria help physicians distinguish between cold and heat syndromes in most cases, but special attention should be paid to the following aspects:

1. Transformation of cold into heat and vice versa

It is common for exogenous cold to be transformed into heat after penetrating the interior of the body. The exterior cold syndrome begins with chills, stuffy nose, headache and general aching, thin white coating of the tongue, and floating, tense pulse. Later, a high fever develops and chills disappear, the tongue is reddened, its coating turns thick and yellow, and the pulse becomes rapid. This is an example of transformation from exterior cold syndrome into interior heat syndrome.

A heat syndrome may be transformed into cold, usually due to improper or undue treatment or due to consumption of genuine *qi* by excessive pathogenic factors. The transformation may be abrupt or gradual. If a patient with high fever suddenly has his body temperature drop to below normal, accompanied by pallor, cold sweat, cold limbs, and exceedingly feeble pulse, it is an abrupt transformation of heat into deficiency-cold (collapse). As an example of gradual transformation, acute dysentery of excess-heat type after a long course without proper treatment may turn into chronic dysentery of deficiency-cold type.

2. Coexistence and interlocking of cold and heat

Complex cases, in which cold and heat syndromes coexist, have four main patterns:

(1) Cold in the exterior and heat in the interior: This is often seen in a patient with internal heat who is affected by exogenous wind-cold or in the transformation of a

syndrome of exterior cold into interior heat while the exterior cold still exists. For example, the patient may have the following symptoms: chills and fever, no sweat, headache, aching of the body, dyspnea, restlessness, thirst, and floating, tense pulse. In this symptom-complex, chills, no sweat, headache, aching of the body and floating, tense pulse indicate affection by exterior cold, while dyspnea, restlessness and thirst suggest the presence of heat in the interior.

(2) Heat in the exterior and cold in the interior: This is often encountered in patients with chronic interior-cold syndrome who are affected by wind-heat. For example, a person with deficiency-cold of the Spleen and the Stomach who gets an upper respiratory infection (wind-heat) may have an exterior heat syndrome manifested by fever, headache, coughing and sore throat, together with an interior cold syndrome manifested by loose stools and cold extremities.

(3) Cold in the upper and heat in the lower: For example, if a patient has epigastric pain aggravated by cold, with vomiting of fluid, and at the same time frequent painful micturition with passage of scanty and dark-colored urine, he is suffering from cold in the Stomach and heat in the Bladder.

(4) Heat in the upper and cold in the lower: For example, if a patient complains of discomfort and a hot feeling in the chest accompanied by diarrhea and abdominal pain which is alleviated by warmth, he is suffering from heat in the upper and cold in the lower.

3. Pseudo-cold and pseudo-heat

When a cold or heat syndrome develops to its extreme, it may be transformed into its opposite, giving a false appearance, i.e., a cold syndrome may appear as a heat syndrome, and a heat syndrome may appear as a cold syndrome. Symptoms of pseudo-cold or pseudo-heat are often misleading, but they require careful identification because patients with such symptoms are usually critically ill.

(1) Heat syndrome with pseudo-cold symptoms: If a patient feels chilly but does not want to be thickly covered, and if the limbs feel cold, but the chest and abdomen feel hot, he or she is suffering from a heat syndrome, even though the symptoms seem to be cold in nature. In such a case, *yin* is kept in the exterior by excessive *yang* in the interior.

(2) Cold syndrome with pseudo-heat symptoms: If a patient feels hot yet wishes to be thickly covered, feels thirsty but drinks little, moves restlessly while being mentally quiescent, and has a tongue coating that is black but moistened, he or she is suffering from a cold syndrome, for these manifestations are false heat symptoms. In such a case, *yang* is kept in the exterior by excessive *yin* in the interior.

The following points are helpful for the differentiation of false symptoms: In heat syndrome with pseudo-cold symptoms the pulse is forceful, the tongue is reddened, the tongue coating is dry, the patient feels thirsty and likes cold drinks, the chest and abdomen are hot, and the urine is deep yellow in color. In a cold syndrome with pseudo-heat symptoms the pulse is weak, the tongue is pale, the tongue coating is moistened, the patient does not like cold drinks or vomits after a cold drink, and the urine is clear.

Deficiency vs. Excess

Deficiency and excess define opposing forces—the pathogenic factors which attack the body and the body's anti-pathogenic factors which resist the pathogenic factors. Deficiency refers to a deficiency in the body resistance; excess refers to an excess of pathogenic factors. When the pathogenic factors are lacking or weak and the body resistance adequate or strong, one is in a healthy state or will soon recover from the illness.

Deficiency syndromes

Deficiency syndromes may be congenital or acquired, but in most instances they are acquired, due to improper diet, emotional influences, stress, overindulgence in sex, chronic diseases or wrong treatment. Since the body's anti-pathogenic factors include *yin*, *yang*, *qi*, blood, essence, fluids and various functions of the internal (*zang-fu*) organs, deficiency syndromes can be classified accordingly—deficiency of *yin*, deficiency of *yang*, deficiency of *qi*, deficiency of blood, and so on. The manifestations of different categories of deficiency syndromes are so diversified that they cannot be summarized adequately, but the following are the common features of most deficiency syndromes: Pallor or sallow complexion, listlessness, lassitude or lack of energy, shortness of breath, spontaneous sweating or night sweating, cold limbs or heat in the palms and soles, no tongue coating or thin coating, and thready or feeble pulse. Deficiency syndromes often occur in long-standing diseases. Determination of a syndrome of the deficiency type only gives a clue to the application of tonics or a reinforcing therapy; concrete treatment should depend upon further diagnosis of the deficiency syndrome in detail, including the deficient element (*yin*, *yang*, *qi*, blood, essence or fluid) and the involved *zang-fu* organ, as well as the cold or heat nature of the syndrome.

Excess syndromes

The word "excess" here is directed at the pathogenic factors. Excess syndromes are syndromes caused by excessive pathogenic factors. The pathogenic factors may be exogenous or endogenous. In most cases of simple excessiveness the pathogenic factors are exogenous. Many endogenous pathogenic factors are products of dysfunctioning *zang-fu* organs, such as retained fluid, phlegm and damp, stagnant *qi* and blood. The related internal organs may be in a deficiency state, for example, insufficiency of the Kidneys with retained fluid, and diminished function of the Spleen producing damp or phlegm. Therefore, syndromes caused by endogenous pathogenic factors may be simply of the excess type, but may also be deficiency syndromes complicated by excess symptoms.

The manifestations of excess syndromes vary greatly in accordance with different pathogenic factors and different portions of the body involved. In most cases, the presence of excessive pathogenic factors is associated with active response of the body resistance. Therefore, if there is fever, it is often high; if there is pain, it is aggravated by pressure or accompanied by tenderness; and if there is coughing, it is harsh. Generally speaking, an excess syndrome is often seen in an acute disease of short duration, particularly in patients with a strong constitution. Thick coating and forceful pulse are the most prominent features indicating excessiveness of the syndrome.

An excess syndrome should be further diagnosed in accordance with the category of the pathogenic factor and the portion of the body or the *zang-fu* organ(s) involved in the disease as well as the cold or heat nature of the syndrome.

In determining deficiency or excessiveness of a syndrome, special attention should be paid to the following points:

1. Intermingling of deficiency and excess

"Excess syndromes occur when evil qi (pathogenic factor) is in abundance, and deficiency syndromes occur when the patient's genuine *qi* (body resistance) is severely damaged." Abundance of evil qi and damage of the genuine *qi* are two separate things, but not infrequently they exist simultaneously in the same disease process. A deficiency syndrome may be complicated with excess, and an excess syndrome may be complicated with deficiency. Sometimes both deficiency and excess coexist as the main conditions.

2. Transformation of excess into deficiency and vice versa

The course of a disease reflects the course of struggle of the body resistance against the pathogenic factors. An excess syndrome may turn into a deficiency one when lingering of the pathogenic factors impairs the genuine *qi* (body resistance). For example, if an excess-heat syndrome manifested by high fever, thirst, sweating, and rapid, full pulse is improperly treated, it may consume the body fluid and *qi*, resulting in emaciation, pallor, anorexia, debility, shortness of breath, scanty or no coating of the tongue, and thready weak pulse. This is a transformation of excess into deficiency. Even though the pathogenic factors may still exist, reinforcing the genuine *qi* should be considered in the treatment.

A deficiency syndrome may be transformed into excess when excessive pathological products of the dysfunctioning *zang-fu* organs such as phlegm, undigested food, stagnant *qi* and blood, and retained fluid in turn become endogenous pathogenic factors. For example, when a patient who has suffered from deficiency of Heart *qi* with cardiac palpitation and shortness of breath for a long time, suddenly feels excruciating precordial pain as a result of obstruction of the Heart vessel due to stagnation of blood resulting from deficiency of *qi*, this is a transformation of deficiency into excess. Even though the deficiency condition still exists, the urgent treatment should be aimed at eliminating the pathogenic factor, namely, to remove the stagnant blood and relieve the pain.

3. Pseudo-deficiency and pseudo-excess

(1) Excess syndrome with pseudo-deficiency symptoms: "If a patient has pathogenic factors accumulated in the interior accompanied by tenderness, flushed face, coarse breathing, coarse, and forceful pulse, the syndrome is naturally an excess one. However, the patient may be indifferent to the circumstances, have no wish to talk or move, or may feel dizzy with blurred vision, or have loose bowels. This can be expressed as 'great excessiveness looking like debilitation'." (*Gu Shi Yi Jing* or *Gu's Mirror of Medicine*, 1718)

The common pseudo-deficiency symptoms are: the patient complains of lassitude but feels better after movement; the patient is morose but his (her) voice is loud when speaking; the patient has loose stools and feels comfortable after emptying the bowels.

(2) Deficiency syndrome with pseudo-excess symptoms: "If one suffers from epigastric pain which can be relieved by pressure, while the complexion is wan and sallow, the voice feeble and the pulse weak, the syndrome is certainly a deficiency one. However, it may be accompanied by constipation and extreme distension and fullness which impairs food intake. This can be expressed as 'extreme insufficiency which gives symptoms of exuberance'." (*Gu Shi Yi Jing* or *Gu's Mirror of Medicine*, 1718)

The common pseudo-excess symptoms are: intermittent abdominal fullness or distension; abdominal pain with no tenderness or even alleviated by pressure.

Besides the symptoms, inspection of the tongue and palpation of the pulse often give important clues to the identification of pseudo-deficiency or pseudo-excess. For pulse-taking, deep palpation is of the utmost significance. Superficial palpation of the pulse may provide false information. A forceful pulse upon deep palpation signifies an excess syndrome. The texture of the tongue is also important. A tender and delicate tongue is usually seen in deficiency syndromes, while a tough and firm tongue is seen in excess syndromes.

Combination of Exterior vs. Interior, Cold vs. Heat, and Deficiency vs. Excess

Since each of the three pairs of parameters reflects one individual aspect of a syndrome, they should be used in combination as the guiding principles of traditional Chinese medical diagnosis. Therefore, syndromes can be classified into the following patterns, if jumbled or complicated cases are excluded.

Exterior deficiency syndromes, which can be further divided into exterior deficiency with exogenous affection and exterior deficiency without exogenous affection.

Exterior excess syndromes, which can be further divided into exterior cold and exterior heat syndromes.

Interior deficiency syndromes, which can be further divided into deficiency-cold and deficiency-heat syndromes.

Interior excess syndromes, which can be further divided into excess-cold and excess-heat syndromes.

The main clinical manifestations of exterior syndromes have already been discussed in this chapter, though some other symptoms may appear if the pathogenic factor is other than cold or heat. It should be noted that in traditional Chinese medicine many terms may have multiple meanings. "Cold" and "heat" as two general parameters in diagnosis denote the nature of a syndrome. However, in etiology they also denote two pathogenic factors, either exogenous or endogenous. When we say "exterior cold syndrome," it means that the disease is in the exterior portion of the body with a syndrome of a cold nature. It does not necessarily mean that the syndrome is caused by cold. If we want to express the cause precisely, we usually say "attack of pathogenic cold on the exterior portion of the body," or more frequently, "exogenous affection by wind-cold." In exogenous affections, besides cold and heat there are other pathogenic factors such as damp and dryness, which may also produce exterior syndromes. These syndromes can also be categorized into cold or heat according to their nature. Therefore, even "exterior cold syndrome" and "exterior heat syndrome" are still two general terms referring to two groups of syndromes. Determination of the pathogenic factors has already been discussed in Chapter IV.

So far as the interior syndromes are concerned, the differentiation is much more complicated, because the interior should be further clarified with respect to the *zang-fu* organs, *qi*, blood or meridians, and the pathogenic factors are no longer limited to the exogenous ones. Therefore, a large number of interior syndromes can be classified, the manifestations of which are to be discussed in detail in the following sections of this chapter. In order to give a general idea about the interior syndromes, the following common clinical features should be borne in mind.

Interior deficiency-cold syndromes are attributed to decline of *yang qi*, and usually manifested by listlessness, pallor, aversion to cold with cold limbs, abdominal pain which is alleviated by pressure, loose stools, diluted urine, lack of energy, pale and flabby tongue, and weak, deep or slow pulse.

Interior deficiency-heat syndromes are attributed to consumption of *yin* fluid, and usually manifested by malar flush, emaciation, afternoon fever with night sweating, heat sensation in the palms and soles, dryness of the throat and mouth, reddened tongue with scanty coating, and rapid and thready pulse.

Interior excess-cold syndromes are attributed to invasion of pathogenic cold or other *yin* pathogenic factors into the interior of the body, and are generally manifested by aversion to cold and preference for warmth, pallor, abdominal pain with tenderness, borborygmi and diarrhea or coughing and dyspnea with thin frothy expectoration, tastelessness in the mouth with profuse saliva, diluted urine, white and moistened tongue coating, and slow or tense pulse.

Interior excess-heat syndromes are attributed to penetration of heat and other *yang* pathogenic factors into the interior of the body, and are commonly manifested by fever, preference for cold, thirst with desire for cold drinks, flushed face and congested eyes, restlessness or delirium, abdominal distension with fullness and tenderness, constipation, concentrated urine, reddened tongue with a dry and yellow coating, and a full, slippery, rapid and replete pulse.

Yin vs. *Yang*

Yin and *yang* are the two most general parameters of syndrome differentiation. Being the key link in the application of the eight overall parameters, *yin* and *yang* are used to summarize the other three pairs of parameters. Generally speaking, interior, cold and deficiency syndromes belong to the category of *yin* syndromes, while exterior, heat and excess syndromes belong to the category of *yang* syndromes. Differentiation of *yin* and *yang* syndromes is of primary importance, as *The Canon of Medicine* states, "One who is good at diagnosing a disease by inspecting the patient's complexion and feeling the patient's pulse first identifies *yin* and *yang*." Zhang Jingyue (1563-1640), a leading physician and the author of the *Lei Jing* (*Classified Canon*), also stressed, "It is the key principle that *yin* and *yang* must be first considered when feeling the pulse and administering treatment." Proper determination of *yin* and *yang* in syndrome differentiation is the very basis of further diagnosis and treatment, but it can only provide a direction of guidance in principle.

Another issue related to *yin* and *yang* is their prosperity and decline. "*Yin* in excess makes *yang* suffer." "*Yang* in excess makes *yin* suffer." "Preponderance of *yin* gives rise to cold syndromes." "Preponderance of *yang* gives rise to heat syndromes." "Deficiency of *yang* brings on external cold." "Deficiency of *yin* brings on internal heat." In all these instances, *yin* and *yang* have their own substantial meanings, and should not be taken as the general parameters of syndrome diagnosis. However, since deficiency of *yin* and deficiency of *yang* are so commonly encountered in clinical practice, it is necessary to know their common manifestations before more detailed discussion with relation to the internal (*zang-fu*) organs.

Deficiency of yin: Its clinical manifestation consists of the symptoms due to deficiency of *yin* fluid or essence and those due to relative preponderance of *yang*, i.e., endogenous heat or fire. The former include dryness of the throat and mouth, dizziness, blurred vision, tinnitus, weakness of the loins and legs, concentrated urine, constipation, dry tongue without coating and thready pulse. The latter include malar flush, afternoon fever with night sweating, dream-disturbed sleep, nocturnal emission, heat in the palms and soles, reddened tongue and rapid pulse.

Deficiency of yang: Its clinical manifestation consists of the symptoms due to diminished functional activities (*yang*) and those due to relative preponderance of *yin*, i.e., endogenous cold and other pathological products. The former include pallor, spontaneous sweating, loose stools, particularly diarrhea daily before dawn, weakness of the legs, impotence, and weak pulse. The latter include edema and aversion to cold with cold limbs.

Two other syndromes related to *yin* and *yang* in their substantial sense are exhaustion of *yin* and exhaustion of *yang*. Both of them are critical conditions manifested by collapse or shock. They may result from gradual worsening of *yin* deficiency and *yang* deficiency, or occur abruptly in acute diseases with high fever, profuse sweating, repeated vomiting, severe diarrhea or massive bleeding.

Exhaustion of yin: Excessive consumption of vital essence and fluid is usually manifested by feverishness of the body, shortness of breath with coarse breathing, sticky sweating, thirst with preference for cold drinks, irritability, restlessness or even delirium, reddened and dry tongue, and a thready, rapid and weak pulse.

Exhaustion of yang: Depletion of *yang qi* is usually manifested by profuse cold sweating, coolness of the body, cold limbs, feeble breathing, listlessness, absence of thirst or preference for hot drinks, pale tongue, and a faint pulse which is scarcely perceptible.

DIFFERENTIATION OF SYNDROMES ACCORDING TO THE STATE OF *QI*, BLOOD AND BODY FLUIDS

Qi, blood and body fluids are the material basis of the functional activities of the *zang-fu* organs, while at the same time the production and circulation of *qi*, blood and body fluids depend on the functional activities of the *zang-fu* organs. Pathological changes in the *zang-fu* organs will cause changes of *qi*, blood and body fluids, and vice versa. Therefore, differentiation of syndromes of *qi*, blood and body fluids is closely related to differentiation of syndromes of *zang-fu* organs. Usually, these two paradigms of syndrome differentiation are used simultaneously and jointly.

Disorders of *Qi*

Disorders of *qi* can be generally classified into four categories: deficiency of *qi*, sinking of *qi*, stagnation of *qi*, and upward perversion of *qi*.

I. Deficiency of *Qi* (Syndrome of *Qi* Deficiency)

Deficiency of *qi* is a group of syndromes due to diminished function of *zang-fu* organs. It is often due to weakness after a long illness, feebleness in old age, or excessive strain or stress. Each *zang-fu* organ needs *qi* for its functional activities. So, *qi* deficiency in individual organs may be manifested diversely in accordance with their different functions, but *qi* deficiency of an individual organ is often associated with generalized deficiency of *qi*, the manifestations of which can be described as follows.

Clinical manifestations: The clinical manifestations of generalized deficiency of *qi* include shortness of breath, taciturnity, lassitude, lack of energy, dizziness, blurring of vision and spontaneous sweating, all of which are aggravated on exertion; in addition, pale tongue with a white coating and feeble pulse may be present.

Syndrome analysis: Deficiency of *qi* and lack of energy are actually synonymous. Shortness of breath, taciturnity and lassitude are all manifestations of lack of energy. If *qi* fail to rise to nourish the head and eyes, dizziness and blurring of vision occur. Defensive *qi* is that part of *qi* which controls the pores. Weakness of defensive *qi* leads to inadequate closing of the pores and thus spontaneous sweating. Because exertion consumes *qi*, it will worsen all the above symptoms. Deficiency of *qi* also implies weakness of *qi* in propelling the normal blood flow, hence the feeble pulse and pale tongue.

II. Sinking of *Qi* (Syndrome of *Qi* Sinking)

One of the functions of *qi* is to hold the internal organs in their normal positions or lift them there. If this function is impaired due to deficiency of *qi*, visceroptosis will occur, as if the internal organs had sunk. Sinking of *qi* is another variety of *qi* deficiency characterized by failure in holding or lifting the internal organs. Since it often occurs in the Middle Energizer, it is also known as "sinking of *qi* of the Middle Energizer" or simply "sinking of the middle *qi.*"

Clinical manifestations: Dizziness, blurring of vision, lassitude, a bearing-down and distending sensation in the abdomen, prolapse of the rectum or uterus, gastroptosis and other visceroptoses; pale tongue and feeble pulse.

Syndrome analysis: Dizziness, blurring of vision, lassitude, pale tongue and feeble pulse are common manifestations of *qi* deficiency. Bearing-down and distending sensation in the abdomen, prolapse of the rectum and uterus, gastroptosis and other visceroptoses are possible outcomes of failure of *qi* in holding the internal organs in their proper places or lifting them there.

III. Stagnation of *Qi* (Syndrome of *Qi* Stagnation)

A syndrome of *qi* stagnation occurs when the flow of *qi* is hindered or obstructed at a certain part of the body or in a certain internal organ. The causes of stagnation of *qi* are multifarious, including obstruction by various pathogenic factors, influence of emotional factors and weakness of *yang,* which fails to promote the flow of *qi.*

Clinical manifestations: The clinical manifestations vary in accordance with the site where the *qi* stagnates. However, the common features of *qi* stagnation are distension and pain.

Syndrome analysis: Hindrance or obstruction of *qi* flow gives rise to local accumulation of *qi*, which produces distension. "Wherever there is obstruction, there is pain." Obstruction of the flow of *qi* also produces pain in addition to distension. In stagnation of *qi*, the distension is usually more severe than the pain, and both distension and pain occur off and on, often not fixed in location.

IV. Upward Perversion of *Qi* (Syndrome of *Qi* Perversion)

Qi should ascend and descend in a normal manner. If *qi* descends abnormally, a sinking syndrome will occur, and if *qi* ascends abnormally, an upward perversion syndrome will occur. Upward perverted flow of *qi* often involves the Lungs, the Stomach and the Liver.

Clinical manifestations: Coughing and dyspnea in upward perversion of Lung *qi*; hiccuping, belching, nausea and vomiting in upward perversion of Stomach *qi*; headache, vertigo, syncope or hematemesis in upward perversion of Liver *qi.*

Syndrome analysis: Upward perversion of Lung *qi* is often due to invasion of exogenous pathogenic factors or due to retention of phlegm in the Lungs. In either case, Lung *qi* fails to descend, but ascends instead, giving rise to coughing and asthmatic breathing.

Retention of fluid, phlegm or food in the Stomach, or invasion of the Stomach by exogenous pathogenic factors may disturb the descent of Stomach *qi*. Upward perversion of Stomach *qi* produces hiccuping, belching, nausea and vomiting.

Injury to the Liver due to anger leads to excessive ascent of Liver *qi*. "Excess of *qi* forms fire." Upward perversion of *qi* and fire causes headache, vertigo or even syncope. In severe cases, blood may surge out of the vessels together with the perverted flow of *qi*, resulting in hematemesis.

Blood Disorders

Disorders of the blood can be roughly classified into four categories: deficiency of blood, stasis of blood, heat in the blood, and cold in the blood.

I. Deficiency of Blood (Syndrome of Blood Deficiency)

Deficiency of blood means insufficient blood to nourish organs and tissues. It includes anemia as well as other pathological conditions with insufficient supply of blood either throughout the body or locally. Deficiency of blood is not exactly equivalent to anemia in Western medicine, because in severe anemia with symptoms of listlessness, lassitude and shortness of breath, the diagnosis is usually deficiency of both *qi* and blood, instead of deficiency of blood alone. Syndromes of blood deficiency are often seen in anemia, chronic consumptive diseases, depressive disorders, menstrual disorders and some neurological disturbances.

Clinical manifestations: Pallor, pale lips, dizziness, blurring of vision, palpitations, insomnia, numbness or tingling sensation of hands and feet, pale tongue and thready pulse.

Syndrome analysis: Pallor, pale lips, dizziness, pale tongue and thready pulse are due to general deficiency of blood. Among the internal organs, the Heart and the Liver are particularly related to blood, as the Heart governs the blood circulation and the Liver stores blood. The Heart also serves as the seat of mental activities, so insufficient supply of blood to the Heart brings about not only palpitation but also insomnia. Deficiency of Liver blood may lead to insufficient blood supply to the eyes, tendons, and Thoroughfare and Conception Vessels, causing blurring of vision, numbness of hands and feet, and menstrual disorders.

II. Stasis of Blood (Syndrome of Blood Stasis)

Blood stasis in traditional Chinese medicine is a term which has a broad meaning. Any pathological change characterized by retarded or impeded blood flow is a condition of blood stasis. Its causes are multifarious, including sprains and contusions, invasion of pathogenic cold or heat on the blood system. More often it is a condition secondary to other pathological changes such as deficiency of *qi*, stagnation of *qi*, and deficiency of blood. From the Western medical perspective, blood stasis refers to a variety of conditions including blood congestion, extravasation, thrombosis and other pathological changes with retarded or impeded blood flow, such as hyperlipemia, hyperglycemia, as well as mass formation and tumors. Clinically, blood stasis is often seen in coronary heart disease, cerebral thrombosis, hepato-splenomegaly, abdominal tumors, thrombo-angiitis obliterans, dysmenorrhea, amenorrhea, ectopic pregnancy, traumatic injuries, and many other diseases with protracted courses.

Clinical manifestations: Local manifestations of blood stasis are pain, mass formation and ecchymosis or petechiae. General manifestations are darkish complexion, scaly dry skin and even cyanosis of lips and nails. The tongue is purple or dark with purple spots, and the pulse thready and hesitant.

Syndrome analysis: The pain occurring as a consequence of obstruction by stagnant blood is fixed in location and stabbing in character. Accumulation of stagnant blood in a local area forms a mass or tumor which has a fixed position and feels firm upon palpation. Stagnation of *qi* may also cause pain and mass formation, but the pain is distending in character, and the mass is soft, without definite shape or fixed position, and often comes and goes.

When a blood vessel is obstructed by stagnant blood, the circulating blood may break out of the vessel, resulting in discharge of blood from the vessel. Therefore, in the treatment of hemorrhage, removing the stagnant blood is sometimes more important than using hemostatics.

Retarded flow of blood impairs the normal nourishment of the skin, so that the complexion becomes darkish, the skin scaly dry, and in severe cases, the lips and nails cyanotic.

III. Heat in Blood (Syndrome of Heat in Blood)

Endogenous heat produced by a dysfunctioning internal organ may cause various hemorrhagic conditions if the heat involves the blood circulation. Clinically, heat in blood often occurs in infectious diseases such as measles, scarlet fever, epidemic cerebrospinal meningitis, and various hemorrhagic diseases such as allergic purpura, thrombocytopenic purpura, aplastic anemia and leukemia.

Clinical manifestations: Hemoptysis, hematemesis, hematuria, epistaxis, and other varieties of hemorrhage, deep red tongue and stringy, rapid pulse.

Syndrome analysis: The diagnosis of heat in blood is based on hemorrhage and heat manifestations. Endogenous heat of the internal organs may injure the blood vessels and drive the circulating blood out of its normal course, resulting in hemorrhage. Deep red tongue and stringy, rapid pulse indicate heat with abundant blood flow.

The blood system may also be invaded by exogenous heat. Syndromes of exogenous heat in blood will be discussed elsewhere.

IV. Cold in Blood (Syndrome of Cold in Blood)

Syndrome of cold in blood refers to local sluggish flow of blood due to pathogenic cold. The syndrome is often encountered in Raynaud's disease and menstrual disorders.

Clinical manifestations: Pain and coldness of hands and feet with cyanosis of the local skin, alleviated by warmth and aggravated by cold; or pain and coldness of the lower abdomen accompanied by cold limbs, delayed menstrual cycle and discharge of dark-colored menstrual blood mixed with clots. Pale and dark tongue with white coating and deep, slow and hesitant pulse.

Syndrome analysis: Cold causes vascular contraction with sluggish flow of blood, giving rise to coldness, pain and cyanosis of hands and feet. In women, exposure to cold or taking too much cold liquid during the menstrual period may lead to cold in the uterus with blood stasis, and hence pain and coldness in the lower abdomen. Because of blood stasis, the menstrual period is delayed and the menstrual flow is mixed with clots. Cold also impedes the blood flow to the tongue, forming a pale and dark tongue with a white coating. A deep pulse points to an interior syndrome, a slow pulse to cold, and a hesitant pulse to blood stasis.

Disorders of Both *Qi* and Blood

Qi and blood are mutually dependent, promoting, and acting. Because of their close interrelationships, disorders of *qi* and blood often occur simultaneously. Common disorders of both *qi* and blood include stagnation of *qi* with blood stasis, deficiency of *qi* with blood stasis, deficiency of both *qi* and blood, failure of *qi* to control blood, and prostration of *qi* after great loss of blood.

I. Stagnation of *qi* with blood stasis

"*Qi* in motion keeps the blood circulating." Lengthy stagnation of *qi* may result in blood stasis.

Clinical manifestation: Distension in the hypochondriac region with unfixed pain, irritability, and hepato-splenomegaly with stabbing pain and tenderness; amenorrhea or dysmenorrhea with discharge of dark blood and clots in women; dark and purple tongue and hesitant pulse.

Syndrome analysis: The key point for the diagnosis of this syndrome is the presence of pain and mass in the areas along the Liver Meridian in a long-standing illness. Either emotional influence or affection by exogenous pathogenic factors causes depressed flow of Liver *qi*, which is usually manifested by distension in the hypochondriac region with unfixed pain and irritability. Long-standing stagnation of Liver *qi* causes disorders of the local blood circulation and finally blood stasis with mass formation. The pain caused by *qi* stagnation and that caused by blood stasis have different features: the latter is severer, stabbing in character and accompanied by tenderness.

The Liver stores blood, serving as the source of menstrual discharge. Stasis of Liver blood leads to impaired menstrual flow and even amenorrhea. The Liver Meridian runs around the genitalia and reaches the lower abdomen. So, stagnation of Liver *qi* and blood is apt to cause pain in the lower abdomen during menstruation. Purple tongue and hesitant pulse are common signs that indicate blood stasis.

II. Deficiency of *qi* with blood stasis

Long-standing deficiency of *qi* may lead to blood stasis.

Clinical manifestations: Pale or darkish complexion, lassitude, shortness of breath, indolence to talk, pectoral or hypochondriac stabbing pain with fixed location and tenderness, pale and darkish tongue or with purple spots, and deep, hesitant pulse.

Syndrome analysis: This is a syndrome of deficiency complicated by excess. Pale complexion, lassitude, shortness of breath and taciturnity are manifestations of *qi* deficiency. Since *qi* is the motive force of blood circulation, the blood flows slowly when *qi* is insufficient. Long-standing deficiency of *qi* will result in blood stasis with the manifestations of darkish complexion, pain with fixed location and tenderness. This syndrome is often seen when the Heart or the Liver is involved, and so there is pectoral or hypochondriac pain. A pale tongue is due to deficiency of *qi,* and a darkish tongue with purple spots due to blood stasis. A deep pulse points to an interior syndrome, and a hesitant pulse to blood stasis.

III. Deficiency of both *qi* and blood

This is a syndrome characterized by simultaneous existence of deficiency of *qi* and deficiency of blood. It is often seen in a chronic illness, either due to deficient *qi*, which fails to generate blood, or deficient blood, which fails to be transformed into *qi*.

Clinical manifestations: Dizziness, blurred vision, shortness of breath, taciturnity, lack of energy, spontaneous sweating, pale or sallow complexion, palpitations, insomnia, pale and flabby tongue, and thready and weak pulse.

Syndrome analysis: The above description of the syndrome is a combination of clinical manifestations of *qi* deficiency and those of blood deficiency. Shortness of breath, taciturnity, lack of energy and spontaneous sweating are common symptoms of *qi* deficiency. Palpitations and insomnia are due to insufficient blood supply to the Heart, which maintains blood circulation through its beating and also serves as the seat of mental activities. Dizziness and blurred vision are usually caused by deficiency of Liver blood. A pale complexion is often related to deficiency of blood, while a sallow complexion to deficiency of *qi*. The manifestations of the tongue and pulse also correspond to deficiency of *qi* and blood.

IV. Failure of *qi* to control blood

Qi keeps the blood circulating normally within the vessels. In a long-standing deficiency of *qi*, this function of *qi* may be impaired, leading to hemorrhage.

Clinical manifestations: Hematochezia, subcutaneous ecchymosis in the lower extremities, or abnormal uterine bleeding, accompanied by shortness of breath, lassitude, lack of energy, pale complexion, pale tongue, and thready, weak pulse.

Syndrome analysis: The *qi* that keeps the blood circulating within the vessels is Spleen *qi*. Failure of *qi* to control blood is actually a variety of Spleen *qi* deficiency. Since deficiency of Spleen *qi* may cause sinking symptoms, hemorrhage in this syndrome is often in the lower parts of the body such as hematochezia and uterine bleeding.

Hemorrhages are more often due to heat in blood. The differences between hemorrhage due to heat in blood and that caused by failure of *qi* to control blood can be listed as follows:

	Failure of *qi* to control blood	**Heat in blood**
Course of disease	mostly chronic	mostly acute
Deficiency/Excess	deficiency	excessive
Location of bleeding	often in the lower parts of the body	any part of the body
Color of blood	pinkish and thin	bright red and thick
Tongue	pale	deep red
Pulse	thready and weak	stringy and rapid

V. Prostration of *qi* after great loss of blood

Clinical manifestations: Sudden presence of pallor, cold limbs, profuse sweating, even fainting; tongue pale, and pulse faint, scarcely perceptible or hollow.

Syndrome analysis: *Qi* and blood are mutually dependent. Great loss of blood deprives *qi* of its carrier, leading to *qi* prostration. Exhausted *qi* fails to send blood upward, resulting in pallor; fails to warm the limbs, resulting in cold limbs; and fails to control the pores, resulting in profuse sweating. Consciousness may also be lost along with the prostration of *qi*. Either a faint and scarcely perceptible pulse or hollow pulse is a critical sign of prostration.

Disorders of Body Fluids

Disorders of body fluids can be generally classified into two groups: insufficiency of fluids and retention of fluids.

I. Insufficiency of Fluids (Syndrome of Fluid Insufficiency)

Insufficiency of fluids belongs to endogenous dryness. It is due either to insufficient production of fluids or to excessive loss of fluids. Diminished function of the Spleen and the Stomach in transportation and transformation, or excessive restriction of fluid intake may result in insufficient production of body fluids. High fever which exhausts fluids, profuse sweating, severe vomiting and severe diarrhea lead to excessive loss of body fluids.

Clinical manifestations: Dryness of the throat, mouth and lips, withered skin, oliguria, constipation, dry reddened tongue, and thready, rapid pulse.

Syndrome analysis: Dryness of the throat, mouth and lips, withered skin, oliguria and constipation are all due to lack of fluids. Insufficiency of fluids (*yin*) may produce endogenous heat, and hence the tongue is dry and reddened, and the pulse thready and rapid.

II. Retention of Water and Fluids (Syndromes of Water-Fluid Retention)

1. Edema

The Lungs, the Spleen and the Kidneys regulate water metabolism. Therefore, edema may be attributed to functional disturbance of any of these organs. Clinically, edema should be first classified according to deficiency and excess. *Yang* edema pertains to excess (of pathogenic factors), while *yin* edema pertains to deficiency (of genuine *qi*).

(1) *Yang* edema

Yang edema or edema of a *yang* nature is an excess syndrome, often caused by exogenous affection of pathogenic wind or overflow of water-damp.

Clinical manifestations: The edema usually has an acute onset, first appearing in the eyelids, then extending downwards to the whole body, and is associated with oliguria. It is often accompanied by aversion to wind, chills, fever, aching joints, thin white tongue coating, and floating, tense pulse. Or it is accompanied by sore throat, reddened tongue, and floating, rapid pulse. Sometimes, anasarca develops gradually, accompanied by heaviness of the limbs, lassitude, oliguria, poor appetite, nausea, white greasy tongue coating and deep pulse.

Syndrome analysis: *Yang* edema with an acute onset is usually due to exogenous affection of the Lungs by pathogenic wind. The Lungs have the function of regulating the water passages, and the normal distribution of fluids will be disturbed if the Lungs are affected by wind. The Lungs are situated in the upper portion of the body and send water downwards. Therefore, edema due to dysfunction of the Lungs first appears in the eyelids and face, accompanied by oliguria. Disturbance in the water passages usually leads to quick accumulation of water, and hence the edema develops rapidly into anasarca. Aversion to wind, chills, fever, aching of joints, and sore throat are symptoms indicating an exterior invasion of exogenous wind, and therefore *yang* edema with such manifestations is also called "wind-edema." Wind-edema is a syndrome of excessiveness, but it may be either cold or hot in nature. If it is a cold syndrome, the tongue coating is thin and white, and the pulse floating and tense, but if it is a heat syndrome, the tongue is reddened, and the pulse is floating and rapid.

An exogenous affection by damp with involvement of the Spleen may also lead to edema of a *yang* nature. When the function of the Spleen in transportation and transformation of water is impaired, endogenous water-damp will be produced, gradually overflowing throughout the body. Since the Spleen is particularly related to the limbs, edema will be more marked in the limbs, accompanied by heaviness sensation and lassitude. Dysfunction of the Spleen with accumulation of damp results in poor appetite. The Spleen and the Stomach are closely correlated, and diseases of the Spleen usually involve the Stomach. Upward perversion of Stomach *qi* causes nausea. A white greasy tongue coating together with deep pulse indicates excess of pathogenic damp in the interior.

(2) *Yin* edema

Yin edema or edema of a *yin* nature is usually a deficiency syndrome due to weakness after a protracted disease, internal injury from excessive strain or stress, or overindulgence in sex.

Clinical manifestations: Pitting edema, more marked in the lower portion of the body below the waist, accompanied by oliguria, abdominal distension, anorexia, loose stools, pale complexion with puffiness, lassitude, pale tongue with white slippery coating and deep pulse. The edema may be exacerbated gradually, accompanied by oliguria, aching and coldness in the loins and knees, cold limbs, aversion to cold, listlessness, pale or dull complexion, pale and plump tongue with a white slippery coating, and deep, slow and weak pulse.

Syndrome analysis: *Yin* edema is characterized by its gradual onset and slow development, starting from the feet and more marked below the waist. It may be due to diminished function of the Spleen in transportation and transformation of water-damp or due to failure of the Kidneys to "send down the turbid" (to secrete urine). In either case, there is disturbance in the water metabolism, which leads to overflow of retained water to the subcutaneous tissue. Since water flows downwards, pitting edema starts from the feet and is more marked below the waist. Hypofunction of the Spleen with endogenous damp causes abdominal distension, anorexia, loose stools and lassitude. Because of hypofunction of the Spleen, *qi* and blood fail to flow upward, and so the complexion and the tongue are pale. Also, because of infiltration of water-damp, the face is puffy, and the tongue coating is white and slippery. A deep pulse indicates an interior syndrome.

A long-standing edema due to diminished function of the Spleen may involve the Kidneys, leading to deficiency of Kidney *yang*. Then the edema will be exacerbated, and aching and coldness in the loins and knees, cold limbs, aversion to cold, and listlessness will appear. Deficiency of Kidney *yang* makes the complexion pale, and hypofunction of the Kidneys with retained water gives the complexion a dull color. A pale and plump tongue with a white slippery coating, and a deep, slow and weak pulse are also due to deficiency of Kidney *yang* with endogenous cold and retained water.

In some cases, deficiency of Kidney *yang* with impaired excretion of water may occur independently, not preceded by diminished function of the Spleen.

2. Retention of Phlegm-Fluid

(1) Phlegm syndrome

Phlegm refers to condensed fluid, thick and viscous, which causes various diseases when retained in internal organs, meridians or other tissues. This is a unique concept in traditional Chinese medicine. Many complicated diseases or symptoms are thought to be caused by phlegm. It is even said that if ordinary pathogenic factors can not explain the cause of a disease, phlegm should be considered.

Phlegm as a pathogenic factor comes from two sources: exogenous (usually due to affection of the Lungs by wind, cold, heat or damp) or endogenous (mostly due to diminished function of the Spleen which produces damp, further accumulated and condensed into phlegm). Exogenous phlegm often leads to an excess syndrome;

endogenous phlegm also causes symptoms indicating excessiveness, but the primary syndrome is deficiency in property.

Clinical manifestations: Coughing, dyspnea, expectoration of sputum and fullness in the chest; distress in the epigastrium with anorexia, nausea, vomiting of thick fluid, and dizziness; loss of consciousness or manic-depressive mental disorders; numbness of limbs and even hemiplegia; scrofula, goiter, or nodules in the breast; feeling of a lump in the throat. Greasy tongue coating, white or yellow in color, and slippery pulse.

Syndrome analysis: Phlegm may have multifarious manifestations based on the internal organs or tissues it affects. When phlegm accumulates in the Lungs, the pathway for air is obstructed, and there results coughing, dyspnea, expectoration of sputum and fullness in the chest. If phlegm is retained in the Stomach, disturbance of the Stomach function leads to distress in the epigastrium, with anorexia, nausea, and vomiting of thick fluid. In addition, phlegm impedes the ascent of clear *yang*, giving rise to dizziness. If the Heart (mind) is clouded by phlegm, there is impairment of consciousness. Mania and depression are also related to phlegm clouding the Heart (mind), but depression is related to phlegm-turbidity, while mania is related to phlegm-fire. When the meridians are blocked by phlegm, there is numbness of the limbs in mild cases and hemiplegia in severe cases. When phlegm is retained subcutaneously, it will become nodules, such as enlarged lymph nodes, goiter and nodules in the breast. Retention of phlegm in the chest combined with stagnant *qi* may produce a smothering sensation as if the throat were obstructed by a lump which can not be swallowed nor spat out (equivalent to "globus hystericus" in Western medicine). Greasy tongue coating and slippery pulse indicate presence of phlegm; phlegm-damp gives rise to a white greasy coating, and phlegm-fire to a yellow greasy coating.

(2) Syndrome of retained fluid

Contrary to phlegm, which is thick and turbid, retained fluid is thin and clear. It may cause four kinds of ailments involving the Lungs, the Stomach and Intestines, the thorax, and the limbs, respectively.

Clinical manifestations:

Retained fluid in the Lungs: Coughing, dyspnea, fullness in the chest, and expectoration of profuse sputum, thin, clear and whitish in color; in severe cases, a gurgling sound in the throat and orthopnea accompanied by palpitation and edema of the lower extremities.

Retained fluid in the Stomach and Intestines: Abdominal distension with a splashing sound in the Stomach or gurgling sound in the intestines.

Retained fluid in the thorax: Chest pain, aggravated by coughing, breathing or turning the body. Retained fluid in the limbs: Edema of the limbs, same as that caused by diminished function of the Spleen.

In all the above conditions, the tongue coating is often white and slippery, and the pulse stringy and/or slippery.

Syndrome analysis: The clinical manifestations vary with the internal organs or tissues in which the fluid is retained. When fluid is retained in the Lungs, upward perversion of the Lung *qi* causes coughing, dyspnea and fullness in the chest, as well as expectoration of profuse sputum, thin, clear and whitish in color. If the air passage is obstructed by retained fluid, there is gurgling in the throat accompanied by orthopnea. A long-standing retention of fluid in the Lungs will impair the function of the Heart and the Spleen, leading to palpitations and edema of the lower extremities. From the Western medical perspective, this may be seen in some cases of chronic bronchitis or bronchiectasis complicated with pulmonary heart disease.

Retention of fluid in the gastro-intestinal tract causes abdominal distension with a splashing sound in the stomach and a gurgling sound in the intestines. From the Western medical perspective, this is analogous to pyloric stenosis or ileus.

Retention of fluid in the thorax with chest pain aggravated by coughing, respiration and turning the body roughly corresponds to pleurisy from the Western point of view.

A white slippery tongue coating and stringy and/or slippery pulse are common signs of retained fluid.

DIFFERENTIATION OF SYNDROMES ACCORDING TO THE PATHOLOGICAL CHANGES OF *ZANG-FU* ORGANS

Traditional Chinese medicine was not founded on the basis of precise anatomy. Internal organs, more accurately called *zang-fu* organs, actually refer to the major functional systems of the human body. In the progress of traditional Chinese medicine, no patho-anatomy was studied. Therefore, the pathological changes of the internal organs should not be misunderstood as the patho-anatomical changes of organs and tissues on which the Western diagnosis of diseases is based. They are the pathophysiological changes of the functional systems recognized in the light of traditional Chinese medical theories.

Diagnosing pathological changes of the internal (*zang-fu*) organs is the most important component of differentiation of syndromes, for it is often a comprehensive analysis of the pathogenesis in a given case, including its location, nature, and the condition of confrontation between the anti-pathogenic and pathogenic factors. In combination with the eight general parameters, determination of the pathogenic factors and the state of *qi*, blood and body fluids, determining the pathological changes of the internal organs usually makes a complete syndrome diagnosis, not only for non-febrile diseases in internal medicine, but also for most diseases in other branches of clinical medicine.

Syndromes of the Heart and the Small Intestine

The Heart rules the blood and houses the mind. Pathological changes of the Heart are often manifested by disturbed blood circulation and abnormal mental activities. The Small Intestine assimilates the essence from food and rejects the dross. Since the Spleen controls the whole process of digestion, pathological changes of the Small Intestine with digestive symptoms are usually included in the disorders of the Spleen. The Heart and the Small Intestine are discussed together because they are closely connected by meridians.

Syndromes of the Heart can be classified into two main groups, according to the conditions of deficiency and excessiveness. The deficiency syndromes include deficiency of *qi* or *yang* and deficiency of blood or yin, and the excess syndromes are often due to accumulation of phlegm, disturbance of fire, congealing of cold, stagnation of blood, and depression of *qi*.

The common symptoms and signs encountered in Heart diseases are: palpitations, precordial pain, insomnia, dream-disturbed sleep, derangement of the mind, and impairment of consciousness.

I. Deficiency of Heart *qi* and Deficiency of Heart *yang*

Both deficiency of Heart *qi* and deficiency of Heart *yang* are characterized by diminished function of the Heart, particularly in controlling blood circulation. They may be encountered in various heart diseases with cardiac insufficiency in Western medicine.

Clinical manifestations: Deficiency of Heart *qi* is manifested by palpitations and shortness of breath aggravated by exertion, oppression in the chest or spontaneous sweating; pale complexion, pale tongue with a white coating, and feeble or irregular pulse. If there is aversion to cold with cold limbs in addition to the above symptoms, and the tongue is pale and plump, with a white and slippery coating, the syndrome is deficiency of Heart *yang*.

Syndrome analysis: Deficiency of Heart *qi* or Heart *yang* implies weakness of the Heart in propelling the blood to circulate, which results in palpitations, shortness of breath, oppression in the chest and feeble pulse. As exertion consumes *qi*, the symptoms become worse with exertion. Spontaneous sweating is due to deficiency of *qi* in controlling the pores. A weakened Heart is unable to propel adequate blood upward, thus causing pale complexion and pale tongue with white coating. Discontinuation of Heart *qi* causes missing or abnormal heart beats and hence an irregular pulse.

Deficiency of Heart *yang* is an aggravation of deficiency of Heart *qi*. Since *yang* deficiency brings on endogenous cold, when Heart *yang* is insufficient, there are cold manifestations such as aversion to cold with cold limbs and corresponding changes to the tongue.

Appendix: Sudden collapse of Heart yang

If Heart *yang* is insufficient to the extreme, there may be a sudden collapse manifested by profuse sweating, impaired consciousness, shortness and faintness of breath, pallor with cyanotic lips, and a scarcely perceptible pulse.

II. Deficiency of Heart blood and Deficiency of Heart *yin*

Yin includes blood, nutrients, essence and fluids. Deficiency of Heart blood can be defined as inadequate blood supply to the Heart (chiefly referring to the seat of the mental activities), and deficiency of Heart *yin* because of inadequate supply of nutrients, essence and fluids. If both blood and other *yin* components are insufficient, it is usually called "deficiency of Heart *yin*-blood." In deficiency of Heart blood or yin, the capacity of the Heart to propel blood may not be impaired, but reduced nourishment of the Heart usually results in mental derangement. These syndromes are most often encountered in mental disorders, particularly anxiety states, but may also occur in cases of anemia and various consumptive diseases.

Clinical manifestations: Palpitations and fidgetiness, insomnia, dream-disturbed sleep, difficulty in concentrating or the mind going blank, and forgetfulness. If the syndrome is accompanied by pallor with a pale tongue and deep, thready pulse, it is deficiency of Heart blood. If it is accompanied by low-grade fever, malar flush, night sweating, heat in the palms and soles, dryness of the mouth, reddened tongue and rapid, thready pulse, it is deficiency of Heart yin.

Syndrome analysis: Insufficiency of *yin*-blood deprives the Heart of nourishment, leading to palpitations. Since the Heart is the seat of the mind, deficiency of *yin*-blood in the Heart also causes fidgetiness, absent-mindedness, poor memory and sleep disturbances. Pallor with a pale tongue and a deep, thready pulse are signs of blood deficiency. Deficiency of Heart *yin* often results in flaming-up of Heart fire, and hence low-grade fever, malar flush, night sweating, heat in the palms and soles, dryness of the mouth, reddened tongue and rapid, thready pulse.

III. Stagnation and obstruction of Heart blood

This often results from insufficiency of Heart *qi* and Heart *yang*, which causes retardation of blood flow in the Heart, and occurs in angina pectoris and myocardial infarction in Western medicine.

Clinical manifestations: Precordial or substernal pain, stabbing or dull in character, often reaching the shoulder and arm, accompanied by palpitations, dark-purplish tongue or purple spots on the tongue, and deep, hesitant or irregular pulse; in severe cases, cyanosis of the face, lips and nails, cold limbs and spontaneous sweating.

Syndrome analysis: Stagnation of blood in the Heart produces cardiac pain and palpitations. As the Heart Meridian of Hand-Shao*yang* traverses the shoulder and the medial aspect of the arm, the above pain occurs. Dark-purplish tongue or purple spots on the tongue, and a deep, hesitant or irregular pulse are signs of blood stagnation. In severe cases, the overall blood circulation is also retarded, leading to cyanosis. Serious deficiency of *qi* and *yang* causes spontaneous sweating and cold limbs.

IV. Hyperactivity of Heart fire

This is often due to mental stress, or excessive indulgence in pungent or hot food, tobacco or alchohol. It may also be due to retention of exogenous pathogenic factors in the interior of the body. It is characterized by inflammation or ulceration of the tongue and urinary disturbances, and so it may be encountered in glossitis, ulcers of the tongue and some urological diseases.

Clinical manifestations: Fidgetiness and insomnia, flushed face, thirst, ulceration and pain of the tongue with reddened tip and yellow coating, and rapid pulse; in severe cases, burning pain in the urethra during micturition, passage of hot and dark urine or even hematuria may occur.

Syndrome analysis: Heart fire disturbs the mind, leading to insomnia and fidgetiness. Consumption of body fluids by fire gives rise to thirst. As the tongue is the "window" of the Heart, the hyperactive Heart fire flares upwards and causes ulceration and pain in the tongue. In severe cases, the fire may also move downwards, resulting in burning pain in the urethra during micturition, passage of hot and dark urine, or even hematuria. Flushed face, reddened tip of the tongue, yellow tongue coating and rapid pulse are signs of hyperactive Heart fire.

Hyperactivity of Heart fire is different from deficiency of Heart *yin* with endogenous fire, although they may have similar manifestations. The former is excess in nature, often seen in an acute condition, while the latter is deficient in nature, and usually chronic.

V. Clouding of the Heart by phlegm

This is characterized by mental derangement or loss of consciousness, and is not infrequently encountered in depressive episode, epilepsy, stroke and the critical stage of a chronic disease.

Clinical manifestations: Impaired consciousness with incoherent speech and rattling of phlegm in the throat, as observed in strokes; or low spiritedness with a feeling of hopelessness, apathy, muttering to oneself, and other abnormal behavior as observed in depression; or sudden loss of consciousness with convulsions and rattling in the throat as observed in epilepsy. A pale tongue with a white greasy coating and a slippery pulse are also the symptoms.

Syndrome analysis: The Heart is in charge of the mental activities. If the Heart is clouded by phlegm, consciousness will be impaired or lost. The formation of phlegm may be related to stagnation of Liver *qi* due to emotional influences. This is often seen in depression, with apathy, muttering to oneself, and other abnormal behavior. In epilepsy, the phlegm is usually derived from dysfunction of *zang-fu* organs and hidden in the Heart Meridian. Once the Liver wind is stirred up, the phlegm will go upward and cloud the Heart, so that the syndrome occurs in paroxysms. In a stroke, loss of consciousness is due to clouding of the Heart by an upsurge of phlegm together with endogenous wind. A pale tongue with a white greasy coating and a slippery pulse are consistent with the presence of turbid phlegm.

VI. Disturbance of the Heart by phlegm-fire

This is often induced by psychic or emotional stimuli. It is mostly encountered in mania, and sometimes in hysteria.

Clinical manifestations: Irritability, insomnia, dizziness, fantalizing, lack of concentration and dangerous raving. These manifestations may be accompanied by a reddened tongue with a yellow greasy coating, and a slippery, rapid pulse.

Syndrome analysis: Mental or emotional stimulation leads to stagnation of *qi*, and the stagnated *qi* is transformed into fire. The fire changes fluids into phlegm. Phlegm and fire in combination disturb the mental activities, resulting in the above-mentioned symptoms. A reddened tongue with a yellow greasy coating, together with a slippery, rapid pulse indicates the presence of phlegm and fire.

VII. Excessive heat of the Small Intestine

This syndrome is included in excessive fire of the Heart.

VIII. Deficiency-cold of the Small Intestine

This syndrome is included in deficiency-cold of the Spleen.

Syndromes of the Lungs and the Large Intestine

The Lungs control respiration, dominate *qi*, take charge of the superficial body resistance and regulate the water passages. The functions have a common feature—disseminating and descending, i.e., disseminating *qi* throughout the body and keeping the inspired air and fluids flowing downward. The Lungs are the only *zang*-organ that communicate with the exterior. This makes the Lungs particularly vulnerable to attacks by exogenous pathogenic factors.

The Large Intestine excretes waste as feces. It is exterior-interiorly related to the Lungs by the connection of their meridians. Thus, many Lung diseases of excess type can be satisfactorily treated with purgatives that act on the Large Intestine.

The syndromes of the Lung can be classified into two main categories according to excessiveness and deficiency. Excess syndromes of the Lung mostly occur in exogenous affections, particularly by pathogenic wind, cold, dryness and heat; deficiency syndromes include deficiency of Lung *qi* and deficiency of Lung *yin*. Deficiency of Lung *yang* is often associated with deficiency of Kidney *yang*, and deficiency of blood in the Lungs is usually a part of general deficiency of blood, so they are not considered separately.

The common symptoms and signs in Lung diseases are coughing and dyspnea due to disturbance of the descending function, expectoration either due to phlegm formed in the Lungs or phlegm formed in the Spleen and stored in the Lungs. Shortness of breath, general weakness and spontaneous sweating are also common when the function of the Lungs in dominating *qi* is reduced. Edema may occur if there is disturbance of the Lungs in regulating the water passages. Diseases of the Large Intestine are manifested by either diarrhea or constipation.

I. Deficiency of Lung *qi*

This is a syndrome due to diminished function of the Lungs in respiration and dominating *qi*. It is usually seen in chronic respiratory diseases such as chronic bronchitis, pulmonary emphysema, and pulmonary tuberculosis in Western medicine.

Clinical manifestations: Feeble cough accompanied by expectoration of thin whitish sputum, dyspnea and shortness of breath aggravated by mild exertion, feeble voice, pale complexion, lassitude, or spontaneous sweating, aversion to wind and vulnerability to colds, pale tongue with a white coating, and feeble pulse.

Syndrome analysis: The syndrome is characterized by feeble coughing, shortness of breath and general weakness. Deficiency of Lung *qi* causes diminished function of the Lungs in respiration and dominating *qi*, so the coughing is feeble and accompanied by shortness of breath. Since physical exertion consumes more *qi* (energy), the above symptoms will be aggravated even by mild exertion. The function of the Lungs in disseminating fluids is also impaired when Lung *qi* is insufficient. Fluids accumulated in the Lungs are coughed up and expectorated as thin, whitish sputum. The voice also depends on Lung *qi*; when the latter is insufficient, the voice becomes feeble. Pale complexion and lassitude are common manifestations of *qi* deficiency. When Lung *qi* is insufficient, distribution of defensive *qi* to the superficial portion of the body is also impaired, so the patient suffers from spontaneous sweating and is averse to wind and apt to catch cold. A pale tongue with a white coating and a feeble pulse are common manifestations of *qi* deficiency.

II. Deficiency of Lung *yin*

This happens when Lung *yin* is consumed by a chronic cough, a chronic Lung disease, or persistent fever. It is often seen in pulmonary tuberculosis, chronic bronchitis and many other chronic respiratory diseases, as well as in febrile diseases in the late stages with depletion of body fluids.

Clinical manifestations: Dry cough with no or scanty sputum, sticky or blood-streaked sputum, dryness in the mouth and throat, hoarseness of voice, afternoon fever, night sweating, malar flush, heat in the chest, palms and soles, dry and reddened tongue, and rapid, thready pulse.

Syndrome analysis: The syndrome is characterized by common symptoms of Lung diseases in combination with manifestations of endogenous heat due to deficiency of *yin*. Deficiency of Lung *yin* leads to the formation of endogenous heat. The heat induces upward perversion of the Lung *qi*, resulting in cough. Owing to deficiency of *yin*-fluid and condensation of the fluid by heat, the cough is dry or accompanied by scanty, sticky sputum. Lack of fluids in combination with endogenous heat brings about dryness in the throat and mouth, and hoarseness. The endogenous heat due to deficiency of *yin* produces afternoon fever and heat sensation in the chest, palms and soles. Effect of the endogenous heat on the nutrient (*ying*) fluid results in night sweating, and upward moving of the endogenous heat gives rise to malar flush. The heat may injure the Lungs, thus causing bleeding and hence blood streaks in the sputum. A dry, reddened tongue with a rapid, thready pulse is a sign of *yin* deficiency with endogenous heat.

III. Invasion of the Lungs by wind-cold

This is an exogenous affection of the Lungs by wind-cold, usually seen in colds and acute bronchitis.

Clinical manifestations: Coughing with expectoration of thin and whitish sputum, chills and mild fever, no sweating, headache, stuffy and runny nose, white coating of the tongue and a floating, tense pulse.

Syndrome analysis: Coughing is the main symptom when the Lungs are invaded by wind-cold. Disturbance of the normal flow of Lung *qi* leads to coughing, and the sputum is thin and whitish because the pathogenic cold impeding the normal distribution of fluid in the Lungs produces phlegm, but does not condense it. The nose is the "specific opening" of the Lungs. Disturbance of the dispersing function of the Lungs results in a stuffed-up nose with watery discharge. The Lungs are also in charge of defensive *qi,* which resists the invading pathogens on the superficial part of the body. When defensive *qi* is restrained by exogenous pathogens, chills occur; and when defensive *qi* resists the pathogens, heat is generated. In addition, the pathogenic cold closes the pores. Therefore, there are chills with fever but no sweating. In comparison with pathogenic heat, pathogenic cold only induces mild fever while pathogenic heat may give rise to high fever. Since the pathogenic factor has not been transmitted into the interior, the tongue coating is still normal. A floating, tense pulse indicates superficial affection by cold.

This syndrome is very similar to exterior cold syndrome (an exterior syndrome caused by wind-cold). The difference lies in the fact that coughing is the chief symptom in this syndrome, while chills and fever are usually mild or even absent; in exterior cold syndrome chills and fever are the main symptoms and coughing is mild or even absent.

IV. Invasion of the Lungs by wind-heat

This is an exogenous affection of the Lungs caused by wind-heat and usually seen in influenza, upper respiratory infections, acute bronchitis and the early stages of general infectious diseases.

Clinical manifestations: Coughing with expectoration of yellow, thick sputum, fever with mild aversion to wind, dryness of the mouth and sore throat, reddened tip and yellow coating of the tongue and a rapid, floating pulse.

Syndrome analysis: The syndrome is characterized by coughing and exterior syndrome of wind-heat. Invasion of the Lungs by exogenous wind-heat impairs the cleansing and descending function of the Lungs, thus causing coughing. By the action of heat, fluids in the Lungs are condensed to phlegm which is thick and yellow. Resistance of defensive *qi* against the invading wind-heat produces fever, and restraint of defensive *qi* by wind at the superficial portion of the body leads to mild aversion to wind. Upward invasion of wind-heat causes sore throat, and impairment of body fluids by heat gives rise to thirst. Reddened tip and yellow coating of the tongue, and rapid, floating pulse indicate the presence of wind-heat.

The difference between this syndrome and exterior heat syndrome (an exterior syndrome caused by wind-heat) lies in the fact that the former is marked by coughing with expectoration of thick, yellow sputum, while in the latter coughing and expectoration is mild or even absent. Fever may be obvious in both syndromes.

V. Invasion of the Lungs by heat (Heat in the Lungs)

This is often caused by direct invasion of the Lungs by exogenous pathogenic heat or heat transformed from wind-cold or wind-heat when the latter enters the interior. It can be encountered in acute and chronic bronchitis, pneumonia and other respiratory infections in Western medicine.

Clinical manifestations: Coughing with expectoration of thick, yellow sputum, dyspnea with coarse breathing or flaring of the nares, high fever with thirst, restlessness, epistaxis, hemoptysis, constipation, scanty concentrated urine, reddened tongue with yellow coating, and a rapid pulse.

Syndrome analysis: The syndrome is characterized by common symptoms of Lung diseases in combination with manifestations of interior heat. Accumulation of pathogenic heat in the Lungs induces upward perversion of Lung *qi*, resulting in coughing. The phlegm is formed due to condensation of fluids by heat, and so is thick and yellow. The pathogenic heat and phlegm impede the descending function of the Lungs, giving rise to dyspnea with coarse breathing. The heat causes fever and impairs the body fluids, resulting in thirst, constipation and scanty, concentrated urine. The heat may also disturb the mind, causing restlessness. If blood vessels are injured by heat, there is epistaxis or hemoptysis. A reddened tongue with a yellow coating and rapid pulse indicates heat in the interior.

VI. Invasion of the Lungs by dryness (Dryness of the Lungs)

This syndrome can be encountered in patients with colds or bronchitis in dry seasons.

Clinical manifestations: Dry cough or cough accompanied by scanty, sticky sputum difficult to expectorate, dry nose, lips, tongue and throat; chills and fever, or chest pain with hemoptysis. Reddened tongue (or tip of the tongue) with thin white or yellow coating, and a rapid pulse.

Syndrome analysis: The syndrome is an exogenous affection characterized by dryness of the respiratory system, and at the early stage it may be accompanied by an exterior syndrome manifested by chills and fever. Dryness is apt to be transformed into heat or fire, which goes deep into the Lungs or injures the blood vessels, thus causing chest pain and hemoptysis. In the early stage, when the pathogenic dryness stays chiefly in the upper portion of the Lungs, only the tip of the tongue is reddened, but when it goes deep into the Lungs, the whole tongue is reddened. The white and yellow colors of the tongue coating depend upon the intensity of the heat into which the pathogenic dryness has been transformed. The rapidity of the pulse also corresponds to the intensity of the heat.

Both invasion of the Lungs by dryness and deficiency of Lung *yin* are characterized by dryness symptoms, but the former is acute while the latter is chronic. If there is any fever in the exogenous affection of the Lungs by dryness, it only persists for a short period and is often accompanied by chills, but in deficiency of Lung *yin* there is usually long-standing afternoon fever accompanied by malar flush and heat sensation in the chest, palms and soles.

VII. Accumulation of phlegm-damp in the Lungs

It may be either acute or chronic. In acute cases, it is due to exogenous affection of cold-damp, and in chronic cases it is related to impaired function of the Spleen or to chronic cough which injures the Lungs. Clinically, it is often seen in asthmatic bronchitis and bronchiectasis diagnosed in Western medicine.

Clinical manifestations: Coughing with expectoration of white and frothy or glutinous sputum, feeling of fullness in the chest, rattling of sputum in the throat, sometimes accompanied by wheezing; white, greasy tongue coating and slippery pulse.

Syndrome analysis: The characteristic feature of this syndrome is coughing with white and frothy sputum or glutinous sputum easy to expectorate. Chronic cases are more frequently encountered than acute ones. In acute cases, the phlegm-damp is produced by the Lungs themselves due to exogenous affection of cold-damp. In chronic cases, the formation of phlegm may be related to the impaired transporting function of the Spleen with accumulation of damp. The damp is condensed to phlegm, which infiltrates into the Lungs. In this case, it is said that the Spleen is the source of phlegm production. On the other hand, the phlegm may also be produced in the Lungs, when chronic cough impairs the dispersing function of the Lungs, bringing about accumulation of fluid. The retained fluid in the Lungs turns into phlegm. Regardless of the different pathogeneses, the common result is coughing. If the air passage is obstructed by phlegm-damp, there will be chest pain, rattling sounds and wheezing. A white, greasy tongue coating with a slippery pulse indicates accumulation of phlegm-damp in the interior.

VIII. Accumulation of heat-phlegm in the Lungs

Combined accumulation of heat and phlegm in the Lungs may be encountered in the following diseases in Western medicine: acute bronchitis, chronic bronchitis with acute exacerbation, bronchiectasis with secondary infection, pneumonia, bronchial asthma and pulmonary emphysema complicated by infection.

Clinical manifestations: Coughing accompanied by dyspnea and expectoration of copious yellow, thick or purulent sputum, fever, thirst, or chest pain; constipation, scanty concentrated urine, reddened tongue with a yellow, greasy coating and a rapid, slippery pulse.

Syndrome analysis: The syndrome is characterized by accumulation of both heat and phlegm in the Lungs. In most cases it is a chronic accumulation of phlegm-damp in the Lungs complicated by an exogenous affection of pathogenic heat, and so there is coughing but the sputum changes from white and frothy to thick and yellow, or even purulent. Fever, thirst, constipation and scanty, concentrated urine are all due to heat in the interior. If heat-phlegm obstructs the blood flow, there will be chest pain. A reddened tongue with a yellow, greasy coating and a rapid, slippery pulse indicate heat and phlegm.

IX. Damp-heat in the Large Intestine

This is due to affection of exogenous damp-heat or improper diet, and is usually seen in bacillary or amebic dysentery, either acute or chronic, and also in colitis.

Clinical manifestations: Abdominal pain, frequent diarrhea with mucous and bloody stools, and tenesmus, or intense, watery diarrhea. A burning feeling in the anus, scanty concentrated urine, thirst, and sometimes chills and fever, or fever alone; a reddened tongue with a yellow greasy coating, and rapid soft or rapid and slippery pulse.

Syndrome analysis: Damp-heat disturbs the activities of the Large Intestine, causing abdominal pain. It injures the Large Intestine and its blood vessels, and so the stools contain mucus, pus and blood. The action of heat on the Large Intestine induces painful straining at stool as well as a burning sensation in the anus. Scanty concentrated urine and thirst are due to excessive discharge of water from the Large Intestine and are also due to impairment of fluids by heat. At the onset, when the exterior portion of the body is affected, there are chills and fever; if the heat is in the interior, there is only fever with no more chills. A reddened tongue with a yellow, greasy coating indicates damp-heat. In diseases caused by damp-heat, the intensity of damp and heat may not be equal. If damp prevails, the pulse is rapid and soft; if heat prevails, the pulse is rapid and slippery.

X. Deficiency of fluid in the Large Intestine

This is a syndrome of *yin* deficiency, either constitutional, or occurring during a chronic disease with impairment of *yin* fluid or after a febrile disease when the consumed fluid has not yet been restored. It may also take place after excessive postpartum hemorrhage. As a constitutional disorder, it is most frequently manifested as habitual constipation.

Clinical manifestations: Hard fecal mass with difficult and infrequent elimination, dryness of the mouth and throat, or accompanied by foul breath and dizziness; dry reddened tongue and thready, hesitant pulse.

Syndrome analysis: Deficiency of fluid in the Large Intestine makes the fecal mass hard and difficult to eliminate. The defecation is often infrequent—once every three or five days or even more than ten days. *Yin* deficiency causes dryness of the mouth and throat. Retention of the fecal mass in the Large Intestine may lead to upward flow of turbid *qi*, resulting in foul breath and dizziness. Deficiency of *yin* is accompanied by relative exuberance of *yang*, and hence the tongue is dry and reddened. Thready and hesitant pulse is due to insufficient fluid in the arteries.

Syndromes of the Spleen and the Stomach

The Spleen digests food, transports, distributes and transforms food essence (nutrients) and replenishes *qi*. The normal function of the Spleen is characterized by ascending *qi*, for it sends nutrients upwards to the Heart and Lungs; it also promotes water metabolism, keeps the blood flowing within blood vessels, and maintains the normal position of visceral organs. So pathological changes of the Spleen are often manifested as digestive and nutritional disorders, deficiency of *qi* and blood, retention of water and damp, bleeding, visceroptosis, etc.

The Stomach receives and digests food. The normal function of the Stomach is characterized by descending *qi*, for it sends its contents downward into the Intestines. Its pathological changes are often manifested as dysfunction in descending and poor appetite.

Since the Spleen and the Stomach are so closely related, they are usually considered together. Their syndromes can also be classified into two main groups, according to deficiency and excessiveness. Their deficiency syndromes include deficiency of *qi*, *yang* and *yin*. However, deficiency of blood in the Spleen and Stomach is seldom considered as an independent syndrome, because it is only a part of general deficiency of blood. Excess syndromes of the Spleen and Stomach are often due to invasion of cold, damp and heat, as well as retention of undigested food.

I. Deficiency of the Spleen *qi*

Deficiency of Spleen *qi* and deficiency of Stomach *qi* may occur jointly or separately. They are characterized chiefly by diminished digestive function, and are often seen in chronic gastritis, peptic ulcers, chronic colitis, functional disorders of the stomach and intestines, chronic hepatitis and other digestive diseases from the Western medical perspective.

Clinical manifestations: Reduced food intake, abdominal distension, loose stools, lassitude, indolence to speak, sallow or pale and puffy complexion, edema or emaciation, pale tongue with a white coating, and relaxed or weak pulse.

Syndrome analysis: The clinical manifestations of deficiency of Spleen *qi* can be classified into two groups: those indicating impaired transporting and transforming functions of the Spleen and those showing deficiency of *qi*. Impaired transporting and transforming functions lead to slowness in digestion and weakness in distribution of food essence, resulting in endogenous dampness, which, in turn, disturbs the Spleen function and causes abdominal distension. The abdominal distension in this case, unlike the distension caused by excessive eating, is deficient in nature. The Stomach is exterior-interiorly related to the Spleen. When Spleen *qi* is insufficient, the Stomach is often weakened, and hence the appetite is impaired and the food intake reduced. The endogenous damp pouring into the Intestines makes the stools loose. The Spleen is in charge of the muscles of the limbs. So there is lassitude or lack of strength with taciturnity when Spleen *qi* is insufficient. Infiltration of dampness into the superficial portion of the body leads to a pale and puffy complexion and even edema. The Spleen provides the material basis of acquired constitution and is the source of nutrients for the generation of *qi* and blood. Prolonged deficiency of Spleen *qi* usually results in insufficiency of nutrients and blood, and hence emaciation and sallow complexion. A pale tongue with a white coating and a relaxed and weak pulse also suggest weakness of Spleen *qi*.

II. Deficiency of Spleen *yang*

Deficiency of Spleen *yang* is characterized by deficiency of Spleen *qi* in association with endogenous cold. It usually develops from deficiency of Spleen *qi*, caused by excessive cold and raw food, or due to deficiency of Kidney *yang* with failure of fire (vital fire) to promote earth (the Spleen).

Clinical manifestations: Abdominal distension with reduced food intake, abdominal pain alleviated by pressure and warmth, loose or even watery stools, cold limbs or heavy sensation in the limbs, or general edema with oliguria, or profuse thin leukorrhea in women; pale and plump tongue with white and slippery coating, and deep, weak and slow pulse.

Syndrome analysis: The clinical manifestations of Spleen *yang* deficiency consist of symptoms indicating diminished function of the Spleen and symptoms showing the presence of cold or damp-cold. Impaired function of the Spleen causes reduced food intake and abdominal distension, as explained above. Deficiency of *yang* is accompanied by relative exuberance of *yin*, giving rise to endogenous cold, which makes the flow of *qi* stagnate by congealing. So there is abdominal pain which can be alleviated by warmth and pressure. Damp is a common pathological product of diminished function of the Spleen. Damp-cold in the Intestines make the bowel movements loose, containing undigested food. The Spleen supplies *qi* to the limbs. Inadequate supply of *yang-qi* from the Spleen makes the limbs cold. Deficiency of Spleen *yang* with accumulation of water and damp may disturb the secretion of urine, resulting in oliguria and edema, which is often generalized and accompanied by a heavy sensation in the limbs. In women, water-damp pour downward, causing profuse thin leukorrhea. A pale and plump tongue with a white and slippery coating and a deep, slow and weak pulse are signs indicating *yang* deficiency with endogenous damp and cold.

Deficiency of Spleen *yang* is usually marked by cold manifestations, and so is also called "deficiency-cold of the Spleen." In addition, it is often accompanied by deficiency of Stomach *yang*, and called "deficiency-cold of the Spleen and Stomach."

III. Sinking of Spleen *qi*

This is also called "sinking of the *qi* of the Middle Energizer" or simply "sinking of middle *qi*." It is often a further development of deficiency of Spleen *qi* and may occur in some cases of chronic colitis, functional disorders of the intestines, prolapse of the rectum or uterus, and probably also in gastroptosis and other visceroptosis in Western medicine.

Clinical manifestations: Deficiency of Spleen *qi* (or *yang*) plus bearing-down sensation in the abdomen, incessant diarrhea, dripping of urine after urination, prolapse of the rectum or uterus.

Syndrome analysis: All the manifestations listed above in addition to deficiency of Spleen *qi* are due to failure of the Spleen in its lifting function.

IV. Failure of the Spleen to control blood

This is characterized by chronic bleeding, particularly in the lower part of the body, and is often seen in functional uterine bleeding, hematochezia, hematuria and hemorrhagic diseases.

Clinical manifestations: Menorrhagia, hematochezia, hematuria, subcutaneous hemorrhage and other chronic hemorrhages, pale tongue, and thready, weak pulse.

Syndrome analysis: The Spleen has the function of keeping the blood flowing within the blood vessels. If deficiency of Spleen *qi* affects this function, blood will escape from the blood vessels. Since the bleeding is due to chronic deficiency of Spleen *qi,* which is often accompanied by loss of its ascending power or lifting function, the bleeding is often chronic and chiefly occurring in the lower part of the body.

V. Weakness of the Spleen with accumulation of damp

In this syndrome, weakness of the Spleen is primary, while accumulation of damp is secondary. Therefore, it is a syndrome of deficiency complicated with excess, and the damp is endogenous. It may be seen in chronic gastritis, chronic colitis, chronic dysentery, chronic hepatitis, liver cirrhosis, edema due to malnutrition, and gynecological diseases with profuse leukorrhea.

Clinical manifestations: It is a combined syndrome of deficiency of Spleen *qi* (or *yang*) with manifestations of damp. Damp manifestations include heavy sensation in the head as if it were wrapped, sticky sensation in the mouth without thirst, or dryness of the mouth with no desire to drink, epigastric fullness and abdominal distension, diarrhea, edema of the legs, excessive leukorrhea with thin, whitish discharge, white slippery or greasy tongue coating, and relaxed pulse.

Syndrome analysis: Diminished function of the Spleen in transporting and transforming fluids leads to accumulation of damp in the body. The accumulated damp, when it is retained in the upper part, produces heavy sensation of the head; when retained in the middle part, it gives rise to a sticky sensation in the mouth without thirst, or dryness of the mouth with no desire to drink, epigastric fullness and abdominal distension; when pouring downwards, causes diarrhea, edema of the legs and excessive leukorrhea. White slippery or greasy tongue coating and relaxed pulse indicate accumulation of damp in the interior.

VI. Disturbance of the Spleen by cold-damp

This is a syndrome of excess, characterized by impairment of Spleen *yang* due to exogenous dampness, such as improper diet with too much raw and cold food, or being drenched in the rain. It may occur in cases of acute gastritis, colitis, and colds with digestive disorders.

Clinical manifestations: Epigastric fullness, distension and pain, reduced food intake, loose stools, nausea, tastelessness in the mouth without thirst, heaviness in the head and body, gloomy complexion or jaundice with a dull facial color, or edema of the limbs with oliguria; pale and plump tongue with white and greasy coating, and soft, relaxed pulse.

Syndrome analysis: The syndrome is characterized by accumulation of cold-damp combined with dysfunction of the Spleen. As the Spleen is intolerant of dampness, when cold-damp invades the Spleen, epigastric fullness, distension and pain ensue, and all kinds of food become insipid. Cold-damp pertains to *yin,* which does not consume fluid, and so there is no thirst. Damp pouring into the Intestines result in loose stools. Dysfunction of the Spleen often involves the Stomach, causing nausea. Dampness makes things heavy, and thus there is heaviness in the head and body. Cold-damp impedes the normal flow of *qi*, making the complexion gloomy. In some cases, it even impedes the normal flow of bile, and thus brings about jaundice. A pale and plump tongue with a white and greasy coating, and a soft, relaxed pulse are consistent with the presence of cold-damp and impairment of the Spleen function.

VII. Accumulation of damp-heat in the Spleen

This is often due to invasion of exogenous pathogenic damp-heat or excessive intake of rich fatty food or alcoholic drinks. It may be encountered in acute icteric hepatitis and acute cholecystitis.

Clinical manifestations: Fullness and distress in the abdomen, anorexia, nausea and vomiting, loose stools, yellow-colored urine, heavy sensation in the limbs, or jaundice with bright yellow discoloration of the skin and sclera accompanied by itching, or fluctuating fever which cannot be relieved by diaphoresis; reddened tongue with yellow greasy coating, and soft, rapid pulse.

Syndrome analysis: The syndrome is characterized by impairment of the transporting and transforming functions of the Spleen and accumulation of damp-heat. Accumulation of pathogenic damp-heat impairs the functions of the Spleen and Stomach, resulting in fullness and distress in the abdomen, anorexia, nausea and vomiting. The Spleen governs the muscles of the limbs, and dampness makes things heavy. So there is a heavy sensation in the limbs. Damp-heat pushing the intestinal contents downward, makes the stools unformed but sticky. Damp-heat in the Spleen and the Stomach forces the bile flow adversely and floods the skin, resulting in itching and jaundice which is bright orange in color. Heat surrounded by damp is difficult to dissipate, and so the fever cannot be relieved by diaphoresis. The reddened tongue with a yellow coating and a rapid pulse indicate heat, and the greasiness of the coating and soft pulse suggest dampness.

VIII. Deficiency of Stomach *yin*

Deficiency of Stomach *yin* may occur in the course of a chronic Stomach disease, at the late stage of a febrile disease with impairment of body fluid, or in people who used to eating spicy and hot food. In addition, it is not infrequently encountered in people who are depressed emotionally because depressed *qi* may be transformed into fire, which impairs Stomach yin. From the Western medical perspective, this syndrome may be found in the cases of chronic gastritis, peptic ulcers and other stomach diseases.

Clinical manifestations: Dull epigastric pain, no desire to eat when feeling hungry, dryness of the mouth and throat, constipation, or fullness and distress in the epigastrium, retching or hiccuping; dry, reddened tongue and thready, rapid pulse.

Syndrome analysis: The syndrome is characterized by common gastric symptoms in combination with symptoms of *yin* deficiency. The relatively exuberant Stomach *yang* during deficiency of Stomach *yin* produces endogenous heat, which, accumulated in the Stomach, disturbs the Stomach function, resulting in dull epigastric pain and no desire to eat though feeling hungry. The digestive function of the Stomach is also impaired by inadequacy of *yin*-fluid, resulting in fullness and distress in the epigastrium. Insufficient Stomach *yin* is unable to go either upwards to moisten the throat or downwards to moisten the Large Intestine, thus bringing about dryness of the mouth and throat, and constipation. The endogenous heat may cause upward adverse flow of Stomach *qi*, leading to retching or hiccuping. A dry, reddened tongue with a thready, rapid pulse indicates endogenous heat due to *yin* deficiency.

IX. Stagnation of food in the Stomach

This is a syndrome caused by impaired digestive function of the Stomach with stagnation of undigested food. In most cases, it occurs in indigestion due to improper diet, particularly due to taking too much food and drink at one meal. It may also be attributed to weakness of the Stomach.

Clinical manifestations: Epigastric fullness, distension or pain, belching with fetid odor, acid eructation or vomiting of sour fetid gastric contents (with alleviation of epigastric distension or pain after vomiting), or flatus and loose bowels with sour fetid stools; thick greasy tougue coating and slippery pulse.

Syndrome analysis: Stagnation of undigested food in the Stomach causes epigastric fullness, distension or pain. Disturbance in the descending function of the Stomach leads to upward perversion, and so there is belching with fetid odor, acid eructation or vomiting of sour fetid undigested food. After vomiting the pathogenic factor (undigested food) is removed, and so the distension and pain are alleviated. Stagnation of undigested food leads to formation of endogenous damp and impairment of the intestinal function, and thus frequent flatus and loose stools with sour fetid odor. Stagnation of undigested food in the Stomach forces the turbid *qi* to ascend, thus forming the thick greasy tongue coating. Slippery pulse in food stagnation suggests excess of the pathogenic factor (undigested food) confronted by powerful *qi* and surging blood.

X. Invasion of the Stomach by cold (Stomach cold)

This is an exogenous affection of the Stomach, often caused by exposure of the abdomen to cold, or to too much cold and raw food.

Clinical manifestations: Epigastric pain, mild in some cases, but severely colicky in others, aggravated by cold and alleviated by warmth; no desire for drink; lassitude, lack of strength, and cold limbs; or gurgling sounds in the Stomach and vomiting of watery fluid; pale tongue with white slippery coating, and slow pulse.

Syndrome analysis: The syndrome is characterized by epigastric pain with cold manifestations. In the early stage, it is an excess syndrome caused by the invasion of pathogenic cold. If the Stomach *yang* is impaired, the syndrome may be complicated by deficiency or even turn into deficiency-cold. Cold has contracting and congealing actions which make *qi* stagnate, giving rise to epigastric pain or even gastric colic. Further exposure to cold naturally aggravates the pain. Cold pertains to *yin*. When cold is in excess, no fluid (*yin*) is consumed, and so there is no desire for drink. If the disease persists, there will be impairment of *yang* with deficiency manifestations, such as lassitude, lack of strength and cold limbs. In some cases, deficiency-cold of the Stomach is so severe that even fluid cannot be digested. Retention of undigested fluid in the Stomach results in gurgling sounds and vomiting of watery fluid. A pale tongue with a white slippery coating and a slow pulse indicate cold.

XI. Fire in the Stomach (Stomach fire)

This is usually due to partiality for spicy hot food which produces heat and fire, emotional depression which leads to transformation of stagnated *qi* into fire, or invasion of the Stomach by exogenous pathogenic heat. Clinically, the syndrome may be seen in gastritis, ulcerative stomatitis, periondontal diseases and diabetes mellitus.

Clinical manifestations: Burning pain in the epigastrium accompanied by acid regurgitation or vomiting right after eating; thirst with desire for cold drinks, polyphagia with frequent hunger; or foul breath, ulceration in the mouth, and swollen, painful and bleeding gums. Constipation and scanty concentrated urine, reddened tongue with a yellow coating, and slippery, rapid pulse.

Syndrome analysis: Fire in the Stomach causes burning pain. It also leads Stomach *qi* adversely upwards, and so there is vomiting right after eating. However, Stomach fire also means hyperactivity of the Stomach, and so in some cases the patient complains of excessive desire for food. The Stomach Meridian sends its branches to the gums. Fire of the Stomach leads to ulceration in the mouth, and swollen, painful, bleeding gums, and forces turbid *qi* in the Stomach to flow upwards, causing foul breath. Fire due to emotional depression usually comes from stagnant *qi* in the Liver (which produces acid according to the five elements theory), and hence causes acid regurgitation. Constipation, scanty, concentrated urine and reddened tongue with a yellow coating are signs indicating the exuberance of fire. Fire expedites blood flow, and so the pulse is not only rapid but also slippery.

Syndromes of the Liver and Gallbladder

The Liver is situated in the upper part of the abdomen on the right side, but it has a pair of meridians branching into the costal and hypochondriac regions on both sides. The Liver stores blood, smoothes and regulates the flow of *qi* and blood, and controls the tendons. The Gallbladder, which stores bile, is attached to the Liver. Since these two organs are closely related, diseases of the Gallbladder are often considered part of the Liver troubles.

Syndromes of the Liver can be classified into two main groups according to the conditions of deficiency and excess. The chief deficiency syndromes are deficiency of Liver blood and deficiency of Liver *yin*, and the excess syndromes of the Liver are often due to invasion of stagnant *qi*, exuberant fire, pathogenic cold and damp-heat.

The common symptoms and signs of Liver diseases are: pain in the lateral pectoral, hypochondriac and lower abdominal regions, irritability and irascibility, dizziness and distending headache, tremors, twitches and even convulsions of the extremities, menstrual disorders, and distending pain of the testis. Those of Gallbladder diseases are: bitterness in the mouth, jaundice, palpitations with fear, and insomnia.

I. Stagnation of Liver *qi* (or "**Liver *qi***" for short)

Stagnation of Liver *qi* is characterized by disturbance in the function of smoothing and regulating the flow of *qi* and blood. It is often induced by emotional depression or violent psychic stimulation, but may also be caused by invasion of certain exogenous pathogenic factors. From the Western medical perspective, this syndrome may occur in anxiety disorders, depression, hepatitis, cholecystitis, and menstrual disorders.

Clinical manifestations: Depressed mood, irritability and irascibility, distension and pain in the lateral pectoral, hypochondriac and lower abdominal regions traversed by the Liver Meridian, discomfort in the chest, frequent sighing, feeling of a lump in the throat, and in women distending pain of the breast, dysmenorrhea, irregular menstruation or even amenorrhea; stringy pulse.

Syndrome analysis: The Liver has the function of smoothing and regulating the flow of *qi*. *Qi* is not confined to energy for bodily activities; it also involves mental activities and emotions. Therefore, when Liver *qi* is depressed and stagnant, there is a depressed or irritable mood. Distension and pain in the lateral pectoral, hypochondriac and lower abdominal regions are symptoms caused by stagnation of Liver *qi* along the Liver Meridian. Stagnant Liver *qi* may also impede the functional activities of the Lungs, leading to discomfort in the chest and frequent sighing. If stagnant Liver *qi* promotes the production of phlegm, and the phlegm together with stagnant *qi* moves upward along the Liver Meridian to the throat, the accumulated phlegm and stagnant *qi* will be felt as a foreign body in the throat ("globus hystericus"). The Liver Meridian is connected with the Thoroughfare Vessel, which controls menstruation in women. Stagnation of Liver *qi* often impairs the normal flow of blood in the Thoroughfare Vessel, thus causing menstrual disorders. A stringy pulse suggests a disease of the Liver.

II. Excessive fire in the Liver Meridian (Liver fire)

This is characterized by upward perversion of *qi* and fire along the Liver Meridian, and is often due to emotional depression with transmission of stagnant Liver *qi* into fire or invasion of the Liver by pathogenic heat. From the Western medical perspective, this syndrome may occur in hypertension, Ménière's syndrome, acute conjunctivitis, acute otitis media, and hemorrhage of the upper digestive tract.

Clinical manifestations: Marked irascibility, headache, vertigo, flushed face, congested eyes, burning pain in the lateral pectoral and hypochondriac regions, insomnia or nightmares, constipation and concentrated urine; in some cases, rumbling in the ear, pain in the ear with purulent discharge, and in some other cases hematemesis, hemoptysis or epistaxis; reddened tongue with a yellow coating, and a stringy, rapid pulse.

Syndrome analysis: The Liver fire usually flames up to the head, face and eyes, resulting in headache, vertigo, flushed face and congested eyes. It disturbs mental activity, causing insomnia and nightmares. Excessive fire in the Liver leads to stagnation of *qi* and blood in the Liver Meridian, and so there is burning pain in the regions where the Liver Meridian passes. The Liver is "a viscus of temperament," and so dysfunction of the Liver makes one apt to get angry. Constipation and concentrated urine are due to consumption of fluids by excessive fire. The Liver and the Gallbladder are interior-exteriorly related. The Liver fire may be shifted to the Gallbladder and flames up along the Gallbladder Meridian which enters the ears. Therefore, excessive Liver fire may induce rumbling in the ears or acute inflammation of the ear with pain, swelling and purulent discharge. In addition, the fire may injure blood vessels or drive the blood to flow adversely. As a result, there is bleeding, such as hematemesis, hemoptysis or epistaxis. Reddened tongue with a yellow coating, and a stringy, rapid pulse are signs indicating excessive fire in the Liver.

III. Deficiency of Liver blood

This is often due to inadequate blood generation by the Spleen and the Kidneys, consumption of Liver blood in chronic diseases, or excessive loss of blood. It may be part of a general deficiency of blood, but deficiency of Liver blood may exist independently without involvement of other internal organs. It is often encountered in anemia, consumptive diseases, menstrual disorders, and some eye diseases and neurological troubles.

Clinical manifestations: Dizziness, dryness of the eyes, diminution of vision or night blindness; numbness or tingling sensation in the limbs and tremors of the extremities; scanty menstrual flow with pinkish discharge or even amenorrhea in women; pale complexion with pale lips, pale tongue with a white coating and a stringy, thready pulse.

Syndrome analysis: The Liver stores blood. Deficiency of Liver blood renders the supply of blood for the head, face and eyes inadequate, causing dizziness, pale complexion, pale lips, dryness of the eyes, diminution of vision or night blindness. The Liver supplies blood to the tendons for the movements of the limbs. Insufficient blood supply leads to numbness or tingling sensation in the limbs and tremors of the extremities. The Liver is connected with the Thoroughfare Vessel, which controls menstruation in women. Thus, deficiency of Liver blood usually causes menstrual disorders characterized by insufficient menstrual discharge. A pale tongue with a white coating and a stringy, thready pulse suggest deficiency of blood in the Liver.

IV. Deficiency of Liver *yin*

Liver *yin* may be consumed in emotional depression with stagnation of *qi* and fire, in some Liver diseases, or in a febrile disease in the late stage. From the Western medical perspective, this syndrome is often seen in hepatitis, anxiety and depressive disorders, and some eye diseases.

Clinical manifestations: Dizziness and tinnitus, dryness of the eyes, hot flushes, costal and hypochondriac pain, heat in the palms and soles, dryness of the throat and mouth, night sweating; reddened tongue with a scanty coating, and a stringy, thready and rapid pulse.

Syndrome analysis: *Yin* is a collective term for various essential substances, including vital essence, blood and fluids. Since deficiency of Liver blood is taken as an independent syndrome, deficiency of Liver *yin* mainly refers to deficient Liver essence and fluids. Inadequte supply of Liver essence to the head causes dizziness, tinnitus and dry eyes. Fluid deficiency explains the dry mouth and throat. Deficiency of *yin* is apt to induce relative exuberance of *yang* or endogenous heat, so there may be night sweating and heat in the palms and soles, and the tongue is reddened instead of being pale due to the deficiency of Liver blood; the pulse is not only stringy and thready, but also rapid.

V. Exuberance of Liver *yang* (or **"Liver *yang*"** for short)

Exuberance of Liver *yang* is usually due to deficiency of Liver *yin*. It differs from Liver fire in the property of the syndromes. In Liver *yang* syndrome, the exuberance of *yang* is relative, and the fundamental property of the syndrome is deficiency. So, the full name of this syndrome should be "deficiency of Liver *yin* with exuberance of Liver *yang*." In excessive fire in the Liver Meridian, there is absolute exuberance of *yang*, and the syndrome is purely excessive in nature. From the Western medical perspective, exuberance of Liver *yang* may be encountered in hepatitis, anxiety disorders, hypertension, and some other psychosomatic diseases.

Clinical manifestations: Dizziness, headache, tinnitus, flushing of the face, redness of the eyes, dryness of the mouth and throat, irritability and irascibility, reddened tongue with a scanty coating and a stringy, thready and rapid pulse.

Syndrome analysis: This syndrome may have some similarities with excessive fire in the Liver Meridian, but the latter often has an acute onset, occurring after an emotional upset, while the former develops on the basis of a deficiency state which usually has run a chronic course. Deficiency of *yin* is often accompanied by relative exuberance of *yang*, which causes an upsurge of *qi* and blood, resulting in dizziness, headache, tinnitus, flushing of the face, and redness of the eyes. The Liver is an "organ of temperament"; exuberance of its *yang* renders one irritable and irascible. A reddened tongue with a scanty coating and a stringy, thready and rapid pulse are signs of deficiency of the Liver *yin* with exuberance of *yang*.

VI. Stirring-up of the Liver wind (or **"Liver wind"** for short)

Syndromes characterized by "shaking" symptoms, such as tremors, convulsions and dizziness as if about to swoon, belong to the condition known as "stirring-up of Liver wind." Clinically, they can be classified into three patterns: (1) transformation of exuberant Liver fire into wind, (2) production of internal wind due to extreme heat, and (3) production of internal wind due to deficiency of *yin*.

(1) Transformation of exuberant Liver *yang* into wind

This often occurs in cases of deficiency of Liver *yin* with exuberant *yang*. The exuberance of Liver *yang* to its extreme may turn into internal wind as seen in cerebrovascular accidents.

Clinical manifestations: Sudden onset of dizziness, fainting, stiffness of the limbs, aphasia, hemiplegia or even total loss of consciousness; reddened tongue with a white or greasy coating, and a stringy, forceful pulse.

Syndrome analysis: The syndrome usually occurs in a case of chronic deficiency of Liver *yin* with exuberant *yang*. Once the exuberant *yang* is transformed into internal wind, a sudden rising of the wind disturbs the normal flow of *qi* and blood, resulting in dizziness and fainting. The Liver Meridian is connected with the root of the tongue. Ascent of the wind along the meridian to the tongue impairs speech. If the Liver wind rises together with phlegm, the Heart will be clouded, and loss of consciousness ensues. Reddening of the tongue is due to *yin* deficiency. Since there is no fire, the coating is still white, but it may be greasy if the wind is combined with phlegm. A stringy and forceful pulse signifies up-stirring of *yang* and wind.

(2) Production of internal wind due to extreme heat

This refers to febrile convulsions.

Clinical manifestations: High fever with delirium or loss of consciousness, convulsions and opisthotonos; reddened or deep-red tongue and stringy, rapid pulse.

Syndrome analysis: In this syndrome the internal wind is derived from extreme heat. treme pathogenic heat often invades the Pericardium[3], leading to delirium or loss of

---

[3]In exogenous affections, since the pathogenic factors come from outside, it is believed that they attack

consciousness. When the heat invades the Liver Meridian, it induces internal wind, resulting in convulsions and opisthotonos. A reddened or deep-red tongue and a stringy and rapid pulse are consistent with invasion of the Liver by heat.

(3) Production of internal wind due to deficiency of blood

This is often encountered in chronic neurological diseases marked by involuntary movements.

Clinical manifestations: Tremors or numbness of the limbs, involuntary head shaking, pale tongue and stringy, thready pulse.

Syndrome analysis: The Liver supplies blood to nourish the tendons. Deficiency of Liver blood impairs the normal functioning of the tendons, resulting in numbness and involuntary movements. A pale tongue with a stringy pulse indicates deficiency of Liver blood.

VII. Stagnation of cold in the Liver Meridian

This syndrome is due to affection of the Liver Meridian by pathogenic cold. It may occur in diseases of the testis and epididymis or in hernia.

Clinical manifestations: Lower abdominal pain, aggravated by cold and alleviated by warmth, with coldness and a bearing-down sensation in the testis or accompanied by contraction of the scrotum; white, slippery tongue coating, and deep, stringy pulse.

Syndrome analysis: The Liver Meridian curves around the external genitalia and passes through the lower abdominal region. Pathogenic cold blocks the *qi* and blood circulation, leading to pain in this region. Cold causes contraction, and so there is bearing-down sensation in the testis or contraction of the scrotum. Warmth disperses cold, and thus alleviates pain; when cold accumulates, the pain becomes worse. A white, slippery tongue coating with a deep pulse indicates cold in the interior; the pulse is often stringy when the Liver is affected.

VIII. Damp-heat in the Liver and Gallbladder

The damp-heat that invades the Liver and Gallbladder may be either exogenous or endogenous. The endogenous damp-heat comes from excessive intake of greasy food. The syndrome often occurs in icteric jaundice, acute cholecystitis and cholelithiasis in Western medicine.

Clinical manifestations: Hypochondriac distension and pain, bitter taste in the mouth, poor appetite, nausea, vomiting, abdominal distension, scanty and dark-yellow urine, yellow sticky or greasy tongue coating and a stringy, rapid pulse. In addition, there may be alternate chills and fever, or yellow discoloration of the sclera and skin. Eczema of the scrotum, swelling and burning pain in the testis or yellow, foul leukorrhea with pruritus of the vulva also suggest damp-heat in the Liver Meridian.

Syndrome analysis: Damp-heat impairs the free flow of *qi* in the Liver and Gallbladder, causing hypochondriac distension and pain. The upward flow of Gallbladder *qi* gives rise to a bitter taste in the mouth. The accumulation of damp-heat also impairs the functions of the Spleen and the Stomach in ascending and descending, causing poor appetite, nausea, vomiting and abdominal distension. Scanty and dark-yellow urine is due to downward infusion of damp-heat into the Bladder. Yellow sticky or greasy tongue

the Pericardium before entering the Heart, and the disturbances of the Pericardium induced by them are the same as those of the Heart, particularly mental disorders.

coating with a stringy and rapid pulse is consistent with damp-heat in the Liver and Gallbladder. When the damp-heat leads to confrontation between the anti-pathogenic and pathogenic factors in the Gallbladder, alternate chills and fever arise. If the normal flow of bile is obstructed by damp-heat, the bile will spread to the exterior portion of the body and result in yellow discoloration of the sclera and skin. Since the Liver Meridian curves around the external genitalia, downward infusion of damp-heat may result in eczema of the scrotum, or swelling of and a burning pain in the testis in men, and yellow, foul leukorrhea with pruritus of the vulva in women.

Syndromes of the Kidneys and the Bladder

The Kidneys are regarded as the "congenital foundation" of the human body. They store essence, dominate reproduction, growth and development, produce marrow, dominate the bones and replenish the brain. As these functions are closely related to Kidney *yin*, when Kidney *yin* is insufficient, there are disorders in reproduction, growth and development, certain activities of the brain, and solidity of the bones and teeth.

Kidneys also govern vital fire, dominate water metabolism, and help the Lungs to take in air. These functions are closely related to Kidney *yang*. If Kidney *yang* is insufficient, there are disorders in the maintenance of body temperature, digestion, respiration, secretion of urine and sexual potency.

The function of the Bladder is temporary storage and eventual excretion of urine. Because of its close relation to the Kidneys, the Kidneys can be regarded as the whole uro-genital system, and some Bladder disorders are attributed to the Kidneys.

I. Deficiency of Kidney *yin*

The common causes of deficient Kidney *yin* include impairment of the Kidneys by a protracted disease, weak constitution or poor natural endowment, sexual overindulgence and excessive use of warming, desiccating drugs. The syndrome is often seen in chronic debility, tuberculosis, diabetes mellitus, chronic nephritis, disorders of the sexual function, sterility, etc.

Clinical manifestations: Soreness and weakness of the loins and knees, impaired hearing, tinnitus; seminal emissions, oligospermia and sterility in men, and amenorrhea and infertility in women; afternoon fever, malar flush, heat sensation in the chest, palms and soles, night sweating, reddened tongue with scanty or no coating, and a deep, thready pulse.

Syndrome analysis: The syndrome is characterized by common symptoms of Kidney disorders and deficiency of *yin* with endogenous heat. Because the Kidneys replenish marrow, which is believed to be the substance that nourishes the bones, and particularly because the loins are where the Kidneys are located, deficiency of Kidney *yin* usually brings about soreness and weakness of the loins and knees. The Kidneys have a specific relationship with the ears, so deficiency of Kidney *yin* often causes tinnitus and impairs the hearing. Since Kidney *yin* includes the reproductive essence, deficiency of Kidney *yin* may be associated with oligospermia and sterility in males, and amenorrhea and infertility in females. Deficiency of Kidney *yin* often leads to exuberance of endogenous heat and "ministerial fire." Afternoon fever, malar flush, and heat in the chest, palms and soles are general manifestations of endogenous heat. Exuberant ministerial fire disturbs the storage of essence, causing seminal emissions. Kidney *yin* deficiency makes the resource of menstrual blood insufficient, resulting in oligomenorrhea or even amenorrhea. A reddened tongue with a scanty or no coating and a deep, thready pulse are signs of *yin* deficiency with endogenous heat.

II. Deficiency of Kidney essence

Kidney essence is a part of Kidney *yin*. Deficiency of Kidney essence is actually a special pattern of deficiency of Kidney *yin*, marked by retarded development, inability of reproduction and premature senility.

Clinical manifestations: Retarded physical and mental development of children, such as delayed closure of fontanel, short and slight stature, and poor intelligence. Oligospermia and sterility in adult male, and amenorrhea, infertility and hyposexuality in adult females. Premature senility, such as loss of hair, reduced solidity of bones, loosening of teeth, impairment of hearing with tinnitus, forgetfulness, and sluggish physical movements and mental responses.

Syndrome analysis: Kidney essence is in charge of reproduction, growth and development. That is why deficiency of Kidney essence causes the above-mentioned disturbances. The growth of hair depends upon Kidney essence, so deficiency of the latter leads to loss of hair. The Kidneys have their specific opening in the ears, and deficiency of Kidney essence brings about impaired hearing and tinnitus. The Kidneys dominate the bones, and the teeth are regarded as the odds and ends of bones. Therefore, deficiency of Kidney essence not only reduces the solidity of the bones, it also causes loosening of the teeth. The Kidneys replenish the brain with vital essence. Deficiency of Kidney essence makes the brain poorly replenished, impairing the memory, physical movements and mental responses.

Theoretically, deficiency of the Kidney essence is just a part of deficiency of Kidney *yin*. The difference between the two syndromes lies in that, if the deficiency is limited to Kidney essence but not other parts of *yin* (such as nutrients and fluids), there is no endogenous heat and the disorders are chiefly related to reproduction, growth, development and aging.

III. Deficiency of Kidney *yang*

This is often due to constitutional weakness, old age, chronic diseases involving the Kidneys and overindulgence in sex. It occurs chiefly in debility after a protracted disease, general weakness in the aged, lumbago, chronic nephritis, adrenocortical insufficiency, hypothyroidism and sexual dysfunction.

Clinical manifestations: Soreness and weakness of the back and loins, aversion to cold with cold limbs, listlessness, hyposexuality, impotence, premature ejaculation, oliguria and edema, chronic diarrhea, pale and puffy or darkened and dull complexion, pale, plump tongue with a thin, white coating, and a deep, thready pulse.

Syndrome analysis: The loins are where the Kidneys are located, and the Kidneys dominate the bones. Decline of Kidney *yang* impairs the nourishment of the bones, causing soreness and weakness in the back, particularly marked in the lumbar region. Kidney *yang* supplies vital fire (heat energy) to warm up the body. Deficient Kidney *yang* leads to slow vital fire, hence the patient is averse to cold and has cold limbs. The Kidneys are in charge of reproduction. The part of vital fire for sexual potency is called "ministerial fire." In deficiency of Kidney *yang*, the "ministerial fire" also declines, and so there is hyposexuality, impotence, or premature ejaculation.

The above are the general manifestations of Kidney *yang* deficiency. The Kidneys are also in charge of water metabolism, and supply vital fire for digestion. Deficiency of Kidney *yang* may give rise to edema and diarrhea as well, but if these disorders are prominent, the diagnosis should be specified as deficiency of Kidney *yang* with water in flood or with chronic diarrhea.

Deficiency of *yang* is usually associated with lack of vigor, and so the patient is listless. Pale and puffy complexion, pale, plump tongue with thin, white coating and deep, thready pulse are common signs consistent with *yang* deficiency. If Kidney *yang* is in a state of extreme deficiency, the turbid *yin* will infiltrate the surface of the body, making the complexion darkened and dull.

IV. Deficiency of Kidney *yang* with water in flood

This is a specific pattern of Kidney *yang* deficiency characterized by disordered water metabolism. It is chiefly encountered in nephrotic syndrome and congestive heart failure.

Clinical manifestations: General manifestations of deficiency of Kidney *yang* combined with anasarca, particularly remarkable below the waist, accompanied by oliguria and abdominal distension. Sometimes edema occurs, accompanied by cardiac palpitations, shortness of breath, orthopnea and expectoration of profuse, thin sputum, plump tongue with a thin, white or thick, greasy coating, and a deep, thready pulse.

Syndrome analysis: The Kidneys dominate the water metabolism. In deficiency of Kidney *yang*, the opening of the "sluice-valve" may be impaired, resulting in oliguria, edema and even ascites with abdominal distension. If the retained water attacks the Heart, cardiac palpitations occur as well as shortness of breath and orthopnea. Retained water may turn into phlegm, leading to profuse expectoration. A plump tongue with a thin, white coating and a deep, thready pulse indicate deficiency-cold, but excessive water-damp may also give rise to a thick, greasy coating.

V. Deficiency of Kidney *yang* with diarrhea

This is a specific pattern of Kidney *yang* deficiency marked by chronic diarrhea. It may be encountered in chronic colitis, chronic dysentery, intestinal tuberculosis, and other intestinal diseases in Western medicine.

Clinical manifestations: General manifestations of Kidney *yang* deficiency combined with chronic diarrhea, usually occurring daily before dawn, aggravated by exposure to cold, and accompanied by a cold sensation and pain in the abdomen and borborygmi, which are alleviated after defecation; pale and plump tongue with a thin, white coating, and a deep, thready and weak pulse.

Syndrome analysis: Spleen digestion needs vital fire (Kidney *yang*) as its motive force. Deficiency of Kidney *yang* may impair the digestion, causing diarrhea with loose stools or stools containing undigested food. Deficiency of *yang* leads to relative exuberance of *yin* with endogenous cold, and so there is a cold sensation in the abdomen. Cold may cause stagnation of *qi* in the intestines, and hence abdominal pain and borborygmi. After defecation the stagnation is reduced, so pain and borborygmi are alleviated. According to the theory of *yin-yang*, day pertains to *yang* and night to *yin*. After nightfall, *yin* is rising and *yang* declining until dawn. At the period just before dawn, *yang* declines to its extreme, and so diarrhea due to Kidney *yang* deficiency usually occurs at this period. A pale and plump tongue with a thin, white coating, and a deep, thready and weak pulse are signs of *yang* deficiency.

VI. Failure of the Kidneys to receive air

This is a deficiency syndrome of Kidney *qi*. Kidney *qi* helps the Lungs receive air. Impairment of this function often happens when Kidney *qi* is injured after chronic coughing, repeated attacks of asthma and other conditions, such as senility. This syndrome may appear in pulmonary emphysema, pulmonary heart disease, and respiratory insufficiency in the aged.

Clinical manifestations: Chronic coughing and asthma, dyspnea characterized by prolonged exhalation and aggravation on mild exertion, accompanied by spontaneous sweating, listlessness, feeble voice, weakness and soreness of the loins and knees, pale tongue with a white coating, and a deep, weak pulse.

Syndrome analysis: The syndrome is *qi* deficiency due to Kidney insufficiency. Although the Lungs are in charge of respiration, the Kidneys help the Lungs receive air. Both impairment of the Lungs and insufficiency of the Kidneys may cause dyspnea. Dyspnea originating from the Lungs is manifested by difficulty in inhalation, while dyspnea due to insufficiency of the Kidneys is marked by prolonged exhalation. Weakness and soreness of the loins and knees is a common symptom caused by insufficiency of the Kidneys. The other symptoms, such as spontaneous sweating, listlessness and a feeble voice are common symptoms indicating general deficiency of *qi*. A pale tongue with a white coating, and a deep, weak pulse are also signs of *qi* deficiency.

VII. Unconsolidation of Kidney qi (Failure of the Kidneys to retain substances)

This is a deficiency syndrome of Kidney *qi* with failure in the retaining function (controlling discharge of urine, sperm, etc.). It happens in the aged with the decline of Kidney *qi*, in children with inadequateness of Kidney *qi*, and in those whose Kidney *qi* is impaired by excessive sexual activity or chronic consumption.

Clinical manifestations: Pallor, listlessness, impaired hearing, weakness and soreness of the loins and knees; frequent discharge of clear urine, dribbling of urine after urination, enuresis, incontinence of urine, or nocturia; spermatorrhea and premature ejaculation in men, and profuse thin leukorrhea and tendency to miscarry in women; pale tongue with a white coating and a deep, weak pulse.

Syndrome analysis: Pallor, listlessness, pale tongue with a white coating and a deep, weak pulse are general symptoms and signs of *qi* deficiency. The Kidneys are closely related to the ears. Supplies of *qi* and blood to the ears will be inadequate when Kidney *qi* is insufficient, and hence the hearing is impaired. Kidney *qi* controls the functions of the Bladder. Weakness of Kidney *qi* gives rise to frequent urination, or incontinence of urine. If the micturition ability is weak, urine cannot be completely discharged, and so dribbling of urine occurs after urination. In children, Kidney *qi* is not well developed, and the brain is not fully replenished by the vital essence. Therefore, infants have enuresis; even teenagers, if their natural endowment is inadequate, may have nocturnal enuresis. At night, *yin* becomes exuberant and *yang* declines, and so those with insufficient Kidney *qi* have nocturia. Storage of essence in the Kidneys is done by Kidney *qi*. If Kidney *qi* is insufficient, the discharge of essence becomes easier, and hence occurs spermatorrhea or premature ejaculation. The Belt and Conception vessels are also controlled and nourished by Kidney *qi*. If the Belt Vessel is out of control, there will be profuse, thin leukorrhea; if the Conception Vessel is poorly nourished, there will be a tendency to miscarry.

Syndromes Involving Two *Zang-fu* Organs

Because of the correlations between *zang-fu* organs, diseases involving two or more organs are not infrequently seen. Following are some of the syndromes involving two organs commonly encountered clinically.

I. Incoordination of the Heart and the Kidneys

This is often caused by impairment of *yin* in chronic diseases, overindulgence in sex, too much worrying or emotional depression. It may be encountered in anxiety states, anemia and chronic consumptive diseases.

Clinical manifestations: Insomnia, palpitations, fidgetiness, dizziness, tinnitus, hypomnesis, soreness of the loins, nocturnal emission, heat in the chest, palms and soles, dryness of the throat and mouth; reddened tongue and a thready, rapid pulse.

Syndrome analysis: Normally, Heart fire (*yang*) comes down to warm the Kidneys and the Kidney water (*yin*) goes up to irrigate the Heart. Breakdown of this balanced condition is called "incoordination of the Heart and the Kidneys," which is characterized by insomnia accompanied by exuberance of Heart fire (manifested by fidgetiness and palpitations) and deficiency of Kidney *yin* (manifested by dizziness, tinnitus and hypomnesis due to inadequate replenishing of the marrow and brain). The basic pathological change of this syndrome is deficiency of *yin* with exuberant fire. Since the fire is of the deficiency type, it causes feverishness in the chest, palms and soles, dryness of the throat and mouth, reddened tongue, and thready, rapid pulse. When the storage of reproductive essence is disturbed by the fire, there is nocturnal emission. The loins are the seat where the Kidneys are located. Soreness of the loins signifies that the Kidneys are involved in the syndrome.

II. Deficiency of both the Heart and the Spleen

This is a combined syndrome of deficient Heart blood and weakened Spleen *qi*. It is usually due to consumption of *qi* and blood in chronic diseases, over-strain, too much worrying and chronic bleeding, and can be encountered clinically in anxiety states, menstrual disorders, anemia and various chronic diseases.

Clinical manifestations: Palpitations, insomnia, dream-disturbed sleep, dizziness, forgetfulness, sallow complexion, anorexia, abdominal distension, loose stools, lassitude, or incessant dripping of small amounts of pink menstrual discharge in women; pale, plump tongue, and a thready, weak pulse.

Syndrome analysis: The Spleen serves as "the source of nutrients for generating *qi* and blood," and has the function of keeping the blood flowing within blood vessels. When Spleen *qi* is deficient, there will be inadequate generation of blood or discharge of blood out of the blood vessels; either of them may cause insufficiency of Heart blood. On the other hand, the Heart governs blood circulation, supplying blood to the Spleen. Deficiency of Heart blood may also bring about deficiency of Spleen *qi*. Therefore, the two pathological conditions may influence each other, forming a combined deficiency of both Heart blood and Spleen *qi*.

Palpitations, insomnia, dream-disturbed sleep, dizziness, and forgetfulness are symptoms indicating deficiency of Heart blood. Sallow complexion, anorexia, abdominal distension, loose stools, and lassitude are manifestations of diminished Spleen function in transportation and transformation, and incessant dripping of small amount of menstrual discharge is due to diminished Spleen function in keeping the blood flowing within the blood vessels. A pale, plump tongue and a thready, weak pulse are signs of deficiency of both *qi* and blood.

III. *Qi* deficiency of the Heart and the Lungs

This is a syndrome of *qi* deficiency involving both the Heart and the Lungs, usually due to chronic cough that consumes *qi* from the two organs, or due to a weak constitution or old age. It may be encountered in pulmonary heart disease, atherosclerotic heart disease, and cardio-pulmonary insufficiency in the aged.

Clinical manifestations: Palpitations, cough, dyspnea and shortness of breath, aggravated by mild exertion; expectoration of thin sputum and feeling of fullness in the chest; pallor, general weakness, dizziness, listlessness, spontaneous sweating, and feeble voice; pale tongue with a white coating, and deep, weak or irregular pulse.

Syndrome analysis: The Lungs are in charge of respiration, and the Heart in charge of blood circulation. Both of them depend on the action of pectoral *qi*. Diminished function of the Lungs leads to inadequate generation of pectoral *qi*, so that Heart *qi* is insufficient. On the other hand, diminished function of the Heart consumes more pectoral *qi*, and Lung *qi* will also be impaired. Either condition will finally result in *qi* deficiency of both organs.

Coughing, dyspnea, and shortness of breath aggravated on mild exertion are manifestations indicating deficiency of Lung *qi*. Palpitations and irregular pulse are caused by deficiency of Heart *qi*. Diminished dispersing function of the Lungs leads to accumulation of fluids, which turn to be phlegm, bringing about fullness sensation in the chest and expectoration of thin sputum. Pallor, general weakness, dizziness, listlessness, spontaneous sweating, feeble voice, pale tongue with a white coating, and a deep, weak pulse are common symptoms and signs of *qi* deficiency.

IV. *Yin* deficiency of the Liver and the Kidneys

This is a combined deficiency syndrome of Liver *yin* and Kidney yin. Clinically, it may be encountered in anemia, hypertension, chronic hepatitis, anxiety states, Ménière's disease, and menstrual disorders.

Clinical manifestations: Vertigo, blurred vision, tinnitus, irritability, irascibility, weakness and soreness of the loins and knees, hypochondriac pain, hot sensation in the chest, palms and soles, malar flush, night sweating, seminal emission in men and oligomenorrhea or amenorrhea in women, reddened tongue with scanty coating, and a thready, rapid pulse.

Syndrome analysis: The mutual promotion of *yin* between the Liver and the Kidneys is so close that the two organs are said to have the same source. If Liver *yin* is abundant, the surplus *yin* is stored in the Kidneys, and if Kidney *yin* is abundant, it constantly nourishes the Liver. In addition, the essence (pertaining to *yin*) stored in the Kidneys and the blood (pertaining to *yin*) stored in the Liver are mutually convertible. Therefore, deficiency of the *yin* of one is often accompanied by deficiency of the *yin* of the other.

Deficiency of Liver *yin* usually leads to exuberance of Liver *yang*, which, going upwards, causes vertigo, blurred vision, tinnitus, and irascibility. It also brings about pain along the Liver Meridian, particularly in the hypochondriac regions. Deficiency of Kidney *yin* leads to generation of endogenous heat and exuberance of endogenous fire ("ministerial fire"), resulting in malar flush, and heat in the chest, palms and soles, and night sweating. If the exuberant ministerial fire agitates the reproductive essence in men, there will be seminal emissions. In women, deficiency of the Liver and Kidney *yin* empties the Thoroughfare and Conception vessels, resulting in oligomenorrhea. A reddened tongue with scanty coating and a thready, rapid pulse are signs of *yin* deficiency.

V. Disharmony of the Liver and the Spleen

This is a combined syndrome of stagnation of Liver *qi* and impaired transporting and transforming function of the Spleen. If stagnation of Liver *qi* is primary, it is usually caused by emotional depression with anger, which injures the Liver; if dysfunction of the Spleen is primary, it is usually due to improper diet or over-strain that injures the Spleen. Clinically, it is often encountered in functional gastro-intestinal disorders, hepatitis, liver cirrhosis, peptic ulcer, chronic gastritis, and other chronic digestive diseases.

Clinical manifestations: Distension, fullness and shifting pain in the chest and hypochondrium, frequent sighing, low spiritedness or irascibility, anorexia, abdominal distension, loose stools, borborygmi with flatus, or abdominal pain which is alleviated after diarrhea; white or greasy tongue coating, and a stringy pulse.

Syndrome analysis: Distension, fullness and shifting pain in the chest and hypochondrium, frequent sighing, low spiritedness or irascibility are caused by stagnation of Liver *qi*. Anorexia, abdominal distension, loose stools, borborygmi with flatus, or abdominal pain which is alleviated after diarrhea indicate impairment of the transporting and transforming function of the Spleen. Abdominal pain is due to stagnation of *qi* in the abdomen. After defecation the stagnated *qi* is removed and hence the abdominal pain is relieved. Stagnated Liver *qi* tends to impair the Spleen function. This is called "wood overchecks earth" according to the five elements theory. On the other hand, dysfunction of the Spleen in transportation and transformation often causes stagnation of *qi* and damp in the Middle Energizer, which may also impair the function of the Liver in smoothing and regulating the flow of *qi*. This is called "earth counterchecks wood." Since there is no marked manifestation of heat or fire, the tongue coating is white, but it may be greasy because of accumulation of damp due to dysfunction of the Spleen. A stringy pulse is a sign showing the stagnation of Liver *qi*.

VI. Disharmony of the Liver and the Stomach

This is a combined syndrome of stagnation of Liver *qi* and dysfunction of the Stomach. It may be caused by emotional depression with transformation of stagnant *qi* into fire, or due to invasion of the Liver and the Stomach by exogenous pathogenic factors. It occurs in hepatitis, cirrhosis of the liver, peptic ulcer and chronic gastritis as well as other gastric diseases.

Clinical manifestations: Epigastric and hypochondriac distension and pain, belching, hiccuping, acid regurgitation, gastric distress, irritability and irascibility, reddened tongue with a thin, yellow coating, and a stringy or stringy and rapid pulse.

Syndrome analysis: When stagnant Liver *qi* is transformed into fire, which impairs the Stomach, epigastric and hypochondriac distension and pain ensue. Disturbance in the descending function of the Stomach leads to upward perversion of Stomach *qi*, manifested by belching and hiccuping. Stagnation of *qi* and fire in the Liver and the Stomach causes gastric distress and acid regurgitation. Dysfunction of the Liver in smoothing and regulating the flow of *qi* is often manifested by irritability and irascibility. A reddened tongue with a thin, yellow coating, and a stringy, rapid pulse indicate stagnation of *qi* with transformed fire.

VII. *Yang* deficiency of the Spleen and Kidneys

This is a syndrome of *yang* deficiency involving both the Spleen and the Kidneys. It occurs in chronic diarrhea or edema either with deficiency of Kidney *yang* or with deficiency of Spleen *yang* as the primary disorder. Over the course of the disease, insufficient Kidney *yang* will fail to warm the Spleen or insufficient Spleen *yang* will fail to nourish the Kidneys, resulting in a combined syndrome with *yang* deficiency of both organs. Clinically, this syndrome is often encountered in chronic colitis, ulcerative colitis, intestinal tuberculosis, nephrotic syndrome, liver cirrhosis with ascites, and other diseases in Western medicine.

Clinical manifestations: Pale and puffy complexion, aversion to cold with cold limbs, lower abdominal pain with cold feeling, chronic diarrhea with mucous or bloody stools, or stools containing undigested food, occurring daily before dawn; or generalized edema with oliguria, and distension of the abdomen with accumulation of fluid. Pale, plump tongue with a white, slippery coating, and a deep, thready pulse.

Syndrome analysis: The Spleen provides the material basis of the acquired constitution. Its transporting and transforming functions depend upon the warming action of the vital fire, i.e., Kidney *yang*. The Kidneys are the foundation of the inborn constitution. All its functions also need supplies of nutrients from the Spleen. Therefore, chronic deficiency of Spleen *yang* will involve the function of the Kidneys, and chronic deficiency of Kidney *yang* will impair the function of the Spleen (the latter is called "failure of fire to promote earth"), thus forming a combined syndrome of *yang* deficiency involving both organs. Pale and puffy complexion and aversion to cold with cold limbs are general manifestations of *yang* deficiency.

VIII. *Yin* deficiency of the Lungs and Kidneys

This is a syndrome of *yin* deficiency involving both the Lungs and the Kidneys. It occurs either due to chronic coughing, which impairs the Lungs, with involvement of the Kidneys, or due to overindulgence in sex, causing deficiency of Kidney *yin* with involvement of the Lungs. Clinically, it may be encountered in pulmonary tuberculosis and other consumptive diseases.

Clinical manifestations: Coughing with scanty expectoration or hemoptysis, emaciation, soreness and weakness of the loins and knees, hectic fever, malar flush, night sweating, dryness of the throat and mouth or hoarseness of voice, seminal emissions in men and menstrual disorders in women, reddened tongue with scanty coating, and thready, rapid pulse.

Syndrome analysis: The Lungs nourish the Kidneys with *yin*-fluid, and vice versa. This is called "metal and water promote each other." Therefore, either deficiency of Lung *yin* or deficiency of Kidney *yin* may develop into *yin* deficiency in both organs. Thus, a combined symptom-complex appears (cf. "Deficiency of Lung yin" and "Deficiency of Kidney *yin*").

IX. *Qi* deficiency of the Spleen and Lungs

This may be due to chronic coughing, which consumes Lung *qi*, with the Spleen involved or due to improper diet or over-strain, which damage the Spleen with inadequate transportation of essence to the Lungs. Clinically, it may occur in chronic bronchitis, pulmonary emphysema and other chronic respiratory diseases.

Clinical manifestations: Chronic coughing and shortness of breath with profuse frothy expectoration, anorexia, abdominal distension, loose stools, lassitude, lack of strength, pale and puffy complexion or even edema; pale tongue with a white coating and a thready, weak pulse.

Syndrome analysis: It is a combined syndrome of deficiency of Lung *qi* and deficiency of Spleen *qi*. Chronic coughing and shortness of breath are caused by deficiency of Lung *qi*, and anorexia, abdominal distension, loose stools, puffy complexion and edema are due to deficiency of Spleen *qi*. A pale tongue with a white coating and a thready, weak pulse are common signs of *qi* deficiency.

The profuse frothy expectoration may come from the diseased Spleen, as damp due to the impaired transporting function of the Spleen may be condensed to phlegm. However, the phlegm may also be formed in the Lungs. When Lung *qi* is insufficient, its dispersing function will be impaired and fluids will accumulate and be condensed to phlegm.

X. Attack on the Lungs by Liver fire

The fire that attacks the Lungs may be due to anger that injures the Liver or heat in the Liver Meridian which rises adversely. It may be encountered in hypertension, bronchitis and anxiety disorders.

Clinical manifestations: Burning pain in the chest and hypochondriac region, irritability and irascibility, dizziness, redness of the eyes, restlessness, bitterness in the mouth, paroxysms of coughing with scanty sticky yellow sputum, or even hemoptysis; reddened tongue with a thin, yellow coating, and a stringy, rapid pulse.

Syndrome analysis: The fire transformed from stagnant Liver *qi* causes a burning pain in the hypochondrium and chest. Irritability and irascibility indicate dysfunction of the Liver in smoothing and regulating the flow of *qi*. Up-flaming of Liver fire gives rise to dizziness, redness of the eyes and bitterness in the mouth. Restlessness is due to stagnation of *qi* and fire in the interior. Liver fire forces Lung *qi* to ascend perversely, resulting in coughing, and condenses the fluid to scanty yellow phlegm. If a blood vessel in the Lungs is injured by fire, there will be hemoptysis. A reddened tongue with a thin, yellow coating, and a stringy, rapid pulse indicate flaming of Liver fire in the interior.

DIFFERENTIATION OF SYNDROMES ACCORDING TO THE AFFECTED MERIDIANS

Exogenous pathogenic factors invading the human body may go through the meridians deep into the internal organs. At the same time, pathological changes in the interior often have their reflection on the superficial portion of the body through the meridians. Determination of the affected meridians can be taken as an additional diagnosis supplementary to the pathological changes of internal (*zang-fu*) organs, and is particularly useful in acupuncture treatment. Each meridian has its own clinical manifestations when it is affected. For example, impairment of the Kidney Meridian is liable to cause the patient to be nervous, flustered and scared, and impairment of the Lung Meridian is marked by a sensation of fullness in the chest and supraclavicular pain. Coughing with dyspnea is a common symptom when the Lung Meridian is affected, but it can also occur when the Kidney Meridian is impaired because the main branch of the Kidney Meridian travels through the liver and diaphragm, enters the lungs and follows the trachea and larynx to the base of the tongue. Therefore, if a person complains of coughing with dyspnea accompanied by a sensation of fullness in the chest, a diagnosis of affection of the Lung Meridian can be made, but if a patient complains of cough and dyspnea associated with terror of his life, impairment of the Kidney Meridian should be considered.

It should be noted that the clinical manifestations in the case of affection of meridians are sometimes quite different from those described under the category of pathological changes of internal organs. The symptoms caused by the affected meridian are not confined to the internal organs that the meridian pertains to, but are more likely to be related to the course along which the meridian runs. For example, in the syndrome differentiation of internal organs, a deficiency condition of the Kidneys is often manifested by dull aching and weakness in the loins as the loins are where the Kidneys are located, but severe lumbago which makes one unable to turn over or sit up is usually attributed to the affection of the Bladder and Liver Meridians, for the Bladder Meridian and a branch of the Liver Meridian meet in the lower back.

I. Affection of the Lung Meridian (the Hand-*Taiyin* Meridian)

Clinical manifestations: Coughing, dyspnea, feeling of oppression and fullness in the chest; pain in the supraclavicular fossa; pain or coldness in the shoulder and back accompanied by shortness of breath, chills, fever, and spontaneous sweating; pain of the antero-lateral aspect of the arm.

II. Affection of the Large Intestine Meridian (the Hand-*Yangming* Meridian)

Clinical manifestations: Toothache, inflammation of the pharynx, swelling of the neck, and epistaxis; pain of the thumb, the index finger and the shoulder.

III. Affection of the Stomach Meridian (the Foot-*Yangming* Meridian)

Clinical manifestations: Fever, more marked in the ventral side of the body; nasal pain, epistaxis, toothache, sore throat and swelling of the neck; facial paralysis; pain along the regions which the Stomach Meridian traverses in the chest, abdomen and lower extremities; and numbness of the middle toe.

IV. Affection of the Spleen Meridian (the Foot-*Taiyin* Meridian)

Clinical manifestations: Epigastric pain and abdominal distension with vomiting after meals and frequent belching; anorexia and loose stools; jaundice; stiffness of the tongue; pain and swelling of the inner aspect of the thigh and knee, and numbness of the great toe.

V. Affection of the Heart Meridian (the Hand-*Shaoyin* Meridian)

Clinical manifestations: Precordial pain with dryness of the throat and thirst; pain of the medial aspect of the arm and in the lateral pectoral region, and burning pain in the palms.

VI. Affection of the Small Intestine Meridian (the Hand-*Taiyang* Meridian)

Clinical manifestations: Sore throat with swelling of the lateral aspect of the neck, which makes it difficult to turn the head; deafness; pain in the neck, shoulder, elbow, and the posterior aspect of the arm.

VII. Affection of the Bladder Meridian (the Foot-*Taiyang* Meridian)

Clinical manifestations: Chills and fever with stuffed-up nose and headache; eye ailments; severe lumbago as if there were a fracture of the lumbar spine, pain in the leg and foot, and numbness of the small toe.

VIII. Affection of the Kidney Meridian (the Foot-*Shaoyin* Meridian)

Clinical manifestations: Feeling hungry but no desire for food, and dark complexion; dyspnea and hemoptysis accompanied by palpitations and liability to be frightened; hot sensation in the mouth, dryness of the tongue and sore throat; pain of the back and inner aspect of the thigh; and feverish sensation in the soles.

IX. Affection of the Pericardium Meridian (the Hand-*Jueyin* Meridian)

Clinical manifestations: Feverish sensation of the palms, muscle spasms in the forearm and elbow, swelling of the axilla; fullness in the chest and lateral pectoral region; palpitations with fidgetiness, incessant laughing, and precordial pain.

X. Affection of the Triple Energizer Meridian (the Hand-*Shaoyang* Meridian)

Clinical manifestations: Abdominal distension, edema and oliguria; deafness; pain in the post-auricular region, and the lateral aspect of the shoulder, arm and elbow; numbness or paralysis of the little finger and ring finger.

XI. Affection of the Gallbladder Meridian (the Foot-*Shaoyang* Meridian)

Clinical manifestations: Bitterness in the mouth; frequent sighing; chest pain aggravated by turning over; migraine, supraclavicular and subaxillary pain, and pain along the regions which the Gallbladder Meridian traverses in the chest, side of the trunk, and lateral aspect of the lower extremities; and numbness in the fourth and little toes.

XII. Affection of the Liver Meridian (the Foot-*Jueyin* Meridian)

Clinical manifestations: Severe lumbago which makes the patient unable to sit up; enuresis or retention of urine; nausea, vomiting and diarrhea; hernia; and gynecological pains.

XIII. Affection of the Governor Vessel

Clinical manifestations: Syncope; headache; lumbago; opisthotonos.

XIV. Affection of the Conception Vessel

Clinical manifestations: Hernia in men, and leukorrhea and mass in the lower abdomen in women.

XV. Affection of the Thoroughfare Vessel

Clinical manifestations: Adverse flow of *qi* from the inguinal region to the chest.

XVI. Affection of the Belt Vessel

Clinical manifestations: Abdominal distension, and aching and weakness in the lower back; leukorrhea in women.

XVII. Affection of the *Yang*-Link and *Yin*-Link Vessels

Clinical manifestations: Chills and fever when the *Yang*-Link Vessel is affected, and precordial pain when the *Yin*-Link Vessel is affected.

XVIII. Affection of the *Yang*-Heel and *Yin*-Heel Vessels

Clinical manifestations: Muscle flaccidity of the medial aspect of the lower extremity with spasm of the lateral aspect when *Yang*-Heel Vessel is affected; muscle flaccidity of the lateral aspect of the lower extremity with spasm of the medial aspect when the *Yin*-Heel Vessel is affected.

DIFFERENTIATION OF SYNDROMES ACCORDING TO *WEI*, *QI*, *YING* AND *XUE*

This paradigm of syndrome differentiation is only available for epidemic febrile diseases. *Wei*, *qi*, *ying* and *xue* are the names of four systems in the human body, arranged from the superficial to the deep portions. *Wei* means superficial defense. In an exogenous affection, this system is first invaded, manifested by an exterior syndrome. *Qi* means energy. When the *qi* system is invaded, the pathogen has already penetrated interiorly and there is usually vigorous resistance of the human body. *Ying* means nutritive or constructive substances, which circulate within the blood vessels, and so *ying* and blood are sometimes called jointly *ying*-blood. When the *ying* system is invaded by pathogens, the condition is serious. *Xue* is blood. Impairment of the blood system is often seen in the severest stage of an epidemic febrile disease.

I. Syndromes of the *wei* (superficial defense) system

Affection of the *wei* system is seen in the initial stage of an epidemic febrile disease when only the superficial defense *qi* is involved, and can be generally classified into the following syndrome patterns according to different pathogens as well as the constitutions of the patient:

(1) Exterior syndrome of wind-heat

This is an exterior syndrome caused by pathogenic wind-heat. The syndrome may appear in the initial stage of influenza, upper respiratory infection, acute tonsillitis, acute pharyngitis, pneumonia and measles.

Clinical manifestations: Fever with mild chills, mild thirst, coughing, sore throat, reddened tip of the tongue with a thin, white or yellowish coating, and a floating, rapid pulse.

Syndrome analysis: Attack of pathogenic wind-heat on the exterior portion of the body causes an exterior heat syndrome, as manifested by fever with mild chills, and a floating, rapid pulse. Mild thirst is due to consumption of body fluids by pathogenic heat even at the beginning of the disease. The Lungs are closely related to superficial defensive *qi*, so there are usually some upper respiratory symptoms such as coughing, sore throat and reddened tip of the tongue.

(2) Exterior syndrome of dryness-heat

This is an exterior syndrome of a febrile disease marked clinically by dryness and heat. Upper respiratory infections or acute bronchitis occurring in a dry season or in patients suffering from *yin* deficiency may show this syndrome in the early stage.

Clinical manifestations: Fever with mild aversion to wind and cold, coughing with no expectoration, dryness of the mouth and throat, thirst, slightly reddened tongue with a thin coating, and a floating, thready and rapid pulse.

Syndrome analysis: Besides the manifestations of exterior heat, symptoms showing dryness (such as dry cough, dry mouth and dry throat) are prominent features. A thready pulse is more frequently found in patients with a constitution marked by *yin* deficiency.

(3) Exterior syndrome of damp-heat

This is an exterior syndrome of an epidemic febrile disease caused by pathogenic damp-heat. It may be encountered in the early stage of influenza in a rainy season, or in cases of Salmonella infection and infectious hepatitis.

Clinical manifestations: Recessive fever, more marked in the afternoon, mild sweating which brings no relief to fever, slight aversion to wind and cold, stuffiness in the chest, heavy sensation in the head and general aching, white and greasy tongue coating, and a thready, soft pulse.

Syndrome analysis: Besides the manifestations of exterior heat, there are symptoms showing dampness. The fever is said to be "recessive," as the patient has a marked feeling of feverishness, but his skin is not so hot to the touch. This is because the spreading of heat to the body surface is stemmed by damp. Sensation of heaviness is another feature of damp affection. Damp also impedes the flow of *qi* in the chest, giving rise to a feeling of stuffiness. Both the greasy tongue coating and the soft pulse are common signs indicating the presence of damp.

II. Syndromes of the *qi* (energy) system

Affection of the *qi* system occurs in the second stage of an epidemic febrile disease when the pathogen has entered the interior of the body: the Lungs, the Stomach and the Large Intestine. At this stage, both the action of the pathogens and the reaction of the body resistance (defensive *qi*) are vigorous. Therefore, there is high fever, and no more chills or aversion to cold. Affection of the *qi* system can be classified into the following syndrome patterns according to the different pathogens and the *zang-fu* organs affected by the pathogens.

(1) Exuberant heat in the *qi* system

Clinical manifestations: High fever, profuse sweating, dire thirst and gigantic (full and forceful) pulse, associated with restlessness, aversion to heat, flushed face, desire for cold drinks, and a dry, yellow tongue coating.

Syndrome analysis: High fever with gigantic pulse is due to vigorous reaction of the human body against the pathogens. High fever persisting with profuse sweating is a characteristic feature showing exuberant heat (*yang*) in the interior, which forces the discharge of body fluid out of the body as sweat. The latter is called "hot sweat" in traditional Chinese medicine in order to distinguish it from "cold sweat"—profuse sweat due to prostration of *yang*, as seen in shock. Both high fever and profuse sweating consume body fluids, and so there is dire thirst with a desire for cold drinks, and a dry, yellow tongue coating.

(2) Accumulation of heat in the Lungs

This is an interior syndrome due to invasion of the Lungs by pathogenic heat, and may be encountered clinically in pulmonary infections such as lobar pneumonia and bronchopneumonia.

Clinical manifestations: Fever with no aversion to cold, chest pain, cough, dyspnea, expectoration of thick, yellow sputum, thirst, concentrated urine, yellow tongue coating with reddened tip and edges of the tongue, and a slippery, rapid pulse.

Syndrome analysis: In an exterior heat syndrome, the upper part of the Lungs may be involved, manifested by coughing and sore throat. In the present syndrome, however, the pathogen has already gone deep into the Lungs, and there is no more exterior syndrome as manifested by aversion to cold. Heat accumulated in the Lungs is apt to condense the fluid into phlegm. Pathogenic heat and phlegm induce coughing, dyspnea and expectoration of thick, yellow sputum. The other symptoms and signs all indicate the presence of pathogenic heat and phlegm.

(3) Impaction of heat in the Stomach and Large Intestine

In this syndrome excessive pathogenic heat induces impaction of fecal masses in the intestines. In some acute infectious diseases, when the fever is accompanied by abdominal pain and tenderness, this syndrome should be considered. In addition, it may also be found in some cases of ileus.

Clinical manifestations: Fever, higher in the afternoon, aversion to heat, flushed face and congested eyes, constipation or fecal impaction with watery discharge, abdominal distension and pain with tenderness, restlessness or even delirium, reddened tongue with a dry, yellow or grey prickle-like coating, and a deep, rapid and forceful pulse.

Syndrome analysis: The syndrome is characterized by excessive pathogenic heat in the interior with fecal impaction in the intestines. Fever, aversion to heat, flushed face, congested eyes, and the changes to the tongue all indicate the presence of excessive heat. Restlessness or delirium is due to disturbance of mental activities by heat. Fecal impaction in the intestines brings about constipation, abdominal distension and pain with tenderness. But in some cases, the constipation is accompanied by discharge of foul liquid, which might be mistaken for diarrhea. In fact, the liquid is produced due to the stimulation of the large intestine by the hard fecal masses. The deep, rapid and forceful pulse signifies an interior heat syndrome of excess type.

(4) Damp-heat in the *qi* system

This is an interior syndrome occurring when the *qi* system is invaded by pathogenic damp-heat which not only causes fever, but also impedes the normal flow of *qi*. Patients with typhoid fever, Salmonella infection, or infectious hepatitis may show this syndrome at a certain stage.

Clinical manifestations: Recessive fever, higher in the afternoon, accompanied by anorexia, lassitude, heaviness feeling of the body, stuffiness sensation in the chest, abdominal distension and fullness, thirst but no desire for drink, reddened tongue with a yellow, greasy coating, and a soft pulse.

Syndrome analysis: In this syndrome, besides manifestations indicating the presence of heat, there are damp symptoms such as lassitude, a feeling of heaviness, greasy tongue coating and soft pulse. As mentioned in the "exterior syndrome of damp-heat," recessive fever is a specific pattern of fever due to damp-heat. Damp is apt to impede the normal flow of *qi*. When this occurs in the chest, a feeling of stuffiness is brought on; when it occurs in the Spleen, there is abdominal distension or fullness. Thirst but no desire for drink is a pathognomonic symptom for damp in the Spleen and the Stomach. Disturbance in distribution of fluids throughout the body or impairment of fluids by heat leads to thirst, but retention of damp in the Spleen and the Stomach makes one unwilling to take more fluid.

III. Syndromes of the *ying* (nutrient) system

In traditional Chinese medicine, *ying* refers to nutritive and constructive substances circulating in the blood vessels. Affection of the *ying* system is either developed from an affection of the *qi* system, or directly transformed from an affection of the *wei* system. In an epidemic febrile disease at this stage, the patient is seriously ill, often with some mental derangement, as *ying* circulates in the blood vessels which connect with the Heart. In some cases, the Pericardium may be directly invaded by the pathogens. Therefore, affection of the *ying* system can be classified into the following two syndrome patterns:

(1) Heat in the *ying* system

This is a syndrome caused by invasion of the *ying* system by heat pathogens. There may be some disturbance of the mental activities, but no direct invasion of the Pericardium by the pathogens. Many acute infectious diseases and some blood diseases such as leukemia and aplastic anemia at the late stage may show this syndrome.

Clinical manifestations: Fever, higher at night, restlessness or delirium, slight thirst, faint skin rashes, crimson tongue with no coating, and a thready, rapid pulse.

Syndrome analysis: *Ying* is a kind of fluid-*yin*. The pathogenic heat entering the *ying* system, steams *ying* up to the mouth, so the patient does not feel very thirsty. Since *ying* circulates in the blood vessels, communicating with the Heart, pathogenic heat in the *ying* system is apt to disturb the normal function of the Heart, leading to restlessness or even delirium. A crimson tongue and a thready, rapid pulse also reflect consumption of *ying* by heat. When the pathogenic heat injures small blood vessels, faint rashes appear.

(2) Heat entering the Pericardium

This syndrome is often due to penetration of heat pathogens directly from the *wei* system into the *ying* system, invading the Heart. But since the Heart is surrounded by the Pericardium for protection, the Pericardium is usually first attacked by the pathogens when they come from the exterior portion of the body (from the *wei* system). Therefore, the name of the syndrome is assigned to the Pericardium. This syndrome may be encountered in epidemic febrile diseases at a very serious stage.

Clinical manifestations: High fever with impaired consciousness, delirium or even coma, dry and retracted crimson tongue, curling and stiff, difficulty in speaking, and a rapid pulse, thready or slippery.

Syndrome analysis: Pathogenic heat deep in the interior may act on the body fluids, transforming them into phlegm. The Pericardium is actually a part of the Heart. Impairment of the Pericardium by phlegm-heat leads to impairment of consciousness and mental confusion, or even coma, as the Heart is in charge of mental activities. The affection may cause retraction of the tongue with difficulty in speaking, for the tongue is specifically related to the Heart. A dry, crimson tongue with a thready rapid pulse indicates affection of the *ying* system by pathogenic heat. If the phlegm is conspicuous, the pulse is rapid and slippery.

The difference between the above two syndromes lies in that the impairment of consciousness is more marked when the Pericardium is invaded by pathogens.

IV. Syndromes of the *xue* (blood) system

Generally speaking, affection of the blood system refers to epidemic febrile diseases at the critical stage developed from affection of the *qi* and *ying* systems when the vital essence, blood and body fluids are all seriously impaired. But in some cases, the pathogens may directly invade the blood system. The following syndrome patterns may be seen in affections of the blood system.

(1) Heat in the blood with bleeding

The syndrome is characterized by high fever with impaired consciousness and bleeding. It may be seen in some acute infectious diseases (e.g., epidemic hemorrhagic fever) and blood diseases.

Clinical manifestations: High fever, purple patches on the skin (ecchymosis or purpura), various kinds of bleeding (such as hemoptysis, hematemesis, epistaxis, hematuria and hematochezia), impaired consciousness or delirium, crimson tongue and thready, rapid pulse.

Syndrome analysis: When pathogenic heat invades the *ying*-blood system, impaired consciousness and bleeding ensue. The latter is due to adverse flow of blood forced by pathogenic heat. Ecchymosis or purpura is also a kind of bleeding—subcutaneous extravasation. Owing to impairment of *ying*-blood by heat, the pulse is rapid and thready.

(2) Heat in the blood with stirring-up of wind

The syndrome is marked by high fever accompanied by wind symptoms (convulsions or opisthotonos). It may be seen in patients with epidemic encephalitis and meningitis, or in infants suffering from high fever.

Clinical manifestations: Fever accompanied by restlessness, thirst, headache, dizziness, crimson tongue and a stringy, rapid pulse, in combination with impaired consciousness and convulsions or opisthotonos.

Syndrome analysis: The Liver stores blood. Extreme heat in blood may impair the Liver, producing wind symptoms, manifested by convulsions or opisthotonos.

(3) Intense heat in both the *qi* (energy) and *xue* (blood) systems

This syndrome appears when the pathogenic heat has already entered the blood system before the heat in the *qi* (energy) system has been relieved.

Clinical manifestations: High fever with sweating, restlessness, thirst, purpura or other kinds of bleeding, crimson tongue with a yellow coating, and a rapid pulse.

Syndrome analysis: This seems to be a combined syndrome of heat in the *qi* and blood systems.

V. Impairment of *yin* by heat

This category of pathological changes may be found during the course of epidemic febrile diseases as complications or in their convalescence period.

(1) Impairment of fluids in the Lungs and Stomach

Clinical manifestations: Dry throat, dry mouth, and dry cough with no expectoration, sometimes accompanied by fever; dry, reddened tongue, and thready, rapid pulse.

Syndrome analysis: Dryness of the throat and mouth is due to impairment of fluids in the Stomach, and dry cough due to impairment of fluids in the Lungs. Deficiency of *yin*-fluid may produce endogenous heat, and hence fever. The changes to the tongue and pulse are also consistent with impairment of *yin*-fluid.

(2) Impairment of *yin* of the Liver and Kidneys

Clinical manifestations: Low-grade fever with feverish sensation in the palms and soles, dryness of the mouth and the tongue, lassitude, malar flush, sometimes impaired hearing; dry, reddened tongue with a scanty coating, and a rapid, large but feeble pulse.

Syndrome analysis: This is a syndrome seen in the late stage of a persistent febrile disease, marked by *yin* deficiency with endogenous heat. The low-grade fever, feverish sensation in the palms and soles and malar flush are all due to endogenous heat. Deficiency of Kidney essence may bring about impairment of hearing. Kidney essence is closely related to genuine *qi*. In the protracted course of a febrile disease with consumption of Kidney essence, *qi* is insufficient, and lassitude with feeble pulse ensues.

(3) Stirring-up of wind of deficiency type

Clinical manifestations: Low-grade fever, tremors or twitching in the extremities, dryness of the mouth and tongue, lassitude, palpitations, crimson tongue and feeble pulse.

Syndrome analysis: This syndrome develops from the impairment of *yin* of the Liver and Kidneys. Consumption of Kidney *yin* further aggravates the impairment of Liver *yin,* which gives rise to wind symptoms, manifested by tremors and twitching. The wind symptoms in this syndrome are of the deficiency type, different from the wind stirred up by extreme heat.

(4) Lingering of pathogens in *yin*

Clinical manifestations: Low-grade fever, alleviated in the morning and aggravated in the evening, accompanied by feverishness in the palms and soles but no sweating when the temperature comes down; reddened tongue and a thready, rapid pulse.

Syndrome analysis: This syndrome should be carefully differentiated from *yin* deficiency with endogenous heat. In this syndrome, the fever is chiefly due to the remanent exogenous pathogenic heat. There is no sweating accompanying the reduction of body temperature. In fever due to *yin* deficiency, however, there is sweating when the body temperature comes down or night sweating.

CHAPTER 7
PRINCIPLES AND METHODS OF TREATMENT

The guiding rules for treatment in traditional Chinese medicine can be described as follows:

I. Prevention first

The significance of prevention has been emphasized since the initial development of Chinese medicine. *The Canon of Medicine* states, "A good doctor treats diseases before they actually occur." Even in the treatment of disease after the onset, prevention of possible deterioration of the disease should be carefully considered. The *Treatise on Febrile and Miscellaneous Diseases* (*Shang Han Za Bing Lun*), the first Chinese book of clinical medicine, written at the beginning of the 3rd century, stresses, "The Spleen should be replenished while treating a Liver disease, because the disease is bound to be transmitted from the Liver to the Spleen."

Therefore, prevention as a medical principle includes prevention of a disease before its onset, and prevention of complications after the onset. For prevention of complications, early diagnosis and appropriate treatment are necessary. For prevention of disease, strengthening the genuine or normal *qi* is of the utmost importance and a variety of preventive methods have been developed. These methods, including lifestyles, are still of significance even today.

II. Treating the fundamental aspect of a disease

A disease has two aspects: the fundamental and the incidental, which can be broadly categorized as follows[1]: (1) the cause or the basic pathogenic state of a disease is regarded as part of the fundamental aspect, while the symptoms are the incidental aspect; and (2) the primary pathological condition is part of the fundamental aspect while the complications are incidental.

Generally speaking, to treat a disease from its fundamental aspect is better than bringing about a relief of symptoms. In this connection, some further discussion is necessary. Since traditional Chinese diagnosis is not based on patho-anatomy, and there is no concept of disease entity in traditional Chinese medicine, a Western medical doctor is apt to consider that the traditional Chinese diagnosis is merely a symptomatic diagnosis. Take peptic ulcer as an example. In Western medicine, the concept of peptic ulcer as a disease entity is based on the occurrence of ulcer(s) in the stomach and the proximal portion of the duodenum. Clinically, the ulceration can be found by X-ray or directly seen by endoscopy. If the patient responds poorly to medical treatment, surgical intervention may be necessary. Surgical intervention, such as partial gastrectomy in the case of gastric

---

[1]Theoretically, the fundamental vs. the incidental also includes the body resistance vs. pathogenic factors, and diseases of the interior vs. those of the exterior. They are not mentioned here because the treatment rules regarding these points are controversial.

ulcer, is often regarded as radical treatment because after the operation the ulcer no more exists. In this case, a traditional Chinese physician has a different way of thinking. The basic pathogenic state in any disease is *yin-yang* imbalance, though there are a great variety of different patterns of *yin-yang* imbalance in different diseases. The "disease" diagnosis in patients with peptic ulcers is most likely "epigastric pain." This is apparently a symptomatic diagnosis, and no proper treatment can be applied merely based on this diagnosis. Differentiation of syndromes or syndrome patterns is required. In some peptic ulcer patients the basic disorder is deficiency-cold in the Spleen and Stomach; in others, disharmony of the Liver and the Stomach, stagnant heat in the Liver and Stomach, or *qi* stagnation and blood stasis in the Stomach. The manifestations of the basic disorder constitute the syndrome pattern, and the treatment should be considered according to the syndrome diagnosis to relieve the basic disorder. All the above-mentioned disorders are actually different patterns of *yin-yang* imbalance. "To treat the fundamental" refers to the correction of the *yin-yang* imbalance and restoration of the normal balance. From the point of view of traditional Chinese medicine, partial gastrectomy in a gastric ulcer patient may be or may not be a radical treatment. This depends on whether the patient's *yin-yang* balance can be totally restored after the operation. On the other hand, a Western medical doctor can hardly believe that the traditional Chinese therapy is really to treat "the fundamental," because the treatment seems to be in no way related to the removal or cure of the basic pathological lesion—the ulceration. Now, the gap between the two different views can be closed by the integration of the two systems of medicine. There is already a considerable amount of data indicating that ulcers really heal after proper treatment with traditional Chinese medicine, though the therapies may be different in different patients.

The rule about treating the fundamental aspect of a disease is very useful both in herbal medication and in acupuncture. Still taking peptic ulcers as an example, in herbal medication there are a number of analgesic drugs, but they are seldom used in the treatment of peptic ulcers unless the epigastric pain is very severe. On the other hand, different herbal formulas should be used for different syndrome patterns or even for different individuals. In acupuncture, different points should be selected according to the syndrome patterns. This is because, no matter whether in herbal medication or in acupuncture, the therapeutic measures should suit the different syndrome patterns: for deficiency-cold in the Spleen and Stomach, to warm and tonify the Spleen and the Stomach; for lack of coordination between the Liver and the Stomach, to soothe the Liver and harmonize the Stomach; for stagnant heat in the Liver and Stomach, to eliminate the stagnant heat from the Liver and Stomach, and for *qi* stagnation and blood stasis in the Stomach, to regulate the flow of *qi* and remove the stagnant blood.

III. Treating the acute symptoms first in emergency cases

Although treatment of the basic or primary pathological condition is of great importance, in emergency cases symptomatic relief must be applied first in order to save the patient's life or relieve severe suffering. For example, in the treatment of liver cirrhosis, if the patient is suffering from a huge amount of ascites with dyspnea and oliguria, the physician should first prescribe diuretics to reduce ascites, and then treat the liver cirrhosis itself. In a chronic disease with little suffering, treatment of the basic or primary condition alone is enough. For example, in a case of *yin* deficiency with low fever and dry cough, use of *yin* tonics alone is preferable. When *yin* is replenished, coughing and fever will naturally disappear.

IV. Strengthening the patient's body resistance and dispelling the invading pathogenic factors

Disease is regarded as a process of confrontation between the patient's body resistance (genuine *qi*) and invading pathogenic factors (evil qi). If genuine *qi* prevails over evil qi, the disease will be cured; but if the evil qi prevails, the disease will aggravate. Therefore, the treatment of the disease is aimed at changing the relative forces of the confronting sides, either to strengthen genuine *qi* or dispel evil qi, which are the two major therapeutic principles in Chinese medicine.

Which principle should be adopted depends on the patient's condition. "Abundance of evil qi forms an excess condition, and consumption of essential *qi* results in a deficiency condition." One of the parameters in syndrome differentiation is the determination of deficiency versus excess. In a deficiency syndrome, use of tonics to strengthen the patient's body resistance is indicated, and in an excess syndrome, methods to dispel the pathogenic factors (such as use of diaphoretics, purgatives, antipyretics, and diuretics) are necessary. Combined use of the two therapeutic principles is appropriate only when the evil qi is exuberant while the genuine *qi* is insufficient.

V. Using routine treatment or treatment contrary to the routine

The routine treatment is to treat cold syndromes with drugs hot or warm in property, to treat heat syndromes with drugs cold or cool in property, to treat excess syndromes with evil-dispelling drugs, and to treat deficiency syndromes with tonics. But on some occasions when false phenomena appear, the treatment will be different: treating pseudo-cold syndromes with drugs cool or cold in property, treating pseudo-heat syndromes with drugs warm or hot in property, treating stuffed conditions with filling methods (e.g., treating abdominal distension or constipation with tonics if the ailment is caused by diminished function of the Spleen), and treating "open" conditions with "opening" methods (e.g., in diarrhea caused by food stagnation, though the bowels are open, purgation should be applied).

VI. Considering treatment according to the climatic and geographical conditions, as well as the patient's personal conditions

This is one of the applications of the holistic concept to medical treatment. Man and the natural environment are taken as an organic whole. Many factors occurring in the natural environment exert impacts on the human body. Therefore, the physician should consider these factors while treating a patient.

1. Season and climate. For treating the same disease, different drugs may be selected during different seasons. In summer, people are apt to sweat, and so large doses of pungent warm drugs that cause diaphoresis should not be used, in order to prevent consumption of body fluids. But in winter when the cold weather checks sweating, a large dose of pungent warm diaphoretic is often necessary for treating an affliction of cold.

2. Geographical conditions. It is not infrequently encountered that an experienced Chinese physician becomes incompetent when he moves to another city with different geographical conditions, if he sticks to his original experience. In a frigid zone with a high altitude and cold, dry air, people are apt to be affected by dryness-cold. Pungent and moistening drugs are often preferred, and drugs cold or cool in property should be used cautiously. In a tropical zone with a low altitude and plentiful rainfall, affliction by damp-heat is common, and so drugs very hot in property or drugs that might aggravate dampness

are often contra-indicated. For treating wind-cold affliction, *Herba Ephedrae* (ephedra), *Ramulus Cinnamomi* (Chinese cinnamon twig) and *Herba Asari* (wild ginger) are usually used in frigid zones, but *Herba Schizonepetae* (schizonepeta) and *Folium Perillae* (perilla leaf) are appropriate in a warm place, and *Rhizoma Notopterygii* (notopterygium rhizome), *Radix Saposhnikoviae* (saposhnikovia root) and *Herba Eupatorii* (eupatorium) are the choice in a damp place.

3. Personal conditions. The treatment of the same disease should be different for patients of different age, sex and constitution. For patients with a constitution of *yang*-heat or used to eating spicy food, it is preferable to administer drugs cool in property; if warming drugs are necessary, they should be used with caution. For patients with a constitution of *yang*-deficiency or used to eating cold, raw food, it is preferable to prescribe drugs warm in property; bitter drugs cold in property should be administered cautiously. In women, caution should also be given when drugs are prescribed during pregnancy, menstruation and lactation. In acupuncture, the manipulation should also be different from individual to individual. For patients with strong constitutions, heavy manipulation may be required, but in those with weak constitutions, similar manipulation may cause fainting.

VII. Applying different treatments to the same disease, and applying the same treatment to different diseases

This is a unique point and also the quintessence of Chinese medical treatment. As *yin-yang* imbalance is the basic pathogenesis, treatment is always aimed at restoring the normal balance of *yin-yang*. Patients suffering from the same disease may have different kinds of *yin-yang* imbalance, no matter whether the word "disease" is used in the traditional Chinese way or according to the Western concept. The application of different kinds of treatment to patients with the same disease has already been discussed in the above example of peptic ulcers. In addition, even in the same patient, the basic disorder may change at different periods, and hence the treatment should also be changed. For example, disharmony of the Liver and the Stomach in peptic ulcer patients may turn into blood stasis in the Stomach if stagnant Liver *qi* has impaired the Stomach for a long time, impeding the latter's blood flow. One more example may be necessary to illustrate that the treatment is not only different, but contradictory in the treatment of the same disease: Colds or flu in patients with strong constitutions usually show exterior excess syndrome and are customarily treated with diaphoretics, while the use of tonics is contra-indicated. But in a weak person, the same disease may be manifested by an exterior deficiency syndrome. In the latter case, drastic diaphoretics are contra-indicated while use of tonics is helpful.

On the other hand, patients with different diseases may show identical syndromes during the whole course or at a certain stage of the course of a disease. Identical syndromes signify that the *yin-yang* imbalances in these patients are the same, and so they should be treated in the same way. For example, patients with chronic diarrhea, prolapse of the uterus, excessive uterine bleeding or gastroptosis may all be diagnosed as suffering from sinking of Spleen *qi*. Therefore, they can be treated with the same therapy, or even with the same formula to reinforce Spleen *qi*, though their these diseases would be diagnosed entirely different from the Western medical point of view.

According to the basic concept of disease in traditional Chinese medicine, in the final analysis all therapeutic methods fall into two major categories: those which strengthen the patient's body resistance and those which dispel the invading pathogenic factors. Corresponding to this classification, the various kinds of acupuncture manipulations can be grouped into two categories: reinforcement and reduction. In herbal medication, this classification is also available, but further classification of the therapeutic methods into eight groups is customarily used. The eight principal therapeutic methods are diaphoresis, emesis, purgation, mediation, warming, febrifugation, tonification, and resolution. Among them, only tonification is purely for the purpose of strengthening the body resistance, while the rest are mostly for dispelling the pathogenic factors.

1. Diaphoresis

Diaphoresis is a therapeutic method for relieving exterior syndromes by dispersing or expelling the exogenous pathogenic factors from the human body. It is indicated in all kinds of exterior excess syndromes, chiefly in exogenous affections at the initial stage, marked by chills and fever, headache, general aching, thin tongue coating and floating pulse. It can be further divided into diaphoretic therapy with pungent warm drugs and diaphoretic therapy with pungent cool drugs. The former is suitable for treating exterior cold syndromes and the latter for exterior heat syndromes.

If an exterior syndrome occurs in patients with deficiency disorders, the treatment should be chiefly to replenish the superficial defensive *qi*. Mild diaphoretics may be used in combination with *qi*, blood, *yin* or *yang* tonics according to the patient's condition, but use of drastic diaphoretics is prohibited.

Even in the case of exterior excess syndromes, diaphoretic therapy can only be used for a short period of time, and should be discontinued as soon as the exterior syndrome is relieved. Excessive diaphoresis must be avoided, for profuse sweating consumes the body fluids and impairs genuine *qi*.

2. Emesis

Emetic therapy is used for expelling pathogenic factors or poisons from the stomach. It is indicated in treating gastric retention of undigested food, accumulation of phlegm in the respiratory tract, or oral intake of poisons. At present, this therapy is only occasionally used.

3. Purgation

Purgation is an important therapy for bringing about evacuation from the bowels, not only for relieving constipation, but particularly for treating accumulation of excessive pathogenic factors (cold, heat, dryness, damp or undigested food) in the intestines and retained water, phlegm and stagnated blood in the body. It is a major therapy for treating interior excess syndromes.

For different conditions of interior excess syndromes, particularly for different pathogenic factors, purgation can be classified into the following classes: purgation with warm-propertied drugs, purgation with cold-propertied drugs, laxation with lubricants, purgation with hydragogues, and purgation of stagnant blood.

Purgation with cold-propertied drugs is used for treating interior excessive heat syndrome, purgation with warm-propertied drugs for accumulation of cold in the intestines, laxation with lubricants for constipation due to deficiency of intestinal fluids, purgation with hydragogues for edema in excess conditions, and purgation of stagnant blood for blood stasis combined with heat in the Lower Energizer.

Purgation with drastic drugs, particularly hydragogues, may impair the genuine *qi* of the human body, and should be used with caution. (Long-term use is prohibited!) It is only effective for patients with fairly sound constitutions, and contra-indicated for women during pregnancy or menstruation, and for weak aged patients.

4. Mediation

Mediation is a therapy involving administering of drugs with regulating or intermediating action to restore normal correlation between the internal organs or eliminate the pathogenic factors from between the exterior and interior of the body. It is indicated in the following conditions: (1) half-exterior half-interior syndrome marked by alternate chills and fever, as seen in hepatitis, cholecystitis or pleurisy; (2) disharmony between the Liver and the Stomach or Spleen, marked by epigastric or abdominal pain accompanied by anorexia or loose stools.

In exogenous affections, mediation therapy is inappropriate if the pathogenic factor is still in the exterior portion of the body, or has already entered the interior.

5. Warming

Warming therapy is also called cold-expelling therapy. It drives away pathogenic cold from the interior and reinforces the *yang-qi* (heat energy) for warming up the internal organ(s) or the whole body. It is indicated in interior cold syndromes, either due to direct invasion of exogenous cold or due to *yang* deficiency with endogenous cold. In the former case warming therapy alone is enough, but in the latter case warming therapy should be used in combination with tonics.

Warming therapy can be further classified into a group of specific therapies: warming the Middle Energizer and expelling cold (for treating deficiency-cold syndrome of the Spleen and/or the Stomach), warming the meridians and dispelling cold (for treating cold-pattern arthralgia), restoring *yang* for resuscitation (in the treatment of collapse or shock), warming the Lungs for phlegmolysis (in the treatment of disorders of the Lungs with profuse thin and whitish expectoration), warming the Kidneys for diuresis (in the treatment of edema caused by deficiency of Kidney *yang*), etc.

It should be noted that warming therapy is chiefly aimed at expelling internal cold. So it is different from tonification of *yang* which reinforces *yang-qi* (heat energy). The drugs used for warming are pungent in flavor and hot in property, so they are apt to induce dryness-heat and are contra-indicated in cases of *yin* deficiency, blood deficiency, and hemorrhages due to heat in the blood.

6. Febrifugation

Febrifugation is a therapy of expelling pathogenic heat from the interior by using drugs cold or cool in property with febrifugal, fire-purging, detoxifying or blood-cooling actions. It is indicated in the treatment of interior excess heat syndromes occurring in exogenous affections when the exterior syndrome has disappeared and the heat stays in the interior (either in the *qi* system or in the *ying* or blood system). In an interior excess heat syndrome with accumulation of heat in the Stomach and Intestines, febrifugation should be used jointly with purgation. Febrifugation can also be used in deficiency heat syndromes (i.e., heat due to deficiency of yin), but *yin* tonics should be the primary treatment, and only some special febrifugals are appropriate.

Febrifugation therapy can be further classified according to the stage of a febrile disease or the different *zang-fu* organs from which the heat is to be removed. For example, fire-purging febrifugation is appropriate for treating heat in the *qi* system, blood-cooling febrifugation for heat in the *ying*-blood system, detoxifying febrifugation for epidemic infectious diseases or pyogenic infections, febrifugation of the Lungs for heat in the Lungs, fire-purging febrifugation of the Heart for fire in the Heart, fire-purging febrifugation of the Liver for fire in the Liver, fire-purging febrifugation of the Stomach for fire in the Stomach, etc.

Drugs used for febrifugation are usually cool or cold in property, and long-term use of these drugs may cause damage to the Spleen and Stomach *yang*.

7. Resolution

Resolution therapy is used for removing undigested food, stagnated *qi* or blood, accumulated phlegm and retained fluid. It is chiefly indicated for the treatment of accumulation of the above-mentioned pathogenic factors. Therefore, the drugs used for resolution include digestants, carminatives, phelgmolytics and diuretics, as well as blood-activating and stasis-eliminating drugs.

It should be noted that this therapy is aimed at removing pathogenic factors which are usually the products of dysfunction of *zang-fu* organs. If the pathogenic factors are produced due to diminished function of the related *zang-fu* organs, tonification should be applied together with resolution therapy.

8. Tonification

Deficiency conditions, that is, deficiency of *qi*, blood, *yin* and *yang* of any *zang-fu* organ all call for tonification. If we say there are only two therapeutic principles in Chinese medicine, namely, to strengthen the genuine or normal *qi* and to eliminate evil qi, the first seven therapies are almost all used for the latter, while tonification is used for the former.

As deficiency conditions are usually divided into four categories—*qi* deficiency, blood deficiency, *yin* deficiency and *yang* deficiency, tonification is also classified into four—tonification of *qi*, blood, *yin* and *yang*. But in clinical practice, it can be further classified according to the tonified *zang-fu* organs, e.g., tonification of Heart yin, tonification of Heart *qi*, tonification of Lung yin, tonification of Liver yin, tonification of Kidney *yang*, etc. In some cases two elements or two organs are in a deficiency state at the same time. In such cases, both elements or organs should be tonified simultaneously. Thus, there are combined tonification therapies such as tonification of both *qi* and blood, tonification of both *qi* and *yin*, tonification of both Liver and Kidney yin, tonification of both Spleen and Kidney *yang*, etc.

There might be some misunderstanding about tonification. Since tonification is explained as a therapy to strengthen the genuine *qi* or body resistance, one might think that tonification can be used everywhere. But, as many Chinese medical books stress, "Misuse of tonification aggravates the illness"; to administer tonics to a patient with a pure excess syndrome is "to close the door and keep the evil in the room (body)." When a patient with normal body resistance is attacked by an excess of pathogenic factors, the body resistance will give adequate reactions, e.g., fever in an exogenous affection. In such as a case, the proper treatment is to dispel or eliminate the pathogenic factors, but not to increase the bodily reactions; tonification gives no benefit but only exacerbates the fever. If the pathogenic factor is in the exterior portion of the body, the illness usually subsides along with sweating. But tonics, especially *qi* tonics, arrest sweating, so they will prolong the course of the disease. If there is excess heat accumulated in the intestines, purgation is the correct therapy. Tonification may cause further accumulation, and hence the patient becomes more seriously ill.

Another important issue is the correct use of different kinds of tonics. Tonification is a very general term; it includes at least four different therapies: tonification of *qi*, blood, yin and *yang*, each of which has its own indications. As any disease is regarded as an imbalance of *yin-yang*, and as the purpose of treatment is to restore the normal balance of *yin-yang*, it will be easy to understand why tonification of *yin* will cause harm to a patient with *yang* deficiency, and vice versa.

PART TWO

TRADITIONAL CHINESE DRUGS

CHAPTER 8

FUNDAMENTAL KNOWLEDGE OF CHINESE DRUGS

THE BASIC ACTIONS OF MEDICINAL SUBSTANCES

In traditional Chinese medicine, the basic actions of medicinal substances include their properties, tastes (or flavors), directions of action (ascending, descending, sinking or floating), and meridian classification. This knowledge is the essence of the experience accumulated in the clinical use of medicinal substances for thousands of years in the light of Chinese natural philosophy and traditional medical theories.

The Four Properties

Medicinal substances can be classified into four categories according to their basic properties, namely, cold, cool, warm and hot. Cold and cool are similar in property, but different in degree; so are hot and warm. Therefore, the four properties are actually two, i.e., cold-cool and warm-hot, or cold and hot for short. This basic classification of Chinese medicines is consistent with the classification of cold and heat syndromes. Generally speaking, medicinal substances cold or cool in property have the effect of relieving heat syndromes, and those hot or warm in property have the effect of treating cold syndromes. Some medicinal substances are neutral in property, neither manifest in coldness nor manifest in heat, but they still might show a tendency to either of the properties. So, it is still said that Chinese medicines have four properties, and not five.

According to modern research, the common actions of cold-propertied medicines and those of heat-propertied medicines can be summarized as follows:

1. Effects on the autonomic nervous activities

One of the different patho-physiological changes in cold and heat syndromes lies in the autonomic nervous system. By determining the balance condition of autonomic nervous activities through basic physiological indices and assaying the levels of catecholamines, 17-hydrocorticosteroid, cAMP vs cGMP, and PGE vs PGF, it has been revealed that heat syndromes occurring in various disease entities is characterized by enhanced activity of the sympathetico-adrenal system, while cold syndromes are characterized by reduced activity of the sympathetico-adrenal system or enhanced parasympathetic activity. Treatment of heat syndromes with drugs cold in property and of cold syndromes with drugs hot in property usually normalizes the activity of the sympathetico-adrenal system along with, or even preceding, the clinical improvement. Experiments in normal animals have also shown that some medicinal substances marked by cold properties, e.g., *Radix Scutellariae* (skullcap root), *Rhizoma Coptidis* (goldthread rhizome) and *Cortex Phellodendri* (phellodendrone bark) have the action of significantly reducing the urine norepinephrine excretion, while those marked by hot properties, e.g., *Radix Aconiti Lateralis* (aconite lateral root) and *Cortex Cinnamomi* (Chinese cinnamon bark) increase it. In addition, the above-mentioned cold-propertied substances have an anti-hypertensive effect, while *Radix Aconiti Lateralis* (aconite lateral root), *Herba Ephedrae* (ephedra) and *Pericarpium Citri Reticulatae Viride* (green tangerine peel), all warm or hot in property, elevate the blood pressure, and are even effective for treating shock. Therefore, it can be concluded that many medicinal substances with cold or hot properties have opposite actions on the autonomic nervous activities.

2. Effects on other central nervous activities

Most tranquilizers, sedatives and anti-convulsives are cool or cold in property.

3. Effects on the endocrine system

Tonics warm or hot in property often have stimulating effects on the endocrine system. For example, *Radix Ginseng* (ginseng) stimulates the pituitary-adrenocortical system, has a gonadotropin-like action, and increases the thyroid function; *Herba Epimedii* (epimedium) enhances the hypothalamic-pituitary-gonadal, hypothalamic-pituitary-adrenocortical, and hypothalamic-pituitary-thymic systems; *Herba Cistanchis* (cistanche) and *Radix Polygoni Multiflori* (fleeceflower root) activate the release of adrenocortical hormone; *Cornu Cervi Pantotrichum* (pilose antler) excites the sexual gland. On the other hand, cold-propertied Gypsum Fibrosum (gypsum), *Rhizoma Anemarrhenae* (anemarrhena rhizome), and *Radix Scutellariae* (skullcap root) when applied for a long time in animal experiments, inhibit the adrenocortical and sexual functions, and reduce the thyrotropin level as well as oxygen consumption.

4. Effects on the cardio-vascular system

Drugs such as *Herba Asari* (wild ginger), *Radix Aconiti Lateralis* (aconite lateral root), *Cortex Cinnamomi* (Chinese cinnamon bark) and *Rhizoma Zingiberis* (ginger), which stimulate the cardiac function and/or promote the blood circulation of the body surface, are hot in property.

5. Effects on the metabolism

Some medicinal substances hot in property, such as *Herba Ephedrae* (ephedra) and *Cornu Cervi Pantotrichum* (pilose antler), increase heat production, while quite a few medicinal substances, such as *Rhizoma Anemarrhenae* (anemarrhena rhizome), *Rhizoma Coptidis* (goldthread rhizome), *Cortex Phellodendri* (phellodendrone bark), *Fructus Gardeniae* (cape-jasmine fruit) and *Radix et Rhizoma Rhei* (rhubarb), decrease heat production by inhibiting the activity of Na^+,K^+-ATPase.

It is worth mentioning that the medicinal substances used in the treatment of bacterial and viral infections are not confined to cold-propertied ones. In the early stage of an acute infectious disease with an exterior cold syndrome, drugs warm in property are often used. Modern research has revealed that although many cold-propertied substances used for treating infectious diseases have antibacterial and/or antiviral effects, quite a few warm-propertied substances also have this kind of effect. Obviously, the cold and hot properties of medicines are determined by their effects on the human body, and not by the pathogens.[1]

---

[1]Although cold and heat are also taken as pathogenic factors, in fact they refer chiefly to the different bodily responses rather than to different pathogens. Otherwise, it will be difficult to explain why a wind-cold affection can easily turn into an interior heat syndrome. It is customarily said that pathogenic wind-cold is transformed into heat after entering the interior. This actually means that the bodily response to the same pathogen has changed from cold symptoms to heat manifestations. Readers should remember that the so-called exogenous pathogenic factors, such as cold, heat, damp and dryness, were merely generalizations of the clinical manifestations; no pathogens such as bacteria had ever been found in the history of Chinese medicine.

The Five Tastes

The "taste" or "flavor" of a medicinal substance is another aspect of its basic action. Just like food, medicinal substances also have different tastes or flavors: pungent (or aromatic), sour, sweet, bitter and salty. They are collectively called "the five tastes." In most instances, the taste or flavor of a medicinal substance is determined by physically tasting or smelling, for example, *Rhizoma Zingiberis Recens* (fresh ginger) tastes pungent, *Radix Glycyrrhizae* (licorice root) tastes sweet, *Radix Sophorae Flavescentis* (light-yellow sophora root) tastes bitter, *Fructus Mume* (black plum) tastes sour and *Thallus Laminariae* (sea tangle) tastes salty. However, the actions of the medicinal substances also help the determination of their tastes. For example, *Scolopendra* (centipede) and *Scorpio* (scorpion) are believed to be pungent in taste because they have the action of dispelling endogenous wind (convulsions). The tastes of medicinal substances related to their effects are illustrated in Table VIII-1.

Why are the tastes of drugs taken as an important part of traditional pharmacology? According to modern research, both the pharmacological action and the taste of a medicinal substance may be associated with its chemical composition. Generally speaking, medicinal substances pungent or aromatic in flavor contain volatile oils which either cause diaphoresis or promote the flow of *qi* and blood. For example, *Rhizoma Zingiberis Recens* (fresh ginger) is a diaphoretic for colds, *Radix Aucklandiae* (costus root) is used for treating abdominal distension by smoothing the stagnated flow of *qi*, *Resina Olibani* (frankincense) relieves pain and swelling in traumatic injuries by invigorating local blood circulation.

Medicinal substances sour in taste usually contain organic acid which has an astringent effect. For example, *Fructus Mume* (black plum) containing citric and malic acid, arrests chronic diarrhea. Some substances such as *Fructus Chebulae* (chebula fruit), *Galla Chinensis* (Chinese gall) and *Catechu* (black catechu) containing large amounts of tannic acid and tannates, have a sour and puckery taste, and have an anti-diarrheal and styptic effect.

Medicinal substances sweet in taste contain saccharides and glycosides. They usually have a tonic effect or an anti-spasmodic action, and are used to replenish or invigorate *qi*, blood, *yin* and *yang* as well as to relieve colic pain. For example, *Radix Ginseng* (ginseng) and *Radix Astragali* (milkvetch root) replenish *qi*, *Colla Corii Asini* (donkey-hide gelatin) and *Radix Rehmanniae Preparata* (prepared rehmannia root) replenish blood, and *Radix Glycyrrhizae* (licorice root) relieve spasms and colic pain. Besides saccharides and glycosides, many medicinal substance sweet in taste and mild in nature contain considerable amounts of proteins, amino acids and vitamins, which may also be related to their tonic effects.

Medicinal substances bitter in taste contain alkaloids and amaroids, with dampness-removing and purging effects. For example, *Cortex Phellodendri* (phellodendron bark) and *Rhizoma Coptidis* (goldthread rhizome) eliminate heat and dampness, *Radix et Rhizoma Rhei* (rhubarb) is a purgative and also eliminates heat.

Medicinal substances salty in taste contain sodium, potassium, calcium, magnesium, iodine and other active components. They often have the effect of softening hard masses and subduing *yang* by replenishing *yin*. For example, *Sargassum* (seaweed) and *Thallus Laminariae* (sea tangle), containing iodine, are effective for preventing and treating endemic goiter; *Plastron Testudinis* (tortoise plastron) and *Carapax Trionycis* (turtle shell) replenish *yin* and subdue *yang*, and are particularly effective for treating low-grade fever and night sweating due to *yin* deficiency.

Table VIII-1. Relations between the Tastes and Effects of Medicinal Substances

Taste	Examples	Actions
Pungent	*Herba Schizonepetae* (schizonepeta)	Dispels exogenous wind (for exterior syndromes)
	Scolopendra (centipede)	Dispels Liver wind (for convulsions)
	Rhizoma Chuanxiong (chuanxiong)	Promotes the flow of *qi* and blood
Bitter	*Radix et Rhizoma Rhei* (rhubarb)	Induces purgation
	Semen Armeniacae Amarum (bitter apricot seed)	Checks the upward perversion of *qi* (for cough and asthma)
	Rhizoma Atractylodis (atractylodes rhizome)	Removes dampness
Sour	*Fructus Rosae Levigatae* (cherokee rose-hip)	Causes astringency for excessive sweating, seminal emission, bleeding, and chronic diarrhea
	Fructus Schisandrae (magnoliavine fruit)	
	Galla Chinensis (Chinese gall)	
Sweet	*Radix Astragali* (Milkvetch root)	Tonifies *qi*
	Radix Rehmanniae Preparata (prepared rehmannia root)	Tonifies blood
	Fructus Lycii(wolfberry)	Tonifies *yin*
	Cornu Cervi Pantotrichum (hairy deerhorn)	Tonifies *yang*
	Radix Glycyrrhizae (licorice root)	Relieves spasms
Salty	*Thallus Laminariae* (sea tangle)	Softens hard masses
Tasteless	*Poria* (Indian bread or fuling)	Promotes diuresis

In addition, some substances have no distinct taste. Most of the tasteless substances, such as *Polyporus* (umbellate polypore), *Poria* (fuling or Indian bread) and *Talcum* (talc), have a diuretic effect; but they are placed in the category of sweet, and so the total number of tastes is still five.

Directions of Effects

This is another unique way of summarizing drug effects. So far as the syndromes are concerned, their manifestations can be classified as upward (e.g., vomiting, belching, and coughing), downward (e.g., diarrhea, menorrhagia, and prolapse of the rectum), inward (e.g., syndrome transmission from the exterior to the interior), and outward (e.g., spontaneous sweating, night sweating, nocturnal emission). Medicinal substances can also be classified in a similar way according to their effects: Those with an ascending (upward) action are usually used for treating syndromes with downward manifestations; those with a floating (outward) action usually have a diaphoretic, cold-dispelling or resuscitating effect. Antitussives, antasthmatics, antiemetics, diuretics and purgatives are considered to be drugs with a descending action, and astringents[2] are usually regarded as drugs with a

[2]The word "astringent" is used in a very broad sense in Chinese medicine. Astringents are drugs that can directly arrest any of the following kinds of abnormal discharge: bleeding, sweating, seminal discharge,

sinking (inward) action.

There seems to be some relationship between the tastes or flavors and the directions of drug effects. Generally speaking, pungent, sweet or tasteless substances often have an ascending action, while bitter, sour or salty substances have a descending action. Medicinal substances warm or hot in property often have a floating action, while those cool or cold in property have a sinking action.

Another interesting issue is that in a compound formula the direction of drug action can be changed by adding some ingredients called "conductants." Conductants are believed to have the action of directing other ingredients to work on the affected site. For example, *Radix Platycodi* (platycodon root) is said to be able to conduct other ingredients upward, particularly to the throat, *Radix Achyranthis Bidentatae* (two-toothed achyranthes root) seems to conduct other ingredients downward to the lower extremities.

Meridian Classification

Medicinal substances different in taste not only have different therapeutic effects; they may also act on different internal organs selectively. The original rule was summarized from clinical practice in the light of the Five Elements theory. As stated in *The Canon of Medicine*, substances bitter, sour, sweet, pungent and salty in taste act on the Heart, Liver, Spleen, Lungs and Kidneys, respectively. This rule, though useful in many instances, is not so precise. For example, *Radix et Rhizoma Rhei* (rhubarb), which is bitter in taste, purges the Stomach, Large Intestine and Liver of heat, but has no direct action on the Heart. Therefore, the meridians on which the drug acts have been determined individually according to their clinical effects. As a diseased Spleen usually leads to diarrhea, drugs to arrest diarrhea are often believed to act on the Spleen Meridian; coughing and expectoration are common manifestations of Lung diseases, and so antitussives and expectorants are usually classified in the category of the Lung Meridian drugs. Among the drugs that eliminate pathogenic heat, *Cortex Mori* (mulberry bark) is classified as a Lung Meridian drug, because it clears the Lungs of heat; *Spica Prunellae* (self-heal spike), as a drug acting on the Liver and Gallbladder Meridians, because it removes heat from the Liver and the Gallbladder; and *Gypsum Fibrosum* (gypsum), as a drug acting on the Lung and Stomach Meridians, because it eliminates heat from the Lungs and the Stomach. Among the tonics, *Radix Rehmanniae Preparata* (prepared rehmannia root) replenishes the Kidneys, and so pertains to the Kidney Meridian; *Rhizoma Atractylodis Macrocephalae* (white atractylodes rhizome) invigorates the spleen, and so pertains to the Spleen Meridian. In our discussion, except for some particular instances, the names of the meridians on which drugs act are generally omitted, because, for instance, "white atractylodes rhizome invigorates the Spleen" already implies that the drug acts on the Spleen Meridian.

PROCESSING OF CHINESE DRUGS

Most Chinese medicinal substances have been processed before use. The purposes of processing are as follows:

1. To remove impurities and useless parts by cleansing, rinsing and maceration.

---

polyuria, protracted diarrhea, and other excessive secretion or excretion. In most cases, astringents are used for the treatment of symptoms.

2. To eliminate or reduce the toxic, irritating and side effects, for example, the processing of *Rhizoma Pinelliae* (pinellia tuber) with ginger juice. (Unprocessed pinellia tuber irritates the mucous membrane of the digestive tract, causing vomiting.)

3. To modify the action and enhance the therapeutic effect. For example, *Radix Rehmanniae* (rehmannia root) is cold in property and has a cooling effect on blood, but after steaming in wine, *Radix Rehmanniae Preparata* (prepared rehmannia root) becomes warm in property and can be used as a blood tonic.

4. By baking to make the medicinal substances dry and easy to store; by macerating or calcining to make the substances easy to cut into pieces or grind into powder.

5. To remove odors from some substances such as by processing *Cortex Ailanthi* (tree-of-heaven bark) by stir-baking with bran.

The following methods are commonly used for processing:

1. Steaming, i.e., preparing a medicinal substance or a substance thoroughly mixed with fluid adjuvant (e.g., wine or vinegar) by steaming in a suitable container.

2. Stir-baking

(1) Stir-baking without any additive: The medicinal substance is baked in a pan with constant stirring to just dry, to cracking, to yellowish, to brown or to the stage of carbonization, according to the requirements for different purposes. Stir-baking to brown is often used for preparing digestants such as *Fructus Crataegi* (hawthorn fruit) and *Fructus Hordei Berminatus* (germinated barley). Stir-baking to the stage of carbonization involves heating the medicinal substance on a strong fire till its outer part is charred while its inner part becomes yellowish-brown, so that its original property is retained. Carbonized substances such as *Radix Sanguisorbae Carbonizatus* (carbonized burnet root) and *Petiolus Trachycarpi Carbonizatus* (carbonized petiole of windmill-palm) have a more hemostatic effect than the original substances.

(2) Stir-baking with bran: chiefly for removing odors.

(3) Stir-baking with earth: for processing *Rhizome Atractylodis Macrocephalae* (bighead atractylodes rhizome) and *Rhizome Dioscoreae* (Chinese yam), to enhance their effect of invigorating the Spleen.

3. Stir-baking with adjuvants: Baking a medicinal substance mixed with a fluid adjuvant such as wine, vinegar, salt water, honey or ginger juice until the latter is absorbed into the medicinal substance.

4. Calcining: burning a medicinal substance on a fire to make it crispy, usually used for processing mineral drugs or shells.

USAGE OF CHINESE DRUGS

Combination of Ingredients

Occasionally, only one single medicinal substance is used in a prescription, which is called a “simple recipe.” In most cases, multiple medicinal substances (ingredients) are used in combination for producing the desired therapeutic effect and reducing toxic or side effects. The following points should be noticed when a compound recipe is prescribed.

1. Mutual reinforcement: two ingredients with a similar action used in combination to reinforce each other's effect.

2. Assistance: two or more ingredients used in combination, one being the principal substance while the rest play a subsidiary role to reinforce the action of the principal one.

3. Mutual restraint: the mutual restraining effect of different ingredients to weaken or neutralize each other's action.

4. Counteraction: the property of one ingredient weakens the action of another ingredient.

5. Neutralization: the property of one ingredient neutralizes the toxicity of another ingredient.

6. Incompatibility: the property of being unsuitable for combination or simultaneous administration.

Incompatibilities and Mutual Restraints

According to the records in ancient materia medica, 18 incompatible medicaments, if given in combination, are believed to have serious side effects: *Radix Glycyrrhizae* (licorice root) being incompatible with *Radix Euphorbiae Pekinensis* (Peking spurge root), *Flos Genkwa* (genkwa flower), *Radix Euphorbiae Kansui* (kansui root), and *Sargassum* (sea weed); *Radix Aconiti* (aconite root) incompatible with *Bulbus Fritillariae* (fritillary bulb), *Fructus Trichosanthis* (snakegourd fruit), *Rhizoma Pinelliae* (pinellia tuber), *Radix Ampelopsis* (ampelopsis root) and *Rhizoma Bletillae* (bletilla tuber); *Radix Veratri Nigri* (black false hellebore) incompatible with *Radix Ginseng* (ginseng), *Radix Salviae Miltriorrhizae* (red sage root), *Radix Adenophorae* (ladybell root), *Radix Scrophulariae* (figwort root), *Herba Asari* (wild ginger) and *Radix Peoniae* (peony root).

Nineteen medicaments of mutual restraint, if used in combination, may restrain or neutralize each other's action: sulphur restrains crude sodium sulphate; mercury restrains arsenic trioxide; *Radix Euphorbiae Ebracteolatae* (unbracteolated spurge root) restrains litharge; *Semen Crotonis* (croton seed) restrains *Semen Pharbitidis* (pharbitis seed); *Flos Caryophylli* (cloves) restrains *Radix Curcumae* (turmeric root); crystalline sodium sulphate restrains *Rhizoma Sparganii* (burreed tuber); *Radix Aconiti* (Sichuan aconite root) and *Radix Aconiti Kuznezoffii* (wild aconite root) restrain *Cornu Rhinoceri* (rhinoceros horn); *Radix Ginseng* (ginseng) restrains *Faeces Trogopterorum* (trogopterus dung); and *Cortex Cinnamomi* (Chinese cinnamon bark) restrains *Halloysitum Rubrum* (red halloysite).

The ancient records on incompatibilities have not been confirmed by modern research. Even in the ancient literature there were conflicting views. For example, Zhu Danxi (1282-1358), one of the most famous physicians of his time, initiated a formula containing both *Radix Glycyrrhizae* (licorice root) and *Flos Genkwa* (genkwa flower) with good effect. In *Yi Zong Jin Jian* (*The Golden Mirror of Medicine*, 1742), one of the best treatises on general medicine, written by a staff of 80 persons at the order of the emperor, *Halloysitum Rubrum* (red halloysite) was recommended to be added to a prescription containing *Cortex Cinnamomi* (Chinese cinnamon bark) for treating chronic diarrhea. Recently, it was reported that *Radix Ginseng* (ginseng) in combination with *Faeces Trogopterorum* (trogopterus dung) showed good effect in treating coronary heart disease. However, for the sake of safety it is better not to make prescriptions with the above-mentioned incom-patibilities.

Contraindications during Pregnancy

Some drugs, such as *Flos Carthami* (safflower) and *Moschus* (musk), may act on the uterus. During pregnancy the uterus becomes extraordinarily sensitive to these drugs, which may cause abortion if taken erroneously. Some other drugs, such as *Venenum Bufonis* (toad venom) and realgar, have no direct action on the uterus, but may impair the normal development of the fetus. According to the degree of endangerment, attention should be paid to the following two groups of herbal drugs: Group I are those definitely contraindicated in pregnancy owing to their strong stimulating effect on the uterus or harmful effect on the development of the fetus. Groups II are those that can only be used with caution.

1. Drugs contraindicated in pregnancy: drastic drugs to remove blood stasis and induce menstrual discharge, such as *Rhizoma Sparganii* (burreed tuber), *Rhizoma Curcumae Zedoariae* (zedoary tumeric), *Hirudo* (leech), *Tabanus* (gadfly), hydragogues such as *Radix Euphorbiae Kansui* (kansui root), *Flos Genkwa* (genkwa flower), *Radix Euphorbiae Pekinensis* (Peking spurge root), *Radix Phytolaccae* (pokeberry root) and *Semen Pharbitidis* (pharbitis seed); strong aromatic stimulants, such as *Moschus* (musk), *Venenum Bufonis* (toad venom), emetics such as *Radix Veratri Nigri* (black false hellebore), and drastic purgatives such as *Semen Crotonis* (croton seed), *Aloe* and *Folium Sennae* (senna leaf).

2. Drugs that can only be used with caution: drastic drugs to relieve *qi* stagnation and blood stasis, herbs pungent in flavor and hot in nature, and those cause catharsis, diuresis and sinking effects, including *Radix et Rhizoma* Rhei (rhubarb), sodium sulphate, *Fructus Aurantii Immaturus* (immature bitter orange), *Semen Persicae* (peach kernel), *Flos Carthami* (safflower), *Pollen Typhae* (cat-tail pollen), *Faeces Trogopterorum* (trogopterus dung), *Semen Vaccariae* (cow-herb seed), *Radix Aconiti Lateralis Preparata* (prepared aconite lateral root), *Rhizoma Zingiberis* (dried ginger), *Cortex Cinnamomi* (Chinese cinnamon bark), *Radix Achyranthis Bidentatae* (two-toothed achyranthes root), *Rhizoma Imperatae* (cogongrass rhizome), *Herba Dianthi* (pink), *Rhizoma Pinelliae* (pinellia tuber), *Rhizoma Arisaematis* (Jack-in-the-pulpit tuber), *Hematitum* (hematite) and *Magnetitum* (magnetite).

Dietary Taboos during Medication

Generally speaking, taking cold and raw food and glutinous food difficult to digest is forbidden during herbal medication. Hot spicy food should be prohibited during the treatment of heat syndromes, and cold raw food in the case of cold syndromes. Fat-rich food is incompatible with drugs for regulating the Spleen and the Stomach; beans are incompatible with *qi*-regulating herbs; fish and shrimps are incompatible with antitussives and antiasthmatics.

Directions for Making Herbal Decoction (Herbal Tea)

Decoction is often considered as most effective preparation method for Chinese drugs, because the ingredients of a set formula can be easily modified in accordance with the patient's condition. The physician may simply give the patients prescriptions, and instruct them to make the decoctions by themselves. The proper way of making a decoction is important, as it guarantees full extraction of the active components and avoids any destruction or loss. The following are the directions:

Use an earthenware or enamelware pot; no utensil made of metal should be used. Put the medicinal substances in the pot and add enough water to cover them. If some of them float on the water surface, get all of them be immersed by stirring lightly. It is better to immerse the substances for a while, and then boil them. After boiling point is reached, turn the fire to low for simmering. Avoid lifting the lid repeatedly, in order to avoid the loss of volatile components. The simmering time varies with different drugs; ordinarily, it takes 20-30 minutes. A simmering time of 10 minutes is enough for making a decoction to relieve an exterior syndrome. But for tonics, a longer simmering time (from 40 to 60 minutes or more) is necessary. Therefore, the amount of water added to the pot varies not only with the quantity of the medicinal substances, but also with the simmering time. It is desirable to get about 100 ml of liquid after straining. Then add an appropriate amount of water to the ingredients and decoct them again in the same way, and another 100 ml of liquid will be obtained. Discarding the dregs, mix the two portions of liquid (decoction). For treating a chronic disease, divide the mixture into two portions, each for one dose, and the total amount of about 200 ml for one day. Several daily doses may be made at once and the decoction kept refrigerated. But it should be taken warm, especially for treating cold syndromes. For treating an acute disease, it is better to take the decoction in extra doses daily. Most decoctions, particularly tonics, are taken before meals, but cathartics should be taken on an empty stomach. Decoctions that might stimulate the stomach should be taken after meals.

In order to get a good effect, some ingredients should be decocted in special ways:

(1) Those with active constituents difficult to extract should be broken into small pieces and decocted at least 30 minutes before other ingredients are added. Most minerals and shells belong to this category, e.g., *Gypsum Fibrosum* (gypsum), *Os Draconis* (dragon's bone), *Haematitum* (hematite), *Concha Haliotidis* (sea-ear shell), *Plastron Testudinis* (tortoise plastron) and *Carapax Trionycis* (turtle shell).

(2) Those with active constituents which easily evaporate should be added when the decoction is nearly done. Herbs containing active volatile components often belong to this category, e.g., *Herba Methae* (peppermint), *Herba Agastachis* (giant-hyssop), *Folium Perillae* (perilla leaf), *Lignum Aquilariae Resinatum* (eagle wood) and *Herba Artemisiae Scopariae* (oriental wormwood).

(3) Downy ingredients, e.g., *Flos Inula* (inula flower); powdered ingredients, e.g., *Pollen Typhae* (cat-tail pollen), *Indigo Naturalis* (natural indigo) and *Talcum* (talc), and ingredients containing glutinous substances, e.g., *Semen Plantaginis* (plantain seed), should be wrapped in a piece of cloth or gauze when the decoction is made.

(4) A decoction without other ingredients is usually made for *Radix Ginseng* (ginseng) and *Cornu Cervi Pantotrichum* (pilose antler).

(5) Gelatin, such as donkey-hide gelatin and deerhorn gelatin, should not be decocted. It is taken after being melted with hot water or in another decoction.

All the above-mentioned ingredients should be specially labeled.

CHAPTER 9
MATERIA MEDICA IN COMMON USE

SUPERFICIES-RELIEVING DRUGS (DIAPHORETICS)

Superficies-relieving drugs are drugs that can expel or disperse exogenous pathogenic factors from the superficies of the body to relieve exterior syndromes. Most drugs in this category are pungent in flavor and diaphoretic in action, for it is believed that the pathogenic factors existing superficially can be expelled or dispersed through perspiration.

Exterior syndromes are syndromes marked by chilliness and fever, headache, general aching, stuffy and runny nose or cough, floating pulse, and thin coating on the tongue, indicating that the external part of the human body is affected by exogenous pathogenic factors. These syndromes are usually encountered in cases of common cold, influenza, upper respiratory infection and the prodromal or early stage of other acute infectious diseases.

Exterior syndromes can generally be divided into two patterns: exterior cold and exterior heat. The former is characterized by more chilliness than fever, floating tense pulse, and no sweating, while the latter, more fever than chilliness, and floating rapid pulse. Therefore, the drugs used for relieving exterior syndromes are classified into two groups respectively: pungent-warm superficies-relieving drugs and pungent-cool superficies-relieving drugs. The former are effective for inducing perspiration, and are used for treating exterior cold syndromes; while the latter, though weak in diaphoresis, have an antipyretic effect, and are used for treating exterior heat syndromes.

Most superficies-relieving drugs are used for treating the general symptoms of exterior syndromes, but some drugs in this category have specific effects. Rhinitis with stuffy and runny nose is a common manifestation of exterior cold syndromes. Some pungent-warm superficies-relieving drugs are specifically useful for treating rhinitis. They can also be used for treating sinusitis. Pharyngitis with sore throat often accompanies exterior heat syndromes. Some pungent-cool superficies-relieving drugs are particularly useful for relieving sore throat.

Since exterior syndromes are usually due to the effect of exogenous wind (exterior cold syndromes due to wind-cold, and exterior heat syndromes due to wind-heat), the drugs for relieving exterior cold syndromes are also called "wind-cold dispersing" drugs, and those for relieving exterior heat syndromes, "wind-heat dispersing" drugs.

Besides general exterior syndromes marked by chilliness and fever, many other disorders or diseases may also be due to wind. Acute nephritis with edema more remarkable in the face and eyelids is considered "wind-edema" (edema caused by wind). Urticaria is marked by its sudden onset, migration of the skin lesions and severe itching. These features are consistent with wind affection, and so urticaria is called "wind-rash" in Chinese medicine. Allergic rhinitis is manifested by the sudden onset of runny nose and paroxysms of sneezing.

It is also considered a kind of wind affection. Arthritis marked by migratory joint pain is believed to be caused by wind. Acute conjunctivitis is considered to be wind-heat affection of the eye. All these disorders can be treated with superficies-relieving drugs. In addition, in the course of measles, eruption is thought to be a process of expelling the pathogens out of the body. Some pungent-cool superficies-relieving (wind-heat dispersing) drugs can promote eruption.

Pungent-Warm Superficies-Relieving Drugs (Wind-Cold Dispersing Drugs)

***Herba Ephedrae*, Ephedra**, 麻黄 (*Mahuang*): the dried herbaceous stem of *Ephedra sinica* Stapf., *Ephedra intermedia* Schrenk et C.A. Mey. or *Ephedra equisetina* Bge. (family Ephedraceae).

[Taste and Properties] Pungent, slightly bitter and warm.

[Effects and Indications] (1) Induces perspiration for relieving exterior-cold syndromes with no sweating; (2) Relieves bronchial asthma; (3) Causes diuresis for treating wind-edema.

[Usage and Dosage] 3-9 g.

[Notes] (1) Ephedra contains ephedrine, psudoephedrine and a small amount of volatile oil. Ephedrine stimulates the central and sympathetic nervous systems, constricts blood vessels, causing elevation of blood pressure, and relieves bronchospasms. Pseudoephedrine has a diuretic action; it also relaxes the bronchial muscle. The volatile oil stimulates the secretion of sweat, and has an inhibitory effect on the influenza virus. Recent research has revealed that *Ephedra sinica* Staph. contains 2,3,5,6-tetramethylpirazine and L-α-terpinenol, which also have an antiasthmatic effect. (2) *Radix Ephedrae* (ephedra root) is anti-hidrotic, and has a hypotensive effect.

***Ramulus Cinnamomi*, Chinese Cinnamon Twig**, 桂枝 (*Guizhi*): the young dried stem of *Cinnamomum cassia* Presl. (family Lauraceae).

[Taste and Properties] Pungent, sweet and warm.

[Effects and Indications] (1) Dispels wind-cold for relieving exterior syndromes, often used together with ephedra in excess cases (characterized by absence of sweat), and together with white peony root in deficiency cases (with sweating); (2) Improves blood circulation for treating angina pectoris, arthralgia and amenorrhea, and also enhances the effect of diuretics in the treatment of edema.

[Usage and Dosage] 3-9 g.

[Notes] Chinese cinnamon twig contains volatile oil, which chiefly consists of cinnamic aldehyde and cinnamic acid. Cinnamic aldehyde dilates cutaneous blood vessels and stimulates the secretion of sweat. In addition, cinnamic oil has stomachic, spasmolytic, analgesic and diuretic effects. Chinese cinnamon twig has been demonstrated to have some bacteriostatic effects on staphylococcus and pneumococcus in vitro, and inhibitory effects on Asian A influenza virus and the ECHO virus. Chinese cinnamon twig also increases the coronary blood flow.

***Folium Perillae*, Perilla Leaf**, 紫苏叶 (*Zisuye*): the dried leaf of *Perilla frutescens* (L.) Britt. (family Labiatae).

[Taste and Properties] Pungent and warm.

[Effects and Indications] (1) Dispels wind-cold for relieving exterior syndromes; (2) Relieves vomiting and diarrhea caused by fish or crab poisoning.

[Usage and Dosage] 4.5-9 g for treating colds; 30-60 g when used as an antidote.

[Notes] *Fructus Perillae* (perilla fruit) is used as an antitussive, antiasthmatic and expectorant; *Caulis Perillae* (perilla stem) is used to regulate the flow of *qi* for relieving oppression feeling in the chest and abdominal distension.

***Herba Schizonepetae*, Schizonepeta Herb**, 荆芥 (*Jingjie*): the dried aerial part of *Schizonepeta tenuifolia* Briq. (family Labiatae).

[Taste and Properties] Pungent and slightly warm.

[Effects and Indications] (1) Induces perspiration for relieving exterior syndromes; (2) Dispels wind for treating urticaria and other pruritic skin diseases.

[Usage and Dosage] 4.5-9 g

[Notes] Schizonepeta herb contains volatile oil that stimulates the secretion of sweat. Decoction of the herb has been shown to have an antiallergic effect.

***Radix Saposhnikoviae*, Saposhnikovia Root**, 防风 (*Fangfeng*): the dried root of *Saposhnikovia divaricata* (Turcz.) Schischk. (family Umbelliferae).

[Taste and Properties] Pungent and warm.

[Effects and Indications] (1) Dispels wind-cold for relieving exterior syndromes; (2) Dispels wind-damp for arthralgia; (3) Relieves convulsions.

[Usage and Dosage] 6-9 g.

[Notes] Its extract shows an antipyretic action in rabbits with experimental fever induced by typhoid vaccine. It also inhibits the influenza virus.

***Radix Angelicae Dahuricae*, Dahurian Angelica Root**, 白芷 (*Baizhi*): the dried root of *Angelica dahurica* (Fisch. ex Hoffm.) Benth. et Hook. f. or *Angelica dahurica* var. *formosana* (Boiss.) Shan et Yuan (family Umbelliferae).

[Taste and Properties] Pungent and warm.

[Effects and Indications] (1) Dispels wind and relieves frontal headache in cases of colds and sinusitis, as well as toothache; (2) Promotes discharge of pus and reduces swelling in boils.

[Usage and Dosage] 3-9 g.

[Notes] It shows antipyretic and local anesthetic effects in animal experiments.

***Herba Asari*, Wild Ginger**, 细辛 (*Xixin*): the dried herb of *Asarum heterotropoides* Fr. var. *mandshuricum* (Maxim.) Kitagawa, *Asarum sieboldii* Miq. var. *seoulense* Nakai (family Aristolochiaceae).

[Taste and Properties] Pungent and warm; toxic at a large dose.

[Effects and Indications] (1) Dispels wind-cold in the case of cold headaches; (2) Dispels cold from meridians for relieving muscle and joint pains; (3) Relieves stuffed nose in cases of rhinitis and sinusitis; (4) Resolves phlegm for treating chronic bronchitis with profuse thin sputum.

[Usage and Dosage] 1-2 g in decoction, and 0.5-1 g in pills.

[Notes] Its volatile oil lowers the body temperature in rabbits with fever induced by typhoid vaccine. It has a local anesthetic effect when used topically. In animal experiments, the volatile oil has a tranquilizing, analgesic and antitussive effect, but in large doses it causes paralysis of the voluntary and respiratory movements. This can explain why it is traditionally held that each dose of wild ginger should not exceed 3 g.

***Fructus Xanthii*, Cocklebur Fruit**, 苍耳子 (*Cang'erzi*): the dried ripe fruit of *Xanthium sibiricum* Patrin. (family Compositae)

[Taste and Properties] Pungent, slightly bitter and warm.

[Effects and Indications] (1) Relieves stuffed nose in cases of rhinitis and sinusitis; (2) Dispels wind-damp for treating urticaria and rheumatism.

[Usage and Dosage] 3-9 g.

***Flos Magnoliae*, Magnolia Flower**, 辛夷 (*Xinyi*): the dried flower bud of *Magnolia biondii* Pamp., *Magnolia denudata* Desr. or *Magnolia sprengeri* Pamp. (family Magnoliaceae)

[Taste and Properties] Pungent and warm.

[Effects and Indications] Relieves nasal obstruction in cases of rhinitis and sinusitis.

[Usage and Dosage] 3-9 g.

[Notes] Its volatile oil has a local astringent effect on the nasal mucosa.

***Rhizoma Zingiberis Recens*, Fresh Ginger**, 生姜 (*Shengjiang*): the fresh rhizome of *Zingiber officinale* (Willd.) Rosc. (family Zingiberaceae).

[Taste and Properties] Pungent and warm.

[Effects and Indications] (1) Induces perspiration and dispels cold in the treatment of colds; (2) Warms the Stomach for treating stomachache and vomiting due to cold.

[Usage and Dosage] 3-9 g or 3 pieces.

[Notes] Fresh ginger contains volatile oil and gingerol. The volatile oil stimulates blood circulation and sweat secretion. Gingerol promotes gastric secretion and intestinal peristalsis, stimulating digestion. Zingiberone and zingiberene isolated from gingerol are the active principles in the antiemetic effect of fresh ginger.

Pungent-Cool Superficies-Relieving Drugs (Wind-Heat Dispersing Drugs)

***Radix Bupleuri*, Thorowax Root**, 柴胡 (*Chaihu*): the dried root of *Bupleurum chinense* DC. or *Bupleurum scorzonerifolium* Willd. (family Umbelliferae).

[Taste and Properties] Bitter, pungent and slightly cold.

[Effects and Indications] (1) Relieves fever in the treatment of common colds and influenza, and in combination with *Radix Scutellariae* (skullcap root) for treating alternate chills and fever in a half-exterior half-interior syndrome; (2) Soothes the Liver in the case of costal and hypochondriac pain, and menstrual disorders due to Liver *qi* stagnation; (3) Elevates Spleen *qi* for treating sinking syndromes.

[Usage and Dosage] 3-9 g.

[Notes] (1) Thorowax root lowers the body temperature in experimental fevers. It can even lower the body temperature in normal animals. The volatile oil contains the main active principles for the antipyretic effect. (2) In vitro, thorowax root is bacteriostatic to *Streptococcus hemolyticus*, *Staphylococcus aureus*, and *Bacillus tuberculosis*; it also inhibits the replication of the influenza virus. Its saponin content, saikoside, has a marked anti-inflammatory effect. The mechanisms of the anti-inflammatory action are complicated.

Saikoside not only stimulates the synthesis and secretion of the adrenocortical hormone, but also by itself suppresses the release of inflammatory transmitters, wandering of leukocytes, and proliferation of connective tissue. (3) Thorowax root is an important drug for "soothing the Liver." In recent years, it has been widely used for treating hepatitis and cholecystitis. In animal experiments, it is effective for treating experimental hepatosis induced by typhoid vaccine, alcohol, or D-aminogalactose. This may be related to the suppression of enzyme activities and the protection of the biomembrane of the liver by saikoside. Saikoside also lowers blood lipids, and this is beneficial for the prevention of fatty liver. In addition, thorowax root is a cholagogue. The root processed with vinegar is more potent than the unprocessed root in increasing the bile flow. (4) Thorowax root and its saponins cause sedation in animal experiments (and sleepiness in patients), and show a marked antitussive effect only slightly inferior to codeine.

Radix Puerariae, **Kudzuvine Root**, 葛根 (*Gegen*): the dried root of *Pueraria lobata* (Willd.) Ohwi or *Pueraria thomsonii* Benth. (family Leguminosae).

[Taste and Properties] Sweet, pungent and cool.

[Effects and Indications] (1) Relieves fever, and particularly neck pain and stiffness resulting from wind-heat affection; (2) Relieves thirst in cases of febrile diseases and diabetes mellitus; (3) Arrests diarrhea in cases of dysentery; (4) Also used as an antianginal and antihypertensive, especially for the relief of headache, tinnitus and neck stiffness in hypertensive patients.

[Usage and Dosage] 9-15 g.

[Notes] It contains flavones, daidzein, puerarin and others. It shows antipyretic effect probably through dilation of cutaneous blood vessels. Its infusion together with daidzein and puerarin can reduce the blood pressure in experimental hypertension and dilate the coronary and cerebral arteries.

Folium Mori, **Mulberry Leaf**, 桑叶 (*Sangye*): the dried leaf of *Morus alba* L. (family Moraceae).

[Taste and Properties] Bitter and slightly cold.

[Effects and Indications] Dispels wind-heat in cases of upper respiratory infections and acute conjunctivitis.

[Usage and Dosage] 4.5-9 g.

Flos Chrysanthemi, **Chrysanthemum Flower**, 菊花 (*Juhua*): the dried flower-head of *Chrysanthemum morifolium* Ramat. (family Compositae).

[Taste and Properties] Pungent, bitter and slightly cold.

[Effects and Indications] (1) Dispels wind-heat in the case of upper respiratory infections and acute conjunctivitis; (2) Soothes the Liver in cases of headache, dizziness and blurred vision due to wind-heat affection of the Liver Meridian or exuberance of the Liver *yang* (as occurring in hypertension).

[Usage and Dosage] 4.5-9 g.

[Notes] In vitro, it inhibits the growth of *Staphylococcus aureus, Streptococcus hemolyticus, Escherichia coli*, and *Salmonella typhi*. It suppresses the vasomotor center and dilates blood vessels, producing a hypotensive effect.

Herba Menthae, **Peppermint**, 薄荷 (*Bohe*): the dried aerial part of *Mentha* *haplocalyx* Briq. (family Labiatae).

[Taste and Properties] Pungent and cool.

[Effects and Indications] (1) Dispels wind-heat in the case of upper respiratory infections with headache and sore throat; (2) Promotes eruption in the case of measles with inadequate eruption, and relieves itching in the case of urticaria and other itchy skin diseases; (4) Soothes the Liver to relieve hypochondriac pain and fullness due to stagnation of Liver *qi*.

[Usage and Dosage] 3-6 g, to be added when the decoction is nearly done.

[Notes] Its volatile oil chiefly contains menthol and methone. A small amount of mentha oil given orally stimulates the thermoregulatory center and dilates cutaneous capillaries, thus promoting the secretion of sweat. Menthol, when applied to the skin and mucous membrane, causes constriction of blood vessels and paralyses the sensory nerve endings, producing a sensation of coolness as well as having analgesic and antipruritic effects.

***Fructus Arctii*, Great Burdock Achene**, 牛蒡子 (*Niubangzi*): the dried ripe fruit of *Arctium lappa* L. (family Compositae).

[Taste and Properties] Pungent, bitter and cold.

[Effects and Indications] (1) Dispels wind-heat and relieves sore throat in the case of upper respiratory infections and other febrile diseases at the initial stage, as well as skin diseases caused by wind-heat; (2) Promotes eruption in the case of measles with inadequate eruption.

[Usage and Dosage] 6-9 g.

[Notes] In vitro, it inhibits the growth of *Diplococcus pneumoniae* and *Staphylococcus aureus*.

***Periostracum Cicadae*, Cicada Slough**, 蝉蜕 (*Chantui*): the slough shed by the nymph of *Cryptotympana pustulata* Fabr. (family Cicadidae).

[Taste and Properties] Sweet and cold.

[Effects and Indications] (1) Dispels wind-heat when treating hoarseness of the voice in the case of upper respiratory infections and relieves skin itching; (2) Arrests convulsions due to high fever or tetanus.

[Usage and Dosage] 3-6 g; for convulsions, 15-30 g.

[Notes] It contains chitin. Experimentally it has antipyretic and sedative effects, and is effective against convulsions induced by strychnine or nicotine. It blocks nerve conduction at the ganglion level.

***Fructus Viticis*, Shrub Chastetree Fruit**, 蔓荆子 (*Manjingzi*): the dried ripe fruit of *Vitex trifolia* L. var. *simplicifolia* Cham. or *Vitex trifolia* L. (family Verbenaceae).

[Taste and Properties] Pungent, bitter and slightly cold.

[Effects and Indications] Dispels wind-heat for relieving headaches in the case of upper respiratory infections.

[Usage and Dosage] 4.5-9 g.

[Notes] Traditionally, shrub chastetree fruit, dahurian angelica root, and wild ginger are drugs commonly used for relieving headaches in the case of exterior syndromes. Shrub chastetree fruit is good for wind-heat headaches, dahurian angelica root for wind-damp headaches, and wild ginger for wind-cold headaches.

Herba Spirodelae, **Common Ducksmeat Herb**, 浮萍 (*Fuping*): the dried whole plant of *Spirodela polyrrhiza* (L.) Schneid. (family Lemnaceae).

[Taste and Properties] Pungent and cold.

[Effects and Indications] (1) Induces perspiration for relieving exterior syndrome in the case of upper respiratory infections; (2) Promotes the secretion of urine for treating edema with exterior syndromes (e.g., acute nephritis in the early stage).

[Usage and Dosage] 3-9 g.

Rhizoma Cimicifugae, **Bugbane Rhizome**, 升麻 (*Shengma*): the dried rhizome of *Cimicifuga heracleifolia* Kom., *Cimicifuga dahurica* (Turcz.) Maxim. or *Cimicifuga foetida* L. (family Ranunculaceae).

[Taste and Properties] Pungent, sweet and slightly cold.

[Effects and Indications] (1) Promotes eruption in measles; (2) Eliminates heat-toxics for relieving pharyngitis and stomatitis; (3) Elevates Spleen *qi* for treating sinking syndromes.

[Usage and Dosage] 3-9 g.

[Notes] The extract of bugbane rhizome shows antipyretic, analgesic and antiphlogistic effect in experimental studies.

According to modern pharmacological research, only a few superficies-relieving drugs are really diaphoretics. Among them, the most potent one is ephedra. Some drugs, such as Chinese cinnamon twig, fresh ginger and kudzuvine root, by dilating the cutaneous blood vessels, can help in diaphoresis.

Besides these, most superficies-relieving drugs have an antipyretic action, but the mechanisms of the action are not clear and may be different in different drugs. Fever is lowered presumably by increasing the heat dissipation from the skin, by affecting the central synthesis of prostaglandin E or by suppressing the inflammatory processes.

Quite a few superficies-relieving drugs show analgesic effects. They are useful for relieving headaches and general aching in the case of exterior syndromes. Many drugs have anti-inflammatory and antiallergic effects, which are also of great significance in the treatment of exterior syndromes. In addition, some of the drugs act on the immune system, enhancing the body's resistance. For example, thorowax root, perilla leaf, dahurian angelica root and bugbane rhizome induce the production of interferon.

Many superficies-relieving drugs have been reported to be bacteriostatic in vitro or inhibit the virus replication. The clinical significance of these data needs further evaluation by pharmacokinetic studies when the drugs are given orally.

The common pharmacological effects of superficies-relieving drugs are summarized in Table IX-1.

ANTITUSSIVE, PHLEGMOLYTIC AND ANTIASTHMATIC DRUGS

Coughing, expectoration and dyspnea (or asthma) are closely related. Clinically, coughing is often accompanied by expectoration of phlegm, while at the same time, the presence of phlegm induces coughing. Coughing and dyspnea (or asthma) may also occur simultaneously. Therefore, in the treatment of coughing or asthma, antitussive, antiasthmatic and phlegmolytic drugs are often used in combination.

Phlegm can be divided into two categories, according to whether it has a cold or hot nature. Cold phlegm is thin, watery or frothy, and whitish in color, accompanied by other cold manifestations. Hot phlegm is thick, sometimes yellow in color, and accompanied by other heat manifestations. Thus, the drugs for resolving phlegm can be classified into two groups accordingly. Warming phlegmolytics are warm in property, and are indicated in the treatment of cold phlegm, but not suitable for hot phlegm or coughing with hemoptysis. Heat-clearing phlegmolytics are cool or cold in property; they are indicated in cases of coughing with yellow thick expectoration and other pathological changes (such as epilepsy and convulsions) due to hot phlegm, but not suitable for cold-phlegm syndromes.

Antitussive and antiasthmatic drugs also have cold and hot properties, for example, bitter apricot seed and coltsfoot flower are warm-propertied, while Dutchman's pipe fruit and mulberry bark are cold-propertied. But, most of them are only slightly warm or cold. In addition, they are often used as auxiliary ingredients for symptomatic relief of cough and asthma in a compound prescription.

Table IX-1. Common Pharmacological Effects of Superficies-Relieving Drugs

	Dia-phoretic	Anti-pyretic	Anal-gesic	Anti-bact.	Anti-viral	Anti-inflam	Anti Allergic
Pungent-warm herbs for relieving exterior syndromes							
Ephedra	+	+	+	+	+	+	+
Cinnamon twig	+	+	+	+	+		+
Schizonepeta		+	+	+	+	+	+
Saposhnikovia root		+	+	+	+	+	+
Perilla leaf			+	+	+		
Wild ginger		+	+	+	+	+	
Fresh ginger	+		+		+	+	+
Dahurian angelica root			+	+			
Pungent-cool herbs for relieving exterior syndromes							
Thorowax root		+	+	+	+	+	
Kudzuvine root		+	+				+
Peppermint		+	+	+	+	+	
Mulberry leaf		+	+	+	+		
Chrysanthemum flower			+				
Great burdock achene		+	+	+			
Bugbane rhizome			+			+	
Ducksmeat herb		+					
Shrub chastetree fruit			+				

Warming Phlegmolytics (Drugs for Resolving Cold Phlegm)

Rhizoma Pinelliae, **Pinellia Tuber**, 半夏 (*Banxia*): the dried root of *Pinellia ternata* (Thunb.) Breit. (family Araceae).

[Taste and Properties] Pungent, warm and toxic.

[Effects and Indications] (1) Resolves phlegm in the case of coughing with profuse thin expectoration; (2) Relieves nausea and vomiting; (3) Dissipates nodulation in the case of boils and scrofula.

[Usage and Dosage] 3-9 g. Unprocessed pinellia is toxic. Only processed pinellia tuber can be taken orally. The toxic compound contained in pinellia tuber cannot be destroyed by boiling, but it can be eliminated by alum. To assist the antiemetic effect, ginger may be added to the processed pinellia tuber (processed pinellia tuber with ginger).

[Warning] Incompatible with aconite and allied drugs.

[Notes] Antitussive effect in animal experiments. Unprocessed pinellia tuber has anemetic action, while processed pinellia tuber is antiemetic by inhibiting the vomiting center.

***Rhizoma Arisaematis*, Jack-in-the-pulpit Tuber**, 天南星 (*Tiannanxing*): the dried tuber of *Arisaema erubescens* (Wall.) Schott., *Arisaema heterophyllum* Bl. or *Arisaema amurense* Maxim. (family Araceae).

[Taste and Properties] Bitter, warm and toxic.

[Effects and Indications] (1) Resolves phlegm in the case of coughing with profuse thin expectoration; (2) Dispels wind-phlegm for treating vertigo, apoplectic hemiplegia and epilepsy.

[Usage and Dosage] 3-6 g.

[Notes] (1) Its saponin content stimulates the gastro-intestinal mucosa, and reflexively increases the bronchial secretion, thus promoting expectoration. It has also revealed sedative, analgesic and anticonvulsive effects in experimental studies.

***Semen Sinapis Albae*, White Mustard Seed**, 白芥子 (*Baijiezi*): the ripe seed of *Sinapis alba* (L.) Boiss. (family Cruciferae).

[Taste and Properties] Pungent and warm.

[Effects and Indications] (1) Eliminates cold phlegm for the treatment of coughing, dyspnea and stuffiness in the chest with profuse thin expectoration, and also for the treatment of arthralgia accompanied by numbness due to obstruction of collaterals by phlegm; (2) Dissipates nodulation for scrofula.

[Usage and Dosage] 3-9 g.

[Notes] It is a stimulant expectorant.

***Flos Inulae*, Inula Flower**, 旋复花 (*Xuanfuhua*): the dried flower-head of *Inula japonica* Thunb. or *Inula britannica* L. (family Compositae).

[Taste and Properties] Bitter, pungent, salty and warm.

[Effects and Indications] (1) Resolves phlegm and relieves asthma, used as an expectorant in cases of asthmatic bronchitis with excessive phlegm; (2) also used as an antiemetic for relieving belching, nausea and vomiting.

[Usage and Dosage] 3-9 g, to be wrapped when making decoction.

[Notes] It is an expectorant and antiemetic, and has shown a mild effect in relaxing bronchospasm in experimental studies.

Heat-clearing Phlegmolytics (Drugs for Resolving Hot Phlegm)

***Fructus Trichosanthis*, Snakegourd Fruit**, 栝蒌 (*Gualou*): the dried ripe fruit of *Trichosanthes kirilowii* Maxim. or *Trichosanthes rosthornii* Hams (family Cucurbitaceae).

[Taste and Properties] Sweet and cold.

[Effects and Indications] (1) Eliminates hot phlegm for treating coughing with thick sputum; (2) Alleviates precordial pain in the case of angina pectoris with a stuffy sensation in the chest; and (3) Relaxes the bowels in the case of constipation.

[Usage and Dosage] 9-15 g.

[Notes] In vitro, it shows a broad-spectrum antibacterial effect. It contains fatty oil, mostly composed of unsaturated fatty acids. It increases coronary blood flow and lowers the blood lipid level in animal experiments.

Bulbus Fritillariae Thunbergii, **Thunberg Fritillary Bulb**, 浙贝母 (*Zhebeimu*): the dried bulb of *Fritillaria thumbergii* Miq. (family Liliaceae).

[Taste and Properties] Bitter and cold.

[Effects and Indications] Clears the Lungs of heat, resolves phlegm, and reduces nodulation, used for treating respiratory infections with thick yellow sputum, and scrofula.

[Usage and Dosage] 4.5-9 g.

[Warning] Incompatible with *Radix Aconiti.*

[Notes] It contains peimine, peiminine and other alkaloids as the main active principles. In animal experiments, peimine and peiminine have an antitussive effect comparable with codeine. Peimine at a low concentration relaxes the smooth bronchial muscle. The alkaloids also decrease bronchial secretion and show sedative and hypotensive effects.

Bulbus Fritillariae Cirrhosae, **Tendrilled Fritillary Bulb**, 川贝母 (*Chuanbeimu*): the dried bulb of *Fritillaria cirrhosa* D. Don, *Fritillaria unibracteata* Hsiao et K. C. Hsia, *Fritillaria przewalskii* Maxim. or *Fritillaria delavayi* Franch. (family Liliaceae).

[Taste and Properties] Bitter, sweet and slightly cold.

[Effects and Indications] Moistens the Lungs and relieves coughing, used as an expectorant and antitussive for treating coughing due to *yin* deficiency or dryness.

[Usage and Dosage] 3-9 g.

[Warning] Incompatible with *Radix Aconiti.*

[Notes] It chiefly contains alkaloids (fritimine and fritillarine) and saponins. They show antitussive and expectorant effects in animal experiments.

Semen Lepidii, **Pepperweed Seed** or **Tansy Mustard Seed**, 葶苈子 (*Tinglizi*): the dried ripe seed of *Lepidium apetalum* Willd. or *Descurainia sophia* (L.) Webb ex Prantl. (family Cruciferae).

[Taste and Properties] Pungent, bitter and very cold.

[Effects and Indications] (1) Purges the Lungs of phlegm and relieves dyspnea, used for treating coughing and asthma with excessive sputum; (2) Causes diuresis for treating edema in pulmonary heart disease.

[Usage and Dosage] 3-9 g.

[Notes] It acts like a cardiac glycoside, increasing the myocardial contractibility and cardiac output.

Caulis Bambusae in Taeniam, **Bamboo shavings**, 竹茹 (*Zhuru*): the dried middle shavings of stem of *Bambusa tuldoides* Munro, *Sinocalamus beecheyanus* (Munro) McClure var. *pubescens* P.F. Li or *Phyllostachys nigra* var. *henonis* Stapf (family Gramineae)

[Taste and Properties] Sweet and slightly cold.

[Effects and Indications] Removes heat, resolves phlegm and arrests vomiting, used for treating coughing due to heat in the Lungs and vomiting due to heat in the Stomach.

[Usage and Dosage] 4.5-9 g.

Semen Sterculiae Lychnophorae, **Boat-fruited Sterculia Seed**, 胖大海 (*Pangdahai*): the dried ripe seed of *Sterculia lychnophora* Hance (family Sterculiaceae).

[Taste and Properties] Sweet and cool.

[Effects and Indications] (1) Clears the Lungs of heat for treating inflammation of the throat and hoarseness; (2) Relaxs the bowels in the case of constipation with headache and bloodshot eyes.

[Usage and Dosage] 2-3 pieces, to be soaked in boiling water.

[Notes] The extract is a bulk laxative. It has also shown strong inhibitory action on influenza virus in experimental studies.

Thallus Laminariae, **Sea Tangle**, 昆布 (*Kunbu*): the dried thallus of *Laminaria japonica* Aresch. (family Laminariaceae).

[Taste and Properties] Salty and cold.

[Effects and Indications] Resolves phlegmy nodules and softens hard masses for treating goiter due to iodine deficiency.

[Usage and Dosage] 9-15 g.

[Notes] It contains iodide.

Sargassum, **Seaweed**, 海藻 (*Haizao*): the dried alga of *Sargassum pallidum* (Turn.) C. Ag. or *Sargassum fusiforme* (Harv.) Setch. (family Sargassaceae).

[Taste and Properties] Salty and cold.

[Effects and Indications] Resolves phlegmy nodules and softens hard masses for treating goiter due to iodine deficiency.

[Usage and Dosage] 9-15 g.

[Notes] It contains iodine, reduces blood cholesterol, and has an anticoagulant effect.

Pseudobulbus Pleiones, **Pleione Pseudobulb**, 山慈菇 (*Shancigu*): the dried pseudobulb of *Cremastra appendiculata* (D. Don) Makino, *Pleione bulbocodioides* (Franch.) Rolfe or *Pleione yunnanensis* Rolfe (family Orchidaceae).

[Taste and Properties] Pungent, sweet and cold; somewhat toxic.

[Effects and Indications] Eliminates heat-toxics and resolves nodules, used as an antiphlogistic and detumescent for treating boils, scrofula, tumors and venomous snake-bite.

[Usage and Dosage] 3-9 g; appropriate quantity for external use.

[Notes] It contains colchicine, which inhibits mitosis.

Antitussive and Antiasthmatic

Semen Armeniacae Amarum, **Bitter Apricot Seed**, 苦杏仁 (*Kuxingren*): the dried ripe seed of *Prunus armeniaca* L. var. *ansu* Maxim., *Prunus sibirica* L., *Prunus mandshurica* (Maxim.) Koehne or *Prunus armeniaca* L. (family Rosaceae).

[Taste and Properties] Bitter, pungent and warm; somewhat toxic.

[Effects and Indications] (1) One of the most commonly used antitussive and antiasthmatic agents; (2) Relaxes the bowels in cases of constipation due to deficiency of *yin* and blood.

[Usage and Dosage] 4.5-9 g.

[Notes] It contains amygdalin. After bitter apricot seed is taken orally, amygdalin is decomposed by digestive enzymes and produces a minute amount of hydrocyanic acid, which slightly inhibits the respiratory center, and induces antitussive and antiasthmatic effects. The seed contains fatty oil (35-50%), which has a laxative effect.

Rhizoma Cynanchi Stauntonii, **Willowleaf Swallowwort Rhizome**, 白前 (*Baiqian*): the dried rhizome and root of *Cynanchum stauntonii* (Decne.) Schltr. ex Levl. or *Cynanchum glaucescens* (Decne.) Hand.-Mazz. (family Asclepiadaceae).

[Taste and Properties] Pungent, bitter and slightly warm.

[Effects and Indications] Eliminates phlegm and relieves coughing, used for treating coughing with copious expectoration and dyspnea.

[Usage and Dosage] 3-9 g.

Radix Platycodi, **Platycodon Root**, 桔梗 (*Jiegeng*): the dried root of *Platycodon grandiflorum* (Jacq.) A. DC. (family Campanulaceae).

[Taste and Properties] Bitter and pungent in taste, and neutral in property.

[Effects and Indications] (1) Expels phlegm and relieves coughing, used as an expectorant for coughing with sticky sputum; (2) Promotes the discharge of pus in cases of pyogenic infection of the Lungs; (3) Relieves sore throat.

[Usage and Dosage] 3-9 g.

[Notes] (1) Its decoction, when given orally in animal experiments, increases the secretion of the respiratory tract, producing a remarkable expectorant effect. This is chiefly due to its saponin content, platycodin. Platycodin is also an antitussive. (2) Its crude saponin, when given orally, has an anti-inflammatory effect, reducing swelling induced by carrageenin or acetic acid. In the treatment of pyogenic infections, platycodon root has no direct antibacterial effect, but it promotes the phagocytosis of macrophages, increases the bacteriocidal action of neutrophils, and elevates the activity of lysozyme. The crude saponin also has antipyretic, sedative and analgesic effects. (3) Platycodon root shows hypoglycemic and hypolipemic effects in animal experiments. It lowers blood sugar level in alloxan-induced rabbits, and reduces the cholesterol content of the liver in mice by increasing the excretion of cholesterol and cholic acid.

Radix Peucedani, **Hogfennel Root**, 前胡 (*Qianhu*): the dried root of *Peucedanum praeruptorum* Dunn or *Peucedanum decursivum* Maxim. (family Umbelliferae).

[Taste and Properties] Bitter, pungent and slightly cold.

[Effects and Indications] Dispels wind-heat, relieves coughing and resolves phlegm for treating coughing and dyspnea with sticky sputum in upper respiratory infections.

[Usage and Dosage] 3-9 g.

[Notes] It contains nodakenin, which stimulates the secretion of the respiratory tract, having an expectorant effect.

Radix Asteris, **Tatarian Aster Root**, 紫苑 (*Ziyuan*): the dried root and rhizome of *Aster tataricus* L. f. (family Compositae).

[Taste and Properties] Bitter, pungent and slightly warm.

[Effects and Indications] Relieves coughing by moistening the Lungs, used as an antitussive for acute cough with sticky phlegm or chronic coughing with blood-streaked sputum.

[Usage and Dosage] 4.5-9 g.

[Notes] It increases the secretion of the respiratory tract, causing dilution of phlegm and facilitating expectoration.

***Flos Farfarae*, Coltsfoot Flower**, 款冬花 (*Kuandonghua*): the dried flower-bud of *Tussilago farfara* L. (family Compositae).

[Taste and Properties] Pungent and warm.

[Effects and Indications] Relieves coughing and resolves phlegm for treating acute and chronic coughing with copious expectoration.

[Usage and Dosage] 4.5-9 g.

[Notes] In animal experiments, it shows a prominent antitussive effect, but no notable expectorant effect.

***Radix Stemonae*, Stemona Root**, 百部 (*Baibu*): the dried root tuber of *Stemona sessilifolia* (Miq.), *Stemona japonica* (Bl.) Miq. or *Stemona tuberosa* Lour. (family Stemonaceae).

[Taste and Properties] Sweet, bitter and slightly warm.

[Effects and Indications] (1) Moistens the Lungs and relieves coughing when treating acute and chronic coughing; (2) its alcoholic infusion (20%) used externally against lice.

[Usage and Dosage] 3-9 g.

[Notes] In animal experiments its alkaloids suppress excitation of the respiratory center, inhibiting the coughing reflex. In vitro, it inhibits *Bacillus tuberculosis hominis*. It kills *Pediculus capitus, P. corporis, Phthirus pubis* and other pests.

***Folium Eriobotryae*, Loquat Leaf**, 枇杷叶 (*Pipaye*): the dried leaf of *Eriobotrya japonica* (Thunb.) Lindl. (family Rosaceae).

[Taste and Properties] Bitter and slightly cold.

[Effects and Indications] (1) Clears the Lungs, used as an expectorant and antitussive for coughing with sticky sputum due to heat in the Lungs or for chronic stubborn coughing; (2) Pacifies the Stomach, used as an antiemetic for vomiting due to heat in the Stomach.

[Usage and Dosage] 4.5-9 g.

***Fructus Aristolochiae*, Dutchmanspipe Fruit**, 马兜铃 (*Madouling*): the dried ripe fruit of *Aristolochia contorta* Bge. or *Aristolochia debilis* Sieb. et Zucc. (family Aristolochiaceae).

[Taste and Properties] Bitter, slightly pungent, and cold.

[Effects and Indications] Clears the Lungs for relieving coughing and asthma due to heat in the Lungs.

[Usage and Dosage] 3-9 g.

***Cortex Mori*, White Mulberry Bark**, 桑白皮 (*Sangbaipi*): the dried root bark, deprived of the external brown corky part, of *Morus alba* L. (family Moraceae).

[Taste and Properties] Sweet and cold.

[Effects and Indications] (1) Clears the Lungs for relieving coughing and asthma caused by heat in the Lungs; (2) Induces diuresis for treating edema with oliguria.

[Usage and Dosage] 6-12 g.

[Notes] In experimental studies it shows diuretic, hypotensive and sedative effects.

***Semen Oroxyli*, India Trumpetflower Seed**, 木蝴蝶 (*Muhudie*): the dried ripe seed of *Oroxylum indicum* (L.) Vent. (family Bignoniaceae).

[Taste and Properties] Bitter and cold.

[Effects and Indications] Clears the Lungs for treating coughing, sore throat and hoarseness due to heat in the Lungs.

[Usage and Dosage] 1.5-3 g.

The results of modern pharmacological studies on the major drugs of this category are summarized in Table IX-2.

Table IX-2. Pharmacological Effects of Antitussive, Phlegmolytic and Antiasthmatic Drugs

	Antitussive	Expectorant	Antiasthmatic	Others
Pinellia tuber	+			antiemetic
Jack-in-the-pulpit tuber	+	+		sedative, anticonvulsive
Thunberg fritillary bulb	+	+	+	hypotensive
Tendrilled fritillary bulb	+	+		hypotensive
Platycodon root	+	+		antipyretic, sedative, anti-inflammatory
Hogfennel root	+			anti-inflammatory, anti-allergic
Bitter apricot seed	+		+	
Coltsfoot flower	+	+	+	
Tatarian aster root	+	+		antibacterial, antiviral

FEBRIFUGALS (DRUGS FOR CLEARING UP INTERNAL HEAT)

Febrifugals are drugs used for clearing up the internal heat or fire in febrile diseases, pyogenic infections and internal injuries. Fire is intense heat; it differs from heat only in degree. Heat-clearing drugs are cool or cold in property. The cool-propertied drugs clear up heat, while the cold-propertied drugs purge fire. Generally, drugs of this category can be classified into five groups: fire-purging febrifugals, detoxifying febrifugals, damp-removing febrifugals, blood-cooling febrifugals and febrifugals for deficiency-type fever.

1. Fire-purging febrifugals: These are febrifugals that directly act on heat or fire in the *qi* (energy) system. They are indicated for treating: (1) excess heat in the *qi* system marked by high fever with thirst, dry yellow tongue coating, and full, replete, forceful and rapid pulse, and (2) excess fire, such as excessive Liver fire marked by redness and swelling of and pain in the eyes (acute conjunctivitis), and excessive Stomach fire with

stomatitis and dipsosis.

2. Detoxifying febrifugals: Pathogenic heat and fire occurring in epidemic diseases and pyogenic infections are believed to be toxic. The toxicity should be removed at the same time as dispelling the heat or fire. Detoxifying febrifugals are drugs used for this purpose.

3. Damp-eliminating febrifugals: These are febrifugals that can eliminate both heat and damp, and are indicated in the treatment of diseases caused by damp-heat, such as acute jaundice, dysentery, acute urinary tract infection, subcutaneous pyogenic infections, otalgia with purulent discharge, etc. In pyogenic infections, toxic heat or toxic fire is considered as the pathogenic factor before suppuration, and damp-heat after suppuration. So there is some overlap between toxic heat and damp-heat affections. Some damp-eliminating febrifugals are at the same time detoxifying febrifugals, e.g., skullcap root, goldthread rhizome, phellodendron bark and Chinese gentian root.

4. Blood-cooling febrifugals: These are febrifugals that can remove heat from the blood system. So they are appropriate for treating heat in the blood system, either marked by hemorrhages or by fever with eruptions. In addition, some of them can also nourish *yin*, and are indicated in the treatment of endogenous heat due to *yin* deficiency.

5. Deficiency-heat febrifugals: The above four categories of febrifugals are generally used for excess-type heat. Febrifugals of this category are indicated for relieving deficiency-heat or asthenic fever, which is often due to *yin* deficiency, marked by low-grade fever, hot sensation in the palms and soles, thirst, night sweats, and fine, rapid pulse.

Fire-purging febrifugals (Drugs for Reducing Intense Heat)

***Gypsum Fibrosum*, Gypsum**, 石膏 (*Shigao*): a plaster stone chiefly composed of hydrated calcium sulphate.

[Taste and Properties] Pungent, sweet and very cold.

[Effects and Indications] (1) Clears up heat, quenches fire and relieves thirst, when treating high fever with dire thirst; (2) Clears the Lungs of heat in cases of coughing and dyspnea due to heat in the Lungs; (3) Clears the Stomach of heat for treating headaches and stomatitis caused by exuberant fire in the Stomach.

[Usage and Dosage] 15-30 g, to be decocted before other ingredients.

[Notes] It contains calcium sulfate and a small amount of other minerals. Its extract lowers the body temperature in rabbits with experimentally induced fever, but calcium sulfate has no such action. Its action against thirst has also been shown in experimental studies.

***Rhizoma Anemarrhenae,* Anemarrhena Rhizome**, 知母 (*Zhimu*): the dried rhizome of *Anemarrhena asphodeloides* Bge. (family Liliaceae).

[Taste and Properties] Bitter and cold.

[Effects and Indications] (1) Clears up heat in cases of high fever and thirst; (2) Nourishs *yin* and reduces fire in cases of low fever and night sweats due to *yin* deficiency; (3) Relieves thirst in cases of diabetes mellitus.

[Usage and Dosage] 6-12 g.

[Notes] (1) The extract of anemarrhena rhizome decreases the heat production by inhibiting the activity of Na^+, K^+-ATPase, and thereby lowers the body temperature of animals with experimentally induced fever. In vitro, anemarrhena decoction shows a broad spectrum of bacteriostatic effects. (2) In animals with experimental "*yin*-deficiency" induced by thyroxin and hydrocortisone, anemarrhena decoction inhibits the activity of the ß-adrenergic receptor and reduces the blood cAMP content. Since modern research has shown that *yin*-deficiency with exuberant fire is characterized by hyperfunction of the ß-adrenergic receptor and cAMP system, the above finding can demonstrate the therapeutic effect of anemarrhena for *yin* deficiency; (3) Anemarrhena contains anemam, which lowers blood sugar in normal animals, and especially in animals with hyperglycemia induced by alloxan or insulin antiserum.

Fructus Gardeniae, **Cape-jasmine Fruit**, 栀子 (*Zhizi*): the dried ripe fruit of *Gardenia jasminoides* Ellis (family Rubiaceae).

[Taste and Properties] Bitter and cold.

[Effects and Indications] (1) Clears up heat and quenches fire for fever with restlessness; (2) Eliminates damp-heat in the case of jaundice and acute urinary tract infections; (3) Removes heat from blood and counteracts toxicity when arresting epistaxis and hemoptysis, and when treating subcutaneous infections.

[Usage and Dosage] 6-9 g.

[Notes] (1) In vitro, it inhibits *Staphylococcus aureus, Diplococcus meningitidis, Diplococcus gonorrheae*, and various dermatophytes. It also kills leptospira and inhibits the hepatitis B virus. (2) It shows cholagogue, antipyretic, sedative and hypotensive effects in experimental studies.

Rhizoma Phragmitis, **Reed Rhizome**, 芦根 (*Lugen*): the fresh or dried rhizome of *Phragmites communis* (L.) Trin. (family Gramineae).

[Taste and Properties] Sweet and cold.

[Effects and Indications] (1) Clears up Stomach heat and promotes the production of body fluids for relieving thirst in febrile diseases, and vomiting and retching due to heat in the Stomach; (2) Clears up Lung heat to relieve coughing and for treating lung abscess.

[Usage and Dosage] 15-30 g.

Herba Lophatheri, **Lophatherum Herb**, 淡竹叶 (*Danzhuye*): the dried aerial part of *Lophatherum gracile* Brongn. (family Gramineae).

[Taste and Properties] Sweet or tasteless, and cold.

[Effects and Indications] (1) Clears the Heart of fire and causes diuresis for treating exuberant fire of the Heart manifested by ulceration of the tongue or dysuria (in acute urinary tract infections); (2) Removes heat and relieves nervousness in the late stage of febrile diseases.

[Usage and Dosage] 6-9 g.

[Notes] Given orally it lowers body temperature in rats with artificially induced fever. It also shows a diuretic effect in the laboratory.

Semen Cassiae, **Cassia Seed**, 决明子 (*Juemingzi*): the dried ripe seed of *Cassia obtusifolia* L. or *Cassia tora* L. (family Legunimosae).

[Taste and Properties] Sweet, bitter and slightly cold.

[Effects and Indications] (1) Clears the Liver of fire for treating excessive Liver fire manifested by acute inflammation of the eye, or headache (in hypertension); (2) Also used as a mild laxative.

[Usage and Dosage] 9-15 g.

[Notes] It contains emodin and carotin. Emodin has a laxative effect, and carotin benefits vision. In addition, the aqueous and ethanol extracts lower the blood pressure and blood cholesterol level.

***Semen Celosiae*, Feather Cockscomb Seed**, 青葙子 (*Qingxiangzi*): the dried ripe seed of *Celosia argentea* L. (family Amaranthaceae).

[Taste and Properties] Bitter and slightly cold.

[Effects and Indications] Clears the Liver of fire for treating acute inflammation of the eye.

[Usage and Dosage] 9-15 g.

***Flos Buddlejae*, Butterfly-bush Flower**, 密蒙花 (*Mimenghua*): the dried flower bud and inflorescence of *Buddleja officinalis* Maxim. (family Loganiaceae).

[Taste and Properties] Bitter and slightly cold.

[Effects and Indications] Removes heat and nourishes the Liver for treating eye diseases due to deficiency of Liver *yin* with endogenous fire.

[Usage and Dosage] 3-9 g.

***Spica Prunellae*, Selfheal Spike**, 夏枯草 (*Xiakucao*): the dried fruit-spike of *Prunella vulgaris* L. (family Labiatae).

[Taste and Properties] Bitter, pungent and cold.

[Effects and Indications] (1) Clears the Liver of fire for treatment of acute inflammation of the eye; (2) Removes heat and dissipates nodules in cases of mastitis, scrofula and goiter.

[Usage and Dosage] 9-15 g.

[Notes] Its aqueous or ethanol extract lowers the blood pressure. In vitro, it inhibits *Mycobacterium tuberculosis, Shigella dysenteriae, Staphylococcus*, and *Streptococcus hemolyticus*. It contains ursolic acid, which has a diuretic effect.

Detoxifying Febrifugals (Drugs for Eliminating Heat-Toxics)

***Flos Lonicerae*, Honeysuckle Flower**, 金银花 (*Jinyinhua*): the dried flower bud of *Lonicera japonica* Thunb., *Lonicera hypoglauca* Miq., *Lonicera confusa* DC. or *Lonicera dasystyla* Rehd. (family Caprifoliaceae).

[Taste and Properties] Sweet and cold.

[Effects and Indications] Eliminates heat-toxics for treating exogenous febrile diseases, as well as for boils and other pyogenic inflammations.

[Usage and Dosage] 6-15 g.

[Notes] (1) In vitro, it shows a broad spectrum of antibacterial Effects on both gram-positive and gram-negative bacteria. It also inhibits various dermatophytes and viruses (such as the influenza, ECHO and herpes simplex viruses). The active principles for the bacteriostatic actions include chlorogenic acid, isochlorogenic acid and luteolin. (2) It is strongly antagonistic to bacterial endotoxins, or even directly destroys them. This action is more important than the bacteriostatic effect in the treatment of infections. (3) It inhibits both the inflammatory exudation and hyperplasia. It also exhibits a marked antipyretic effect in experimental fevers. (4) It promotes the phagocytosis of leukocytes, and activates

T lymphocytes, enhancing the transformation of lymphocytes. (5) It reduces the intestinal absorption of cholesterol, lowering the plasma cholesterol level.

***Fructus Forsythiae*, Forsythia Fruit**, 连翘 (*Lianqiao*): the dried fruit of *Forsythia suspensa* (Thunb.) Vahl (family Oleaceae).

[Taste and Properties] Bitter and slightly cold.

[Effects and Indications] (1) Eliminates heat-toxics for treating exogenous febrile diseases; (2) Causes subsidence of swelling in pharyngitis, mastitis and other pyogenic inflammations.

[Usage and Dosage] 6-15 g.

[Notes] (1) It is bacteriostatic to *Salmonella typhi, Staphylococcus aureus, Streptococcus hemolyticus* and *Shigella dysenteriae* in vitro. It also inhibits the influenza virus. (2) It has anti-inflammatory, antipyretic and antiemetic effects. (3) It contains a considerable amount of rutin, which reduces the permeability of the capillaries.

***Radix Isatidis*, Isatis Root** or **Woad Root**, 板蓝根 (*Banlangen*): the dried root of *Isatis indigotica* Fort. (family Cruciferae).

[Taste and Properties] Bitter and cold.

[Effects and Indications] (1) Eliminates heat-toxics for influenza and other viral infections, and also for pyogenic inflammations; (2) Reduces heat in blood for eruptive epidemic diseases.

[Usage and Dosage] 9-15 g.

[Notes] Isatis root has a broad spectrum of bacteriostatic actions, and kills Leptospira in vitro. It also inhibits the influenza virus. It is particularly worth noting that isatis root is effective against endotoxin released by gram-negative bacteria, and is effective for treating toxemia. This may partly explain the detoxifying effect.

***Folium Isatidis*, Woad Leaf**, 大青叶 (*Daqingye*): the dried leaf of *Isatis indigotica* Fort. (family Cruciferae).

[Taste and Properties] Bitter and cold.

[Effects and Indications] Same as *Radix Isatidis*, particularly good for eruptive diseases.

[Usage and Dosage] 9-15 g.

[Notes] It has a broad spectrum of bacteriostatic effects; its tryptanthrin content is the active antibacterial principle. It inhibits encephalitis B, mumps and the influenza virus. It also shows antipyretic and anti-inflammatory effects in experimental studies.

***Indigo Naturalis*, Natural Indigo**, 青黛 (*Qingdai*): the deep-blue powder prepared from the leaf of *Baphicacanthus cusia* (Nees) Bremek. (family Acanthaceae), *Polygonum thinctorium* Ait. (family Polygonaceae) or *Isatis indigotica* Fort. (family Cruciferae)

[Taste and Properties] Bitter and cold.

[Effects and Indications] Eliminates heat-toxics and reduces heat in blood for treating eruptive epidemic diseases and high fever in children, also used externally for boils and ulcerative stomatitis.

[Usage and Dosage] 1.5-3 g, used for making pills or powder; appropriate quantity for external use.

***Herba Taraxaci*, Dandeleon**, 蒲公英 (*Pugongying*): the dried herb of *Taraxacum mongolicum* Hand.-Mazz., *Taraxacum sinicum* Kitag. or several other species of the same genus (family Compositae).

[Taste and Properties] Bitter, sweet and cold.

[Effects and Indications] (1) Eliminates heat-toxics and induces subsidence of swelling for mastitis, boils and other pyogenic inflammations; (2) also used as a detoxicant for food poisoning.

[Usage and Dosage] 9-30 g.

[Notes] Its aqueous extract has a strong bacteriostatic action on *Staphylococcus aureus*.

***Herba Violae*, Violet Herb**, 紫花地丁 (*Zihuadiding*): the dried herb of *Viola yedoensis* Makino (family Violaceae).

[Taste and Properties] Bitter, pungent and cold.

[Effects and Indications] Eliminates heat-toxics and reduces heat in blood for boils, carbuncles and other pyogenic inflammations.

[Usage and Dosage] 9-30 g.

[Notes] It inhibits *Shigella dysenteriae, Klebsiella pneumoniae* and *Pseudomonas aeruginosa* in vitro. It also shows antipyretic and anti-inflammatory effects.

***Herba Houttuyniae*, Houttuynia**, 鱼腥草 (*Yuxingcao*): the dried aerial part of *Houttuynia cordata* Thunb. (family saururaceae).

[Taste and Properties] Pungent and slightly cold.

[Effects and Indications] (1) Eliminates heat-toxics and promotes the drainage of pus for treating pyogenic pulmonary infections; (2) Relieves dysuria in case of acute urinary tract infections.

[Usage and Dosage] 15-30 g, to be decocted briefly.

[Notes] (1) Houttuynia has a broad spectrum of bacteriostatic actions. The juice of the fresh herb is more potent than the decoction of the dried herb, but the action is weakened after heating. A synergetic antibacterial effect is shown when houttuynia is used together with methoxybenzyl aminopyrimidine (TMP). The main active principle against bacteria is decanoylacetaldehyde. (2) Houttuynia promotes the immune function, increasing the phagocytosis of leukocytes and macrophages, and elevating the serum properdin level.

***Herba Patriniae*, Patrinia**, 败酱草 (*Baijiangcao*): the dried herb of *Patrinia scabiosaefolia* Fisch. or *Patrinia villosa* Juss. (family Valerianaceae).

[Taste and Properties] Pungent, bitter and slightly cold.

[Effects and Indications] Eliminates heat-toxics and promotes pus discharge for treating abscesses and acute appendicitis.

[Usage and Dosage] 9-15 g.

[Notes] (1) It inhibits streptococcus and staphylococcus in vitro. (2) It prevents the liver cells degenerating and necrosis, and promotes their regeneration. (3) It has a mild sedative effect.

***Radix Pulsatillae*, Pulsatilla Root**, 白头翁 (*Baitouweng*): the dried root of *Pulsatilla chinensis* (Bge.) Regel (family Ranunculaceae).

[Taste and Properties] Bitter and cold.

[Effects and Indications] Used as an antidysenteric agent for treating bacillary and amebic dysentery.

[Usage and Dosage] 9-15 g.

[Notes] In vitro, it only shows a mild antiamebic effect and bacteriostatic action on *Shigella dysenteriae*.

***Herba Andrographitis*, Andrographis Herb**, 穿心莲 (*Chuanxinlian*): the dried aerial part of *Andrographis paniculata* (Burm. f.) Nees (family Acanthaceae).

[Taste and Properties] Bitter and cold.

[Effects and Indications] Eliminates heat-toxics for treating acute respiratory infections, boils, and acute urinary tract infections.

[Usage and Dosage] 9-15 g.

[Notes] (1) It shows a broad spectrum of antibacterial actions, particularly active against *Diplococcus pneumoniae* and *Streptococcus hemolyticus*. (2) It delays the deterioration of embryonic renal cells caused by $ECHO_{11}$ virus; (3) It increases the phagocytosis of leukocytes.

***Herba Oldenlandiae*, Oldenlandia**, 白花蛇舌草 (*Baihuasheshecao*): the dried herb of *Oldenlandia diffusa* (Willd.) Roxb., *Oldenlandia corymbosa* L. and other related species (family Rubiaceae).

[Taste and Properties] Slightly bitter, sweet and cold.

[Effects and Indications] (1) Eliminates heat-toxics for treating acute appendicitis, pelvic inflammation, urinary tract infection, and venomous snake bite; (2) also used as an antineoplastic agent for cancers of the gastro-intestinal tract.

[Usage and Dosage] 15-60 g.

[Notes] In vitro, it only slightly inhibits *Staphylococcus aureus* and *Shigella dysenteriae*, but can enhance the bacteriocidal action of the serum, increase the phagocytosis of the leukocytes, and promote the adrenocortical function. It also shows an antineoplastic action in cases of leukemia, ascites carcinoma and sarcoma in experimental studies.

***Herba Lobeliae Chinensis*, Chinese Lobelia**, 半边莲 (*Banbianlian*): the dried herb of *Lobelia chinensis* Lour. (family Campanulaceae).

[Taste and Properties] Sweet or tasteless, and slightly cold.

[Effects and Indications] Eliminates heat-toxics and induces diuresis for treating tonsillitis, ascites in liver cirrhosis and nephritic edema.

[Usage and Dosage] 9-15 g.

[Notes] It has a persistent diuretic action, increasing the urinary volume as well as the excretion of sodium and chlorides. The main active principle is radicanin.

***Herba Scutellariae Barbatae*, Barbated Skullcap**, 半枝莲 (*Banzhilian*): the dried whole plant of *Scutellaria barbata* D. Don (family Labiatae).

[Taste and Properties] Slightly bitter, and cold.

[Effects and Indications] (1) Eliminates heat-toxics and induces diuresis when treating hepatitis and liver cirrhosis with ascites; (2) also used as an antineoplastic agent for cancers of the Lungs, liver and rectum.

[Usage and Dosage] 15-30 g.

***Radix Sophorae Tonkinensis*, Vietnamese Sophora Root**, 山豆根 (*Shandougen*): the dried root and rhizome of *Sophora tonkinensis* Gapnep. (family Leguminosae).

[Taste and Properties] Bitter and cold.

[Effects and Indications] (1) Eliminates heat-toxics for treating sore throat and painful swollen gums due to toxic heat of the Lungs or the Stomach; (2) also used as an antineoplastic agent for cancers of the Lungs, larynx and bladder.

[Usage and Dosage] 3-9 g.

[Warning] Contraindicated in patients with deficiency syndromes of the Spleen.

[Notes] It shows an inhibitory action on malignant tumors in animal experiments. It inhibits the growth of dermatophytes in vitro.

Damp-eliminating Febrifugals (Drugs for Eliminating Heat and Dampness)

***Radix Scutellariae*, Skullcap Root**, 黄芩 (*Huangqin*): the dried root of *Scutellaria baicalensis* Georgi (family Labiatae).

[Taste and Properties] Bitter and cold.

[Effects and Indications] (1) Eliminates damp-heat in the Large Intestine in cases of acute enteritis and dysentery; (2) Eliminates heat-toxics in cases of boils and other pyogenic inflammations; (3) Clears the Lungs of fire in cases of coughing with yellow thick sputum; (4) Removes heat from the fetus when there is a danger of abortion.

[Usage and Dosage] 3-9 g.

[Notes] (1) Skullcap root has a broad spectrum of bacteriostatic actions, and also inhibits Asian influenza virus and hepatitis B virus antigens (HBsAg, HBcAg and HBeAg). The main antibacterial constituents are baicalein and wogonin. (2) Skullcap root shows anti-inflammatory and antiallergic effects in experimental studies. Baicalein and baicalin inhibit the activity of the SH enzyme, thereby reducing the release of transmitters for the allergic reaction. Baicalin also inhibits the activity of lipo-oxygenase in blood platelets, suppressing the release of the slow-reacting substance. (3) Skullcap root decoction and baicalin show sedative, hypotensive and cholagogue effects in animal experiments, and baicalein and wogonin stimulate the secretion of urine.

***Rhizoma Coptidis*, Goldthread Rhizome**, 黄连 (*Huanglian*): the dried rhizome of *Coptis chinensis* Franch., *Coptis deltoidea* C. Y. Cheng et Hsiao or *Coptis teeta* Wall. (family Ranunculaceae).

[Taste and Properties] Bitter and cold.

[Effects and Indications] (1) Eliminates damp-heat in case of dysentery; (2) Eliminates heat-toxics in cases of boils and other pyogenic infections; (3) Clears the Heart of fire in cases of restlessness and insomnia due to exuberant fire of the Heart.

[Usage and Dosage] 1.5-6 g.

[Notes] (1) Goldthread rhizome contains berberine as its main antibacterial constituent. In vitro, both goldthread rhizome and berberine show a broad spectrum of bacteriostatic actions, particularly on Flexner's and Shiga's bacilli, staphylococcus, streptococcus, pneumococcus, gonococcus and *Vibro cholerae*. When used alone, either goldthread or berberine is apt to induce drug-resistant strains. But if berberine is used in combination with other febrifugal drugs or antibiotics, its antibacterial action will be doubled or redoubled, and there is no cross-resistance between berberine and penicillin or streptomycin. Goldthread rhizome and berberine also inhibit leptospira, dermatophytes and various strains of influenza A and B viruses, as well as amebas, *Trichomonas vaginalis* and trypanosome. (2) Goldthread rhizome or berberine can improve toxemia in many kinds of bacterial infections. Even below the bacteriostatic concentration, goldthread rhizome can still inhibit the bacteria to form coagulase, reducing their virulence. (3) Goldthread rhizome exhibits an obvious antipyretic effect in leukocytic pyrogen-induced fever, probably by its action on the nerve center. (4) Goldthread rhizome has marked anti-inflammatory actions. It also enhances the phagocytosis of leukocytes and reticulo-endothelial cells, thus raising the body's resistance. (5) Berberine suppresses ventricular and supraventricular arrhythmias by blocking the calcium channel. It also has a positive inotropic action and is a vasodilator. (6) Berberine inhibits platelet aggregation induced by various agents, particularly by collagen. (7) Goldthread rhizome and berberine lower the blood sugar level in normal and hyperglycemic animals. This is probably due to suppression of glyconeogenesis and promotion of glycolysis.

***Cortex Phellodendri*, Phellodendron Bark**, 黄柏 (*Huangbai*): the dried bark of *Phellodendron chinense* Schneid. or *Phellodendron amurense* Rupr. (family Rutaceae).

[Taste and Properties] Bitter and cold.

[Effects and Indications] (1) Eliminates damp-heat for dysentery, urinary tract infection and eczema; (2) Reduces endogenous fire due to deficiency of Kidney *yin* manifested by low fever, night sweats and seminal emission; (3) Eliminates heat-toxics in case of pyogenic inflammation.

[Usage and Dosage] 3-12 g.

[Notes] It contains berberine and has similar pharmacological actions as goldthread rhizome.

***Radix Gentianae*, Chinese Gentian Root**, 龙胆 (*Longdan*): the dried root and rhizome of *Gentiana manshurica* Kitag., *Gentiana scabra* Bge., *Gentiana triflora* Pall. or *Gentiana rigescens* Franch. (family Gentianaceae).

[Taste and Properties] Bitter and cold.

[Effects and Indications] Eliminates damp-heat and quenches fire in the Liver and the Gallbladder when treating acute conjunctivitis, sore throat, hypochondriac pain, or acute otitis media caused by excess fire; and jaundice, urodynia, swelling and itching of the vulva, and eczema of the scrotum caused by damp-heat.

[Usage and Dosage] 3-6 g.

[Notes] (1) It shows anti-inflammatory and antipyretic effects in experimental studies. (2) It contains gentiopicrin and gentianine, which stimulate gastric secretion and promote digestion. (3) It reduces serum glutamic-pyruvic transaminase level in hepatosis.

***Radix Sophorae Flavescentis*, Light-yellow Sophora Root**, 苦参 (*Kushen*): the dried root of *Sophora flavescens* Ait. (family Leguminosae).

[Taste and Properties] Bitter and cold.

[Effects and Indications] (1) Eliminates damp-heat in cases of dysentery, jaundice, eczema, and morbid leukorrhea; (2) Kills parasites and relieve itching for scabies, ringworm and pruritus of vulva caused by *Trichomonas vaginalis*.

[Usage and Dosage] 4.5-9 g.

[Notes] (1) Light-yellow sophora root contains matrine and oxymatrine, which has a marked inhibitory effect on inflammatory reactions, with a potency comparable with hydrocortisone, but with a mechanism unrelated to the pituitary-adrenal system. Probably the effect is due to the action on the lysosome membrane, decreasing the release of inflammatory transmitters. (2) Light-yellow sophora root has an antiallergic action. Oxymatrine inhibits all types I-IV of allergic reactions. (3) The decoction of light-yellow sophora root and its alkaloids shows antineoplastic Effects in experimental studies. (4) Either the decoction or matrine has a diuretic effect, with increase of urine volume and sodium chloride excretion. (5) Matrine exhibits a positive inotropic action on the heart, and a quinidine-like effect on arrhythmia.

***Herba Artemisiae Scopariae*, Oriental Wormwood**, 茵陈 (*Yinchen*): the dried seedling of *Artemisia scoparia* Waldst. et Kit. or *Artemisia capillaris* Thunb. (family Compositae).

[Taste and Properties] Bitter and slightly cold.

[Effects and Indications] Eliminates damp-heat from the Liver and Gallbladder when treating jaundice (e.g., icteric hepatitis).

[Usage and Dosage] 6-15 g.

[Notes] Traditionally it is an important drug for treating jaundice. Modern research has revealed its cholagogue effect. Its decoction increases the bile secretion and relaxes Oddi's sphincter. It also has preventive and therapeutic effects on liver damage caused by carbon tetrachloride or acetaminophenol in animal experiments.

***Herba Abri*, Canton Love-pea Vine**, 鸡骨草 (*Jigucao*): the dried whole plant of *Abrus cantoniensis* Hance (family Leguminosae) deprived of pods.

[Taste and Properties] Sweet and cool.

[Effects and Indications] Eliminates damp-heat in cases of acute and chronic hepatitis, cirrhosis of the liver, and urinary tract infection.

[Usage and Dosage] 15-30 g.

***Cortex Dictamni*, Dittany Bark**, 白藓皮 (*Baixianpi*): the dried root-bark of *Dictamnus dasycarpus* Turcz. (family Rutaceae).

[Taste and Properties] Bitter and cold.

[Effects and Indications] Eliminates damp-heat, dispels wind and relieves itching when treating skin diseases such as ulceration, eczema and urticaria, and also acute rheumatic arthritis.

[Usage and Dosage] 4.5-9 g.

[Notes] (1) It shows an antipyretic effect in the laboratory. (2) In vitro, it inhibits various fungi, including trichophytons.

Blood-cooling Febrifugals (Drugs for Reducing Heat in Blood)

***Cornu Bubali*, Buffalo Horn**, 水牛角 (*Shuiniujiao*): the horn of *Bubalus bubalis* L. (family Bovidae), used to replace *Cornu Rhinoceri* (rhinoceros horn).

[Taste and Properties] Bitter and cold.

[Effects and Indications] Reduces heat in blood in cases of high fever with delirium and eruptions in cases of acute infectious diseases and for treating bleeding due to blood heat.

[Usage and Dosage] 15-30 g, to be decocted for more than 3 hours before other ingredients.

[Notes] It shows cardiotonic Effects in experimental studies.

Radix Rehmanniae, **Dried Rehmannia Root** (unprocessed), 生地黄 (*Shengdihuang*), the dried tuberous root of *Rehmannia glutinosa* Libosch (family Scrophulariaceae).

[Taste and Properties] Sweet, bitter and cold.

[Effects and Indications] (1) Reduces heat in blood and nourishes *yin* when treating febrile diseases at the *ying*-blood stage (manifested by fever, thirst, reddened tongue and eruptions), and *yin* deficiency with endogenous heat (manifested by persistent low fever); (2) also used for arresting bleeding due to heat in blood.

[Usage and Dosage] 9-15 g.

[Notes] (1) It shows a prominent sedative effect in animal experiments. (2) It inhibits inflammation, presumably by increasing the synthesis of adrenocortical hormone. It also enhances the phagocytosis of reticulo-endothelial system, and increases the peripheral T lymphocyte count. (3) It has a styptic effect, shortening the bleeding and coagulation times.

Cortex Moutan, **Tree Peony Bark**, 牡丹皮 (*Mudanpi*): the dried root-bark of *Paeonia suffruticosa* Andr. (family Ranunculaceae).

[Taste and Properties] Bitter, pungent and slightly cold.

[Effects and Indications] (1) Reduces heat in blood in the case of febrile diseases at the *ying*-blood stage, and *yin* deficiency with endogenous heat; (2) Invigorates blood circulation and removes stasis for amenorrhea and dysmenorrhea, sores and carbuncles, and traumatic injuries.

[Usage and Dosage] 6-12 g.

[Warning] Contraindicated in pregnancy.

[Notes] (1) In vitro, tree peony bark shows bacteriostatic Effects on *Staphylococcus aureus, Shigella dysenteriae, Salmonella typhi* and dermatophytes. (2) Tree peony bark contains peonol, which has sedative, antipyretic, analgesic, anti-inflammatory, antiallergic and spasmolytic effects. (3) Tree peony bark inhibits platelet aggregation, and protects the heart from ischemia. (4) It has an abortifacient action.

Radix Scrophulariae, **Figwort Root**, 玄参 (*Xuanshen*): the dried root of *Scrophularia ningpoensis* Hemsl. (family Scrophulariaceae).

[Taste and Properties] Bitter, salty and cold.

[Effects and Indications] (1) Reduces heat in blood for febrile diseases at the *ying* stage marked by fever with thirst, dry crimson tongue and delirium; (2) Replenishes *yin* and subdues fire in case of deficiency of Lung *yin* with dryness and fire manifested by coughing with scanty expectoration, hemoptysis or sore throat; (3) Softens hard nodules (e.g., scrofula and goiter).

[Usage and Dosage] 9-15 g.

Radix Arnebiae seu Lithospermi, **Arnebia Root** or **Gromwell Root**, 紫草 (*Zicao*): the dried root of *Arnebia euchroma* (Royle) Johnst. or *Lithospermum erythrorhizon* Sieb.

et Zucc. (family Boraginaceae).

[Taste and Properties] Sweet and cold.

[Effects and Indications] Reduces heat in blood and promotes eruption for treating measles without adequate eruption and other eruptive diseases.

[Usage and Dosage] 4.5-9 g.

[Notes] (1) It shows some antibacterial, antiviral and antifungal effects in the laboratory. (2) It has antipyretic and anti-inflammatory effects. (3) It stimulates the cardiac activity and peripheral blood circulation, and helps in the excretion of toxins. This may in part explain its function of promoting eruption.

Deficiency-heat Febrifugals (Drugs for Relieving Asthenic Fever)

***Cortex Lycii*, Wolfberry Bark**, 地骨皮 (*Digupi*): the dried root bark of *Lycium chinense* Mill. or *Lycium barbarum* L. (family Solanaceae).

[Taste and Properties] Sweet and cold.

[Effects and Indications] (1) Reduces heat in blood for treating hemoptysis and epistaxis; (2) Relieves consumptive fever due to *yin* deficiency.

[Usage and Dosage] 9-15 g.

[Notes] It shows antipyretic, hypotensive and hypoglycemic effects in the laboratory.

***Radix Stellariae*, Starwort Root**, 银柴胡 (*Yinchaihu*): the dried root of *Stellaria dichotoma* L. var. *lanceolata* Bge. (family Caryophyllaceae).

[Taste and Properties] Sweet and slightly cold.

[Effects and Indications] Reduces consumptive fever due to *yin* deficiency in phthisis and infantile malnutrition.

[Usage and Dosage] 3-9 g.

***Rhizoma Picrorhizae*, Figwortflower Picrorhiza Rhizome** or **Tibet Bitterroot**, 胡黄连 (*Huhuanglian*): the dried rhizome of *Picrorhiza scrophulariiflora* Pennell (family Scrophulariaceae).

[Taste and Properties] Bitter and cold.

[Effects and Indications] (1) Reduces consumptive fever in phthisis and infantile malnutrition; (2) Eliminates damp-heat in cases of dysentery and jaundice.

[Usage and Dosage] 1.5-9 g.

[Notes] It is a bitter stomachic, improves digestion and has a cholagogue effect.

***Herba Artemisiae Annuae*, Sweet Wormwood**, 青蒿 (*Qinghao*): the dried aerial part of *Artemisia annua* L. (family Compositae).

[Taste and Properties] Bitter and cold.

[Effects and Indications] (1) Reduces heat in blood in cases of epidemic febrile diseases involving *yin*, manifested by night fever with no sweating in the morning when the fever subsides; (2) Reduces consumptive fever due to deficiency of *yin*; (3) Also used as an antimalarial agent.

[Usage and Dosage] 4.5-9 g.

[Notes] (1) In vitro, sweet wormwood shows some bacteriostatic actions. It also inhibits various dermatophytes and influenza A virus. (2) Sweet wormwood strongly acts against plasmodia. A new antimalarial, *qinghaosu*, was developed from the herb in the 1970s. *Qinghaosu* directly kills the plasmodia at the erythrocytic stage, but does not affect them at the pre-erythrocytic and exo-erythrocytic stages. (3) Sweet wormwood has antipyretic, analgesic and anti-inflammatory effects. It suppresses some immune functions, such as the release of interleukin and induction of interferon.

Modern research has demonstrated that most febrifugals have an antipyretic action. But the action seems to be different from that of diaphoretics, because no sweating can be observed clinically when the fever is brought down by febrifugals.

Since the febrifugals are effective in the treatment of acute infectious diseases, they were once considered to be antimicrobial drugs. Although many febrifugals show bacteriostatic actions in vitro, proof of their clinical use as bacteriostatic agents is only available in a few of them. For the majority of them, it is doubtful whether the required concentration in the blood can be reached when a routine dose is taken orally, and therefore further studies are necessary. Some febrifugals show antiviral or antiprotozoal (antimalarial, antiamebic) effects.

Many Effects other than direct inhibition of the pathogens may be helpful for the control of infection. Anti-inflammatory and immune-enhancing actions are of great significance. Most febrifugals show anti-inflammatory actions, though the mechanisms of Effects may be different in different febrifugals. Forsythia fruit inhibits inflammatory exudation by reducing the capillary permeability; andrographis herb acts against the inflammatory processes by stimulating the pituitary-adrenal system; skullcap root, houttuynia and gromwell root suppress the activity of epoxidase and lipoxidase in the production of inflammatory transmitters.

Quite a few febrifugals have immune-stimulating or immune-enhancing effects. For example, goldthread rhizome, skullcap root, honeysuckle flower, dandeleon, houttuynia, pulsatilla root, rehmannia root and tree peony bark enhance the phagocytosis of the leukocytes and reticulo-endothelial system; houttuynia elevates the activity of lysozyme and the plasma properdin level; dandelion, honeysuckle flower, goldthread rhizome, skullcap root and Vietnamese sophora root promote lymphocyte transformation. However, some febrifugals are immune-suppressors. Dittany bark suppresses cellular immunity. Dittany bark and phellodendron bark inhibit humoral immunity.

The action of febrifugals against toxins is worthy of special discussion. Not all bacteria but only pathogenic bacteria are harmful to the human body. Their pathogenicity or virulence is often due to the toxins they possess. In infections, many local lesions are actually caused by the toxins, and severe general symptoms by toxemia. Although antibiotics may be bacteriostatic or even bacteriocidal, most of them have no effect on endotoxins. Polymyxin, is an exception, but owing to its severe side effects, it is impractical to use polymyxin as an anti-endotoxin drug. A potent antibiotic may even induce a transient aggravation of toxemia due to the sudden release of endotoxin from the bacteria killed by the antibiotic. Such phenomena seldom occur in the course of Chinese herbal treatment.

Among the febrifugals, some have direct actions against toxins. Honeysuckle flower, forsythesia fruit, dandelion and patrinia degrade the bacterial endotoxins. Berberine (an active principle contained in goldthread root and phellodendron bark) is antagonistic to the exotoxin of *Vibro cholerae*. Some other febrifugals act against toxins indirectly. For example, tree peony bark, skullcap root and anemarrhena rhizome at a very low concentration (below the bacteriostatic level) inhibit the formation of coagulase of *Staphylococcus aureus*, reducing the latter's virulence and alleviating its damage to the tissues.

Malignant tumors may lead to heat and toxic syndromes. Therefore, detoxifying febrifugals have often been used in the treatment of malignant tumors. Experimental studies have also shown that some of the febrifugals can notably inhibit cancer cells.

In Table IX-3 are listed the common pharmacological actions of febrifugals. Each febrifugal may have other actions which are not included in the table.

Table IX-3 Common Pharmacological Effects of Febrifugals

	Anti-Bact.	Anti-Viral	Anti-toxic	Anti-protoz.	Anti-Inflam.	Anti-Pyretic	Immuno-Enhanc.	Anti-Neopl.
Fire-purging febrifugals								
Gypsum						+	+	
Anemarrhena rhizome	+					+		+
Cape-jasmine fruit	+					+		
Detoxifying fegrifugals								
Honeysuckle flower	+	+	+	+	+	+	+	+
Forsythesia fruit	+	+			+	+		
Wosd root	+	+		+	+	+	+	
Woad leaf	+	+		+	+	+	+	
Natural indigo	+				+		+	+
Dandelion	+							+
Violet herb	+				+			
Houttuynia	+	+			+		+	+
Pulsatilla root	+	+		+				
Andrographis herb	+		+		+	+	+	+
Vietnamese sophora root	+				+			
Damp-eliminating febrifugals								
Skullcap root	+	+	+		+	+		+
Goldthread rhizome	+	+	+	+	+	+	+	+
Phellodendron bark	+	+	+		+	+		
Chinese gentian root					+		+	
Light-yellow sophora root	+			+	+	+		+
Blood-cooling febrifugals								
Rehmannia root	+		+		+			
Tree peony bark	+				+	+	+	+
Figwort root	+					+		
Gromwell root	+	+	+		+	+		+
Deficiency-heat febrifugals								
Wolfberry bark	+	+				+		+
Starwort bark								
Tibet better-root	+							
Sweet wormwood	+	+	+	+			+	

WIND-DAMP DISPELLING DRUGS (ANTIRHEUMATIC DRUGS)

The term "rheumatism" used here embraces a variety of disorders that have in common pain and stiffness referable to the musculo-skeletal system. It is equivalent to "wind-damp affection" in Chinese medicine. Antirheumatic drugs are those that can dispel wind and damp, and relieve rheumatic pains and/or muscular contraction. Some of them have the effect of strengthening the tendons and bones as well. Therefore, they can generally be divided into three groups: anti-rheumatic drugs with analgesic effect, antirheumatic drugs with collateral-activating effect[1] (to relieve muscular contraction), and antirheumatic drugs with tonic effect (to strengthen the tendons and bones).

Among the antirheumatic drugs, notopterygium rhizome, pubescent angelica root, climatis root, large-leaf gentian root and tetrandra root are commonly used for relieving rheumatic pains; flowering-quince flower, siegesbeckia herb, kadsura pepper stem, orientvine and longnoded pit viper are used for relieving muscular contraction; homalomena rhizome, mulberry mistletoe and acanthopanax bark have the effect of strengthening tendons and bones.

Most antirheumatics are pungent in flavor and warm in property. So caution should be exercised when antirheumatics are used in arthritic patients with *yin* deficiency or blood deficiency.

Rhizoma seu Radix Notopterygii, **Notopterygium Rhizome** or **Root**, 羌活 (*Qianghuo*): the dried rhizome or root of *Notopterygium incisum* Ting ex H.T. Chang or *Notopterygium forbesii* Boiss. (family Umbelliferae).

[Taste and Properties] Pungent, bitter and warm.

[Effects and Indications] Dispels wind-damp for rheumatalgia, especially that of the upper part of the body, and headaches associated with common colds.

[Usage and Dosage] 3-9 g.

[Notes] It shows diaphoretic, antipyretic and analgesic effects in the laboratory.

Radix Angelicae Pubescentis, **Pubescent Angelica Root**, 独活 (*Duhuo*): the dried root of *Angelica pubescens* Maxim. f. *biserrata* Shan et Yuan (family Umbellifereae).

[Taste and Properties] Pungent, bitter and slightly cold.

[Effects and Indications] Relieves rheumatic conditions for arthralgia, especially that of the lower part of the body.

[Usage and Dosage] 3-9 g.

[Notes] It is anti-inflammatory, analgesic and antipyretic. It also has a hypotensive effect by dilating blood vessels.

Radix Clematidis, **Clematis Root**, 威灵仙 (*Weilingxian*): the dried root and rhizome of *Clematis chinensis* Osbeck, *Clematis hexapetala* Pall. or *Clematis manshurica* Rupr. (family Ranunculaceae).

[Taste and Properties] Pungent and warm.

[Effects and Indications] Relieves rheumatic conditions for arthralgia, especially for

[1]Muscular contraction is taken as a manifestation due to obstruction of *qi* flowing in the collaterals. When the obstruction is removed and the flow of *qi* in the collaterals is activated, the contraction will be relieved.

wandering pain all over the body.

[Usage and Dosage] 6-9 g.

[Notes] It has diuretic, analgesic and antipyretic effects, and can make uric acid soluble. It is also used in treating gout.

***Radix Gentianae Macrophyllae*, Large-leaf Gentian Root**, 秦艽 (*Qinjiao*): the dried root of *Gentiana macrophylla* Pall., *Gentiana crassicaulis* Duthie ex Burk. or *Gentiana straminea* Maxim., *Gentiana dahurica* Fisch. (family Gentianaceae).

[Taste and Properties] Pungent, bitter slightly cold.

[Effects and Indications] (1) Relieves rheumatic conditions for arthralgia; (2) Reduces consumptive fever due to deficiency of *yin*.

[Usage and Dosage] 4.5-9 g.

[Notes] It contains gentianine, which shows inhibitory action against the inflammation induced by formaldehyde or egg white in animal experiments, probably through its stimulation of the pituitary to increase ACTH secretion. Gentianine also exhibits tranquilizing, analgesic and antipyretic effects in experimental studies, and alleviates histamine-induced asthma.

***Radix Stephaniae Tetrandrae*, Fourstamen Stephania Root**, 防己 (*Fangji*): the dried root of *Stephania tetrandria* S. Moore (family Menispermaceae).

[Taste and Properties] Bitter, pungent and cold.

[Effects and Indications] (1) Relieves rheumatic conditions for acute arthralgia; (2) Induces diuresis for edema with oliguria.

[Usage and Dosage] 4.5-9 g.

[Notes] Its main active principle is tetrandrine. Tetrandrine shows marked anti-inflammatory, antiallergic, antipyretic, analgesic and hypotensive effects. Tetrandrine suppresses arrhythmias and has a negative inotropic action on the heart. The antiarrhythmic mechanisms are the blockage of the calcium channel and the suppression of intracellular calcium release. Tetrandrine dilates the coronary artery, and protects the myocardium from ischemia. Tetrandrine can remarkably improve experimental pneumonosilicosis in rats.

***Fructus Chaenomelis*, Flowering-quince Fruit**, 木瓜 (*Mugua*): the dried ripe fruit of *Chaenomeles speciosa* (Sweet) Nakai (family Rosaceae).

[Taste and Properties] Sour and warm.

[Effects and Indications] (1) Lessens contraction for treatment of arthritis with ankylosis, and for systremma; (2) Dispels damp and regulates the Stomach for relieving vomiting, diarrhea and indigestion.

[Usage and Dosage] 4.5-9 g.

[Notes] It shows a marked anti-oncotic effect in protein-induced arthritis in animal experiments.

***Herba Siegesbeckiae*, Siegesbeckia Herb**, 豨莶草 (*Xiqiancao*): the dried aerial part of *Siegesbeckia orientalis* L., *Siegesbeckia pubescens* Makino or *Siegesbeckia glabrescens* Makino (family Compositae).

[Taste and Properties] Bitter and cold.

[Effects and Indications] Relieves rheumatic conditions for arthralgia.

[Usage and Dosage] 9-12 g.

[Notes] It is anti-inflammatory. It lowers blood pressure by dilating blood vessels. It also has some anti-malarial effect.

***Caulis Piperis Kadsurae*, Kadsura Pepper Stem**, 海风藤 (*Haifengteng*): the dried stem of *Piper kadsura* (Choisy) Obwi. (family Piperaceae).

[Taste and Properties] Pungent, bitter and slightly cold.

[Effects and Indications] Dispels wind-damp for treatment of rheumatalgia with contraction.

[Usage and Dosage] 6-12 g.

***Caulis Sinomenii,* Orientvine**, 青风藤 (*Qingfengteng*): the dried lianoid stem of *Sinomenium acutum* (Thunb.) Rehd. et Wils. (family Menispermaceae).

[Taste and Properties] Bitter in taste and neutral in property.

[Effects and Indications] Relieves rheumatic conditions for treatment of arthralgia with swelling.

[Usage and Dosage] 6-12 g.

[Notes] It shows anti-inflammatory, analgesic, sedative and hypotensive effects in the laboratory.

***Radix, Folium et Flos Tripterygii Wilfordii,* Tripterygium,** 雷公藤 (*Leigongteng*): the root, leaf and flower of *Tripterygium wilfordii* Hook.f. (family Celastraceae).

[Taste and Properties] Bitter and toxic.

[Effects and Indications] Relieves rheumatic conditions for treating rheumatoid arthritis.

[Usage and Dosage] 6-12 g.

[Notes] It has been reported to be effective for treating rheumatoid arthritis only in recent decades. It is a non-steroid anti-inflammatory and at the same time an immune-suppressor. It may cause side effects such as disordered menstruation or amenorrhea, reduction in sperm count, skin eruptions, decrease of white blood cell and platelet counts, and abdominal pain with diarrhea. The side effects usually disappear soon after discontinuance of the therapy.

***Rhizoma Homalomenae*, Homalomena Rhizome**, 千年健 (*Qiannianjian*): the dried rhizome of *Homalomena occulta* (Lour.) Schott (family Araceae).

[Taste and Properties] Bitter, pungent and warm.

[Effects and Indications] Relieves rheumatic conditions and strengthens the bones for rheumatoid arthritis with contraction and for musculo-skeletal disorders in the aged.

[Usage and Dosage] 4.5-9 g.

***Cortex Acanthopanacis*, Acanthopanax Bark**, 五加皮 (*Wujiapi*): the dried root-bark of *Acanthopanax gracilistylus* W. W. Smith (family Araliaceae).

[Taste and Properties] Pungent and warm.

[Effects and Indications] (1) Dispels wind-damp in treating rheumatalgia; (2) Induces diuresis for treatment of edema with oliguria.

[Usage and Dosage] 4.5-9 g.

[Notes] (1) It inhibits carrageenin-, egg-white-, and formaldehyde-induced swelling, adjuvant arthritis, and allergic inflammation type I, III and IV. Its anti-inflammatory action is mainly due to its suppression of the release of inflammatory transmitters such as leukocyte chemotactic factor and prostaglandins. It inhibits the passive cutaneous allergic reaction by suppressing the production of IgE. (2) It shows sedative, analgesic and hypoglycemic effects in experimental studies. It also enhances the body's resistance to high temperature, hypoxia and stress.

DAMP-ELIMINATING DRUGS

Damp-eliminating drugs are used for treating diseases or syndromes caused by damp. According to the different damp-eliminating mechanisms, the drugs of this category can be classified into three groups—aromatic damp-resolving drugs, diuretic drugs and febrifuging diuretic drugs.

Aromatic Damp-resolving Drugs

Aromatic damp-resolving drugs are pungent in flavor and warm in property. They have a drying action to remove damp and invigorate the function of the Spleen. They are often used in the treatment of accumulation of damp with dysfunction of the Spleen manifested by epigastric fullness, stuffy sensation in the chest, vomiting, diarrhea, reduced food intake, sweetness in the mouth and white greasy coating of the tongue. These drugs contain volatile oils which send forth fragrance, and the active components usually exist in the volatile oils. Therefore, when making a decoction, these drugs should be simmered only for a short time.

***Herba Pogostemonis*, Cablin Patchouli**, 广藿香 (*Guanghuoxiang*): the dried aerial part of *Pogostemon cablin* (Blanco) Benth. (family Labiatae).

[Taste and Properties] Pungent and slightly warm.

[Effects and Indications] (1) Removes turbid damp for treating nausea, vomiting and anorexia due to accumulation of dampness; (2) Dispels summer-damp for treating damp affections in summer, marked by lassitude and stuffiness in the chest or abdominal pain, vomiting and diarrhea.

[Usage and Dosage] 3-9 g.

[Notes] (1) Its antiemetic and antidiarrheal effects are presumably attributed to its action on the vagus nerve. It contains volatile oil, which stimulates gastric secretion, promoting digestion. (2) It shows an antipyretic action, probably by relaxing the peripheral capillaries.

***Herba Agastachis*, Giant-hyssop**, 藿香 (*Huoxiang*): the dried aerial part of *Agastache rugosus* (Fisch. et Mey.) O. Ktze. (family Labiatae).

[Taste and Properties] Pungent and slightly warm.

[Effects and Indications] Same as *Herba Pogostemonis*.

[Usage and Dosage] 3-9 g.

***Herba Eupatorii*, Eupatorium**, 佩兰 (*Peilan*): the dried aerial part of *Eupatorium fortunei* Turcz. (family Compositae).

[Taste and Properties] Pungent in taste and neutral in property.

[Effects and Indications] Resolves damp and invigorates the Spleen for treating epigastric fullness and anorexia due to summer-damp or disturbance of the Spleen by dampness.

[Usage and Dosage] 3-9 g.

[Notes] Its volatile oil inhibits the influenza virus in the laboratory.

***Rhizoma Atractylodis*, Atractylodes Rhizome**, 苍术 (*Cangzhu*): the dried rhizome of *Atractylodes lancea* (Thunb.) DC. or *Atractylodes chinensis* (DC.) Koidz. (family Compositae).

[Taste and Properties] Pungent, bitter and warm.

[Effects and Indications] (1) Resolves dampness and invigorates the Spleen for anorexia, nausea, vomiting and diarrhea in damp affections; (2) Dispels wind-damp for rheumatalgia; (3) Improves vision for night blindness.

[Usage and Dosage] 3-9 g.

[Notes] It contains considerable amounts of vitamins A and D.

***Fructus Amomi Rotundus*, Round Cardamom Fruit**, 豆蔻 (*Doukou*): the dried ripe fruit of *Amomum kravanh* Pirre ex Gagnep, or *Amomum compactum* Soland ex Maton (family Zingiberaceae).

[Taste and Properties] Pungent and warm.

[Effects and Indications] (1) Resolves dampness for treating anorexia, nausea and vomiting due to accumulation of turbid damp in the Spleen and the Stomach; (2) Removes stagnation of food for treating indigestion.

[Usage and Dosage] 3-6 g, to be added when the decoction is nearly done.

[Notes] Its volatile oil has stomachic and antiemetic effects, stimulating gastric secretion and intestinal peristalsis, and inhibiting abnormal fermentation in the intestines.

***Fructus Amomi*, Spiny Amomum Fruit**, 砂仁 (*Sharen*): the dried ripe fruit of *Amomum villosum* Lour., *Amomum villosum* var. *xanthioides* T.L. Wu et Senjen or *Amomum longiligulare* T.L. Wu (family Zingiberaceae).

[Taste and Properties] Pungent and warm.

[Effects and Indications] (1) Resolves dampness for treating epigastric stuffiness and anorexia due to accumulation of damp in the Spleen and the Stomach; (2) Warms the Spleen to check diarrhea of deficiency-cold type; (3) Prevents miscarriage.

[Usage and Dosage] 3-6 g, to be added when the decoction is nearly done.

[Notes] Its volatile oil regulates the motility of the gastro-intestinal tract, promoting normal peristalsis and evacuation, while inhibiting excessive motility and relieving entero-spasm.

Diuretic Drugs

Endogenous damp is abnormally retained fluid. When retained subcutaneously, it forms edema. Diuretic drugs are drugs used to promote urine secretion for treating edema. Most of them are slightly sweet in taste or tasteless. Prolonged administration of diuretic drugs may consume body fluids, so caution should be used when they are administered to patients with *yin* deficiency. If the edema is due to diminished function of the Spleen, diuretics are usually used in combination with tonics to invigorate the Spleen function.

***Poria*, Fuling** or **Indian Bread**, 茯苓 (*Fuling*): the dried sclerotinum of the fungus,

Poria cocos (Schw.) Wolf (family Polyporaceae).

[Taste and Properties] Sweet or tasteless, and neutral in property.

[Effects and Indications] (1) Induces diuresis for treating edema with oliguria; (2) Invigorates the Spleen for treating anorexia and diarrhea due to retention of damp in the Spleen; (3) Eases the mind for treating palpitations and insomnia.

[Usage and Dosage] 9-15 g.

[Notes] (1) Poria shows a diuretic effect in chronic experiments. The active principle is poriatin, which is presumed to be antagonistic to aldosterone receptor. In addition, poria activates Na^+-K^+-ATPase, thus regulating the water-electrolyte metabolism. (2) The polysaccharide contents of poria (pachyman and its derivatives) enhance the immune function, including the activity of macrophages, the number of peripheral leukocytes, and the cellular immune reactions. Pachyman and poriatin also show some antineoplastic activity, chiefly by activating the immunosurveillance. (3) The polysaccharides show some sedative effect in animal experiments. (4) Poria acts on the digestive system, reducing the gastric acidity in experimental gastric ulcer, relaxing the intestinal muscle, protecting the liver against chemical damage, and accelerating the regeneration of the liver cells.

***Polyporus*, Chuling** or **Umbellate Polypore**, 猪苓 (*Zhuling*): the dried sclerotinum of the fungus, *Polyporus umbellatus* (Pers.) Fries (family Polyporaceae).

[Taste and Properties] Sweet or tasteless, and neutral in property.

[Effects and Indications] Induces diuresis and removes dampness for treating edema with oliguria, diarrhea, and excessive leukorrhea.

[Usage and Dosage] 6-12 g.

[Notes] (1) The decoction given orally has a diuretic effect in animal experiments, mainly by inhibiting the water and electrolyte reabsorption of the renal tubules. (2) The polysaccharide content of polyporus (glucan) enhances the immune functions, including the phagocytosis of reticulo-endothelial system, B cell's reaction to antigen, the number of antibody-forming cells and lymphocyte transformation. (3) Besides strengthening the immunosurveillance, glucan directly suppresses the growth of certain malignant tumors, probably by inhibiting the synthesis of DNA of the tumor cells. (4) Glucan protects the liver against chemical damage, and promotes regeneration of the liver cells.

***Rhizoma Alismatis*, Oriental Water-plantain Rhizome**, 泽泻 (*Zexie*): the dried tuber of *Alisma orientalis* (Sam.) Juzep. (family Alismataceae).

[Taste and Properties] Sweet or tasteless, and cold.

[Effects and Indications] Induces diuresis and removes dampness for treating edema with oliguria, diarrhea, and urinary disturbances.

[Usage and Dosage] 6-9 g.

[Notes] (1) The decoction shows a marked diuretic effect with increased excretion of electrolytes and urea. (2) The alcoholic extract reduces blood cholesterol and prevents atherosclerosis in experimental hypercholesterolemia. The effect is comparable to that of clofibrate. The rhizome also improves fat metabolism in the liver and prevents fatty liver. (3) The rhizome has mild hypoglycemic and hypotensive effects.

***Semen Plantaginis*, Plantain Seed**, 车前子 (*Cheqianzi*): the dried seed of *Plantago asiatica* L. or *Plantago depressa* Willd. (family Plantaginaceae).

[Taste and Properties] Sweet and cold.

[Effects and Indications] (1) Induces diuresis and removes dampness for treating edema with oliguria, diarrhea, and dysuria with painful urination; (2) Reduces Liver heat for treating inflammation of the eye.

[Usage and Dosage] 9-15 g, to be wrapped for making a decoction.

[Notes] It has a diuretic effect with increased excretion of sodium, urea and uric acid, as well as a hypoglycemic effect. It contains a large amount of mucilaginous substance, and so wrapping is necessary for making a decoction.

***Herba Plantaginis*, Plantain Herb**, 车前草 (*Cheqiancao*): the dried herb of *Plantago asiatica* L. or *Plantago depressa* Willd. (family Plantaginaceae).

[Taste and Properties] Sweet and cold.

[Effects and Indications] (1) Induces diuresis and removes dampness for treating edema with oliguria, diarrhea, and dysuria with painful urination; (2) Eliminates heat-toxics for treatment of boils and other pyogenic inflammations; (3) Promotes expectoration for cough caused by phlegm-heat.

[Usage and Dosage] 9-30 g.

[Notes] It has less marked diuretic effect than plantain seed, but it inhibits a spectrum of bacteria in vitro, including *Salmonella typhi, Salmonella paratyphi, Shigella dysenteriae* and *Staphylococcus aureus*. In addition, it stimulates the secretion of the respiratory tract to facilitate expectoration, and acts on the respiratory center to alleviate coughing.

***Talcum*, Talc**, 滑石 (*Huashi*): a very soft mineral composed mainly of hydrous magnesium silicate.

[Taste and Properties] Sweet or tasteless, and cold.

[Effects and Indications] (1) Induces diuresis and reduces heat in cases of urinary tract infection; (2) Removes summer damp-heat by inducing diuresis, used for treating thirst, oliguria and watery diarrhea caused by heatstroke; (3) Used externally as an astringent agent for eczema and miliaria.

[Usage and Dosage] 9-24 g, to be wrapped for making a decoction; appropriate quantity for external use.

***Semen Coicis*, Coix Seed**, 薏苡仁 (*Yiyiren*): the dried ripe kernel of *Coix lacryma-jobi* L. var. *ma-yuen* (Roman.) Stapf (family Graminae).

[Taste and Properties] Sweet or tasteless, and slightly cold.

[Effects and Indications] (1) Invigorates the Spleen and induces diuresis for treating edema with oliguria, and diarrhea due to insufficiency of the Spleen with accumulation of damp; (2) Removes heat and promotes pus discharge for treating lung abscesses and appendicitis; (3) Relieves rheumatic conditions for acute arthralgia.

[Usage and Dosage] 9-30 g.

[Notes] It contains coixenolide which inhibits the growth of certain cancers (e.g., ascites cancer) in animal experiments.

***Rhizoma Dioscoreae Hypoglaucae*, Hypoglaucous Yam**, 萆薢 (*Bixie*): the dried rhizome of *Dioscorea hypoglauca* Palibin (family Dioscoreaceae).

[Taste and Properties] Bitter in taste and neutral in property.

[Effects and Indications] (1) Removes turbid damp for chyluria and urinary tract infection with turbid urine; (2) Dispels wind-damp for rheumatalgia.

[Usage and Dosage] 9-15 g.

***Herba Lysimachiae*, Loosestrife**, 金钱草 (*Jinqiancao*): the dried herb of *Lysimachia christinae* Hance (family Primulaceae).

[Taste and Properties] Bitter and slightly cold.

[Effects and Indications] (1) Removes damp-heat and relieves dysuria in cases of acute urinary tract infection; (2) Expels calculi for treating biliary and urinary stones.

[Usage and Dosage] 15-60 g.

[Notes] It shows diuretic and cholagogue effects in experimental studies. The decoction stimulates bile secretion and relaxes Oddi's sphincter.

***Spora Lygodii*, Japanese Climbing-fern Spore**, 海金沙 (*Haijinsha*): the dried spores of *Lygodium japonicum* (Thunb.) Sw. (family Lygodiaceae).

[Taste and Properties] Sweet and cold.

[Effects and Indications] Removes damp-heat and expel calculi for treating urinary stone and urinary tract infection with painful urination.

[Usage and Dosage] 6-15 g, to be wrapped for making a decoction.

***Semen Phaseoli*, Rice Bean**, 赤小豆 (*Chixiaodou*): the dried ripe seed of *Phaseolus calcalatus* Roxb. or *Phaseolus angularis* Wight (family Leguminosae).

[Taste and Properties] Sweet and sour in taste and neutral in property.

[Effects and Indications] (1) Induces diuresis for edema with oliguria; (2) Promotes the discharge of pus for treatment of boils and other pyogenic inflammations.

[Usage and Dosage] 9-30 g.

Febrifuging Diuretic Drugs

This group of drugs can dispel damp-heat through diuresis, and are indicated in the treatment of acute urinary tract infections and other damp-heat affections manifested by diarrhea or eczema. If the heat is exuberant, febrifugals are usually added; if the damp is exuberant, aromatic damp-dispelling drugs are used in combination. Most of them are bitter in taste and cold in property. Caution should be used when they are administered to patients with *yin* deficiency or deficiency type edema.

***Caulis Clematidis Armandii*, Clematis Stem**, 木通 (*Mutong*): the dried lianoid stem of *Clematis armandii* Franch. or *Clematis montana* Buch.-Ham. (family Ranunculaceae).

[Taste and Properties] Bitter and cold.

[Effects and Indications] (1) Removes heat and induces diuresis for treatment of acute urinary tract infection; (2) Stimulates menstrual discharge for treatment of amenorrhea; (3) Promotes lactation.

[Usage and Dosage] 3-9 g.

[Warning] Overdosage may cause damage to the renal function.

[Notes] It shows diuretic and cardiotonic effects in animal experiments. In vitro, it inhibits *Salmonella typhi, Shigella dysenteriae* and various dermatophytes.

***Folium Pyrrosiae*, Pyrrosia Leaf,** 石韦 (*Shiwei*): the dried leaf of *Pyrrosia sheareri* (Bak.) Ching, *Pyrrosia lingua* (Thunb.) Farwell or *Pyrrosia petiolosa* (Christ) Ching (family Polypodiaceae).

[Taste and Properties] Bitter, sweet and slightly cold.

[Effects and Indications] (1) Removes heat, induces diuresis and relieves dysuria for acute urinary tract infection and urinary calculi, also used for treating nephritic albuminuria; (2) Clears the Lungs, resolves phlegm and relieves coughing for the treatment of acute and chronic bronchitis.

[Usage and Dosage] 6-12 g.

[Notes] It shows expectorant, antitussive and antiasthmatic effects in experimental studies.

***Herba Polygoni Avicularis,* Common Knotgrass,** 萹蓄 (*Bianxu*): the dried aerial part of *Polygonum aviculare* L. (family Polygonaceae).

[Taste and Properties] Bitter in taste and neutral in property.

[Effects and Indications] (1) Removes heat, induces diuresis and relieves dysuria for acute urinary tract infections; (2) Removes damp-heat for jaundice and exudative skin lesions.

[Usage and Dosage] 9-15 g.

[Notes] It has a marked diuretic effect with increased excretion of sodium. It shows a hypotensive effect in experimental hypertension. In vitro, it inhibits *Shigella dysenteriae, Microsporum lanosum* and fungi.

***Herba Dianthi,* Lilac Pink,** 瞿麦 (*Qumai*): the dried aerial part of *Dianthus superbus* L. or *Dianthus chinensis* L. (family Caryophyllaceae).

[Taste and Properties] Bitter and cold.

[Effects and Indications] (1) Removes damp-heat and relieves dysuria for treatment of acute urinary tract infection and prostatitis with difficult and painful urination; (2) Stimulates menstrual discharge for treatment of amenorrhea.

[Usage and Dosage] 9-15 g.

[Warning] Contraindicated in pregnancy.

[Notes] It shows a diuretic effect with increased excretion of chlorides in the laboratory.

***Fructus Kochiae,* Broom Cypress Fruit** or **Belvedere Fruit,** 地肤子 (*Difuzi*): the dried ripe fruit of *Kochia scoparia* (L.) Schrad. (family Chenopodiaceae).

[Taste and Properties] Bitter and cold.

[Effects and Indications] Removes damp-heat and induces diuresis for treating dysuria and itchy skin lesions caused by damp-heat.

[Usage and Dosage] 9-15 g; for external use, appropriate quantity to be decocted for fuming and washing.

[Notes] It shows a diuretic effect in experimental studies. It inhibits various dermatophytes in vitro.

INTERIOR-WARMING DRUGS (DRUGS FOR DISPELLING INTERNAL COLD)

Drugs warm or hot in property, used for dispelling internal cold are called interior-warming drugs. There are two patterns of internal cold: one comes from outside (exogenous), and the other is endogenous. Exogenous pathogenic cold may directly invade the interior of the body, resulting in vomiting, diarrhea, abdominal coldness and pain. The treatment is to warm the interior and dispel the pathogenic cold. Endogenous cold originates from decline of *yang*, manifested by aversion to cold, cold limbs, pale complexion, dilute urine, pale tongue with whitish coating, and deep, thready pulse, or even from exhaustion of *yang* with cold sweating and scarcely perceivable pulse (collapse). The treatment should be to restore the normal *yang*. In both cases, interior-warming drugs are indicated. In addition, interior-warming drugs also dispel cold from the meridians and collaterals. So, they are also often used in the treatment of arthralgia due to cold affection.

Interior-warming drugs are hot in property and pungent in flavor. They are contraindicated in heat syndromes of either excess type or deficiency type (endogenous heat due to *yin* deficiency).

Radix Aconiti Lateralis Preparata, **Prepared Aconite Lateral Root**, 附子 (*Fuzi*): the processed daughter root of *Aconitum carmichaeli* Debx. (family Ranunculaceae).

[Taste and Properties] Pungent, very hot, and toxic.

[Effects and Indications] (1) Restores Heart *yang* for treating collapse or shock; (2) Dispels cold in the case of gastric or abdominal pain and diarrhea due to invasion of cold and arthralgia due to cold-damp; (3) Reinforces *yang* for all internal organs, particularly the Kidneys.

[Usage and Dosage] 3-9 g, to be boiled for one hour (in order to minimize its toxicity) before other ingredients are added for making a decoction.

[Warning] Contraindicated in pregnancy.

[Notes] (1) The root contains aconitine, which is toxic for the heart. After boiling for a long time, aconitine is hydrolyzed and the toxicity is minimized. (2) The root is a cardiac tonic, increasing the myocardial contractibility, heart rate and cardiac output. The main active principle is demethylcoclaurine. In addition, the root dilates the coronary, cerebral and peripheral arteries, and improves capillary circulation

Cortex Cinnamomi, **Chinese Cinnamon Bark**, 肉桂 (*Rougui*): the dried bark of *Cinnamomum cassia* Presl. (family Lauraceae).

[Taste and Properties] Pungent, sweet, and very hot.

[Effects and Indications] (1) Reinforces Kidney *yang* for treating edema with oliguria, and chronic diarrhea with cold limbs; (2) Dispels cold for relieving abdominal pain and dysmenorrhea.

[Usage and Dosage] 1-3 g.

[Warning] Contraindicated in *yin* deficiency with endogenous heat, hemorrhagic diseases and pregnancy.

[Notes] It mainly contains cinnamic oil, which dilates peripheral blood vessels, increases blood circulation, and causes mild stimulation of the gastro-intestinal tract, promoting digestion, expelling gas and relieving gastro-entero-spasm.

***Rhizoma Zingiberis*, Dried Ginger**, 干姜 (*Ganjiang*): the dried rhizome of *Zingiber officinale* (Willd.) Rose. (family Zingiberaceae).

[Taste and Properties] Very pungent and hot.

[Effects and Indications] (1) Warms the Spleen and the Stomach for treating nausea, vomiting, abdominal pain and diarrhea; (2) Warms the Lungs for chronic bronchitis with frothy expectoration.

[Usage and Dosage] 3-9 g.

[Warning] Contraindicated in cases of fever, *yin* deficiency and pregnancy.

[Notes] (1) It reflexively stimulates the vasomotor center and the sympathetic nervous system, elevating the blood pressure. (2) When given orally, it dilates the blood vessels and increases the blood circulation of the gastro-intestinal tract, improving digestion and arresting vomiting and diarrhea. It can check the vomiting caused by copper sulfate, but has no effect on vomiting caused by digitalis or apomorphine. This indicates that the antiemetic effect is directly due to the local action, and is not related to inhibition of the vomiting center. (3) It contains shogaol, which has an antitussive effect.

***Fructus Evodiae*, Evodia Fruit**, 吴茱萸 (*Wuzhuyu*): the dried nearly mature fruit of *Evodia rutaecarpa* (Juss.) Benth., *Evodia rutaecarpa* var. *officinalis* (Dode) Huang or *Evodia rutaecarpa* var. *bodinieri* (Dode) Huang (family Rutaceae).

[Taste and Properties] Bitter, pungent and very hot.

[Effects and Indications] (1) Warms the Stomach for relieving gastric and abdominal pain; (2) Relieves nausea, vomiting and acid regurgitation (for acid regurgitation, goldthread root is often used in combination).

[Usage and Dosage] 1.5-6 g.

[Warning] Contraindicated in cases of fever. Overdosage may cause visual disturbances.

[Notes] It shows an analgesic effect, and slightly elevates the body temperature in animal experiments.

***Rhizoma Galangae*, Galangal Rhizome**, 高良姜 (*Gaoliangjiang*): the dried rhizome of *Alpinia officinarum Hance* (family Zingiberaceae).

[Taste and Properties] Pungent and very warm.

[Effects and Indications] Warms the Stomach for relieving gastric pain and vomiting.

[Usage and Dosage] 3-6 g.

[Notes] Traditionally, both galangal rhizome and dried ginger are used for warming the Spleen and the Stomach. Dried ginger is more frequently used to warm the Spleen for checking diarrhea, and galangal to warm the Stomach for relieving epigastric pain.

***Flos Caryophylli*, Clove,** 丁香 (*Dingxiang*): the dried flower bud of *Eugenia caryophyllata* Thunb. (family Myrtaceae).

[Taste and Properties] Pungent and warm.

[Effects and Indications] (1) Warms the Spleen and the Stomach for relieving hiccups, vomiting and diarrhea; (2) Reinforces Kidney *yang* for treating impotence.

[Usage and Dosage] 1.5-5 g.

[Notes] (1) Modern studies have shown that clove increases the local blood circulation, and the secretion and motility of the gastro-intestinal tract. (2) Traditionally, clove, kaki calyx and inula flower are all the principal agents for treating hiccups. Clove is indicated for cold-type hiccups, kaki calyx for heat-type hiccups and inula flower for hiccups due to phlegm-damp.

***Fructus Foeniculi*, Fennel**, 小茴香 (*Xiaohuixiang*): the dried fruit of *Foeniculum vulgare* Mill (family Umbelliferae).

[Taste and Properties] Pungent and warm.

[Effects and Indications] (1) Dispels cold, regulates the flow of *qi* and relieves pain for relieving cold pain in the lower abdomen, and distending pain of the testis; (2) Improves appetite.

[Usage and Dosage] 5-10 g.

[Notes] Its volatile oil increases the motility of the gastro-intestinal tract, and thus expels the gas.

***Folium Artemisiae*, Argyi Wormwood Leaf** or **Argyi Leaf**, 艾叶 (*Aiye*): the dried leaf of *Artemisia argyi* Levl. et Vant. (family Compositae).

[Taste and Properties] Bitter, pungent and warm.

[Effects and Indications] (1) Warms the uterus for treating infertility and dysmenorrhea due to deficiency-cold; (2) Arrests uterine bleeding of the deficiency-cold type.

[Usage and Dosage] 3-9 g.

The main pharmacological actions of the major interior-warming drugs according to modern studies are summarized in Table IX-4.

Table IX-4 Main Pharmacological Effects of Interior-Warming Drugs

	cardio-tonic	vascular dilating	anti-shock	stom-achic	carmin-ative	sed-ative	anal-gesic
Aconite lateral root	+	+	+	+		+	+
Dried ginger	+	+	+	+	+		+
Cinnamon bark		+		+	+	+	+
Evodia fruit		+		+	+	+	+
Cloves				+	+		

QI-REGULATING DRUGS (DRUGS FOR REGULATING THE FLOW OF *QI*)

Qi is the dynamic force for the physiological functions of the internal organs. Disorders of the *qi* flow will bring about various functional disturbances. The common patterns of disordered *qi* flow are stagnation and perversion of the flow. Stagnated *qi* flow may induce a sensation of fullness in mild cases, distension in moderate cases and mass formation in severe cases. The mass formed by stagnated *qi* is soft, movable and of no fixed shape. Perverted flow of *qi* is actually another kind of *qi* stagnation which interferes with the normal ascending or descending of *qi*. Upward perverted flow of Lung *qi* leads to cough and asthma, and upward perverted flow of Stomach *qi* causes belching, hiccups, nausea and vomiting. Transverse perverted flow of Liver *qi* may give rise to fullness or distension in the chest and hypochondriac regions. If the Stomach is attacked by perverted Liver *qi*, there will be epigastric distension and pain; if the Spleen is involved, there will be abdominal distension, pain and diarrhea. *Qi*-regulating drugs are drugs that restore and smooth the normal flow of *qi* for relieving the stagnation and perversion of *qi* flow. Carminatives are included in this category, but in Chinese medicine regulating the *qi* flow has a much broader sense than relieving flatulence.

According to the different conditions of *qi* stagnation, the actions of the *qi*-regulating drugs can be further classified as (1) adjusting the *qi* flow (for mild stagnation of *qi*), (2) promoting the *qi* flow (for sluggish flow of *qi*), (3) smoothing Liver *qi* flow (also called "soothing the Liver" for relieving the depressed flow of Liver *qi*), (4) directing the *qi* flow downward (for checking the upward perverted flow of *qi*), and (5) dissipating the accumulated *qi* (for treating masses).

Qi-regulating drugs are mostly pungent in flavor, warm in property and desiccating in action. Long-term use of this kind of drug may consume both *qi* and yin. So caution should be exercised if they are administered to patients with *yin* deficiency or *qi* deficiency. In addition, since they contain volatile constituents, they should not be decocted too long.

Pericarpium Citri Reticulatae, **Tangerine Peel,** 陈皮 (*Chenpi*): the dried pericarp of the ripe fruit of *Citrus reticulata* Balanco or its cultivated varieties (family Rutaceae).

[Taste and Properties] Pungent, bitter and warm.

[Effects and Indications] Regulates the flow of Spleen and Stomach *qi* and resolves phlegm, used as a carminative, stomachic and expectorant for epigastric and abdominal distension, vomiting and coughing with profuse phlegm.

[Usage and Dosage] 6-9 g.

[Notes] (1) It relaxes the smooth muscle of the gastro-intestinal tract, increases normal gastric secretion, but inhibits gastric secretion in experimental peptic ulcer. It also has a cholagogue effect, and its volatile oil can dissolve cholesterol calculus. (2) It contains limonene (a part of the volatile oil) which is a stimulant expectorant. The alcoholic extract relieves bronchospasms induced by histamine.

Pericarpium Citri Reticulatae Viride, **Green Tangerine Peel,** 青皮 (*Qingpi*): the dried green unripe exocarp of *Citrus reticulata* Balanco or its cultivated varieties (family Rutaceae).

[Taste and Properties] Pungent, bitter and warm.

[Effects and Indications] Dissipates stagnated Liver *qi* and restores its normal flow for treating costal and hypochondriac pain, gastrointestinal distension and mastitis.

[Usage and Dosage] 3-9 g.

[Notes] (1) It shows a marked spasmolytic effect on the gastro-intestinal tract as well as a cholagogue effect in experimental studies. (2) Its extract relieves bronchospasms induced by histamine. It contains limonene, which is an expectorant.

Semen Citri Reticulatae, **Tangerine Seed,** 橘核 (*Juhe*): the dried ripe seed of *Citrus reticulata* Balanco or its cultivated varieties (family Rutaceae).

[Taste and Properties] Bitter in taste and neutral in property.

[Effects and Indications] Restores the normal flow of Liver *qi* for treating mastitis and painful swollen testis.

[Usage and Dosage] 6-9 g.

***Exocarpium Citri Rubrum*, Red Tangerine Peel**, 橘红 (*Juhong*): Its use is the same as that of *Chenpi* (tangerine peel), but with more potent effect.

***Fructus Aurantii Immaturus*, Immature Bitter Orange**, 枳实 (*Zhishi*): the dried small immature fruit of *Citrus aurantinum* L. and its cultivated varieties with a diameter under 2.5 cm (family Rutaceae).

[Taste and Properties] Bitter, pungent and slightly cold.

[Effects and Indications] (1) Eliminates stagnation of *qi* and resolves phlegm for relieving sensations of stuffiness in the chest and abdominal pain due to enterospasm; (2) Also used for treating dyspepsia, gastroptosis, prolapse of the rectum and prolapse of the uterus.

[Usage and Dosage] 3-9 g.

[Warning] Use with caution during pregnancy.

[Notes] (1) Immature bitter orange shows bi-directional regulatory actions on the gastro-intestinal tract and the uterus; relaxing them when they are in tonic contraction, and stimulating them when their tonicity is low. This may explain why the drug can be used in the treatment of dyspepsia due to diminished tonus of the gastro-intestinal tract, gastroptosis and prolapse of the uterus on the one hand, and gastro-enterospasm on the other hand. (2) Immature bitter orange contains synephrine and N-methyl-tyramine, which strengthen the vascular and cardiac contraction, increase the cardiac output and elevate the blood pressure, and so the drug has been used for treating shock and heart failure in recent years.

***Fructus Aurantii*, Bitter Orange**, 枳壳 (*Zhiqiao*): the dried immature fruit of *Citrus aurantinum* L. and its cultivated varieties with a diameter between 3-5 cm (family Rutaceae). It has the same indications and usage as Zhishi (immature bitter orange), but with a milder effect.

***Cortex Magnolia Officinalis*, Officinal Magnolia Bark**, 厚朴 (*Houpo*): the dried stem bark, root bark or branch bark of *Magnolia officinalis* Rehd. et Wils. or *Magnolia officinalis* var. *biloba* Rehd. et Wils. (family Magnoliaceae).

[Taste and Properties] Bitter, pungent and warm.

[Effects and Indications] (1) Directs the flow of *qi* downward, used as a carminative for treating abdominal distension with pain due to food stagnation; (2) Removes damp from the Spleen for arresting vomiting and diarrhea; (3) Relieves coughing and asthma.

[Usage and Dosage] 3-9 g.

[Notes] (1) The decoction stimulates the digestive tract, promoting its motility and secretion. The volatile oil content (1%) of magnolia bark possesses carminative and stomachic effects. (2) The extract prevents passive cutaneous anaphylaxis in animal experiments.

***Caulis Perillae*, Perilla Stem**, 紫苏梗 (*Zisugeng*): the dried stem of *Perilla frutescens* (L.) Britt. (family Labiatae).

[Taste and Properties] Pungent and slightly warm.

[Effects and Indications] (1) Regulates the flow of *qi* for treating stuffiness in the chest and distension of the abdomen; (2) Prevents abortion.

[Usage and Dosage] 4.5-9 g.

***Radix Auklandiae*, Costus Root**, 木香 (*Muxiang*): the dried root of *Aucklandia lappa* Decne. (family Compositae).

[Taste and Properties] Pungent, bitter and warm.

[Effects and Indications] Regulates the flow of *qi*, improves digestion and checks diarrhea for relieving abdominal distension due to stagnation of *qi* of the Stomach and Intestines, indigestion with anorexia, and abdominal pain and tenesmus in cases of dysentery.

[Usage and Dosage] 1.5-6 g.

[Notes] It relieves enterospasms and bronchospasms in animal experiments.

***Rhizoma Cyperi*, Cyperus Tuber**, 香附 (*Xiangfu*): the dried tuber of *Cyperus rotundus* L. (family Cyperaceae).

[Taste and Properties] Pungent, slightly bitter, and warm.

[Effects and Indications] Regulates the flow of Liver *qi* for relieving epigastric, hypochondriac and abdominal distension and pain, as well as menstrual disorders and dysmenorrhea due to Liver *qi* stagnation.

[Usage and Dosage] 6-9 g.

[Notes] (1) It reduces the tonicity and contraction of the uterus. It contains cyperene I, which acts like estrogen. (2) It relaxes the intestines, and prevents bronchospasms induced by histamine. (3) It shows analgesic and antipyretic effects.

***Radix Linderae*, Spicebush Root**, 乌药 (*Wuyao*): the dried tuberous root of *Lindera aggregata* (Sims) Kosterm. (family Lauraceae).

[Taste and Properties] Pungent and warm.

[Effects and Indications] (1) Regulates the flow of *qi* for relieving epigastric and lower abdominal pain with cold sensation; (2) Warms the Kidneys for arresting frequent urination or enuresis.

[Usage and Dosage] 3-9 g.

[Notes] It increases intestinal peristalsis, expelling gas.

***Bulbus Allii Macrostemonis*, Longstamen Onion**, 薤白 (*Xiebai*): the dried bulb of *Allium macrostemon* Bge. (family Liliaceae).

[Taste and Properties] Pungent, bitter and warm.

[Effects and Indications] (1) Promotes the flow of *qi* in the chest for relieving angina pectoris; (2) Also used as an antidysenteric agent.

[Usage and Dosage] 3-9 g.

[Notes] It inhibits the smooth muscle contraction after a transient stimulation.

***Pericarpium Arecae*, Areca Peel**, 大腹皮 (*Dafupi*): the dried pericarp of *Areca catechu* L. (family Palmae).

[Taste and Properties] Pungent and slightly warm.

[Effects and Indications] Promotes the descending of *qi* and induces diuresis for treating abdominal distension, ascites and edema with oliguria.

[Usage and Dosage] 4.5-9 g.

Lignum Dalbergiae Odoriferae, **Rose Wood**, 降香 (*Jiangxiang*): the heart-wood of trunk and root of *Dalbergia odorifera* T. Chen (family Leguminosae).

[Taste and Properties] Pungent and warm.

[Effects and Indications] (1) Promotes the flow of *qi* for relieving angina pectoris and stomachache; (2) Promotes blood circulation and arrests bleeding in the case of traumatic injuries.

[Usage and Dosage] 3-6 g, to be added later in making a compound decoction.

Lignum Aquilariae Resinatum, **Eagle Wood**, 沉香 (*Chenxiang*): the resinous wood of *Aquilaris sinensis* (Lour.) Gilg (family Thymelaeaceae).

[Taste and Properties] Pungent and slightly warm.

[Effects and Indications] (1) Regulates the flow of *qi* for relieving distension and pain in the chest and abdomen, and for arresting vomiting and hiccups; (2) Also used for relieving asthma.

[Usage and Dosage] 1-3 g, to be made into powder and taken directly with liquid or added later in making a compound decoction.

Calyx Kaki, **Persimmon Calyx**, 柿蒂 (*Shidi*): the dried persistent calyx of *Diospyros kaki* L. f. (family Ebenaceae).

[Taste and Properties] Puckery in taste and neutral in property.

[Effects and Indications] Checks upward perverted flow of Stomach *qi* for arresting hiccups.

[Usage and Dosage] 3-9 g.

Fructus Toosendan, **Szechwan Chinaberry**, 川楝子 (*Chuanlianzi*): the dried ripe fruit of *Media toosendan* Sieb. et Zucc. (family Meliaceae).

[Taste and Properties] Bitter and cold.

[Effects and Indications] (1) Smooths the flow of Liver *qi* for relieving hypochondriac, epigastric and lower abdominal pain; (2) Also used as an anthelmintic for intestinal ascariasis.

[Usage and Dosage] 6-9 g.

[Notes] It contains toosendanin, which is anthelmintic.

According to modern pharmacological studies, most drugs of this category, particularly green tangerine peel, tangerine peel, immature bitter orange and bitter orange, have an antispasmodic action on the gastro-intestinal tract. This is probably due to the action of synephrine, an alpha receptor stimulant contained in the above-mentioned drugs. On the other hand, immature bitter orange and bitter orange increase gastro-intestinal peristalsis in animal experiments. This may explain their clinical effect of relieving flatulence and assuaging distending pain. The bi-directional actions depend chiefly upon the functional states of the stomach and intestines, and also upon the drug concentration. Immature bitter orange has bi-directional actions on the uterus as well.

Some *qi*-regulating drugs are used as digestants clinically. They have been shown to stimulate gastric secretion in experimental studies. The cholagogue action of "Liver-soothing" drugs demonstrated experimentally can partially explain their effect in smoothing the flow of Liver *qi*.

Some *qi*-regulating drugs for checking the upward perversion of Lung *qi* are used in the treatment of coughing and asthma. Their antasthmatic effect is attributed to the relaxation of the bronchial smooth muscle, and their antitussive effect to facilitated expectoration by stimulating the bronchial secretion.

The main pharmacological actions of the commonly-used *qi*-regulating drugs are summarized in Table IX-5.

Table IX-5 Main Pharmacological Effects of *Qi*-Regulating Drugs

	G-I motility	G-I secretion	Broncho-relaxant	Chola-gogue	Others
Immature bitter orange	↑ ↓			±	Cardiotonic and uterine timulant
Bitter orange	↑ ↓			+	ditto
Tangerine peel	↓	↑	+	+	expectorant
Green tangerine peel	↓		+	+	expectorant
Spicebush root	↑ ↓	↑			antineoplastic
Costus root	↑ ↓		+		
Cyperus tuber	↓			+	inhibits uterine contraction
Areca peel	↑				
Magnolia bark	↑ ↓				

↑ = stimulates ↓ = inhibits

BLOOD-REGULATING DRUGS

Drugs that are used for treating bleeding and blood stasis are called blood-regulating drugs. They can be classified into three groups: hemostatics (to arrest bleeding), blood-activating drugs (to improve local blood circulation), and stasis-eliminating drugs. The latter two groups will be discussed jointly because of overlappings.

Hemostatic Drugs

The common causes of bleeding include traumatic injury, heat in the blood, and failure of *qi* to control the blood flow. In addition, bleeding may also be a complication of blood stasis or due to the congealing of blood due to cold. Therefore, hemostatics can also be classified into the following groups: (1) astringent hemostatics, such as agrimony, bletilla tuber and carbonized petiole of windmill palm; (2) blood-cooling hemostatics, such as Japanese thistle, small thistle, pagodatree flower and cogongrass rhizome; (3) blood stasis-removing hemostatics, such as notoginseng, cat-tail pollen and madder root; and (4) warming hemostatics, such as argyi leaf and baked ginger.

Although the hemostatics are classified according to the cause of bleeding, they can only be used to relieve symptoms. For example, blood-cooling hemostatics are suitable for arresting bleeding due to heat in the blood, but they have not much effect for eliminating heat. Therefore, hemostatics should be used in combination with other drugs to cure primary conditions, e.g., blood-cooling febrifuges for heat in the blood, *qi*-tonics for failure of *qi* to control the blood flow. It is emphasized in Chinese medicine that blood stasis should be carefully examined when astringent hemostatics are administered, for the use of astringent hemostatics alone may aggravate blood stasis.

Herba Agrimoniae, **Agrimony**, 仙鹤草 (*Xianhecao*): the dried aerial part of *Agrimonia pilosa* Ledeb. (family Rosaceae).

[Taste and Properties] Bitter and puckery in taste and neutral in Properties.

[Effects and Indications] Used as an astringent hemostatic for various types of hemorrhages.

[Usage and Dosage] 10-30 g.

Radix Notoginseng, **Notoginseng**, 三七 (*Sanqi*): the dried root of *Panax notoginseng* (Burk.) F.H. Chen (family Araliaceae).

[Taste and Properties] Sweet, slightly bitter and warm.

[Effects and Indications] (1) Arrests bleeding and dissipates stagnated blood for treatment of various types of hemorrhages; (2) Causes subsidence of swelling and alleviates pain in the case of traumatic injuries.

[Usage and Dosage] 1.5-6 g, to be ground into powder and taken with water; appropriate quantity for external use.

[Notes] (1) It is said traditionally that "notoginseng arrests bleeding, but does not leave stagnated blood." Modern pharmacological studies have revealed that it contracts the blood vessels, shortens the bleeding time and promotes coagulation. The active principle is dencichine. On the other hand, it contains panaxatriol, which reduces the production of thromboxane (TXA_2), thus inhibiting the platelet aggregation. The latter action becomes manifest only after 20 days of oral administration. In addition, notoginseng accelerates the absorption of intraocular extravasated blood both clinically and in animal experiments. Since dencichine can be destroyed by boiling, for arresting bleeding, notoginseng should be used in powder form instead of a decoction. When it is used for treating thrombotic diseases, long-term administration is necessary. (2) Notoginseng shows anti-inflammatory and analgesic effects in animal experiments. (3) The saponin content of notoginseng is similar to that of ginsenoside in chemical structure and pharmacological actions. Therefore, notoginseng possesses similar tonic effects as ginseng does (e.g., regulating the immune function, counteracting peroxidation, improving memory, and promoting the anabolism of proteins and nucleic acid).

Pollen Typhae, **Cat-tail pollen**, 蒲黄 (*Puhuang*): the dried pollen of *Typha angustifolia* L., *Typha orientalis* Presl. or related species (family Typhaceae).

[Taste and Properties] Sweet in taste and neutral in property.

[Effects and Indications] Invigorates blood circulation for relieving dysmenorrhea and traumatic pain; carbonized cat-tail pollen arrests bleeding.

[Usage and Dosage] 3-9 g; for external use, appropriate quantity to be applied topically.

[Warning] Use with caution during pregnancy.

[Notes] (1) Topical application of the powder has a hemostatic effect. The decoction given orally shortens blood coagulation time in animal experiments. Carbonized cat-tail pollen is more effective. The active hemostatic principle is isorhamnetin. However, it also contains a flavonoid substance which inhibits platelet aggregation. (2) It dilates peripheral and coronary arteries, protects the heart from ischemia, lowers serum cholesterol in experimental hypercholesterolemia, and prevents the formationn of experimental atherosclerosis. (3) It stimulates the uterus, increasing the uterine tonus and contraction.

***Rhizoma Bletillae*, Bletilla Tuber**, 白及 (*Baiji*): the steamed and dried tuber of *Bletilla striata* (Thunb.) Reichb. f. (family Orchidaceae).

[Taste and Properties] Bitter, sweet and puckery in taste, and neutral in property.

[Effects and Indications] Arrests bleeding in case of hemoptysis and hematemesis; are applied externally for traumatic injuries.

[Usage and Dosage] 6-9 g for making a decoction; 1-3 g to be powdered for direct taking with liquid; appropriate quantity for external use.

[Notes] Its hemostatic effect is probably due to its mucilage content, which promotes blood coagulation.

***Herba Cirsii Japonici*, Japanese Thistle**, 大蓟 (*Daji*): the dried aerial part or root of *Cirsium japonicum* (family Compositae).

[Taste and Properties] Sweet, bitter and cool.

[Effects and Indications] (1) Arrests bleeding for hemorrhages due to heat in the blood; (2) Promotes the subsidence of swelling for boils and sores; (3) Used as an antihypertensive agent recently.

[Usage and Dosage] 9-15 g; for external use, appropriate quantity of the fresh herb to be pounded into paste and applied topically.

[Notes] (1) The charred herb has a more hemostatic effect than the unprepared herb. (2) The aqueous extract lowers blood pressure in animal experiments.

***Herba Cirsii*, Field Thistle**, 小蓟 (*Xiaoji*): the dried aerial part of *Cirsium setosum* (Willd.) (family Compositae).

[Taste and Properties] Sweet, bitter and cool.

[Effects and Indications] (1) Arrests bleeding in cases of hemorrhages due to heat in the blood; (2) Used as an antihypertensive agent recently.

[Usage and Dosage] 4.5-9 g; for external use, appropriate quantity of the fresh herb to be pounded into paste and applied topically.

***Radix Rubiae*, Madder Root**, 茜草 (*Qiancao*): the dried root and rhizome of Indian madder, *Rubia cordifolia* L. (family Rubiaceae).

[Taste and Properties] Bitter and cold.

[Effects and Indications] (1) Arrests bleeding in cases of hemorrhages due to heat in the blood; (2) Removes blood stasis for treating traumatic injuries and amenorrhea.

[Usage and Dosage] 6-9 g.

***Radix Sanguisorbae*, Burnet Root**, 地榆 (*Diyu*): the dried root of *Sanguisorba officinalis* L. or *Sanguisorba officinalis* var. *longifolia* (Bert.) Yu et Li (family Rosaceae).

[Taste and Properties] Bitter, puckery and slightly cold.

[Effects and Indications] Arrests bleeding in cases of hemorrhages in the Lower Energizer (hematochezia, hematuria and uterine bleeding).

[Usage and Dosage] 6-15 g.

Flos Sophorae, **Pagodatree Flower**, 槐花 (*Huaihua*): the dried flower or flower-bud of *Sophora japonica* L. (family Leguminosae).

[Taste and Properties] Bitter and cold.

[Effects and Indications] (1) Arrests bleeding by dispelling heat from blood for treating bleeding hemorrhoids and hematochezia; (2) Also used as an antihypertensive.

[Usage and Dosage] 6-15 g.

[Notes] (1) It contains a considerable amount of rutin (10-25%), which reduces vascular permeability. (2) It shows a hypotensive effect in animal experiments.

Rhizoma Imperatae, **Lalang Grass Rhizome** or **Cogongrass Rhizome**, 白茅根 (*Baimaogen*), the dried rhizome of *Imperata cylindrica* Beauv. var. *major* (Nees) C. E. Hubb. (family Graminae).

[Taste and Properties] Sweet and cold.

[Effects and Indications] (1) Arrests bleeding by dispelling heat from blood for treatment of epistaxis and hematuria; (2) Removes damp-heat for treating jaundice and acute urinary tract infection; (3) Causes diuresis for treating edema.

[Usage and Dosage] 9-15 g.

[Notes] (1) It has a diuretic effect, probably because it contains a large amount of potassium. (2) It shows a hemostatic effect, probably by reducing vascular permeability.

Petiolus Trachycarpi Carbonizatus, **Carbonized Windmill-palm Petiole**, 棕榈炭 (*Zonglütan*): the carbonized petiole of *Trachycarpus fortunei* H. Wendl. (family Palmae).

[Taste and Properties] Bitter and puckery in taste and neutral in property.

[Effects and Indications] Used as an astringent hemostatic for hemoptysis, epistaxis, hematochezia and uterine bleeding.

[Usage and Dosage] 6-12 g.

According to modern scientific research, the mechanism of hemostatic action may be different in different drugs, as shown in Table IX-6. Notoginseng, field thistle and Japanese thistle cause local vascular contraction; pagodatree flower and lalang grass rhizome reduce the vascular fragility and capillary permeability; agrimony increases the number of blood platelets and promotes the platelet adhesion and aggregation; bletilla tuber enhances the activity of the platelet factor III; cat-tail pollen and notoginseng increase blood thrombin; madder root has an anti-heparin action; bletilla tuber, field thistle, Japanese thistle and burnet root inhibit the conversion of profibrinolysin into fibrinolysin, and hence fibrinolysis.

It is worth noting that notoginseng and cat-tail pollen, though effective for arresting bleeding, contain some constituents that inhibit platelet aggregation. So they can also be used for the prevention of thrombosis.

Blood-activating and Stasis-eliminating Drugs

This category of drugs was first used in the treatment of trauma (particularly with

Table IX-6. Mechanisms of the Hemostatic Effect of Herbal Drugs

	Vascular contraction	Ascular resistance	Blood coagulation	Fibrinolysis
Stasis-eliminating hemostatics				
Notoginseng	↑		↑	
Cat-tail pollen			↑	
Madder root			↑	
Blood-cooling hemostatics				
Field thistle	↑			↓
Japanese thistle	↑			↓
Burnet root				↓
Pagodatree flower		↑		
Cogongrass rhizome		↑		
Astringent hemostatics				
Agrimony			↑	↓
Bletilla tuber			↑	↓
Warm-propertied hemostatics				
Argyi leaf				↓
Baked ginger				↓

ecchymosis and pain) and gynecological diseases (such as dysmenorrhea, amenorrhea, and pelvic mass formation), but later their indications were widely expanded. To date, blood activation and stasis elimination is a very important therapy for treating a large variety of diseases covering almost all fields of medicine.

Blood stasis is usually a secondary change. Its primary pathology includes stagnation of *qi*, deficiency of *qi*, and deficiency of blood. In addition, many pathogenic factors such as heat, cold or phlegm may obstruct the normal flow of blood, resulting in blood stasis. Blood stasis may bring about various manifestations, among which pain, mass formation and bleeding are most commonly encountered. Therefore, drugs in this category can be further divided into the following groups:

(1) Blood-nourishing and blood-activating drugs, such as red sage root, red peony root and spathologus stem.

(2) Blood-activating and stasis-eliminating drugs, such as chuanxiong, safflower and motherwort.

(3) Stasis-eliminating and pain-relieving drugs, such as corydalis tuber, frankincense, myrrh, corydalis tuber, dragon's blood and turmeric root.

(4) Stasis-eliminating drugs and mass-dissipating drugs, such as burreed tuber, zedoary and peach seed.

(5) Stasis-eliminating hemostatics such as notoginseng and cat-tail pollen (see Hemostatic Drugs).

There is also some difference between blood activation and stasis elimination. Generally, the blood-activating drugs are mild in action, while stasis-eliminating drugs have a more potent effect, and mass-dissipating drugs are drastic in action.

***Radix Salviae Miltiorrhizae*, Red Sage Root,** 丹参 (*Danshen*): the dried root and rhizome of *Salvia miltiorrhiza* Bge. (family Labiatae).

[Taste and Properties] Bitter and slightly cold.

[Effects and Indications] (1) Invigorates blood circulation and removes stasis in cases of angina pectoris, dysmenorrhea, amenorrhea and abdominal mass (including hepatosplenomegaly) due to blood stasis; (2) Calms the mind in cases of fidgetiness and insomnia accompanying febrile diseases.

[Usage and Dosage] 6-15 g.

[Notes] (1) Intravenous dripping dilates the coronary artery, improves the heart function and increases myocardial contractility, but does not augment the myocardial oxygen consumption. This serves as the pharmacological basis for its recent use in the treatment of myocardial infarction. (2) It inhibits blood platelet aggregation, elevates the activity of fibrolysin, and improves capillary circulation. This is the reason for its wide use in the treatment of ischemic and thrombotic diseases. (3) It promotes tissue renovation and regeneration, and also protects the liver from chemical damage. This may explain why it can be used for treating chronic hepatitis and early cirrhosis with hepatosplenomegaly.

***Radix Paeoniae Rubra*, Red Peony Root**, 赤芍 (*Chishao*): the root of *Paeonia lactiflora* Pall. or *Paeonia veitchii* Lynch (family Ranunculaceae).

[Taste and Properties] Bitter and slightly cold.

[Effects and Indications] (1) Invigorates blood circulation for menstrual disorders and angina pectoris; (2) Reduces heat from blood and induces subsidence of swelling for boils and carbuncles.

[Usage and Dosage] 6-9 g.

[Notes] (1) Both red peony root and white peony root are obtained from *Paeonia lactiflora* Pall. In ancient times, they were identified according to the color of the flower, but in modern usage, the white peony root refers to the root with its bark removed, while the red peony root refers to the entire root. (2) In vitro, the red peony root inhibits *Staphylococcus aureus, Streptococcus hemolyticus* and *Shigella dysenterie*. (3) It shows tranquilizing, analgesic and antispasmodic effects in experimental studies. It also dilates the coronary artery.

***Caulis Spatholobi*, Spatholobus Stem**, 鸡血藤 (*Jixueteng*): the dried lianoid stem of *Spatholobus suberectus* Dunn (family Leguminosae).

[Taste and Properties] Bitter and warm.

[Effects and Indications] (1) Invigorates blood circulation and nourishes blood in cases of menstrual disorders due to blood deficiency; (2) Clears the meridians of obstructions for relieving numbness and arthralgia.

[Usage and Dosage] 9-15 g.

[Notes] (1) It inhibits the uterus in vitro, but stimulates the uterus in vivo, strengthening the rhythmic uterine contraction. (2) Its alcoholic extract, when given orally, shows a marked therapeutic effect for experimental arthritis.

***Radix Cyathulae;* Cyathula Root**, 川牛膝 (*Chuanniuxi*): the dried root of *Cyathula officinalis* Kuan (family Amaranthaceae).

[Taste and Properties] Bitter and sour in taste and neutral in property.

[Effects and Indications] (1) Eliminates blood stasis and stimulates menstruation for treating amenorrhea; (2) Dispels wind-damp for rheumatalgia.

[Usage and Dosage] 4.5-9 g.
[Warning] Contraindicated in pregnancy.
[Notes] It stimulates uterine contraction.

Rhizoma Chuanxiong, **Szechwan Lovage Rhizome (Chuanxiong)**, 川芎 (*Chuanxiong*): the dried rhizome of *Ligusticum chuanxiong* Hort. (family Umbelliferae).

[Taste and Properties] Pungent and warm.

[Effects and Indications] (1) Promotes the flow of *qi* and blood for treating menstrual disorders and other ailments due to *qi* stagnation and blood stasis. (2) Dispels wind and relieves pain in cases of headache and general aching accompanying exogenous affections.

[Usage and Dosage] 3-9 g.

[Notes] (1) *Chuanxiong* dilates the coronary and cerebral arteries and the arteries of the extremities. The active principles are ligustrazine and ferulic acid. In experimental studies ligustrazine prevents and relieves spasms of the vascular smooth muscle induced by adrenalin and barium chloride. It also reduces the severity and area of myocardial infarction caused by ligation of the descending anterior branch of the coronary artery in rabbits. Pharmacokinetic studies have revealed that ligustrazine can rapidly penetrate the blood-brain barrier, improving the cerebral microcirculation and inhibiting platelet aggregation. Ferulic acid also increases the coronary blood flow and protects the myocardium against ischemia. It has an α-receptor blocking action. In addition, *chuanxiong* shows an antithrombotic action with prolonged blood coagulation time, and reduced length and weight of the thrombus. Both ligustrazine and ferulic acid inhibit blood platelet aggregation. Ligustrazine is now widely used for treating coronary disease, thromboarteritis and ischemic cerebral disease. (2) Aqueous extract of *chuanxiong* shows a marked spasmolytic action on the uterus. This may partly explain its effect in the treatment of dysmenorrhea.

Herba Leonuri, **Motherwort**, 益母草 (*Yimucao*): the dried aerial part of *Leonurus heterophyllus* Sweet (family Labiatae).

[Taste and Properties] Pungent, slightly bitter and somewhat cold.

[Effects and Indications] (1) Regulates menstruation by invigorating blood circulation, used in the treatment of menstrual disorders due to blood stasis, also used for treating postpartum hemorrhage and subinvolution of the uterus; (2) Induces diuresis for edema in acute nephritis.

[Usage and Dosage] 9-30 g.

[Warning] Contraindicated in pregnancy.

[Notes] (1) The herb causes strong and persistent stimulation to the uterus, increasing the uterine tonus and contractibility. The active principle is leonurine, a heat-stable and water-soluble alkaloid. (2) The herb protects the myocardium against ischemia, inhibits blood platelet aggregation, and acts against thrombosis.

Flos Carthami, **Safflower**, 红花 (*Honghua*): the dried flower of *Carthamus tinctorius* L. (family Compositae).

[Taste and Properties] Pungent and warm.

[Effects and Indications] (1) Invigorates blood circulation and regulates menstruation for treating amenorrhea, dysmenorrhea and abdominal masses due to blood stasis; (2) Removes blood stasis and relieves pain in the case of traumatic injuries.

[Usage and Dosage] 3-9 g.

[Warning] Used with caution in pregnancy.

[Notes] (1) It dilates blood vessels, probably due to its α-adrenergic blocking action. (2) It markedly prolongs blood coagulation time. It contains safflor yellow, which inhibits blood platelet aggregation and enhances the activity of fibrinolysin. (3) The decoction causes contraction of the uterus, particularly in pregnancy.

***Faeces Trogopterorum*, Trogopterus Dung**, 五灵脂 (*Wulingzhi*): the dried feces of *Trogopterus xanthipes* Milne-Edwards (family Petauristidae).

[Taste and Properties] Sweet and warm.

[Effects and Indications] Eliminates stagnated blood and relieves pain due to blood stasis (e.g., postpartum abdominal pain, and dysmenorrhea).

[Usage and Dosage] 4.5 g.

[Warning] Use with caution in pregnancy.

[Notes] It relieves spasms in smooth muscles.

***Sanguis Draconis*, Dragon's Blood**, 血竭 (*Xuejie*): a red resin secreted from the fruit of *Daemonorops draco* Bl. (family Palmae).

[Taste and Properties] Sweet and salty in taste and neutral in property.

[Effects and Indications] Dissipates stagnated blood, promotes tissue regeneration and relieves pain due to traumatic injuries, also used topically to check traumatic bleeding.

[Usage and Dosage] 1-1.5 g. For external use, appropriate quantity to be applied topically.

[Notes] It shows hemostatic effect in animal experiments.

***Resina Olibani*, Frankincense**, 乳香 (*Ruxiang*): a gum-resin obtained from *Boswellia carterii* Birdwood and possibly other species of *Boswellia* (family Burseraceae).

[Taste and Properties] Pungent, bitter and warm.

[Effects and Indications] Relieves pain and swelling by eliminating blood stasis in traumatic injuries.

[Usage and Dosage] 3-9 g; appropriate quantity ground into powder for external use.

[Warning] Contraindicated in pregnancy. A large dose taken orally may cause adverse effects on the stomach.

[Notes] Frankincense and myrrh are often used in combination. Both of them relieve pain and swelling by eliminating blood stasis, but frankincense eliminates blood stasis by promoting the flow of *qi*, while myrrh directly dissipates the stagnated blood. They are synergetic in action.

***Resina Myrrhae*, Myrrh**, 没药 (*Moyao*), a gum-resin obtained from the stem of *Commiphora molmol* Engler and probably other species (family Burseraceae).

[Taste and Properties] Bitter in taste and neutral in property.

[Effects and Indications] Eliminates blood stasis in cases of amenorrhea, and also in cases of pain and swelling resulting from traumatic injuries.

[Usage and Dosage] 3-9 g; appropriate quantity ground into powder for external use.

***Rhizoma Corydalis*, Corydalis Tuber (Yanhusuo)**, 延胡索 (*Yanhusuo*): the steamed and dried tuber of *Corydalis yanhusuo* W.T. Wang (family Papaveraceae).

[Taste and Properties] Pungent, bitter and warm.

[Effects and Indications] Invigorates blood circulation and *qi* flow for relieving pain (such as hypochondriac, gastric and abdominal pain, and dysmenorrhea) caused by *qi* stagnation and blood stasis.

[Usage and Dosage] 3-9 g; or 1.3-3 g of powder to be swallowed at a time.

[Notes] (1) The analgesic effect of *yanhusuo* has been demonstrated in the laboratory. The analgesic potency of its total alkaloids is about 40% of that of morphine. The most active principle is tetrahydropalmatine, which, though less potent than morphine, is non-addictive and has no such side-effects as respiratory inhibition and constipation. Tetrahydropalmatine has a tranquilizing effect comparable with that of phenothiazine. (2) *Yanhusuo* improves the coronary blood flow. The active principle is dehydrocorydaline. In addition, dehydrocorydaline protects the stomach from gastric ulcers in animal experiments.

***Radix Curcumae*, Turmeric Root,** 郁金 (*Yujin*): the steamed and dried tuberous root of *Curcuma wenyujin* Y.H. Chen et C. Ling, *Curcuma longa* L., *Curcuma kwangsiensis* S.G. Lee et C.F. Liang, or *Curcuma phaeocaulis* Val. (family Zingiberaceae).

[Taste and Properties] Pungent, bitter and cold.

[Effects and Indications] (1) Promotes the flow of *qi* and blood for relieving hypochondriac distension, pectoral and abdominal pain, and dysmenorrhea; (2) Reduces heat from blood for arresting bleeding; (3) Increases the flow of bile for treating jaundice; (4) Calms the mind for treating depression-mania.

[Usage and Dosage] 3-9 g.

[Notes] It contains essential oil and curcumin, which stimulate the secretion of bile.

***Rhizoma Sparganii*, Burreed Tuber,** 三棱 (*Sanleng*): the peeled and dried tuber of *Sparganium stoloniferum* Buch.-Ham. (family Sparganiaceae).

[Taste and Properties] Pungent and bitter in taste, and neutral in property.

[Effects and Indications] Drastically eliminates blood stasis for treating amenorrhea, hepatosplenomegaly and other abdominal masses.

[Usage and Dosage] 3-9 g.

[Warning] Contraindicated in pregnancy and excessive menstruation.

[Notes] Burreed tuber and zedoary are often used in combination. Both of them drastically eliminate blood stasis. Burreed tuber is more potent in this action, but zedoary also promotes the flow of *qi*. Their combined use gives a synergetic effect.

***Rhizoma Curcumae Zedoariae*, Zedoary,** 莪术 (*Ezhu*): the steamed and dried rhizome of *Curcuma zedoaria* Rosc., *Curcuma phaeocaulis* Valeton, or *Curcuma kwangsiensis* S.G. Lee et C.F. Liang or *Curcuma wenyujin* Y.H. Chen et C. Ling (family Zingiberaceae).

[Taste and Properties] Pungent, bitter and warm.

[Effects and Indications] (1) Drastically eliminates blood stasis and promotes the flow of *qi* for treating amenorrhea, hypochondriac and abdominal pain, and masses in the abdomen; (2) Removes retained food with epigastric distension and pain.

[Usage and Dosage] 3-9 g.

[Warning] Contraindicated in pregnancy and excessive menstruation.

[Notes] (1) It inhibits the growth of various malignant tumors in experimental studies, probably due to its action of enhancing the immunogenicity of the tumor cells. (2) It has an action against progesterone, and may cause abortion in early pregnancy.

Semen Persicae, **Peach Seed**, 桃仁 (*Taoren*): the dried ripe seed of *Prunus persica* (L.) Batsch or *Prunus davidiana* (Carr.) Franch. (family Rosaceae).

[Taste and Properties] Bitter and sweet in taste and neutral in property.

[Effects and Indications] (1) Drastically eliminates blood stasis for treating amenorrhea, masses in the abdomen and traumatic pain; (2) Causes mild laxation for constipation.

[Usage and Dosage] 6-9 g.

[Warning] Use with caution in pregnancy.

[Notes] It increases the cerebral blood flow and inhibits blood coagulation. It also shows a laxative effect in the laboratory.

Semen Vaccariae, **Cowherb Seed**, 王不留行 (*Wangbuliuxing*): the dried ripe seed of *Vaccaria segetalis* (Neck.) Garcke (family Caryophyllaceae).

[Taste and Properties] Bitter in taste and neutral in property.

[Effects and Indications] (1) Stimulates menstrual discharge and milk secretion, used as an emmenagogue and galactagogue for amenorrhea and galactostasis; (2) Promotes blood circulation and reduces swelling for treatment of masses due to blood stasis and also for treating boils.

[Usage and Dosage] 6-15 g.

[Warning] Use with caution in pregnancy.

[Notes] The decoction causes uterine contraction.

Eupolyphaga, **Ground Beetle**, 土鳖虫 (*Tubiechong*): the dried female insect of *Eupolyphaga sinensis* Walk. or *Steleophaga plancyi* (Bol.) (family Corydiidae).

[Taste and Properties] Salty, cold, and slightly toxic.

[Effects and Indications] Removes stagnated blood and promotes the healing of bone fracture, used for bone fracture, amenorrhea and formation of mass in the abdomen due to blood stasis.

[Usage and Dosage] 3-9 g.

According to modern studies, blood stasis in Chinese medicine chiefly refers to pathological processes related to the following disturbances of blood circulation: (1) Abnormal hemorheological changes, including increased blood concentration, viscosity, coagulability and cellular aggregation; (2) Microcirculatory disturbances, including retarded blood flow, stasis or even thrombosis, distortion of the capillaries, peri-capillary extravasation, and microvascular constriction or occlusion; (3) Hemodynamic abnormalities with decreased volume of local blood flow, as seen in coronary heart disease, thromboangitis, ischemic apoplexy, and chronic hepatitis.

Therefore, drugs for relieving blood stasis usually have the following actions: (1) Improving blood rheological conditions (including the blood lipid level, which influences the blood viscosity) and counteract the formation and development of thrombus (chiefly by inhibiting platelet aggregation and enhancing the activity of fibrinolysin); (2) Improving microcirculation (to increase microcirculatory flow, to restore the normal appearance of the capillaries, and to reduce peri-capillary extravasation); (3) Improving hemodynamics by dilating the local blood vessels.

In addition, some blood-activating and stasis-eliminating drugs used to stimulate menstruation have the action of increasing the uterine contraction, those used to relieve pain due to blood stasis usually show an analgesic effect in experimental studies.

The main pharmacological actions of blood-activating and stasis-eliminating drugs are summarized in the Table IX-7.

AROMATIC STIMULANTS

Aromatic stimulants are pungent or fragrant in flavor. They have resuscitating effects and are usually used for treating loss of consciousness, delirium and convulsions in acute febrile diseases, epilepsy and apoplexy. Most of them are only for emergency use.

Borneolum, **Borneol**, 冰片 (*Bingpian*): a crystalline organic compound ($C_{10}H_{18}O$) obtained synthetically or from natural sources.

[Taste and Properties] Pungent, bitter and slightly cold.

[Effects and Indications] (1) Used as a stimulant for impaired consciousness and convulsions in febrile diseases; (2) As an antiphlogistic and analgesic for inflammation of the throat, oral ulcers, boils and sores.

[Usage and Dosage] 0.15-0.3 g, used in preparation of pills or powder; for external use, approporiate quantity to be ground into powder and applied topically.

Calculus Bovis, **Bezoar (Ox gallstone)**, 牛黄 (*Niuhuang*): the dried gallstone of domestic cattle, *Bos taurus domesticus* Gmelin (family Bovidae).

[Taste and Properties] Bitter and cool.

[Effects and Indications] (1) Used as a stimulant and anticonvulsive for impaired consciousness and convulsion in cases of febrile diseases; (2) As an antiphlogistic and analgesic for inflammation of the throat, oral ulcers, boils and sores.

[Usage and Dosage] 0.15-0.3 g, mostly used in the preparation of pills or powder; for external use, approporiate quantity to be ground into powder and applied topically.

[Notes] (1) Bezoar has sedative and anticonvulsive effects, counteracting the central stimulation and convulsion induced by caffeine, camphor, picrotoxin and metrazol. (2) Bezoar has a marked antipyretic effect, probably due to its taurine content. The mechanisms of the antipyretic effect of taurine include its action on serotonin in the brain, its combination with the thermogenic carriers, and its direct regulation of the body temperature. (3) Bezoar directly inactivates the encephalitis B virus, but has no action on the virus replication in the brain. This indicates that bezoar is effective only during the period of virusemia. (4) Bezoar has the capacity to dramatically relieve the manifestations of inflammation. It alters the vascular response to injury by limiting the increased capillary permeability that normally occurs. Thus, fewer polymorphonuclear leukocytes leave the vessels at the site of injury. Bezoar is much more potent than hydrocortisone in this action. (5) Bezoar is cardiotonic and relieves experimental arrhythmia. (6) Bezoar protects the liver from chemical damage in experimental studies.

Table IX-7 Pharmacological Effects of Blood-Activating and Stasis-Eliminating Drugs

	Hemodynamics		Inhibits platelet aggregation and thrombosis	Improves microcir Culation	Others
	Dilates blood vessels	Increases Coronary Flow			
Drugs for Nourishing Blood and Promoting Circulation					
Red sage root	+	+	+	+	Sedative
Red peony root	+	+	+	+	Sedative, analgesic, anti-inflammatory
Spatholobus stem	+	+	+		
Drubs for Promoting Blood Circulation and Removing Stasis					
Chuanxiong	+	+	+	+	Sedative
Safflower	+	+	+	+	Uterotonic, hypolipemic
Motherwort	+	+	+	+	Uterotonic, diuretic, anti- hypertensive
Cat-tail pollen	+	+	±*	+	Uterotonic, sedative, hypolipemic
Drugs for Eliminating Blood Stasis and Relieving Pain					
Frankincense	+				Analgesic, increasing vascular permeability
Myrrh	+				Analgesic, anti-inflammatory
Corydalis tuber	+	+			Sedative, analgesic, anti-ulcerative
Dragon's blood					Analgesic
Trogopterus dung					Analgesic, increasing vascular permeability
Drastic Drugs for Eliminating Blood Stasis and Dissipating Masses					
Burreed tuber	+		+		
Turmeric root	+				Cholagogue, hypolipemic, anti-neoplastic
Zedoary					anti-neoplastic, terminating early pregnancy
Peach seed					Uterotonic, anti-tussive, anti-inflammatory

*Cat-tail pollen inhibits platelet aggregation, but its carbonized preparation hastens blood coagulation.

***Rhizoma Acori Tatarinowii*, Grass-leaved Sweetflag Rhizome,** 石菖蒲 (*Shichangpu*): the dried rhizome of *Acorus tatarinowii* Schott. (family Araceae).

[Taste and Properties] Pungent and warm.

[Effects and Indications] (1) Eliminates turbid phlegm for treating impaired consciousness in epilepsy and dementia; (2) Nourishes the Heart and improves memory; (3)

Removes dampness for relieving anorexia and abdominal distension.

[Usage and Dosage] 3-9 g.

[Notes] It shows a central inhibitory action in experimental studies. The decoction also relieves spasms of the gastro-intestinal smooth muscles.

***Styrax*, Storax,** 苏合香 (*Suhexiang*): purified, semi-fluid, viscid balsam obtained from the trunk of *Liquidambar orientalis* Miller (family Hamamelidaceae).

[Taste and Properties] Pungent and warm.

[Effects and Indications] Induces resuscitation and relieves pain, used as a stimulant for treating loss of consciousness in apoplexy, and also for relieving angina pectoris.

[Usage and Dosage] 0.3-1 g, used in pills or powder, but not in decoction.

[Notes] (1) It increases coronary blood flow and reduces oxygen consumption of the myocardium in experimental myocardial infarction. It also protects the heart from ischemia induced by pitressin. (2) It prevents thrombosis by inhibiting platelet aggregation, reducing the plasma fibrinogen level and increasing the activity of fibrinolysin.

***Moschus*, Musk,** 麝香 (Shexiang): the dried secretion obtained from the musk sac of the adult male musk deer, *Moschus berezovskii* Flerov, *Moschus sifanicus* Przewalski or *Moschus moschiferus* L. (family Cervidae).

[Taste and Properties] Pungent and warm.

[Effects and Indications] (1) Induces resuscitation, used as a stimulant for treatment of loss of consciousness in high fever and apoplexy; (2) Invigorates blood circulation and reduces inflammation in boils and sores.

[Usage and Dosage] 0.03-0.1 g, mostly used in making pills or powder, but not in decoction; appropriate quantity for external use.

[Warning] Contraindicated in pregnancy.

[Notes] (1) It shows a dual action on the central nervous system, exciting at a smaller dose and inhibiting at a larger dose. It increases the brain's tolerance of oxygen deficit. (2) It dilates the coronary artery, increases coronary blood flow and reduces myocardial oxygen consumption. It also inhibits platelet aggregation and reduces the action of thrombin. (3) It counteracts inflammation at all the stages of increased capillary permeability, wandering of leukocytes, and formation of granulation. (4) It stimulates the uterus, particularly in pregnancy.

TRANQUILIZING DRUGS

Drugs in this category are used to allay excitement (mental instability, irritability, anxiety, fidgeting and insomnia). They are classified as heavy-weighted tranquilizers and Heart-nourishing tranquilizers.

Heavy-weight tranquilizers, possessing high specific gravity, are usually minerals or shells, and are indicated in excess syndromes. Heart-nourishing tranquilizers are botanical drugs with tonic actions to nourish blood or replenish *yin* in addition to tranquilization. So the latter are usually used in deficiency cases.

Heavy-Weight Tranquilizers

***Cinnabaris*, Cinnabar**, 朱砂 (*Zhusha*): a mineral containing mainly mercuric sulfide (HgS).

[Taste and Properties] Sweet, slightly cold, and toxic.

[Effects and Indications] (1) Induces tranquilization for anxiety, maniac-depressive syndrome, and insomnia with palpitations; (2) Counteracts toxins for treating boils and sores.

[Usage and Dosage] 0.3-1.5 g. used in making pills or powder for oral administration; appropriate quantity for external use.

[Warning] Long-term administration should be avoided.

***Os Draconis*, Dragon's Bone**, 龙骨 (*Longgu*): fossil bone of large ancient mammals, such as *Stegodon orientalis* and *Rhinocerus sinensis*.

[Taste and Properties] Sweet and puckery in taste and neutral in property.

[Effects and Indications] (1) Calms the mind for treating insomnia, irritability, anxiety and forgetfulness; (2) Also used as an astringent for night sweating, seminal emission or excessive leukorrhea.

[Usage and Dosage] 15-30 g, to be decocted before other ingredients.

Heart-Nourishing Tranquilizers

***Semen Ziziphi Spinosae*, Spiny Date Seed**, 酸枣仁 (*Suanzaoren*): the dried ripe seed of *Ziziphus jujuba* var. *spinosa* (Bunge) Hu ex H.F. Chou (family Rhamnaceae).

[Taste and Properties] Sweet and sour in taste, and neutral in property.

[Effects and Indications] (1) Calms the mind by nourishing Heart and Liver blood for treating insomnia and palpitations; (2) Arrests excessive sweating due to debility.

[Usage and Dosage] 9-15 g.

[Notes] (1) It shows sedative and hypnotic effects in animal experiments. It counteracts the convulsions induced by metrazol or strychnine, but has no effect on electrofit. It also has an analgesic effect, and lowers the body temperature in normal rats.

***Radix Polygalae,* Milkwort Root**, 远志 (*Yuanzhi*), the dried root of *Polygala tenuifolia* Willd. or *Polygala sibirica* L. (family Polygalaceae).

[Taste and Properties] Bitter and warm.

[Effects and Indications] (1) Harmonizes the coordination between the Heart and the Kidneys for treating insomnia; (2) Eliminates phlegm for treating coughing with profuse expectoration and psychic disorders caused by phlegm.

[Usage and Dosage] 3-9 g.

[Notes] It shows sedative, anticonvulsive and expectorant effects in the laboratory.

***Caulis Polygoni Multiflori*, Fleece-flower Stem**, 首乌藤 (*Shouwuteng*): the dried lianoid stem of *Polygonum multiflorum* Thunb. (family Polygonaceae).

[Taste and Properties] Sweet in taste and neutral in property.

[Effects and Indications] Induces tranquilization by nourishing the Heart for treating insomnia with fidgetiness.

[Usage and Dosage] 9-15 g.

***Semen Platycladi*, Arborvitae Seed**, 柏子仁 (*Baiziren*): the dried ripe kernel of *Platycladus orientalis* (L.) Franco (family Cupressaceae).

[Taste and Properties] Sweet in taste and neutral in property.

[Effects and Indications] (1) Induces tranquilization by nourishing the Heart for treating insomnia with palpitations; (2) Also used as a mild laxative for treating constipation.

[Usage and Dosage] 6-12 g.

***Cortex Albiziae*, Silktree Bark**, 合欢皮 (*Hehuanpi*): the dired bark of *Albizia julibrissin* Durazz. (family Leguminosae).

[Taste and Properties] Sweet in taste and neutral in property.

[Effects and Indications] Eases the mind and induces tranquilization for treating melancholy and insomnia.

[Usage and Dosage] 6-12 g.

SEDATIVES AND ANTICONVULSIVES (DRUGS FOR SUBDUING HYPERACTIVITY OF THE LIVER AND EXTINGUISHING ENDOGENOUS WIND)

There are two kinds of wind as pathogenic factors, one is exogenous, and the other endogenous. Exogenous wind usually attacks the exterior of the body, and is treated by wind-dispelling drugs, as mentioned in the section on diaphoretics and antirheumatics. Endogenous wind, existing in the interior, is induced by hyperactivity of the Liver (exuberance of Liver *yang*) and manifested by vertigo, convulsions and trembling symptoms. For extinguishing endogenous wind, sedatives and anticonvulsives are indicated.

Hyperactivity of the Liver (exuberance of Liver *yang*) may be due to harassment by excessive pathogenic heat or due to deficiency of *yin* and blood. In either case, the use of sedatives or anticonvulsives merely treats the symptoms. In cases of excess, they should be used in combination with febrifuges, and in cases of deficiency, *yin* tonics and/or blood tonics should be administered jointly.

Endogenous wind as a pathogenic factor is apt to combine with phlegm, forming wind-phlegm. Serious cases of endogenous wind are often accompanied by phlegm symptoms, as for example, when an epileptic patient usually loses consciousness during convulsions. In such a case, both anticonvulsives and phlegmolytics should be administered.

***Rhizoma Gastrodiae*, Gastrodia Tuber**, 天麻 (*Tianma*): the dried tuber of *Gastrodia elata* Bl. (family Orchidaceae).

[Taste and Properties] Sweet in taste and neutral in property.

[Effects and Indications] Subdues Liver wind for treating headache, dizziness, numbness of the limbs and premonitory symptoms of stroke.

[Usage and Dosage] 3-9 g.

[Notes] (1) It shows sedative, anticonvulsive and analgesic effects in animal experiments. (2) It lowers blood pressure and inhibits blood platelet aggregation. It protects the heart from acute ischemia and arrhythmia induced by pitressin.

***Ramulus Uncariae cum Uncis*, Uncaria Stem**, 钩藤 (*Gouteng*): the dried hook-bearing branch of *Uncaria rhynchophylla* (Miq.) Lacks., *Uncaria macrophylla* Wall., *Uncaria hirsuta* Havil., *Uncaria sinensis* (Oliv.) Havil. or *Uncaria sessilifructus* Roxb. (family Rubiaceae).

[Taste and Properties] Sweet and slightly cold.

[Effects and Indications] Clears heat and extinguishes endogenous wind for treating headache and dizziness due to Liver heat or exuberant Liver *yang*, and also for convulsions due to high fever.

[Usage and Dosage] 6-15 g.

[Notes] It lowers the blood pressure in experimental hypertension, causes sedation and relieves smooth muscle spasm of the bronchus, intestine and uterus.

***Cornu Saigae Tataricae*, Antelope's Horn**, 羚羊角 (*Lingyangjiao*): the horn of *Saiga tatarica* L. (family Bovidae).

[Taste and Properties] Salty and cold.

[Effects and Indications] To be ground into powder and 0.3-0.6 g taken each time.

[Usage and Dosage] Extinguishes endogenous wind for arresting convulsions.

[Notes] (1) It shows sedative and hypnotic effects and counteracts the convulsions caused by strychnine, metrazole or caffeine and electrofit in animal experiments. (2) It has a marked antipyretic effect in experimental fevers. Its alcoholic extract lowers the body temperature by more than 0.5°C in normal mice. (3) It also has a hypotensive effect.

***Lumbricus*, Earthworm**, 地龙 (*Dilong*): the dried body of *Pheretima aspergillum* (Perrier) (family Megascolecidae), or *Allolobophora caliginosa* (Savigny) *trapezoides* (Ant. Duges) (family Lumbricidae).

[Taste and Properties] Salty and cold.

[Effects and Indications] (1) Used as an antipyretic and anticonvulsive for hyperpyretic convulsion; (2) As an antirheumatic for rheumatalgia; (3) As an antiasthmatic for bronchial asthma and asthmatic bronchitis.

[Usage and Dosage] 6-9 g.

[Notes] (1) Earthworm extract shows a prominent antipyretic effect in rabbits with fever induced by colitoxin, milder but more lasting than that of pyramidon. The effect is due to its action on the thermoregulatory center, increasing the heat dissipation. The active principle is lumbrofebrine. (2) The extract causes sedation, and counteracts the convulsions induced by metrazole or caffeine, and electrofit. The active principle is succinic acid. (3) The extract partly relieves histamine-induced asthma and passive allergic reaction of the skin in animal experiments. This is probably due to its competitive combination with the histamine receptor. (4) The extract shows marked antithrombotic action by promotion of fibrinolysis, inhibition of platelet aggregation, and enhancement of the stability of the red blood cell membrane. (5) The extract is also a hypotensor, acting on the vasomotor center.

***Scolopendra*, Centipede**, 蜈蚣 (*Wugong*): the dried body of *Scolopendra subspinipes mutilans* L. Koch (family Scolopendridae).

[Taste and Properties] Pungent, warm and toxic.

[Effects and Indications] (1) Extinguishes endogenous wind for relieving convulsions; (2) Removes obstructions from the collateral meridians for relieving pain, used in the treatment of stubborn migraine and arthralgia.

[Usage and Dosage] 2.5-4.5 g.

[Warning] Contraindicated in pregnancy.

[Notes] (1) Centipede possesses two apisin-like poisons, one hemolytic and the other acting as histamine. (2) Centipede shows sedative and anticonvulsive effects in animal experiments.

***Scorpio*, Scorpion**, 全蝎 (*Quanxie*): the boiled and dried body of *Buthus martensii* Karsch (family Buthidae).

[Taste and Properties] Pungent in taste and neutral in property; toxic.

[Effects and Indications] (1) Extinguishes endogenous wind for relieving convulsions; (2) Removes obstruction from the collateral meridians for relieving pain, used in the treatment of stubborn migraine and arthralgia.

[Usage and Dosage] 2.5-4.5 g.

[Notes] (1) Scorpion shows anticonvulsive and hypotensive effects in animal experiments. (2) The scorpion venom is destroyed by heating to 100°C for 30 minutes.

***Bombyx Batryticatus*, White-stiff Silkworm**, 僵蚕 (*Jiangcan*): dried silkworm larva, *Bombyx mori* L. (family Moniliaceae) died of infection of *Beauveria bassiana* (Bals.) Vuill.

[Taste and Properties] Salty and pungent in taste and neutral in property.

[Effects and Indications] (1) Extinguishes endogenous wind for relieving headache, dizziness, and convulsions; (2) Resolves phlegmy nodules (e.g., scrofula).

[Usage and Dosage] 4.5-9 g.

[Notes] It shows sedative and anticonvulsive effects in the laboratory.

***Haematitum*, Hematite**, 赭石 (*Zheshi*): a mineral containing mainly ferric oxide (Fe_2O_3).

[Taste and Properties] Bitter and cold.

[Effects and Indications] (1) Checks exuberant Liver *yang* for headaches and dizziness (e.g., in hypertension); (2) Suppresses the reverse flow of Stomach or Lung *qi* for treating belching, vomiting and asthma.

[Usage and Dosage] 9-30 g, to be decocted before other ingredients.

Concha Haliotidis, Sea-ear Shell, 石决明 (*Shijueming*): the shell of *Haliotis diversicolor* Reeve, *Haliotis discus hanai* Ino or *Haliotis ovina* Gmelin, *Haliotis ruber* (Leach), *Haliotis asinina* L., or *Haliotis laevigata* (Donovan) (family Haliotidae).

[Taste and Properties] Salty and slightly cold.

[Effects and Indications] (1) Checks exuberant Liver *yang* for treating headaches and dizziness (e.g., in hypertension); (2) Clears the Liver of heat for treating glaucoma.

[Usage and Dosage] 9-30 g, to be decocted before adding other ingredients.

TONICS

Tonics are used to replenish or tonify *qi*, blood, *yin* and *yang* of the human body for treating deficiency syndromes. Therefore, they can be roughly classified into four groups: *qi* tonics, blood tonics, *yin* tonics and *yang* tonics.

Qi Tonics

Qi tonics are used for treating *qi* deficiency. Generalized *qi* deficiency is manifested by lassitude, lack of strength, spontaneous sweating and feeble pulse. *Qi* deficiency of a *zang-fu* organ is marked by diminished function of that organ, e.g., reduced food intake in deficiency of Stomach *qi*, indigestion in deficiency of Spleen *qi*, cardiac palpitation in deficiency of Heart *qi*, and shortness of breath in deficiency of Lung *qi*. In all these conditions, *qi* tonics are indicated. In addition, generation of blood depends upon the action of *qi*. Therefore, *qi* tonics are often used together with blood tonics in the treatment of blood deficiency.

Generation of *qi* in the human body is closely related to the function of the Lungs and the Spleen. So, most *qi* tonics chiefly tonify the Lungs and the Spleen, but some *qi* tonics also tonify the Stomach, the Heart and the Kidneys. (Table IX-8)

Qi tonics generally are sweet in taste and slightly warm in property. The actions and indications of individual *qi* tonics are as follows:

Table IX-8 Action Sites of *Qi* Tonics

	General	Heart	Spleen	Stomach	Lungs	Kidneys
Ginseng	+ (original *qi*)	+	+		+	+
Tangshen			+		+	
Milkvetch root	+ (defensive *qi*)		+		+	
White atractylodes rhizome			+		+	
Thorny acantho-panax root	+	+	+			+
Chinese yam			+	+	+*	+
Solomonseal rhizome			+		+*	
Chinese date			+	+		
Licorice root		+	+			

*also nourishes Lung *yin*

***Radix Ginseng*, Ginseng**, 人参 (*Renshen*): the dried root of *Panax ginseng* C. A. Mey. (family Araliaceae).

[Taste and Properties] Sweet, somewhat bitter, and slightly warm.[Effects and Indications] (1) Replenishes original *qi* and promotes the production of body fluid in cases of general weakness, diabetes mellitus, impotence or frigidity, heart failure, and cardiogenic shock; (2) Replenishes Spleen and Lung *qi* for treating anorexia, diarrhea, coughing and shortness of breath.

[Usage and Dosage] 3-9 g.

[Notes] (1) Ginseng has a dual action on the central nervous system, stimulation in small doses and inhibition in large doses. It improves memory in animal experiments. (2) Ginseng enhances the immune function in various respects, phagocytosis of the reticulo-endothelial cells, activity of natural killer lymphocytes (NK cells), formation of IgG, IgA and IgM, transformation of lymphocytes, and production of leukocytes. (3) Ginseng is cardiotonic, increasing the myocardial contractibility and reducing the heart rate. The active principle is ginsenoside, which has similar effects to cardiac glycoside (i.e., promoting the release of catecholamines and inhibiting the activity of Na^{+}-K^{+}-ATPase of the myocardial cell membrane). Ginsenoside improves the electrocardiographic changes in cardiac ischemia induced by norepinephrine. Ginseng dilates the coronary, cerebral and pulmonary arteries, improving the blood circulation in these organs, and has a bi-directional regulatory effect on blood pressure, lowering it in cases of hypertension, and raising it in cases of hypotension or shock. (4) Ginsenoside prevents blood coagulation, promotes fibrinolysis, inhibits the clustering of erythrocytes and aggregation of platelets, increases the fluidity of blood and improves tissue perfusion. Ginseng extract stimulates hemopoiesis of the bone marrow, increasing the white and red blood cell counts as well as the hemoglobin level. (5) Ginseng stimulates the hypothalamic-pituitary-adrenocortical axis, increasing the release of ACTH and then the secretion of corticosteroids. Ginseng also stimulates the adenohypophysis to release gonadotropic hormones. In female animals, ginseng accelerates sexual maturity, shortens the proestrum and prolongs the estrum. In young male animals, ginseng increases the weight of the testes and epididymides, and the amount of sperm in the testis. (6) Ginseng stimulates the islets of Langerhans to release insulin, but ginseng itself also has an effect on carbohydrate metabolism different from insulin. It lowers blood sugar and liver glycogen simultaneously in hyperglycemia, while it elevates blood sugar in hypoglycemia. It also affects protein and lipid metabolism, promoting the biosynthesis of protein, DNA and RNA, and preventing hypercholersterolemia and atherosclerosis. (7) Ginseng retards the aging process of the tested animals and cells. In old animals, it inhibits the activity of monoamine oxidase in the brain stem, reduces the tissue lipofuscin and serum lipid peroxide, increases the activity of superoxide dismutase (SOD), and eliminates the free radicals that cause senility. In conclusion, ginseng shows “adaptogen” effects, strengthening the adaptability, enhancing the body’s resistance to harmful stimulation and stress, and restoring disordered functional activities to normal.

***Radix Codonopsis*, Tangshen**, 党参 (*Dangshen*): the dried root of *Codonopsis pilosula* (Franch.) Nannf., *Codonopsis pilosula* var. *modesta* (Nannf.) L. T. Shen or *Codonopsis tangshen* Oliv. (family Campanulaceae).

[Taste and Properties] Sweet and slightly warm.

[Effects and Indications] Replenishes Spleen and Lung *qi* for anorexia, loose stools, general weakness and shortness of breath.

[Usage and Dosage] 9-30 g.

[Notes] (1) Tangshen enhances the immune function and the resistance to harmful stimulation and stress. The latter is related to, but not confined to, the excitation of the hypothalamic-pituitary-adrenocortical axis, for tangshen still shows the effect of counteracting hypoxia in animals with bilateral adrenal glands extirpated. (2) Tangshen improves digestion and has a regulatory effect on the motility of the gastro-intestinal tract. (3) Tangshen is cardiotonic, increasing the myocardial contractibility and cardiac output by inhibiting the activity of phosphodiesterase of the myocardial cells (a mechanism different from that of ginseng). It counteracts myocardial ischemia and regulates blood pressure. (4) Tangshen markedly increases red blood cell counts and hemoglobin level, restores the white blood cell counts in leukopenia caused by chemotherapy and radiotherapy. Tangshen inhibits platelet aggregation, and reduces blood viscosity. (5) Tangshen improves intelligence (ability of learning and memory) and induces tranquilization. (6) Tangshen promotes the growth of *Staphylococcus aureus* and *Bacillus coli*, and increases the mortality of mice with septicemia caused by staphylococcus. This explains why tangshen is contraindicated in the treatment of "exogenous affections with excessive pathogens."

***Radix Astragali*, Milkvetch Root**, 黄芪 (*Huangqi*): the dried root of *Astragalus membranaceus* (Fisch.) Bge. or *Astragalus membranaceus* var. *mongholicus* (Bge.) Hsiao (family Leguminosae).

[Taste and Properties] Sweet and slightly warm.

[Effects and Indications] (1) Replenishes Spleen and Lung *qi* in cases of lack of strength, sinking syndromes and bleeding due to *qi* deficiency; (2) Arrests excessive perspiration in cases of spontaneous sweating and night sweats; (3) Dispels pus and promotes the healing of chronic ulcers; (4) Induces diuresis in cases of nephritic edema.

[Usage and Dosage] 9-30 g. For replenishing *qi*, milkvetch root processed with honey is better.

[Notes] (1) Milkvetch root enhances non-specific immunity, increasing blood leukocyte count, promoting phagocytosis and bacteriocidal power of neutrophils and macrophages, augmenting the activity of natural killer lymphocytes (NK cells), and facilitating the production of interferon induced by viruses. It also enhances specific immune functions, including cellular immunity and humoral immunity. It acts like interleukin-II (IL-2), increasing the activity of lymphokine-activated killer (LAK) cells, and also restores the normal production of IL-2 in animals with insufficient production. It markedly increases the production of antibodies as well. (2) Milkvetch root prolongs the lifespan of fruit flies and increases the replicative lifespan of cultivated human diploid fibroblasts. It reduces the activity of monoamine oxidase in the brain of old mice, increases the central catecholamine level and minimizes the production of free radicals. (3) Milkvetch root shows cardiotonic effects by inhibiting the activity of phosphodiesterase of the myocardial cells. It dilates peripheral, cerebral, coronary and renal arteries, improves microcirculation, lowers blood pressure. It also inhibits platelet aggregation. (4) Milkvetch root stimulates hemopoiesis of the bone marrow, promoting the generation, development and maturation of all kinds of blood cells. (5) Milkvetch root promotes the anabolism of RNA, DNA and protein in animal experiments. It has a bi-directional regulatory effect on carbohydrate metabolism, showing no effect on normal blood sugar, but counteracting both hyperglycemia and hypoglycemia experimentally. (6) Besides its action on the induction of interferon and the activity of NK cells, milkvetch root has a direct antiviral effect (on Coxsackie virus).

***Rhizoma Atractylodis Macrocephalae*, Largehead or White Atractylodes Rhizome**, 白术 (*Baizhu*): the dried rhizome of *Atractylodes macrocephala* Koidz. (family

Compositae).

[Taste and Properties] Sweet, somewhat bitter, and warm.

[Effects and Indications] (1) Invigorates the Spleen and replenishes *qi* for treating weakness of the Spleen and the Stomach with anorexia, abdominal distension, lassitude and loose stools; (2) Removes dampness and induces diuresis for treating diarrhea and edema due to diminished Spleen function; (3) Prevents miscarriages.

[Usage and Dosage] 6-12 g.

[Notes] (1) It promotes gastric secretion and lowers the blood sugar content. (2) It protects the liver against chemical damage. (3) It induces diuresis by inhibiting the reabsorption of sodium.

***Radix Acanthopanacis Senticosis*, Thorny Acanthopanax Root**, 刺五加 (*Ciwujia*): the dried root and rhizome of *Acanthopanax senticosus* (Rupr. et Maxim.) Harms (family Araliaceae).

[Taste and Properties] Pungent, slightly bitter, and warm.

[Effects and Indications] Replenishes *qi*, tonifies the Spleen and the Kidneys, and induces tranquilization for general weakness, anorexia, soreness of the back and knees, and insomnia.

[Usage and Dosage] 3-9 g.

[Notes] (1) Thorny acanthopanax root not only improves the excitatory process of the central nervous system; it also strengthens the inhibitory process. (2) It enhances the body's resistance to harmful stimulation, stress and fatigue. (3) It shows bi-directional regulatory effects on the endocrine system: It prevents adrenal hyperplasia caused by ACTH on the one hand, and reduces adrenal atrophy caused by cortisone on the other. It prevents both thyroid enlargement caused by thyroxin and thyroid atrophy by methylthiouracil. It lowers the blood sugar to normal in alloxan-induced diabetes mellitus, and raises the blood sugar in hypoglycemia caused by insulin. (4) It enhances immune functions, including phagocytosis of reticulo-endothelial system, production of interleukin-II and IgG and IgM antibodies, and induction of interferon. (5) It dilates cerebral vessels, improving cerebral blood supply. It also increases coronary blood flow, and markedly inhibits platelet aggregation. Therefore, it has been used recently in the treatment of coronary heart disease and cerebral thrombosis.

***Rhizoma Dioscoreae*, Chinese Yam**, 山药 (*Shanyao*): the dried rhizome of *Dioscorea opposita* Thunb. (family Dioscoreaceae).

[Taste and Properties] Sweet in taste and neutral in property.

[Effects and Indications] (1) Invigorates the Spleen and the Stomach for treating anorexia, loose stools and leukorrhagia; (2) Replenishes Lung and Kidney *yin* in cases of dry coughing and diabetes mellitus.

[Usage and Dosage] 9-30 g.

***Rhizoma Polygonati*, Solomonseal Rhizome**, 黄精 (*Huangjing*): the steamed and dried rhizome of *Polygonatum kingianum* Coll. et Hemsl., *Polygonatum sibiricum* Red., or *Polygonatum cyrtonema* Hua (family Liliaceae).

[Taste and Properties] Sweet in taste and neutral in property.

[Effects and Indications] (1) Replenishes Spleen *qi* for treating lassitude and anorexia; (2) Nourishes Lung *yin* for relieving dry coughing in cases of chronic bronchitis and phthisis.

[Usage and Dosage] 9-15 g.

[Notes] It shows hypoglycemic and hypotensive effects in animal experiments.

***Fructus Jujubae*, Chinese Date**, 大枣 (*Dazao*): the dried ripe fruit of *Ziziphus jujuba* Mill. (family Rhamnaceae).

[Taste and Properties] Sweet in taste and neutral in property.

[Effects and Indications] (1) Replenishes Spleen *qi* and harmonizes the Stomach for treating lassitude, anorexia and diarrhea; (2) Moderates the drastic effects of other ingredients.

[Usage and Dosage] 6-15 g (4-10 pieces)

***Radix Glycyrrhizae,* Licorice Root**, 甘草 (*Gancao*): the dried root and rhizome of *Glycyrrhiza uralensis* Fisch., *Glycyrrhiza inflata* Bat. or *Glycyrrhiza glabra* L. (family Leguminosae).

[Taste and Properties] Sweet in taste and neutral in property.

[Effects and Indications] (1) Replenishes Heart and Spleen *qi*; (2) Arrests coughing due to heat in the Lungs; (3) Relieves spasms in cases of abdominal colic; (4) Moderates drastic and toxic effects of other ingredients.

[Usage and Dosage] 1.5-9 g.

[Notes] (1) Licorice has adrenocortical hormone-like effects: It promotes retention of sodium and water, and excretion of potassium, acting like mineralocorticoid. It causes atrophy of the thymus gland, increases the weight of the adrenal gland, and reduces blood eosinophils and lymphocytes, acting like glucocorticoid. (2) Licorice counteracts peptic ulcers by inhibiting acid secretion and phosphodiesterase of the gastric mucosa. It inhibits the motility of the intestines, relieving enterospasms. It also protects the liver from chemical damage. (3) Licorice shows anti-inflammatory and antiallergic effects, as adrenocortico-steroid does. (4) Licorice contains glycyrrhizin (6-14%), which inhibits the proliferation of hepatitis, varicella and herpes zoster viruses. (5) Licorice removes the toxic quality of various drugs (e.g., urethane, histamine, pilocarpine, barbital), animal toxins (snake venom, tetrodotoxin) and bacterial toxins (diphtherotoxin, tetanus toxin). (6) Licorice extract is an antitussive and also an expectorant.

Blood Tonics

Blood tonics are used for treating blood deficiency. Since the Heart governs blood, the Liver stores blood, and the Kidney essence can be converted into blood, blood tonics are usually tonics acting on the Heart, Liver and Kidneys. The Spleen is the source of *qi* and blood production, so Spleen tonics are certainly of significance in the treatment of blood deficiency. But those tonics are classified as *qi* tonics, and not blood tonics.

Blood deficiency in Chinese medicine is roughly equivalent to anemia in Western medicine, particularly in moderate and mild cases. Just like anemia, blood deficiency may be general or local, either in quality or in quantity (though blood deficiency in quantity is more precisely called oligemia, and local deficiency of blood, ischemia in Western medicine). General blood deficiency is manifested by pallor or sallow complexion, dizziness, pale lips, pale tongue, and thready pulse. Blood deficiency of the Heart is marked by cardiac palpitation and insomnia; blood deficiency of the Liver by blurred vision, numbness of the limbs, and oligomenorrhea or amenorrhea in women. These are the common indications for blood tonics.

Yin in its broader sense includes blood. So, some blood tonics are at the same time *yin* tonics, and some *yin* tonics may also have the effect of replenishing blood.

***Radix Angelicae Sinensis*, Chinese Angelica Root**, 当归 (*Danggui*): the dried root of *Angelica sinensis* (Oliv.) Diels (family Umbelliferae).

[Taste and Properties] Sweet, pungent and warm.

[Effects and Indications] (1) Tonifies blood, activates blood circulation, regulates menstruation and relieves pain. Used for treating anemia, menstrual disorders and dysmenorrhea; (2) Relaxes the bowels in cases of constipation due to blood deficiency in the aged or debilitated.

[Usage and Dosage] 4.5-9 g.

[Notes] (1) Chinese angelica root promotes hemopoiesis, increasing the red blood cell count and hemoglobin in experimental anemia, and the white blood cells and blood platelets in leukopenia induced by cyclophosphamide. (2) Chinese angelica root inhibits blood platelet aggregation, and shows marked antithrombotic effects in experimental studies. The main active principle is ferulic acid. (3) Chinese angelica root, by improving the myocardial blood supply, relieves myocardial ischemia, and by dilating peripheral arteries, lowers the blood pressure and improves microcirculation. (4) Chinese angelica root has a bi-directional effect on the uterus, stimulating and inhibiting the uterine smooth muscle. This can explain its wide use in the treatment of menstrual disorders. In addition, it relieves experimental asthma by relaxing bronchospasm. (5) Chinese angelica root enhances immune functions, non-specific phagocytosis, cellular immunity and humoral immunity.

***Radix Rehmanniae Preparata*, Prepared Rehmannia Root**, 熟地黄 (*Shudihuang*): the steamed and dried tuberous root of *Rehmannia glutinosa* Libosch. (family Scrophulariaceae).

[Taste and Properties] Sweet and slightly warm.

[Effects and Indications] (1) Tonifies blood and regulate menstruation for blood deficiency with dizziness, palpitation and menstrual disorders; (2) Replenishes Kidney *yin* for treating tidal fever, night sweating, low back pain and diabetes mellitus due to Kidney *yin* deficiency.

[Usage and Dosage] 9-15 g.

[Notes] It shows cardiotonic, diuretic and hypoglycemic effects in the laboratory.

***Radix Paeoniae Alba*, White Peony Root**, 白芍 (*Baishao*): the peeled and dried root of *Paeonia lactiflora* Pall. (family Ranunculaceae).

[Taste and Properties] Bitter, sour and slightly cold.

[Effects and Indications] (1) Nourishes blood and regulates menstruation in cases of menstrual disorders due to blood deficiency; (2) Soothes the Liver for relieving headache, abdominal pain and spasm of the calf muscles due to stagnation of Liver *qi*.

[Usage and Dosage] 6-15 g.

[Notes] (1) In experimental studies it shows a remarkable antispasmodic effect on the stomach, intestines and uterus, as well as sedative and analgesic effects. This may explain its action of "soothing the liver and relieving pain." (2) It has immuno-modulating effects. The active constituents in the immune function are its glycosides. (3) Peoniflorin, one of its glycosides, dilates the coronary and peripheral arteries, and can prevent peptic ulcers induced by stress.

***Colla Corii Asini*, Donkey-hide Glue,** 阿胶 (*Ejiao*): solid glue prepared from the skin of asses, *Equus asinus* L. (family Equidae).

[Taste and Properties] Sweet in taste and neutral in property.

[Effects and Indications] (1) Nourishes blood and arrests bleeding in cases of blood deficiency and various hemorrhages; (2) Replenishes *yin* for treating insomnia and dry cough.

[Usage and Dosage] 3-9 g, to be melted as a hot decoction.

[Notes] In animal experiments it accelerates the hemopoiesis in anemia induced by blood loss.

***Arillus Longan*, Longan aril,** 龙眼肉 (*Longyanrou*): the dried aril of *Dimocarpus longan* Lour. (family Sapindaceae).

[Taste and Properties] Sweet in taste and neutral in property.

[Effects and Indications] Replenishes the Heart and the Spleen, nourishes blood and induces tranquilization for treating palpitations, insomnia and forgetfulness due to deficiency of *qi* and blood.

[Usage and Dosage] 9-15 g.

***Placenta Hominis*, Human Placenta,** 紫河车 (*Ziheche*): the dried human placenta.

[Taste and Properties] Sweet, salty and warm.

[Effects and Indications] Nourishes blood and replenishes *qi* for general weakness and anemia.

[Usage and Dosage] 1.5-3 g, to be ground into powder for oral administration.

[Notes] (1) It contains estrogen and chorionic gonadotropin, stimulating the development of the uterus and ovaries, and the secretion of milk. (2) It enhances the body's immunity and has antiallergic effects. Its globulin content acts as an antibody against measles.

Yin Tonics

Yin tonics are used for the treatment of *yin* deficiency. A simple *yin* deficiency syndrome is characterized by endogenous dryness symptoms such as dryness of the mouth and throat, constipation, concentrated urine, scanty tongue coating and thready pulse. But serious *yin* deficiency is usually accompanied by relative exuberance of *yang*, manifested by feverishness in the chest, palms and soles, malar flush, night sweating, reddened tongue and rapid pulse. If a given organ is particularly affected by *yin* deficiency, there will be some other manifestations, e.g., fidgetiness and insomnia in deficiency of Heart *yin*, blurred vision, dizziness or oligomenorrhea in deficiency of Liver *yin*, dry coughing in deficiency of Lung *yin*, and aching and weakness of the loins and legs in deficiency of Kidney *yin*. All these conditions call for *yin* tonics. *Yin* tonics may act on different organs, and their sites of action are shown in Table IX-9.

Table IX-9. Action Sites of *Yin* Tonics

	Replenishing *yin* of					Nourish-ing blood
	Heart	Lungs	Stomach	Liver	Kidneys	
American ginseng		+	+			
Dendrobium		+	+	+	+	
Lilyturf root	+	+	+			
Asparagus root		+			+	
Glehnia root		+	+			
Figwort Root		+	+			
Wolfberry fruit				+	+	+
Dogwood fruit				+	+	
Fleeceflower root				+	+	+
Twotoothed Achyranthes root				+	+	
Glossy privet fruit				+	+	
Mulberry mistletoe				+	+	+
Tortoise Plastron	+			+	+	
Turtle shell				+		
Mulberry fruit				+	+	+

***Radix Ginseng Americana*, American Ginseng**, 西洋参 (*Xiyangshen*): the dried root of *Panax quinquefolium* L. (family Araliaceae).

[Taste and Properties] Bitter, sweet and cool.

[Effects and Indications] Replenishes *yin*, reduces internal heat and promotes the production of body fluid for relieving low-grade fever, spontaneous or night sweating, thirst, chronic coughing and lassitude in consumptive diseases.

[Usage and Dosage] 3-6 g.

[Notes] It causes tranquilization of the cerebral cortex, but moderately stimulates the vital centers. It contains ginsenoside Rg_1 which helps to relieve fatigue.

***Herba Dendrobii*, Dendrobium**, 石斛 (*Shihu*): the fresh or dried stem of *Dendrobium loddigesii* Rolfe., *Dendrobium chrysanthum* Wall., *Dendrobium fimbriatum* var. *oculatum* Hook., *Dendrobium nobile* Lindl. or *Dendrobium candidum* Wall. ex Lindl. (family Orchidaceae).

[Taste and Properties] Sweet or tasteless, and slightly cold.

[Effects and Indications] (1) Replenishes Lung and Stomach *yin*, reduces heat and promotes the production of body fluids for relieving dry coughing, thirst and retching; (2) Replenishes Kidney *yin* for treating blurred vision due to deficiency of Liver and Kidney *yin*.

[Usage and Dosage] 6-12 g.

[Notes] The decoction given orally stimulates gastric secretion and promotes intestinal peristalsis to help digestion. It also has mild analgesic and antipyretic effects.

***Radix Ophiopogonis*, Lilyturf Root**, 麦冬 (*Maidong*): the dried tuberous root of *Ophiopogon japonicus* (Thunb.) Ker.-Gawl. (family Liliaceae).

[Taste and Properties] Sweet but somewhat bitter, and slightly cold.

[Effects and Indications] Replenishes Stomach, Lung and Heart *yin* for treating thirst due to consumption of body fluid, dry coughing, hemoptysis or palpitations.

[Usage and Dosage] 6-12 g.

[Notes] (1) It shows antipyretic, antitussive, expectorant and diuretic effects in the laboratory. (2) It lowers blood sugar in both normal and alloxan-induced diabetic rabbits.

***Radix Asparagi*, Asparagus Root**, 天冬 (*Tiandong*): the dried tuberous root of *Asparagus conchinchinensis* (Lour.) Merr. (family Liliaceae).

[Taste and Properties] Sweet but somewhat bitter, and cold.

[Effects and Indications] Replenishes Lung and Kidney *yin* and promotes the production of body fluid for relieving dipsosis, dry throat, coughing with sticky phlegm, and constipation.

[Usage and Dosage] 6-12 g.

***Radix Glehniae*, Glehnia Root**, 北沙参 (*Beishashen*): the dried root of *Glehnia littoralis* Fr. Schmidt ex Miq. (family Umbelliferae).

[Taste and Properties] Sweet and slightly cold.

[Effects and Indications] Replenishes Stomach *yin* for relieving thirst due to deficiency of body fluids.

[Usage and Dosage] 6-9 g.

***Fructus Lycii*, Wolfberry Fruit**, 枸杞子 (*Gouqizi*): the dried ripe fruit of *Lycium barbarum* L. (family Solanaceae).

[Taste and Properties] Sweet in taste and neutral in property.

[Effects and Indications] Replenishes Liver and Kidney *yin* for treating aching and weakness of the back and legs, impotence, seminal emission, dizziness and blurred vision.

[Usage and Dosage] 6-12 g.

[Notes] (1) It enhances the immune function, increasing the number and activity of C_3b and Fc receptors, promoting the production of interleukin-2, and stimulating the lymphokine-activated killer (LAK) cells. (2) It increases leukocyte count in normal mice and in cyclophosphamide-induced leukopenic mice. It also promotes the proliferation of marrow cells. (3) It retards senility by increasing cAMP and the cAMP/cGMP ratio as well as the plasma testosterone level. Experimentally, it prolongs the life span of fruit flies and diminishes lipofuscin. (4) It reduces blood cholesterol, prevents the liver damage caused by chemicals, inhibits deposition of lipids in liver, and promotes the regeneration of the liver cells.

***Fructus Corni*, Dogwood fruit**, 山茱萸 (*Shanzhuyu*): the dried ripe sarcocarp of *Cornus officinalis* Sieb. et Zucc. (family Cornaceae).

[Taste and Properties] Sweet, sour and slightly warm.

[Effects and Indications] Replenishes Liver and Kidney *yin* and arrests discharges for treating dizziness, seminal emission, menorrhagia, polyuria and excessive sweating.

[Usage and Dosage] 6-12 g.

[Notes] (1) It promotes the proliferation of antigen-combining cells in the spleen at the early stage of an immune reaction, and the phagocytosis of macrophages, and inhibits the delayed allergy in mice. (2) It significantly increases the count of white blood cells in experimental leukopenia caused by cyclophosphamide. (3) It contains ursolic acid, which lowers blood sugar in experimental diabetes, but has no hypoglycemic effect in normal animals.

***Radix Polygoni Multiflori*, Fleeceflower Root**, 何首乌 (*Heshouwu*): the dried tuberous root of *Polygonum multiflorum* Thunb. (family Polygonaceae).

[Taste and Properties] Sweet, puckery and slightly warm.

[Effects and Indications] (1) Processed fleeceflower root replenishes Liver and Kidney *yin* and nourishes blood for treating premature greying of the hair and sluggishness in motion as well as anemia; (2) The unprocessed root is a laxative.

[Usage and Dosage] 6-12 g.

[Notes] (1) Fleeceflower root promotes hemopoiesis of the bone marrow in animal experiments. (2) It enhances the body's immune function related to thymus-dependent T cells. (3) It reduces blood lipids, counteracts atherosclerosis, and retards the aging process. (4) It prevents fatty liver and liver damage caused by peroxidized zeistic oil. (5) It contains anthraquinone, which causes laxation.

***Radix Achyranthis Bidentatae*, Twoteethed Achyranthes Root**, 怀牛膝 (*Huainiuxi*): the dried root of *Achyranthes bidentata* Bl. (family Amaranthaceae).

[Taste and Properties] Bitter and sour in taste and neutral in property.

[Effects and Indications] Replenishes Liver and the Kidney *yin,* and strengthens the tendons and bones for relieving aching in the back and knees and weakness of the legs.

[Usage and Dosage] 4.5-9 g.

[Warning] Use with caution in pregnancy.

[Notes] (1) It shows an analgesic effect in animal experiments. (2) It causes uterine contraction in pregnancy.

***Fructus Ligustri Lucidi*, Glossy Privet Fruit**, 女贞子 (*Nüzhenzi*): the dried ripe fruit of *Ligustrum lucidum* Ait. (family Oleaceae).

[Taste and Properties] Sweet, bitter and cool.

[Effects and Indications] Replenishes Liver and Kidney *yin* for treating premature senility with early greying of the hair, blurred vision, impaired hearing, tinnitus and loosening of teeth.

[Usage and Dosage] 6-12 g.

[Notes] It contains oleanolic acid, which has cardiotonic actions, and mannitol, which acts as a laxative.

***Ramulus Loranthus*, Mulberry Mistletoe**, 桑寄生 (*Sangjisheng*): the dried leaf-bearing stem and branch of *Loranthus parasiticus* (L.) Merr. (family Loranthaceae).

[Taste and Properties] Bitter in taste and neutral in property.

[Effects and Indications] (1) Replenishes Liver and Kidney *yin*, and dispels wind-damp for treating rheumatalgia and weakness of the legs; (2) Nourishes blood and prevents miscarriage when treating abortion danger due to blood deficiency.

[Usage and Dosage] 10-30 g.

[Notes] (1) It lowers blood pressure by inhibiting the medullary vasomotor center. (2) It lowers blood cholesterol. (3) Its constituent avicularin has a marked diuretic effect.

***Plastrum Testudinis*, Tortoise Plastron**, 龟板 (*Guiban*): the ventral shell of fresh-water tortoise, *Chinemys reevesii* (Gray) (family Testudinidae).

[Taste and Properties] Salty, sweet and cold.

[Effects and Indications] (1) Replenishes *yin* and subdues *yang* for treating dizziness, tidal fever and night sweats due to *yin* deficiency with exuberant *yang* or fire, and also for relieving excessive thirst due to fluid consumption after a febrile disease; (2) Tonifies the Kidneys and strengthens the bones for treating weakness of the legs in adults and retarded closure of fontanel in infants.

[Usage and Dosage] 9-24 g, to be decocted before other ingredients.

***Carapax Trionycis*, Turtle Shell**, 鳖甲 (*Biejia*): the dorsal shell of *Trionyx sinensis* Wiegmann (family Trionychidae).

[Taste and Properties] Salty and cold.

[Effects and Indications] (1) Replenishes *yin* and subdues *yang* for treating fever and night sweats due to deficiency of *yin*; (2) Softens hard masses such as splenohepatomegaly.

[Usage and Dosage] 9-24 g.

[Notes] It contains gelatin, keratin, vitamin D and iodine. It inhibits hyperplasia of connective tissue and elevates the plasma albumin level.

***Fructus Mori,* Mulberry Fruit,** 桑椹 (*Sangshen*): the dried fruit-spike of *Morus alba* L. (family Moraceae).

[Taste and Properties] Sweet and cold.

[Effects and Indications] Replenishes *yin* and nourishes blood for treating dizziness, tinnitus, and blurred vision due to deficiency of *yin* with exuberant *yang*, and also for treating constipation due to deficiency of blood.

[Usage and Dosage] 9-15 g.

Yang Tonics

Drugs that reinforce *yang* are called *yang* tonics. *Yang* includes *qi* and fire (in their physiological senses). *Qi* deficiency can be treated with *qi* tonics. So *yang* tonics are usually used for treating deficiency of vital fire as well as some functional disorders related to deficient vital fire. Since the Kidneys control the vital fire, reinforcing *yang* is chiefly referred to as strengthening Kidney *yang*. Common disorders or symptoms due to deficiency of Kidney *yang* are as follows: (1) Aversion to cold; (2) Aching and weakness in the lower back and legs; (3) Hyposexuality (including impotence and frigidity); (4) Chronic diarrhea; (5) Chronic asthma; and (6) Urinary disturbances (e.g., incontinence of urine and frequent urination). Different Kidney *yang* tonics are effective for treating different disorders, as shown in Table IX-10. Other *zang-fu* organs may also suffer from *yang* deficiency. As *yang* deficiency of an organ is manifested by *qi* deficiency (diminished function) of that organ plus cold symptoms, it is usually treated by using *qi* tonics together with warming drugs (e.g. aconite lateral root, cinammon twig and dried ginger to warm the Heart and the Spleen, and galangal rhizome, evodia fruit and fresh ginger to warm the Stomach).

Table IX-10 Different Effects of *Yang* Tonics on the Kidneys

	Aversion to cold	Back-ache	Hypo-sexuality	Chronic diarrhea	Chronic asthma	Urinary distur-bance
Pilose antler	+	+	+	+	+	+
Cistanche		+	+			
Curculigo rhizome		+	+			+
Epimedium		+	+			
Morinda root		+	+			+
Psoralea fruit		+	+	+		+
Dodder seed		+	+			+
Eucommia bark		+	+			
Cibot rhizome		+				+
Teasel root		+		+		
Drynaria rhizome		+		+		
Cordyceps		+	+		+	
Tokay (Gecko)			+		+	
Cnidium fruit			+			

***Cornu Cervi Pantotrichum*, Pilose Antler (Hairy Deerhorn),** 鹿茸 (*Lurong*): the hairy, unossified young horns of male sika deer, *Cervus nippon* Temminck, or red deer, *Cervus elaphus* L. (family Cervidae).

[Taste and Properties] Sweet, salty and warm.

[Effects and Indications] (1) Reinforces Kidney *yang*, promotes virility and strengthens the bones and muscles for treating intolerance of cold, lack of strength, impotence, spermatorrhea, leukorrhagia and other symptoms of *yang* deficiency in chronic diseases; (2) Promotes the bursting of abscesses and drainage of pus for treating chronic sores difficult to heal.

[Usage and Dosage] 1-2 g, to be ground into powder and taken with liquid or made into pills.

[Notes] (1) Hairy deerhorn promotes the anabolism of proteins and nucleic acids, and hemopoiesis of the bone marrow. (2) The ethanol extract, pantocrine, enhances the phagocytosis of the reticulo-endothelial system, and elevates the serum hemolysin antibody level. This may explain the use of hairy deerhorn in the treatment of chronic sores. (3) Pantocrine given by injection stimulates the growth of the prostate and seminal vesicle in immature male animals. On the other hand, it promotes the development of the uterus. Therefore, it possesses both androgen-like and estrogen-like actions. (4) Hairy deerhorn improves the learning ability, memory, and the body's resistance to stress and harmful stimulation in animal experiments. It also helps to relieve fatigue. (5) Extract of hairy deerhorn given orally to mice inhibits monoamine oxidase in the brain and the liver, reduces the heart lipofuscin, and increases the brain and liver superoxide dismutase contents. These effects may be beneficial for retarding senility.

***Herba Cistanches*, Cistanche,** 肉苁蓉 (*Roucongrong*): the dried fleshy stem with scales of *Cistanche deserticola* Y. C. Ma (family Orobanchaceae).

[Taste and Properties] Sweet, salty and warm.

[Effects and Indications] (1) Reinforces Kidney *yang* for treating impotence and premature ejaculation; (2) Induces mild laxation for constipation in the debilitated or the aged.

[Usage and Dosage] 9-15 g.

***Rhizoma Curculiginis*, Curculigo Rhizome**, 仙茅 (*Xianmao*): the dried rhizome of *Curculigo orchioides* Gaertn. (family Amaryllidaceae).

[Taste and Properties] Pungent, warm and slightly toxic.

[Effects and Indications] Reinforces Kidney yang for treating impotence, backache with cold sensation, and urorrhea in the aged.

[Usage and Dosage] 3-9 g.

***Herba Epimedii*, Epimedium**, 淫羊藿 (*Yinyanghuo*): the dried aerial part of *Epimedium brevicornum* Maxim., *Epimedium sagittatum* (Sieb. et Zucc.) Maxim., *Epimedium wushanense* T. S. Ying or *Epimedium koreanum* Nakai (family Berberidaceae).

[Taste and Properties] Pungent, sweet and warm.

[Effects and Indications] (1) Reinforces Kidney *yang* for treating impotence; (2) Dispels wind-damp for treating rheumatalgia of the lower extremities.

[Usage and Dosage] 3-9 g.

[Notes] (1) Epimedium has an androgen-like action in stimulating the production of semen. (2) Epimedium enhances both the cellular and humoral immunity. The active principles are mainly its flavones and polysaccharide. They stimulate the induction and differentiation of T helper cells, and also act on the B cells. The polysaccharide promotes the formation of antibodies, increases the number of peripheral leukocytes and induces the production of interferon. (3) The flavones enhance the activity of superoxide dismutase, decrease the formation of lipid peroxide and lipofuscin, and so may retard senility. (4) Epimedium increases the coronary and cerebral blood flow, and has a hypotensive effect.

***Radix Morindae Officinalis*, Morinda Root**, 巴戟天 (*Bajitian*): the dried root of *Morinda officinalis* How (family Rubiaceae).

[Taste and Properties] Pungent, sweet and slightly warm.

[Effects and Indications] Reinforces Kidney *yang* for treating impotence and premature ejaculation in men, and frigidity in women.

[Usage and Dosage] 3-9 g

***Fructus Psoraleae*, Scurfpea Fruit**, 补骨脂 (*Buguzhi*): the dried ripe fruit of *Psoralea corylifolia* L. (family Leguminosae).

[Taste and Properties] Pungent, bitter and warm.

[Effects and Indications] Reinforces Kidney *yang* for treating impotence and nocturnal emission in male adults, urorrhea in the aged, and diarrhea daily before dawn due to *yang* deficiency of the Spleen and the Kidneys.

[Usage and Dosage] 6-9 g.

[Notes] (1) It dilates the coronary arteries. (2) It contains psoralen, which induces photosensitization for the treatment of vitiligo.

***Semen Cuscutae*, Dodder Seed**, 菟丝子 (*Tusizi*): the dried ripe seed of *Cuscuta chinensis* Lam. (family Convolvulaceae).

[Taste and Properties] Pungent and sweet in taste, and neutral in property.

[Effects and Indications] (1) Reinforces Kidney *yang* for treating urorrhea, impotence and nocturnal emission; (2) Prevents miscarriage in cases of abortion dangers.

[Usage and Dosage] 6-12 g.

***Cortex Eucommiae*, Eucommia Bark**, 杜仲 (*Duzhong*): the dried stem-bark of *Eucommia ulmoides* Oliv. (family Eucommiaceae).

[Taste and Properties] Sweet, pungent and slightly warm.

[Effects and Indications] (1) Tonifies the Kidneys and Liver, and strengthens the muscles and bones for treating backache and weakness of the legs; (2) Prevents miscarriage; (3) Reduces high blood pressure.

[Usage and Dosage] 6-9 g.

[Notes] (1) It lowers the blood pressure in experimental hypertension. (2) It has immune-enhancing, anti-inflammatory, sedative and analgesic effects. (3) It inhibits the stimulating action of pituitrin and acetylcholine on isolated uterus, and restores the contracted uterus to normal.

***Rhizoma Cibotii*, Cibot Rhizome**, 狗脊 (*Gouji*): the dried rhizome of *Cibotium barometz* (L.) J. Sm. (family Dicksoniaceae).

[Taste and Properties] Sweet, bitter and warm.

[Effects and Indications] (1) Tonifies the Kidneys and Liver, and strengthens the muscles and bones for relieving aching and weakness in the back and knees; (2) Dispels wind-damp for treating rheumatalgia, especially rhachialgia.

[Usage and Dosage] 6-12 g.

***Radix Dipsaci*, Teasel Root**, 续断 (*Xuduan*): the dried root of *Dipsacus asperoides* C.Y. Cheng et T. M. Ai (family Dipsacaceae).

[Taste and Properties] Bitter and slightly warm.

[Effects and Indications] (1) Tonifies the Kidneys and Liver, and strengthens the muscles and bones for treating aching in the back and knees, and traumatic injuries; (2) Facilitates the healing of bone fractures; (3) Stops uterine bleeding and prevents miscarriage.

[Usage and Dosage] 9-15 g.

***Rhizoma Drynariae*, Drynaria Rhizome**, 骨碎补 (*Gusuibu*): the dried rhizome of *Drynaria fortunei* (Kunze) J. Sm. or *Drynaria baranii* (Christ) Diels (family Polypodiaceae).

[Taste and Properties] Bitter and warm.

[Effects and Indications] Reinforces the Kidneys, strengthens the bones, promotes blood circulation and relieves pain for treating traumatic injuries, bony and lumbar pains, and tinnitus and chronic diarrhea due to Kidney insufficiency.

[Usage and Dosage] 3-9 g.

***Cordyceps*, Chinese Caterpillar Fungus**, 冬虫夏草 (*Dongchongxiacao*): a composite consisting of the dried stroma of the fungus, *Cordyceps sinensis* (Berk.) Sacc.

(family Hypercreaceae) growing on the larva of certain insects (family Hepialidae) and dead caterpillars.

[Taste and Properties] Sweet and warm.

[Effects and Indications] Reinforces the Kidneys and the Lungs for treating impotence and seminal emission due to insufficiency of the Kidneys, and chronic coughing and asthma due to insufficiency of the Lungs.

[Usage and Dosage] 3-9 g.

[Notes] (1) It enhances the immune functions, strengthening the phagocytosis of monocytes and macrophages, increasing the number of Fc receptors, and facilitating the production of interleukin-II. (2) It stimulates the function of the adrenocortex, and has androgen-like actions. (3) It markedly dilates the bronchi, and helps adrenalin and aminophylline to relieve bronchospasms.

***Gecko*, Tokay**, 蛤蚧 (*Gejie*): the dried body, with the viscera removed, of a lizard, *Gekko gecko* L. (family Geckonidae).

[Taste and Properties] Salty in taste and neutral in property.

[Effects and Indications] Reinforces the Kidneys and the Lungs for treating chronic asthma.

[Usage and Dosage] 3-6 g, used in making pills, powders or medicinal wines.

***Fructus Cnidii*, Cnidium Fruit**, 蛇床子 (*Shechuangzi*): the dried ripe fruit of *Cnidium monnieri* (L.) Cuss. (family Umbelliferae).

[Taste and Properties] Pungent, bitter and warm.

[Effects and Indications] (1) Reinforces Kidney *yang* for treating impotence and leukorrhagia; (2) Destroys parasites and relieves itching, used externally for eczema, itchy skin diseases, particularly for pruritus vulvae and trichomonal vaginitis.

[Usage and Dosage] 3-9 g; appropriate quantity to be made into hot decoction for fuming and washing, or ground into powder for topical application after mixing with liquid.

[Notes] (1) It has sex hormone-like actions, prolonging the copulative period of mice, increasing the weight of the uterus and ovaries in the female and that of the prostate and seminal vesicles in the male. (2) It inhibits the growth of various dermatophytes in vitro, and shows astringent action on cutaneous exudation. (3) It inhibits the activity of trichomonas in vitro.

According to modern research, the pharmacological actions of tonics in Chinese medicine chiefly involve the following aspects:

1. Effects on the immune functions. Most tonics enhance the non-specific immune function by increasing the peripheral white blood cell counts and the phagocytosis of the reticulo-endothelial system.

On specific immunity, many tonics reinforce the function of T cells. For example, milkvetch root and glossy privet fruit suppress the suppressor T lymphocytes and thus enhance the action of T helper lymphocytes. Ginseng, white peony root, Chinese angelica and thorny acanthopanax root promote the release of interleukin-II.

Qi tonics as well as many *yin* tonics and *yang* tonics enhance or regulate the humoral immunity, including the production of antibodies. Milkvetch root, epimedium and thorny acanthopanax root promote the production of interferon induced by viruses or directly induce the production of interferon.

2. Effects on the nervous system. Intelligence chiefly refers to the ability to learn and memories, in which the following factors are involved: (1) Proper concentration of neurotransmitters (e.g., acetylcholine, norepinephrine and dopamine) in the central nervous system; (2) Sufficient synthesis of nucleic acids and proteins in the brain; (3) Adequate supply of oxygen and heat energy to the brain; and (4) Appropriate excitation. Many tonics may have the capacity to improve the intelligence through different approaches. For example, ginseng, milkvetch root, tangshen, fleeceflower root and wolfberry regulate the cerebral contents of neurotransmitters; ginseng, milkvetch root and thorny acanthopanax root improve the protein anabolism; Chinese angelica increases the cerebral blood flow and improves the cerebral microcirculation; hairy deerhorn and ginseng cause moderate excitation of the central nervous system.

3. Effects on the metabolism. Many *qi* tonics, particularly ginseng and milkvetch root, promote the anabolism of nucleic acids and protein. Some *yin* tonics, such as wolfberry fruit and lilyturf root regulate the protein metabolism.

Many tonics act on carbohydrate metabolism. The effect is often bi-directional, namely, to reduce the blood sugar content in hyperglycemia and elevate the blood sugar content in hypoglycemia.

Some tonics such as ginseng, fleeceflower root, wolfberry and cordyceps have hypolipemic functions, and show beneficial effects on the prevention of atherosclerosis.

4. Effects on the endocrine system. Many tonics have beneficial effects on the endocrine system, particularly on the adrenal and sex glands.

Ginseng stimulates the hypothalamus or pituitary to secrete ACTH, increasing the synthesis and secretion of corticosteriods. Other *qi* tonics such as milkvetch root, *tangshen* and thorny acanthopanax also have such effects.

Many tonics, particularly *yang* tonics such as epimedium, cordyceps, dodder seed, morinda root and cistanche promote the secretion of sex hormones. Since they can be effectively used in both males and females, it is presumed that their effect is not directly on the sex glands, but on the regulatory centers of the sex glands.

5. Effects on the cardiovascular system. Ginseng, milkvetch root and lilyturf root are cardiotonics. Chinese angelica, lilyturf root, epimedium, scurfpea fruit and cordyceps dilate the coronary arteries, and increase the coronary blood flow. Ginseng and cordyceps have some effect against arrhythmia. Most tonics are not countraindicated in hypertension, and some can even be used as hypotensives, but they often have a bi-directional action, i.e., lowering the blood pressure in hypertension, and raising the blood pressure in hypotension.

6. Effects on the hematopoietic system. Blood tonics promote hemopoiesis, but many other tonics also have such an effect.

7. Effects on the digestive system. Most *qi* tonics act on the digestive system, improving digestion, relieving gastro-enterospasm or regulating the motility of the gastro-intestinal tract.

8. Anti-senility effects. Ginseng and milkvetch root prolong the life-span in animal experiments and cell culture. Many other tonics are presumed to have anti-senility effects because of their antiperoxidation by eliminating the free radicals.

The pharmacological actions of individual tonics, according to modern studies, are summarized in Table IX-11.

Table IX-11 Pharmacological Effects of Tonics

	Robo	Adapt.	Immunity		Blood			Pituit.	Sex	Prot.	Cardio
	rant		cell.	humor.	Rbc	Hb	Wbc	adren.	gl	Anab	tonic
Qi tonics											
Ginseng	+	↑	↑	↑	↑	↑	↑	↑	↑	↑	+
Thorny acantho-Panax root	+	↑	↑	↑			↑	↑	↑		
Milkvetch root		↑	↑	↑	↑	↑	↑			↑	+
Tangshen		↑	↑	↑	↑	↑		↑			
White atracty-Lodes root	+		↑	↑			↑	↑		↑	
Licorice root								↑			
Blood tonics											
Chinese angelica Root			↑		↑	↑					
Prepared rheman-Nia root		↑									
White peony root			↑			↑					+
Donkey-hide Gelatin		↑		↑	↑	↑					
Yin tonics											
Lilyturf root		↑					↑	↑			+
Wolfberry			↑	↑			↑				
Glossy privet Fruit	+		↑	↑			↑				+
Dogwood fruit				↑			↑				
Fleeceflower root			↑					↑			+
Yang tonics											
Hairy deer horn	+						↑		↑		
Epimedium			↑				↑		↑		
Scurfpea fruit			↑	↑			↑		↑		+

ASTRINGENT DRUGS

Drugs that arrest discharges are called astringents. In Chinese medicine, the term astringent has a broader sense, as it arrests sweating, diarrhea, seminal emission, urination, bleeding, leukorrhea and even chronic coughing. Usually, it is only used for relief of symptoms. Most astringent drugs are sour or puckery in taste.

***Fructus Tritici Levis*, Light wheat,** 浮小麦 (*Fuxiaomai*): dried light grains of *Triticum aestivum* L. (family Graminae).

[Taste and Properties] Sweet and cool.

[Effects and Indications] Arrests excessive perspiration in cases of spontaneous or night sweating.

[Usage and Dosage] 10-15 g in a compound decoction; 30-60 g if used alone

***Radix Ephedrae*, Ephedra Root,** 麻黄根 (*Mahuanggen*): the dried root and rhizome of *Ephedra sinica* Stapf. or *Ephedra intermedia* Schrenk et C. A. Mey (family Ephedraceae).

[Taste and Properties] Sweet in taste and neutral in property.

[Effects and Indications] Arrests excessive perspiration in cases of spontaneous or night sweating.

[Usage and Dosage] 3-9 g.

[Notes] It contains pseudoephedrine, which arrests sweating.

***Galla Chinensis*, Chinese Gall,** 五倍子 (*Wubeizi*): the gall produced mainly by parasitic aphids of *Melaphis chinensis* (Bell) Baker on the leaf of *Rhus chinensis* Mill., *Rhus potaninii* Maxim. or *Rhus punjabensis* Stew. var. *sinica* (Diels) Regd. et Wils. (family Anacardiaceae).

[Taste and Properties] Sour, salty and cold.

[Effects and Indications] (1) Used as an antihidrotic for excessive sweating; (2) As an antidiarrheal for chronic diarrhea; (3) As an antitussive for persistent cough; (4) Externally as a styptic in cases of bleeding.

[Usage and Dosage] 1.5-6 g; appropriate quantity for external use.

[Notes] (1) It contains a large amount of tannic acid, which causes protein coagulation of the skin, mucous membrane or surfaces of ulcers, and stimulates blood coagulation, producing the astringent effects. (2) In vitro, it has antibacterial, antiviral and antifungal functions.

***Fructus Chebulae*, Chebula Fruit,** 诃子 (*Hezi*): the dried ripe fruit of *Terminalia chebula* Retz. or *Terminalia chebula* var. *tomentella* Kurt. (family Combretaceae).

[Taste and Properties] Bitter, sour and puckery in taste, and neutral in property.

[Effects and Indications] (1) Astringes the Intestines for checking chronic diarrhea; (2) Astringes the Lungs for treating persistent coughing and hoarseness.

[Usage and Dosage] 3-9 g.

[Notes] It contains tannin, which is responsible for the astringent effects. It also contains chebulin, which has an antispasmodic effect like that of papaverine.

***Halloysitum Rubrum*, Red Halloysite,** 赤石脂 (Chishizhi): a mineral, hydrated aluminium silicate, in red color due to the presence of iron oxides.

[Taste and Properties] Sweet, sour, puckery and warm.

[Effects and Indications] (1) Arrests discharge in cases of chronic diarrhea and leukorrhagia; (2) Also used as a styptic in cases of menorrhagia.

[Usage and Dosage] 9-12 g.

[Notes] It absorbs toxic substances in the intestines and protects the intestinal mucosa, producing an antidiarrheal effect. It also shortens the blood coagulation time.

***Semen Nelumbinis*, Lotus Seed**, 莲子 (*Lianzi*): the dried ripe seed of *Nelumbo nucifera* Gaertn. (family Nymphaeaceae).

[Taste and Properties] Sweet and puckery in taste, and neutral in property.

[Effects and Indications] (1) Invigorates the Spleen and checks diarrhea for treating chronic diarrhea due to insufficiency of the Spleen; (2) Replenishes the Kidneys for arresting seminal emission.

[Usage and Dosage] 6-15 g.

***Semen Euryales*, Gordon Euryale Seed**, 芡实 (*Qianshi*): the dried kernel of ripe seed of *Euryale ferox* Salisb. (family Nymphaeaceae).

[Taste and Properties] Sweet and puckery in taste, and neutral in property.

[Effects and Indications] (1) Invigorates the Spleen and checks diarrhea for treating chronic diarrhea due to insufficiency of the Spleen; (2) Tonifies the Kidneys for arresting seminal emission, as well as urorrhea and leukorrhagia.

[Usage and Dosage] 9-15 g.

***Fructus Mume*, Smoked Plum**, 乌梅 (*Wumei*): the dried nearly ripe fruit of *Prunus Mume* (Sieg.) Sieb. et Zucc. (family Rosaceae).

[Taste and Properties] Sour and puckery in taste and neutral in property.

[Effects and Indications] (1) Astringes the Lungs and replenishes the Kidneys, used for treating persistent coughing and asthma due to insufficiency of both the Lungs and the Kidneys; (2) Arrests discharge in cases of seminal emission and chronic diarrhea; (3) Promotes the production of body fluids and arrests perspiration in cases of thirst and night sweating due to deficiency of Liver and Kidney *yin*; (4) Nourishes the Heart for treating palpitations and insomnia.

[Usage and Dosage] 6-12 g.

***Semen Myristicae*, Nutmeg**, 肉豆蔻 (*Roudoukou*): the dried kernel of *Myristica fragrans* Houtt. (family Myristicaceae).

[Taste and Properties] Pungent and warm.

[Effects and Indications] Warms the Spleen and the Stomach, and checks diarrhea as an astringent, used in cases of chronic diarrhea, epigastric pain, abdominal distension and anorexia due to deficiency-cold of the Spleen and the Stomach.

[Usage and Dosage] 3-9 g.

***Fructus Schisandrae*, Magnoliavine Fruit**, 五味子 (*Wuweizi*): the ripe fruit of *Schisandra chinensis* (Turcz.) Baill. or *Schisandra sphenanthera* Rehd. et Wils. (family Magnoliaceae).

[Taste and Properties] Sour in taste and warm in property.

[Effects and Indications] (1) Astringes the Lungs and nourishes the Kidneys for relieving dry coughing, dyspnea and night sweating; (2) Arrests discharge in cases of seminal emission and chronic diarrhea daily before dawn; (3) Calms the Heart in cases of palpitations and insomnia.

[Usage and Dosage] 1.5-6 g.

[Notes] (1) It has a regulatory effect on the cerebral cortex. It causes excitation of various parts of the central nervous system, improving the latter's efficiency (particularly intellectual activities and endurance), but it also has a tranquilizing effect as shown by the prolongation of sleeping time induced by barbital. (2) It exhibits a cardiotonic effect in experimental studies, causing stronger contraction and more complete relaxation. (3) It retards senility in old rats, probably by inhibiting the activity of monoamine oxidase (MAO) and enhancing the activity of superoxide dismutase (SOD) in the brain and the liver. (4) It contains schizandrin, which potently protects the liver against chemical poisons, inhibiting the release of transaminase. The mechanisms of the liver-protective effect include accelerated renovation and regeneration of the liver cells, reduction in the permeability of the liver cell membrane, and inhibition on oxidation. (5) In animal experiments, the decoction stimulates respiration. The acid content decreases the mucopolysaccharides in the tracheal glands, thus reducing phlegm secretion and coughing.

***Fructus Rosae Laevigatae*, Cherokee Rose Fruit**, 金樱子 (*Jinyingzi*): the dried ripe fruit of *Rosa laevigata* Mickx. (family Rosaceae).

[Taste and Properties] Sour and puckery in taste and neutral in property.

[Effects and Indications] Arrests discharge in cases of seminal emission, leukorrhagia, urorrhea, frequent micturition, and chronic diarrhea.

[Usage and Dosage] 6-12 g.

[Notes] It contains tannins, which possess astringent effects.

***Fructus Rubi*, Raspberry**, 覆盆子 (*Fupenzi*): the steamed and dried fruit of *Rubus chingii* Hu (family Rosaceae).

[Taste and Properties] Sweet, sour and slightly warm.

[Effects and Indications] Arrests discharge in cases of frequent micturition, urorrhea and seminal emission.

[Usage and Dosage] 6-12 g.

DIGESTANT DRUGS

Digestant drugs assist digestion and promote appetite. They are used for treating dyspepsia manifested by epigastric distension, anorexia, belching with fetid odor, acid regurgitation, nausea and vomiting. Dyspepsia may be due to over-eating or to diminished function of the Spleen and the Stomach. In the former case, it is appropriate to use digestants alone. But in the latter case, digestants should be used in combination with tonics to invigorate the functions of the Spleen and the Stomach.

***Fructus Crataegi*, Hawthorn Fruit**, 山楂 (*Shanzha*): the dried ripe fruit of *Crataegus pinnatifida* Bge. var. *major* N. E. Br. or *Crataegus pinnatifida* Bge. (family Rosaceae).

[Taste and Properties] Sour, sweet and slightly warm.

[Effects and Indications] (1) Charred hawthorn fruit improves digestion and eliminates stagnated meat; (2) Unprocessed hawthorn fruit removes stagnated blood for treating amenorrhea and postpartum pain due to blood stasis.

[Usage and Dosage] 9-12 g.

[Notes] (1) Hawthorn fruit contains cratagic acid, ascorbic acid (vitamin C) and lipase. Lipase helps the digestion of fat, and cratagic acid increases the activity of pepsin for the digestion of protein. (2) Hawthorn fruit, particularly its hydrolyzate, increases the coronary blood flow, reduces the myocardial oxygen consumption, strengthens the cardiac actions and lowers blood pressure. (3) The extract shows blood cholesterol-lowering effect and prevents atherosclerosis in experimental hyperlipemia. (4) The decoction inhibits various species of *Bacillus dysenteriae* in vitro. (5) Hawthorn fruit stimulates the uterus, facilitating its involution and the discharge of intrauterine blood clots.

***Fructus Hordei Germinatus*, Germinated Barley**, 麦芽 (*Maiya*): the dried germinated ripe fruit of *Hordeum vulgare* L. (family Gramineae).

[Taste and Properties] Sweet in taste and neutral in property.

[Effects and Indications] (1) Assists digestion, used for treating indigestion, particularly indigestion caused by food containing starch and infantile dyspepsia; (2) Checks the secretion of milk for weaning.

[Usage and Dosage] 9-15 g; for checking the secretion of milk, 60 g.

[Notes] (1) It contains amylase and vitamin B group, which promote digestion. The decoction also stimulates gastric acid secretion. (2) It contains ergotoxin, which inhibits the secretion of prolactin.

***Massa Fermentata Medicinalis*, Medicated Leaven**, 神曲 (*Shenqu*): the dried mass of a fermented mixture of wheat flour, fresh aerial parts of *Artemisia annua*, *Xanthium sibiricum*, and *Polygonum hydropiper*.

[Taste and Properties] Sweet, pungent and warm.

[Effects and Indications] Improves digestion for treating dyspepsia and food stagnation with abdominal distension.

[Usage and Dosage] 6-12 g.

[Notes] It contains amylase and protease to promote digestion and lactobacillus to inhibit excessive fermentation in the intestines for relieving abdominal distension. The decoction also stimulates the secretion of digestive juices.

Charred triplet, 焦三仙 (*Jiaosanxian*): a mixture consisting of equal parts of Charred Medicated Leaven, Charred Hawthorn Fruit and Charred Germinated Barley.

[Effects and Indications] Improves digestion, with a comprehensive effect on various kinds of food.

[Usage and Dosage] 15-30 g.

***Endothelium Corneum Gigeriae Galli*, Chicken's Gizzard-skin**, 鸡内金 (*Jineijin*): the dried lining membrane of the gizzard of common fowl.

[Taste and Properties] Sweet in taste and neutral in property.

[Effects and Indications] (1) Invigorates the Spleen and promotes digestion for treating dyspepsia with anorexia, particularly in children; (2) Used as an astringent for seminal emission in adults and enuresis in children; (3) Also used for eliminating urinary and biliary stones.

[Usage and Dosage] 3-9 g.

[Notes] When given orally, it promotes the secretion and motility of the stomach. One of its active principles is ventriculin.

***Semen Raphani*, Radish Seed**, 莱菔子 (*Laifuzi*): the dried ripe seed of *Raphanus sativus* L. (family Cruciferae).

[Taste and Properties] Pungent and sweet in taste, and neutral in property.

[Effects and Indications] (1) Improves digestion and expels gas downward for relieving abdominal distension; (2) Eases expectoration in cases of chronic bronchitis.

[Usage and Dosage] 4.5-9 g.

[Notes] (1) It promotes the rhythmic contractions of the ileum, relieving abdominal distension caused by diminished intestinal motility. (2) It shows antitussive and expectorant effects in the laboratory.

According to modern pharmacological studies, the mechanisms of digestant actions of the above-mentioned drugs include: (1) Assisting digestion with enzymes (e.g., hawthorn fruit contains lipase and organic acids that promote the activity of pepsin, germinated barley contains amylase, medicated leaven containes amylase and protease); (2) Activating digestion by its content of vitamin B group; (3) Stimulating secretion of digestive juices; and (4) Accelerating the gastro-intestinal peristalsis and evacuation.

The pharmacological effects on the gastro-intestinal tract of individual digestant drugs are shown in Table IX-12.

Table IX-12 Pharmacological Effects of Digestant Drugs

	Digestive enzymes	Vitamin B group	G-I tract motility	Digestive secretion
Hawthorn fruit	+	+		+
Germinated barley	+	+		+
Medicated leaven	+	+		+
Chicken's gizzard-skin	+		+	+
Radish seed			+	

PURGATIVE DRUGS

Purgative drugs cause evacuation from the bowels. They are divided chiefly according to the severity of their action, into several classes: laxative, drastic and hydragogue.

Laxatives are aperient drugs, most of which are seeds containing oils with lubricant action to facilitate evacuation from the bowels. They are particularly useful for constipation due to blood or fluid deficiency, as occurring in the aged and in women after childbirth.

Drastic purgatives, bitter in taste and cold in property, are used for purging retention of undigested food and excessive heat in the intestines (interior excess syndromes). They are contraindicated in aged and debilitated persons, and women in pregnancy or during menstruation.

Hydragogues are cathartics which cause watery purgation. They are chiefly used for treating severe edema, ascites or hydrothorax. As they are apt to consume body fluids, they should be used with caution, and are contraindicated in debility or pregnancy.

***Semen Pruni*, Bush-cherry seed,** 郁李仁 (*Yuliren*): the dried ripe seed of *Prunus* *humilis* Bge. *Prunus japonica* Thunb. or *Prunus pedunculata* Maxim. (family Rosaceae).

[Taste and Properties] Pungent, bitter and sweet in taste, and neutral in property.

[Effects and Indications] Used as a laxative and diuretic for constipation and edema.

[Usage and Dosage] 3-9 g.

[Notes] It is an emollient laxative containing fatty oils (58-74%).

Fructus Cannabis, **Hemp Seed**, 火麻仁 (*Huomaren*): the dried ripe fruit of *Cannabis sativa* L. (family Moraceae).

[Taste and Properties] Sweet in taste and neutral in property.

[Effects and Indications] Used as a laxative for constipation in the debilitated or the aged (due to deficiency of blood and intestinal fluid).

[Usage and Dosage] 9-15 g.

[Notes] It contains fatty oils (30%) which soften the stools and lubricate the intestines.

Radix et Rhizoma Rhei, **Rhubarb**, 大黄 (*Dahuang*): the dried root and rhizome of *Rheum palmatum* L., *Rheum tanguticum* Maxim. ex Balf. or *Rheum officinale* Baill. (family Polygonaceae).

[Taste and Properties] Bitter and cold.

[Effects and Indications] Unprepared rhubarb causes catharsis, purges heat, eliminates stagnated blood and stimulates menstrual discharge; used for treating fever with constipation and abdominal pain, jaundice caused by damp-heat, amenorrhea due to blood stasis and hemorrhage from the upper gastro-intestinal tract.

Rhubarb stir-fried in wine removes toxic heat from the blood in the upper portion of the body, used for treating inflammation of the eye and painful swelling of the throat and gums.

Prepared rhubarb purges heat and removes toxic substances; used for treating boils, sores and abscesses.

Carbonized rhubarb removes stagnated blood and arrests bleeding; used for treating hemorrhage with blood stasis.

[Usage and Dosage] 3-12 g, not to be decocted for a long time if it is used for purgation.

[Warning] Use with caution in pregnancy.

[Notes] (1) Rhubarb is a stimulant purgative. It contains anthraquinone. When rhubarb is given orally, most of anthraquinone is not absorbed by the small intestine, and reaches the colon, where it is hydrolyzed and reduced into emodin anthrone. Emodin anthrone stimulates the intestinal peristalsis and increases the intra-intestinal osmotic pressure, thus resulting in purgation. Among the preparations of rhubarb, unprepared rhubarb has the most potent purgative effect, while processing or long-time decocting makes the effect weaker due to hydrolysis of anthraquinone. (2) Rhubarb is a cholagogue by stimulating the secretion of bilirubin and bile acid, and inducing contraction of the gallbladder and relaxation of Odds's sphincter. Rhubarb also protects the liver against chemical damage. In vitro, rhubarb markedly inhibits hepatitis B surface antigen (HBsAg), and in vivo, it activates the production of interferon. (3) Rhubarb accelerates the secretion and discharge of pancreatic juice and markedly inhibits the activity of trypsin, chymotrypsin, pancreatic amylase, and pancreatic lipase. This can explain why rhubarb can be effectively used in the treatment of acute pancreatitis. (4) Rhubarb counteracts gastric and duodenal ulcers in experimental studies. (5) Rhubarb possesses a definite hemostatic effect. The active principles are α-catechin and gallic acid, which promote adhesion and aggregation of blood platelets, shorten the coagulation time and reduce the activity of antithrombin III. In addition, rhubarb causes constriction of injured local blood vessels, reduces vascular permeability and shortens bleeding time. On the other hand, rhubarb is also used to activate blood circulation and remove stagnated blood in traditional Chinese medicine. Modern research has revealed that rhubarb, when taken orally, reduces blood viscosity and hematocrit and increases plasma osmotic pressure, thus inducing transfer of interstitial fluid into blood, expanding the blood volume and improving microcirculation. (6) Rhubarb markedly lowers the level of blood lipids (including total cholesterol, triglyceride, low-density lipoprotein and lipid peroxide) in experimental hyperlipemia. (7) Rhubarb improves the renal function in cases of chronic renal failure, mitigating hyperazotemia. (8) Rhubarb shows a broad spectrum of bacteriostatic actions in vitro. It also inhibits influenza, ECHO, herpes simplex, hepatitis B and poliomyelitis viruses, as well as ameba, *Trichomonas vaginalis* and *Leptospira*. The active principles are mainly rhein, emodin and aloe-emodin. The bacteriostatic effect is due to restraint on the enzyme system of folic acid and then the biosynthesis of nucleic acids and proteins of the bacteria. (9) Rhubarb shows marked anti-inflammatory and antipyretic effects in experimental studies. The antipyretic effect is due to the reduction of the central pyrogenic neuro-transmitters, and the anti-inflammatory effect is related chiefly to the inhibition of epoxidase activity and reduction of prostaglandin synthesis.

Folium Sennae, **Senna**, 番泻叶 (*Fanxieye*): the dried leaflets of *Cassia angustifolia* Vahl or *Cassia acutifolia* Delile (family Leguminosae).

[Taste and Properties] Sweet, bitter and cold.

[Effects and Indications] (1) Purges away heat and relaxes the bowels for treating constipation due to accumulation of heat; (2) induces diuresis for ascites and edema.

[Usage and Dosage] 3-9 g, often use alone and made into water infusion.

[Warning] Use with caution in pregnancy.

[Notes] (1) Senna has a definite purgative effect, with defecation occurring 4-8 hours after it is taken orally. The active principle is sennoside. (2) Senna has a broad-spectrum bacteriostatic effect in vitro, including the inhibition of *Bacillus coli* and *Shigella dysenteriae*. (3) When given orally, senna has a hemostatic effect, increasing the blood platelets and fibrinogen, and shortening the coagulation time and clot retraction time. Under gastroscopy, the aqueous infusion sprayed on the hemorrhagic lesions of the gastric mucosa can immediately stop bleeding.

Natrii Sulfas, **Sodium Sulfate**, 芒硝 (*Mangxiao*): a crystallin substance containing hydrated sodium sulfate ($Na_2SO_4 \cdot 10H_2O$).

[Taste and Properties] Salty, bitter and cold.

[Effects and Indications] (1) Softens dry feces, relaxes the bowels and purges heat; used for treating constipation with abdominal pain caused by excessive heat; (2) Reduces inflammatory swelling and is used externally for treating mastitis.

[Usage and Dosage] 6-18 g; appropriate quantity for external use.

[Warning] Contraindicated in pregnancy.

[Notes] It is a nonabsorbable saline cathartic which holds water in the intestines in amounts sufficient to maintain an isotonic concentration, and soft or liquid bowel movements will follow. It also has a cholagogue effect by stimulating the ampulla to reflexively induce contraction of the gallbladder and relaxation of Oddi's sphincter.

***Radix Euphorbiae Kansui*, Kansui Root**, 甘遂 (*Gansui*): the dried tuberous root of *Euphorbia kansui* T. N. Liou ex T. P. Wang (family Euporbiaceae).

[Taste and Properties] Bitter, cold, and toxic.

[Effects and Indications] Causes drastic purgation and expels retained water; used for treating anasarca, hydrothorax and ascites.

[Usage and Dosage] 0.6-1.5 g, mostly used for making pills or powder.

[Warning] Contraindicated in pregnancy. Incompatible with licorice root.

[Notes] It causes intense stimulation on the intestinal mucosa, resulting in hyperactivity of intestinal peristalsis and severe diarrhea.

***Flos Genkwa*, Genkwa Flower**, 芫花 (*Yuanhua*): the dried flower-bud of *Daphne genkwa* Sieb. et Zucc. (family Thymelaeaceae).

[Taste and Properties] Pungent, warm and toxic.

[Effects and Indications] Causes drastic purgation and expels retained water; used for treating anasarca, hydrothorax and ascites.

[Usage and Dosage] 0.6-1.5 g, mostly used for making pills or powder.

[Warning] Contraindicated in pregnancy. Incompatible with licorice root.

[Notes] It stimulates the intestinal mucosa, causing severe diarrhea. It also shows a diuretic effect in the laboratory.

***Radix Euphorbiae Pekinensis*, Peking Euphorbia Root**, 京大戟 (*Jingdaji*): the dried root of *Euphorbia pekinensis* Rupr. (family Euphorbiaceae).

[Taste and Properties] Bitter, cold and toxic.

[Effects and Indications] Causes drastic purgation and expels retained water; used for treating anasarca, hydrothorax and ascites.

[Usage and Dosage] 0.6-1.5 g, mostly used for making pills or powder.

[Warning] Contraindicated in pregnancy. Incompatible with licorice root.

[Notes] It induces severe purgation in animal experiments.

CHAPTER 10

HERBAL FORMULAS

In Chinese medicinal drugs are usually prescribed in formulas with medicinal substances serving as the ingredients. Most formulas are composed of more than one ingredient. How to properly combine the ingredients to make the formula effective is a part of the fundamental knowledge of traditional Chinese medicine. Through thousands of years of practice, a large number of herbal formulas have been initiated and tested. The number of herbal formulas considered to be clinically effective and recorded in the Chinese medical literature is much greater than that of medicinal substances. For example, in Li Shizhen's *Ben Cao Gang Mu* (*Compendium of Materia Medica*), 1,892 medicinal substances are listed, while more than 10,000 formulas are described. Selection of the proper formula for a given patient is of the utmost importance for successful treatment. The following are the key points for the selection.

I. Correct diagnosis of the syndrome pattern

In Chinese medicine, most formulas are used for treating syndrome patterns instead of the disease entities. Even in patients with the same disease, if they have different syndromes, they should receive different prescriptions. Take chronic atrophic gastritis as an example. Patients with similar endoscopic findings may have different syndrome patterns. Some patients complain of dull epigastric pain, abdominal distension, anorexia and general weakness, accompanied by pale and plump tongue with white coating and soft pulse. They are suffering from a syndrome of weakness (*qi*-deficiency) of the Spleen and the Stomach, and can be treated with *Xiang Sha Liujunzi Wan* (Pill of Six Noble Ingredients with Costus and Amomum) to invigorate the Spleen and pacify the Stomach. But some other patients complain of burning pain in the epigastrium, dryness of the mouth and constipation, accompanied by a reddened tongue with scanty coating and rapid thready pulse. In this case, the syndrome diagnosis is deficiency of Stomach *yin*, and the formula recommended is *Yiwei Tang* (Stomach-Replenishing Decoction). The two formulas are composed as follows:

Xiang Sha Liujunzi Wan (Pill of Six Noble Ingredients with Costus and Amomum): *Radix Ginseng* (ginseng), *Rhizoma Atractylodis Macrocephalae* (white atractylodes root), *Poria* (fuling or poria), *Radix Glycyrrhizae Preparata* (prepared licorice root), *Rhizoma Pinelliae* (pinellia rhizome), *Pericarpium Citri Reticulatae* (tangerine peel), *Radix Aucklandiae* (costus root), and *Fructus Amomi* (amomum fruit).

Yiwei Tang (Stomach-Replenishing Decoction): *Radix Glehniae* (glehnia root), *Radix Ophiopogonis* (lilyturf root), *Radix Rehmanniae* (rehmannia root), *Rhizoma Polygonati Odorati* (fragrant solomonseal rhizome), *Radix Bupleuri* (thorowax root), and *Cortex Lycii* (wolfberry bark).

A comparison between the two formulas will show big differences. They are composed of entirely different ingredients, none of which overlaps. The formula used for treating chronic atrophic gastritis with a syndrome of *qi*-deficiency of the Spleen and the Stomach is not at all suitable for the same disease with a syndrome of deficiency of Stomach *yin*. In the Pill of Six Noble Ingredients, *qi* tonics such as ginseng and atractylodes rhizome are the main ingredients. Deficiency of Stomach *yin* should be treated with *yin* tonics, and so glehnia root and lilyturf root are used. If ginseng is used to treat deficiency of Stomach *yin*, it gives no help but aggravates the symptoms, because its warming action will further impair Stomach *yin*. Similarly, if the *yin* tonics glehnia and lilyturf are given to patients with weakened Spleen and Stomach, they may also cause adverse effects, because deficiency of Spleen *qi* often leads to accumulation of damp, and *yin* tonics replenishing fluids will accelerate the formation of damp. Not only a disease entity (in the Western sense), but even a symptom should also be treated following the syndrome diagnosis. Rhubarb is a well-known purgative, but it is not always suitable for constipation. First of all, constipation should be classified into excess and deficiency types, and then into cold and heat types. Only for constipation due to excessive heat is rhubarb indicated. If constipation is due to deficiency of *qi* or blood as occurring in the aged or in women after delivery, rhubarb is contraindicated, and the formulas used are entirely different. Milkvetch root should be the principal ingredient for constipation due to deficiency of *qi*, and Chinese angelica root for constipation due to deficiency of blood. Some lubricant laxatives can be added to the prescription.

The above examples illustrate the importance of syndrome differentiation in the selection of formulas.

II. Reasonable combination of the ingredients

1. Composition of a compound formula

Although some of the medicinal substances are used singly (e.g., ginseng, pilose antler), most of them are prescribed in combination. Administration of a compound prescription usually has the advantages of exerting a better therapeutic effect and causing fewer side effects than taking a single substance.

As a rule, a compound formula is composed of the following four kinds of ingredients: the principal, adjuvant, auxiliary and conductant (or moderator).

The principal ingredient provides the principal curative action for the major problem.

The adjuvant may have two kinds of actions: one is to help strengthen the principal curative effect, and the other is to exert the principal curative effect on a combined or complicated condition.

The auxiliary ingredients have three different kinds of effects: (1) Relief of secondary symptoms; (2) Tempering of drastic action of the principal ingredient; (3) Acting as a corrigent (e.g., use of an ingredient with an opposite nature in order to favorably modify the action of a principal ingredient which might be too powerful or harsh, namely, adding a small amount of cool-natured ingredient to a prescription of a very hot nature, or adding a small amount of a warm-natured ingredient to a prescription of very cold nature).

The conductant or moderator directs the drug's effect to the affected meridian or moderates the drug's effect.

Take *Ma Huang Tang* (Decoction of Ephedra) as an example. This formula may be used for the treatment of exterior cold syndrome marked by chills and fever with no sweating, accompanied by headache, general aching, stuffed-up nose, coughing or asthma, thin white tongue coating and floating tense pulse. The formula is composed of four ingredients: *Herba Ephedrae* (ephedra), *Ramulus Cinnamomi* (cinnamon twig), *Semen Armeniacae Amarum* (bitter apricot seed) and *Radix Glycyrrhizae* (licorice root), among which ephedra is the principal ingredient which causes diaphoresis to relieve exterior-cold syndrome and also has the effect of relieving coughing and asthma. Cinnamon twig plays an adjuvant role. It dilates peripheral blood vessels, assisting ephedra in diaphoresis. Apricot seed is an auxiliary for relieving coughing and asthma; and licorice serves as a moderator of all other ingredients.

In any formula there must be a principal ingredient, but the adjuvant, auxiliary and conductant (or moderating) ingredients may not be all available. For example, *Zuo Jin Wan* (Pill of Goldthread and Evodia) which is indicated in treating attacks on the Stomach by Liver fire, only contains two ingredients, i.e., goldthread root and evodia fruit. In this formula, goldthread root is the principal ingredient which clears the Stomach of fire, and evodia fruit, the auxiliary which eases the Liver and relieves regurgitation or vomiting.

Some complicated formulas are composed of multiple ingredients, each of which has its own particular effects. In such instances, it may be difficult to divide the ingredients into the above four categories. A more practical way is to divide them into the major and minor ones.

2. Basic combinations

Medicinal substances are generally used in combination for the purpose of strengthening the curative effects and minimizing the side effects. The following pairs are some basic combinations. Though simple, they usually serve as the fundamental elements for the composition of complicated formulas.

(1) To strengthen the curative effect by combining two ingredients of the same kind:

Radix Codonopsis (tangshen) + *Radix Astragali* (milkvetch root): to replenish *qi*;

Radix Glehniae (glehnia root) + *Radix Ophiopogonis* (lilyturf root): to replenish *yin* and promote fluid secretion;

Semen Biotae (arborvitae seed) + *Semen Ziziphi Spinosae* (spiny date seed): to nourish the Heart for tranquilization;

Radix Aconiti Lateralis Preparata (prepared aconite lateral root) + *Cortex Cinnamomi* (cinnamon bark): to warm up the Kidney (reinforce *yang*);

Rhizoma Cimicifugae (bugbane rhizome) + *Radix Bupleuri* (thorowax root): to elevate the middle *qi*;

Radix Angelicae Sinensis (Chinese angelica root) + *Rhizoma Chuanxiong*: to nourish blood, promote blood circulation and eliminate stasis;

Semen Persicae (peach seed) + *Flos Carthami* (safflower): to promote blood circulation and eliminate stasis;

Pollen Typhae (cat-tail pollen) + *Faeces Trogopterorum* (trogopterus dung), forming a formula called *Shi Xiao San* (Wonderful Powder for Relieving Pain of Blood

Stasis): to eliminate blood stasis and relieve pain;

Resina Olibani (frankincense) + *Resina Myrrhae* (myrrh): to regulate the flow of *qi*, dissipate stagnated blood and relieve pain;

Rhizoma Sparganii (burreed tuber) + *Rhizoma Curcumae Zedoariae* (zedoary): to eliminate blood stasis and dissipate masses;

Fructus Cannabis (hemp seed) + *Fructus Trichosanthis* (snakegourd fruit): to cause laxation;

Herba Pogostemonis (cablin patchouli herb) + *Herba Eupatorii* (eupatorium): to clear up summer-damp;

Folium Mori (mulberry leaf) + *Flos Chrysanthemi* (chrysanthemum flower): to dispel wind-heat;

Rhizoma Notopterygii (notopterygium rhizome) + *Radix Angelicae Pubescentis* (pubescent angelica root): to dispel wind-damp;

Flos Lonicerae (honeysuckle flower) + *Fructus Forsythiae* (forsythia fruit): to eliminate toxic-heat;

Herba Taraxaci (dandelion) + *Herba Violae* (violet): to eliminate toxic-heat;

Radix Scutellariae (skullcap root) + *Rhizoma Coptidis* (goldthread rhizome): to purge fire and eliminate toxins;

Cortex Phellodendri (phellodendron bark) + *Rhizoma Arnemarrhenae* (anemarrhena rhizome): to eliminate damp-heat and clear up fire due to *yin* deficiency;

Thallus Laminariae (sea tangle) + *Sargassum* (seaweed): to soften hard masses and resolve phlegmy nodules.

All the above examples are combined uses of two ingredients similar in effect. They are very frequently used in making compound formulas, based on empirical experience. Whether such pairs of ingredients have merely an additive action or have a synergetic action is worth further investigation.

(2) To improve the curative effect by combining two ingredients of different kinds:

Radix Astragali (milkvetch root) + *Radix Angelicae Sinensis* (Chinese angelica root), forming a formula called *Danggui Buxue Tang* (Blood Tonic Decoction with Chinese Angelica): to replenish *qi* for generation of blood;

Radix Aucklandiae (costus root) + *Fructus Amomi* (spiny amomum fruit): to regulate the flow of *qi* and remove dampness from the Spleen and the Stomach;

Rhizoma Atractylodis (atractylodes rhizome) + *Cortex Magnoliae Officinalis* (officinal magnolia bark): to clear up dampness and relieve fullness;

Rhizoma Pinelliae (pinellia tuber) + *Pericarpium Citri Reticulatae* (tangerine peel): to resolve phlegm and regulate the flow of *qi*;

Semen Armeniacae Amarum (bitter apricot seed) + *Bulbus Fritillariae* (fritillary bulb): to relieve coughing and resolve phlegm (ease expectoration);

Rhizoma Coptidis (goldthread rhizome) + *Radix Aucklandiae* (costus root), forming a formula called *Xiang Lian Wan* (Pill of Goldthread and Costus): to treat dysentery;

Rhizoma Atractylodis (atractylodes rhizome) + *Cortex Phellodendri* (phellodendron bark), forming a formula called *Ermiao San* (Powder of Two Wonderful Ingredients): to eliminate damp-heat from the Lower Energizer;

Flos Inulae (inula flower) + *Hematitum* (hematite): to send the Stomach *qi* downward to arrest vomiting;

Fructus Aurantii Immaturus (immature bitter orange) + *Caulis Bambusae in Taeniam* (bamboo shavings): to clear the Stomach of heat to arrest vomiting;

Rhizoma Cyperi (cyperus tuber) + *Rhizoma Galagae* (galangal rhizome), forming a formula called *Liang Fu Wan* (Pill of Galangal and Cyperus): to warm up the Stomach for the relief of pain;

Radix Ginseng (ginseng) + *Radix Aconiti Lateralis* (aconite lateral root), forming a formula called *Shen Fu Tang* (Decoction of Ginseng and Aconite): to cause resuscitation from collapse or shock.

(3) To achieve a new curative effect by combining two ingredients with opposite actions (cold vs. heat, tonification vs. elimination, floating action vs. sinking action, etc.):

Ramulus Cinnamomi (cinnamon twig) + *Radix Paeoniae Alba* (white peony root): to harmonize the *Ying* (nutritive or constructive) and *Wei* (defensive) systems;

Fructus Toosendan (Szechwan chinaberry) + *Rhizoma Corydalis* (corydalis tuber): to regulate *qi* flow, promote blood circulation and relieve pain;

Fructus Trichosanthis (snakegourd fruit) + *Bulbus Allii Macrostemonis* (longstamen onion): to free the flow of *yang-qi* in the chest for relieving pectoral pain;

Rhizoma Atractylodis Macrocephalae (white atractylodes rhizome) + *Fructus Aurantii Immaturus* (immature bitter orange): to invigorate the Spleen and relieve abdominal distension;

Rhizoma Coptidis (goldthread rhizome) + *Fructus Evodiae* (evodia fruit), forming a formula called *Zuojin Wan* (Pill of Goldthread and Evodia): to purge Liver fire for inhibiting acid regurgitation;

Rhizoma Coptidis (goldthread rhizome) + *Cortex Cinnamomi* (cinnamon bark), forming a formula called *Jiao Tai Wan* (Pill of Goldthread and Cinnamon): to restore normal coordination between the Heart and the Kidneys;

Radix Astragali (milkvetch root) + *Radix Saposhnikoviae* (saposhnikovia root): to consolidate the superficies for arresting excessive sweating;

Radix Astragali (milkvetch root) + *Radix Stephaniae Tetrandrae* (*fourstamen stephania* root): to replenish *qi* and relieve edema.

3. Appropriate modification of the formula

Because of the complexity of human beings and their diseases, herbal formulas though numerous in number may still be inadequate to meet all the variations in patients' constitutions and morbid conditions. Decoction is often the first choice in Chinese medicine, for the ingredients can be changed in accordance with the patient's conditions, and formulas are only taken as general guidelines for making prescriptions. The disadvantage of decoction is its inconvenience, and so more and more ready-to-use preparations have come into being. Even with these preparations (pills, tablets, granules, etc.) modification of the composition is still possible in some instances. For example, in the treatment of influenza with an exterior heat syndrome, *Yin Qiao San* (Powder of Honeysuckle and Forsythia) is almost routinely used. But in recent years it has been found that *Radix Isatidis* (woad root) has an anti-viral effect, and so in the prescription this ingredient is often added. With ready-to-use preparations this may also be achieved by using *Banlangen Chongji* (Isatis-Root Granules) in combination with *Yin Qiao Jiedu Wan*[1] (Detoxicant Pill of Honeysuckle and Forsythia).

Among ready-to-use preparations, a basic formula may have some derivatives, so that the therapeutic action is somewhat modified to match the patient's condition. For example, *Lizhong Wan* (Pill for Regulating the Middle Energizer) is effective for treating deficiency of Spleen and the Stomach *yang* marked by epigastric pain with cold feeling, dyspepsia and chronic diarrhea. If the cold manifestations are remarkable, it is better to add some more ingredients to warm the Spleen and the Stomach. In this case, *Fuzi Lizhong Wan* (Aconite Pill for Regulating the Middle Energizer) can be selected, for aconite lateral root, a potent warming ingredient, is added to the basic formula, *Lizhong Wan.*

FORMULAS FOR RELIEVING EXTERIOR SYNDROMES

Pungent-Warm Formulas for Relieving Exterior Syndromes

***Mahuang Tang* (Decoction of Ephedra)**: *Herba Ephedrae* (ephedra) 9 g, *Ramulus Cinnamomi* (cinnamon twig) 6 g, *Semen Armeniacae Amarum* (bitter apricot seed) 9 g, and *Radix Glycyrrhizae* (licorice root) 3 g, to be made into a decoction.

[Effects] Induces diaphoresis, dispels cold, and relieves coughing and asthma.

[Indications] Wind-cold affection with exterior excess syndrome marked by chills and fever but no sweating, accompanied by headache, general aching, coughing or asthma, thin white tongue coating, and floating and tense pulse.

[Analysis] The principal ingredient is ephedra, which is diaphoretic and at the same time antiasthmatic. Cinnamon twig serving as an adjuvant, markedly enhances the diaphoretic action of ephedra by increasing peripheral blood flow. In addition, cinnamon twig also warms up the meridians, thus relieving headaches and general aching due to attack on the meridians by cold. Bitter apricot seed is an auxiliary to relieve coughing and asthma. Licorice root moderates the actions of other ingredients.

[Clinical Applications] Common cold, influenza, chronic bronchitis and bronchial asthma with an exterior excess syndrome.

***Guizhi Tang* (Decoction of Cinnamon Twig)**: *Ramulus Cinnamomi* (cinnamon twig) 9 g, *Radix Paeoniae Alba* (white peony root) 9 g, *Radix Glycyrrhizae* (licorice root) 6 g, *Rhizoma Zingiberis Recens* (fresh ginger) 9 g, and *Fructus Ziziphi Jujubae* (Chinese date) 4pc; to be made into a decoction.

[Effects] Induces diaphoresis by harmonizing the *ying* (constructive) and *wei* (superficial defensive) systems.

[Indications] Wind-cold affection with exterior deficiency syndrome marked by chilliness, fever and headaches with sweating, aversion to wind, joint and muscle pain, thin white tongue coating, and floating, relaxed pulse.

---

[1] *Yin Qiao Jiedu Wan* (*Pian*) is the name of *Yin Qiao San* when the latter is made into pills or tablets.

[Analysis] This is a formula for relieving exterior cold syndrome of deficiency type, i.e., chilliness (or aversion to wind) and fever with sweating. Sweating is closed related to the *ying* (constructive) system and *wei* (superficial defensive) system, of which the former is in charge of sweat secretion, and the latter is responsible for sweat excretion. The two systems function in harmony, and there is normal sweating to adapt the human body to the environmental changes. Sweating in an exterior syndrome is usually due to "disharmony between *Ying* (constructive system) and *wei* (superficial defensive system)." There are two kinds of derangement hampering their harmonious effects: one is weakened *ying* (constructive) system which results in sweating only during fever, the other is weakened *wei* (superficial defensive) system which leads to spontaneous sweating without fever. The traditional explanation can be described as follows: At the initial stage of an exogenous cold affection, *wei* (superficial defensive energy) closes the sweating pores to protect the body against the invasion of exogenous pathogenic factors, and fights against the pathogenic factors, resulting in fever (heat at the superficies). If *ying* is weakened, it will be unable to hold the secretion, and the sweat will be forced out by the heat. In this case sweating occurs only during fever, and Decoction of Cinnamon Twig is suitable for the treatment because it contains white peony root to consolidate *ying* (constructive system). However, if *wei* is weakened, it will be unable to close the pores to hold the sweat excretion and there is an exterior deficiency syndrome marked by sweating without fever. In the latter case, Decoction of Cinnamon Twig is not preferable. Another formula, *Yupingfeng San* (Jade Screen Powder) is indicated, because it contains milkvetch root to strengthen the defensive energy.

As reflected by the name of the decoction, Cinnamon twig is the principal ingredient, inducing mild diaphoresis and expelling the pathogens. White peony root is used to consolidate *ying* (constructive system). Combined use of these two ingredients can achieve the purpose of relieving the exterior syndrome and restoring the harmonious actions of *ying* and *wei*. Fresh ginger and Chinese date form another pair of ingredients to give similar effects: They help cinnamon twig and white peony root respectively. Licorice root is used to moderate the actions of other ingredients.

Probably a question will be raised in this connection. Since the patient is already sweating, why is diaphoresis still necessary? Sweating during fever is considered a symptom of the disease, but not a process of recovery. Mild sweating caused by the decoction is different. It is a therapeutic approach to expelling the pathogenic factors from the body and relieving the exterior syndrome.

[Modern Pharmacology] (1) Antiviral and anti-inflammatory actions: The decoction markedly inhibits the pulmonary infection caused by the influenza virus in mice. Tests on each individual ingredient show that white peony root is the principal ingredient suppressing the replication of the virus. The decoction also counteracts inflammation. Among the ingredients, cinnamon twig has the most prominent anti-inflammatory effect. (2) Effect on the body temperature: The decoction given orally has a bi-directional effect on the body temperature. It shows a prominent antipyretic effect on experimentally induced fever and restores the body temperature to normal when hypothermia is induced by compound aminopyrine injection. (3) Effect on sweating: The decoction has a mild diaphoretic effect, but it markedly inhibits the excessive sweating induced by aminopyrine; on the other hand, it promotes the secretion of sweat when the latter is suppressed by atropine. This may in part illustrate the harmonizing effect on *ying* and *wei*. (4) Sedative and analgesic actions: The decoction shows sedative and analgesic effects in the laboratory, and the effects have a circadian rhythm, i.e., more marked at the active hours. (5) Effect on the immune function: The decoction has a marked inhibitory effect on delayed hypersensitivity.

[Clinical Applications] (1) Common cold, influenza and respiratory tract infections with an exterior deficiency syndrome, as described above; (2) hyperhidrosis; (3) allergic diseases such as allergic rhinitis, urticaria and erythema multiforme.

***Jing Fang Baidu San* (Antiphlogistic Powder of Schizonepeta and Saposhnikovia)**[2]: *Herba Schizonepetae* (schizonepeta) 9 g, *Radix Saposhnikoviae* (saposhnikovia root) 9 g, *Rhizoma seu Radix Notopterygii* (notopterygium rhizome or root) 9 g, *Radix Angelicae Pubescentis* (pubescent angelica root) 9 g, *Radix Chuanxiong* (*chuanxiong*) 6 g, *Radix Bupleuri* (thorowax root) 6 g, *Radix Peucedani* (hogfennel root) 6 g, *Radix Platycodi* (platycodon root) 6 g, *Fructus Aurantii* (bitter orange) 6 g, *Poria* (fuling or poria) 9 g, *Radix Glycyrrhizae* (licorice root) 3 g, and *Herba Menthae* (peppermint) 3 g; to be made into a decoction.

[Effects] Disperses wind-cold and expel damp.

[Indications] Exterior syndrome due to affection by wind-cold and damp, marked by chills and fever with no sweating, accompanied by severe headache, musculo-articular pain, and white greasy tongue coating.

[Analysis] The principal ingredients, schizonepeta, saposhnikovia and notopterygium, are pungent warm diaphoretics for relieving exterior wind-cold. As auxiliaries, pubescent angelica root which warms the meridians and collaterals, and *chuanxiong*, which promotes the blood circulation and also dispels wind, and arrests severe headaches and general aching. Thorowax root and peppermint are adjuvants, assisting the principal ingredients to relieve the exterior syndrome. Hogfennel root and platycodon root are beneficial to the Lungs, and bitter orange to the Spleen. Poria expels damp, and licorice moderates the drug effects.

[Clinical Applications] Common cold, influenza, bronchitis, rheumatism and skin diseases with above-mentioned manifestations.

***Xiao Qinglong Tang* (Minor Decoction of Blue Dragon)**[3]: *Herba Ephedrae* (ephedra) 9 g, *Ramulus Cinnamomi* (cinnamon twig) 6 g, *Herba Asari* (wild ginger) 3 g, *Rhizoma Zingiberis* (dried ginger) 3 g, *Rhizoma Pinelliae Preparata* (prepared pinellia rhizome) 9 g, *Fructus Schisandrae* (magnoliavine fruit) 3 g, *Radix Paeoniae Alba* (white

---

[2]In traditional Chinese formularies, *san* (powder) may be a dosage form of patent medicines, but more frequently it is just a crude preparation for making a decoction. Decocting the powdered medicinal substances may facilitate a complete extraction of the active principles.

[3]The name of the formula needs some explanation. According to an ancient Chinese myth, the Blue Dragon was the god of the wood, residing in the East Sea. Dragons could raise storms with drastic actions, and stir up waves with mild movements. Drastic Decoction of Blue Dragon induces profuse sweating like a heavy rainstorm, and Mild Decoction of Blue Dragon removes the retained fluid in waves.

peony root) 9 g, and *Radix Glycyrrhizae* (licorice root) 6 g, to be made into a decoction.

[Effects] Dispels wind-cold, warms the Lungs and resolves retained fluid.

[Indications] Wind-cold affection with retained fluid in the interior, manifested by chills, fever without sweating or thirst, accompanied by coughing and asthma with profuse frothy expectoration, white moistened tongue coating and floating pulse.

[Analysis] In the formula, ephedra and cinnamon twig relieve the exterior syndrome by diaphoresis. Furthermore, ephedra is antitussive and antiasthmatic; cinnamon twig and white peony root in combination harmonize *ying* (constructive energy) and *wei* (defensive energy). Wild ginger and dried ginger warm the Lung to resolve the retained fluid. Pinellia eliminates damp and phlegm. Magnoliavine fruit is an astringent which prevents consumption of Lung *qi* by other ingredients. Licorice root is used for moderating the actions of other ingredients, and is itself also an expectorant and antitussive.

[Clinical Applications] Chronic bronchitis and bronchial asthma at acute episodes precipitated by colds.

Pungent-Cool Formulas for Relieving Exterior Syndromes

Sang Ju Yin **(Decoction of Mulberry Leaf and Chrysanthemum)**: *Folium Mori* (mulberry leaf) 8g, *Flos Chrysanthemi* (chrysanthemum flower) 6 g, *Herba Menthae* (peppermint) 3 g, *Semen Armeniacae Amarum* (bitter apricot seed) 6 g, *Radix Platycodi* (platycodon root) 6 g, *Radix Glycyrrhizae* (licorice root) 3 g, *Fructus Forsythiae* (forsythia fruit) 6 g, and *Rhizoma Phragmitis* (reed rhizome) 6 g, to be made into a decoction.

Its ready-to-use preparation is called ***Sang Ju Ganmao Pian*** **(Anti-Flu Tablet of Mulberry and Chrysanthemum)**.

[Effects] Dispels wind-heat and relieves coughing.

[Indications] Wind-heat affection with exterior syndrome manifested by moderate fever, coughing, slight thirst, thin whitish tongue coating, and floating pulse.

[Analysis] Mulberry leaf and chrysanthemum flower are the principal ingredients which dispel wind-heat and also clear the Lungs of heat. Peppermint helps dispel wind-heat, bitter apricot seed relieves cough, and platycodon root removes obstruction of Lung *qi*, being adjuvants. Forsythia fruit also relieves exterior syndrome, and reed rhizome reduces heat and promotes production of fluid to relieve thirst, serving as auxiliaries. Licorice root moderates the actions of other ingredients, and it also relieves sore throat when used in combination with platycodon root.

[Clinical Applications] Influenza, acute tonsillitis and epidemic conjunctivitis with exterior heat syndrome.

Yin Qiao San **(Powder of Honeysuckle and Forsythia)**: *Flos Lonicerae* (honeysuckle flower) 9 g, *Fructus Forsythiae* (forsythia fruit) 9 g, *Fructus Arctii* (great burdock achene) 6 g, *Herba Schizonepetae* (schizonepeta) 6 g, *Herba Menthae* (peppermint) 6 g, *Semen Sojae Preparatum* (prepared soybean) 6 g, *Radix Platycodi* (platycodon root) 6 g, *Radix Glycyrrhizae* (licorice root) 6 g, *Herba Lophatheri* (lophatherum) 6 g, and *Rhizoma Phragmitis* (reed rhizome) 6 g, to be made into decoction.

Its ready-to-use preparations include ***Yin Qiao Jiedu Wan*** **(Detoxicant Pill of**

Honeysuckle and Forsythia), ***Yin Qiao Jiedu Pian*** (**Detoxicant Tablet of Honeysuckle and Forsythia**) and ***Yin Qiao Jiedu Chongji*** (**Detoxicant Granules of Honeysuckle and Forsythia**).

[Effects] Relieves exterior syndrome and eliminate toxic heat.

[Indications] Epidemic febrile diseases at the onset, marked by fever with mild chills, headache, thirst, cough, sore throat, reddened tongue tip, thin and white tongue coating, and floating, rapid pulse.

[Analysis] In the formula honeysuckle flower and forsythia fruit are the principal ingredients. They expel pathogens and clear up toxic heat. Prepared soybean, peppermint and schizonepeta dispel pathogens from the exterior, serving as adjuvants. Lophatherum and reed rhizome reduce heat and promote production of fluid to relieve thirst. Platycodon root, burdock achene and licorice root alleviate sore throat and reduce cough. All of them are auxiliaries. Licorice root also moderates the actions of other ingredients.

[Modern Pharmacology] (1) Antipyretic action: The decoction and the granules possess a marked antipyretic effect chiefly by acting on the temperature sensitive neurons. (2) Anti-inflammatory action: The decoction and granules inhibit inflammations in the laboratory, particularly inflammation induced by histamine. (3) Antibacterial and antiviral actions: In vitro, the tablet shows a bacteriostatic action on Staphylococcus aureus (including penicillin-resistant species) and other bacteria, but it is unable to prevent the death of the mice infected by Staphylococcus aureus.

[Clinical Applications] Influenza, upper respiratory infection and other acute infectious diseases with the above-mentioned manifestations.

Ma Xing Shi Gan Tang (**Decoction of Ephedra, Apricot seed, Gypsum and Licorice root**): *Herba Ephedrae* (ephedra) 6 g, *Gypsum Fibrosum* (gypsum) 24 g, *Semen Armeniacae Amarum* (bitter apricot seed) 9 g, and *Radix Glycyrrhizae* (licorice root) 6 g, to be made into a decoction.

Ready-to-use preparations of this formula are available, but with different names.

[Effects] To clear the Lungs of heat and relieve dyspnea.

[Indications] Transformation of wind-cold or wind-heat into the interior (the Lungs) marked by fever with or without sweating, accompanied by cough, dyspnea, thirst, thin white or yellow tongue coating, and floating, slippery and rapid pulse.

[Analysis] In the formula, gypsum is the principal ingredient, which clears the Lungs of heat. Ephedra is an adjuvant, which relieves exterior syndrome and reduces coughing and dyspnea. Although ephedra is pungent in flavor and warm in nature, a large dose of gypsum, which is also pungent in flavor but very cold in nature, makes the formula pungent and cool. Bitter apricot seed is also an antitussive and antiasthmatic, serving as an auxiliary. Licorice root moderates the actions of other ingredients, but it also protects the Stomach from the side effects of gypsum, and so it is used in a larger dose in this formula than in Decoction of Ephedra.

[Clinical Applications] Acute bronchitis, pneumonia and bronchial asthma marked by heat in the Lungs with or without an exterior sydrome.

ANTITUSSIVE, PHLEGM-RESOLVING AND ANTIASTHMATIC FORMULAS

***Erchen Tang* (Decoction of Pinellia Tuber and Tangerine Peel)**: *Rhizoma Pinelliae Preparata* (prepared pinellia rhizome) 9 g, *Pericarpium Citri Reticulatae* (tangerine peel) 9 g, *Poria* (fuling or poria) 6 g, and *Radix Glycyrrhizae* (licorice root) 3 g, to be made into decoction.

Its ready-to-use preparation is called ***Erchen Wan* (Pill of Tangerine Peel and Pinellia Tuber)**.

[Effects] Removes damp-phlegm and regulates the middle *qi*.

[Indications] Phlegm in the Lungs manifested by coughing and expectoration of profuse white sputum, or phlegm in the Stomach manifested by nausea and vomiting. In either case, the tongue coating is white and greasy, and the pulse slippery.

[Analysis] This is the basic formula for resolving damp-phlegm. According to traditional Chinese medicine, phlegm is produced due to retention of water-damp caused by impaired flow of *qi*. In this formula, the principal ingredient, pinellia tuber, eliminates damp-phlegm from the Spleen and the Stomach, and also arrests vomiting by harmonizing the Stomach function. Tangerine peel as the adjuvant, regulates the flow of *qi* and eliminates damp. Since the Spleen is the source from which phlegm is produced, poria is used to invigorate the Spleen function and remove damp through diuresis. Licorice root moderates the actions of other ingredients, and also helps poria to invigorate and harmonize the Spleen and the Stomach.

[Clinical Applications] Chronic bronchitis and chronic gastritis with phlegm syndrome.

Since phlegm may cause a variety of diseases, this formula is more frequently used as the basis for forming more complicated ones. The following are some examples.

***Ditan Tang* (Decoction for Cleansing the Heart from Phlegm)** = Decoction of Pinellia Tuber and Tangerine Peel + *Rhizoma Arisaematis* (Jack-in-the-pulpit tuber), *Fructus Aurantii Immaturus* (immature bitter orange), *Rhizoma Acori Tatarinowii* (grass-leaved sweetflag rhizome) and *Radix Ginseng* (ginseng). It is used for treating aphasia due to misting of the Heart by phlegm.

***Qingqi Huatan Wan* (*Qi*-Clearing and Phlegm-Resolving Pill)** = Decoction of Pinellia Tuber and Tangerine Peel—*Radix Glycyrrhizae* (licorice root) + *Rhizoma Arisaematis* (Jack-in-the-pulpit tuber), *Fructus Trichosanthis* (snakegourd fruit) + *Semen Armeniacae Amarum* (bitter apricot seed), *Radix Scutellariae* (skullcap root) and *Fructus Aurantii Immaturus* (immature bitter orange). It is used for treating chronic bronchitis with excessive heat manifested by sticky yellow expectoration.

***Banxia Baizhu Tianma Tang* (Decoction of Pinellia, White Atractylodes and Gastrodia)** = Decoction of Pinellia Tuber and Tangerine Peel + *Rhizoma Atractylodis Macrocephalae* (white atractylodes rhizome) and *Rhizoma Gastrodiae* (gastrodia tuber). It is used for treating upward attacks of wind-phlegm marked by vertigo and headache with stuffiness in the chest, white and greasy tongue coating, and stringy, slippery pulse. In modern studies this formula has been proved effective for the treatment of Ménèire's syndrome.

***Sanzi Yangqin Tang* (Decoction of Three Kinds of Seeds for the Aged)**: *Semen Sinapis Albae* (white mustard seed) 6 g, *Semen Perillae* (perilla seed) 9 g, and *Semen Raphani* (radish seed) 9 g, to be made into a decoction.

[Effects] Resolves cold-phlegm, regulates the flow of *qi*, and promotes digestion.

[Indications] Weakness of the Spleen in the aged with accumulation of phlegm and stagnated *qi*, manifested by cough, asthma, profuse expectoration, stuffy sensation in the chest, reduced food intake, white greasy tongue coating, and slippery pulse.

[Analysis] White mustard seed warms up the Lungs, facilitates the flow of Lung *qi*, and eliminates phlegm. Perilla seed checks the upward flow of *qi* to relieve asthma. Radish seed promotes digestion and removes stagnated food.

[Clinical Applications] This formula is widely used as the basic formula for treating chronic bronchitis, asthmatic bronchitis and pulmonary emphysema with profuse expectoration but no infection.

FORMULAS FOR CLEARING UP INTERNAL HEAT

Internal heat or heat in the interior syndromes can be exogenous or endogenous, generalized or only involving a certain *zang-fu* organ. Therefore, formulas for clearing up internal heat can be classified into the following categories: (1) formulas for clearing up heat of the *qi* system, (2) formulas for clearing up heat of the *ying*-blood system, (3) formulas for clearing up toxic-heat, (4) formulas for clearing up heat of a certain *zang-fu* organ, (5) formulas for clearing up damp-heat, and (6) formulas for clearing up endogenous heat of deficiency type.

***Baihu Tang* (White Tiger Decoction)**[4]: *Gypsum Fibrosum* (gypsum) 30 g, *Rhizoma Anemarrhenae* (anemarrhena rhizome) 9 g, *Radix Glycyrrhizae* (licorice root) 3 g, and *Oryza* (nonglutinous rice)[5] 9 g, to be made into a decoction.

[Effects] Clears heat and promotes fluid secretion.

[Indications] Excessive heat in the *qi* system, marked by high fever, profuse sweating, dire thirst and gigantic pulse.

[Analysis] Gypsum is the principal ingredient, which has a strong antipyretic action, clearing heat from the Lungs and the Stomach and also promoting fluid secretion to relieve thirst. Anemarrhena rhizome clears heat, and at the same time nourishes *yin*, serving as an

---

[4]The name of the decoction comes from mythology. The White Tiger is the god of metal, residing in the west, and representing autumn. Once autumn comes, the hot summer is naturally at an end. So the name is a metaphor for its antipyretic action on high fever.

[5]Nowadays, the rice is usually not added, and the other three ingredients are used as the basic ingredients to compound decoctions.

adjuvant in this formula. Licorice and rice are used to protect the Stomach for preventing the side effects of gypsum and anemarrhena on the Stomach.

[Clinical Applications] Epidemic encephalitis B, lobar pneumonia and epidemic hemorrhagic fever with heat in the *qi* system.

Baihu Jia Renshen Tang **(White Tiger Decoction Plus Ginseng)**: *Gypsum Fibrosum* (gypsum) 30 g, *Rhizoma Anemarrhenae* (anemarrhena rhizome) 9 g, *Semen Oryzae Nonglutinosae* (nonglutinous rice) 9 g, *Radix Glycyrrhizae* (licorice) 3 g, and *Radix Ginseng* (ginseng) 9 g, to be made into a decoction.

This formula is derived from *Baihu Tang* (White Tiger Decoction), and so it has a similar effect as the latter. In addition, it invigorates the Spleen and the Stomach, and replenishes *qi* by adding ginseng. It is used for treating high fever with consumption of *qi* and fluids, and also for diabetes mellitus.

Baihu Jia Guizhi Tang **(White Tiger Decoction with Cinnamon twig)**: *Gypsum Fibrosum* (gypsum) 30 g, *Rhizoma Anemarrhenae* (anemarrhena rhizome) 9 g, *Radix Glycyrrhizae* (licorice) 3 g, *Semen Oryzae Nonglutinosae* (nonglutinous rice) 3 g, and *Ramulus Cinnamomi* (cinnamon twig) 3 g, to be made into a decoction.

This is also a formula derived from *Baihu Tang* (White Tiger Decoction), which clears away heat. Since cinnamon twig, an antirheumatic, is added, the formula is good for heat-type arthralgia.

Qingying Tang **(Decoction for Clearing up Heat from the *Ying* System)**: *Cornu Rhinoceri* (rhinoceros horn)* 2g, *Radix Rehmanniae* (rehmannia root) 15 g, *Radix Scrophulariae* (figwort root) 9 g, *Herba Lophatheri* (lophatherum) 3 g, *Radix Ophiopogon* (lilyturf root) 9 g, *Radix Salviae Miltiorrhizae* (red sage root) 6 g, *Rhizoma Coptidis* (goldthread rhizome) 4.5 g, *Flos Lonicerae* (honeysuckle flower) 9 g, and *Fructus Forsythiae* (forsythia fruit) 6 g, to be made into a decoction.

(*Rhinoceros horn should be replaced by concentrated powder of buffalo horn, and the dosage increased.)

[Effects] Clears the *ying* system of heat, counteracts toxins and nourishes *yin*.

[Indications] Excessive heat in the *Ying* system, marked by fever higher at night, accompanied by delirium, restlessness, faint skin rashes, and dry crimson tongue.

[Analysis] The principal ingredient in the formula is rhinoceros horn (replaced by water buffalo horn) which clears away heat from the *ying* and blood systems, and also induces tranquilization. Figwort, lilyturf and rehmannia roots all have the effect of nourishing *yin* and reducing heat, being adjuvants. Goldthread rhizome purges fire and removes toxins, lophatherum clears the Heart of fire, honeysuckle flower and forsythia fruit eliminate toxic heat, and red sage root activates blood circulation and prevents blood stasis in rashes, all acting as auxiliaries. Red sage root is also a conductant in this formula, because it directs all the ingredients to the *ying* system for clearing heat.

[Clinical Applications] Epidemic encephalitis, Epidemic meningitis, septicemia, and other febrile diseases with invasion of heat into the *ying* system.

***Xijiao Dihuang Tang* (Decoction of Rhinoceros Horn and Rehmannia)**: *Cornu Rhinoceri* (rhinoceros horn)* 1.5-3 g, *Radix Rehmanniae* (rehmannia root) 30 g, *Radix Paeoniae Rubra* (red peony root) 12 g, and *Cortex Moutan* (moutan bark) 9 g, to be made into a decoction.

(*Rhinoceros horn should be replaced by concentrated powder of buffalo horn, and the dosage increased.)

[Effects] Clears the blood of heat and toxins, and removes blood stasis.

[Indications] Heat in blood system manifested by fever with epistaxis, hematuria, hematochezia and dark purpura, crimson and prickled tongue.

[Analysis] Rhinoceros horn (replaced by water buffalo horn) is the principal ingredient, which clears the blood of heat. Rehmannia root is the adjuvant, which reduces heat from blood and nourishes *yin*. *Moutan* bark and red peony root act as the auxiliary ingredients, which help stop bleeding and prevent stagnation of the extravasated blood.

[Clinical Applications] Epidemic hemorrhagic fever, thrombocytopenic purpura and some other hemorrhagic diseases caused by heat in the blood.

***Huanglian Jiedu Tang* (Detoxicant Decoction of Goldthread)**: *Rhizoma Coptidis* (goldthread rhizome) 9 g, *Radix Scutellariae* (skullcap root) 6 g, *Cortex Phellodendri* (phellodendron bark) 6 g, and *Fructus Gardeniae* (cape-jasmine fruit) 9 g, to be made into a decoction.

[Effects] Purges fire and counteracts toxins.

[Indications] Excessive toxic-heat syndromes in all the three Energizers manifested by high fever, thirst, delirium, reddened tongue with yellow coating and rapid, forceful pulse.

[Analysis] In the formula, goldthread rhizome clears the Heart and the Middle Energizer of fire, skullcap root clears the Upper Energizer, phellodendron bark clears the Lower Energizer, and cape-jasmine fruit clears the Triple Energizer. All the four ingredients eliminate heat toxins.

[Modern Pharmacology] (1) Antibacterial and antitoxic actions: In vitro, the decoction inhibits a variety of bacteria including Staphylococcus aureus and Shigella dysenteriae. The ingredients are synergetic in the bacteriostatic action, and the formula is much more effective than goldthread root alone. The decoction also has a prominent effect against bacterial toxins, such as hemolysin and coagulase of Staphylococcus aureus, and endotoxins. (2) Sedative and antipyretic actions: The decoction has a mild sedative effect and a potent antipyretic effect, slow-acting but persistent. (3) Anti-inflammatory effects: The decoction notably suppresses inflammation and enhances the activity of reticulo-endothelial cells. (4) Hypotensive action: The decoction lowers the blood pressure in experimental hypertension chiefly by stimulating the ß-adrenergic receptor. (5) Effect on the cerebral circulation: The decoction, given orally for 2-4 weeks, can markedly increase the cerebral blood flow in experimental cerebral ischemia. It can also improve the intelligence in presenile dementia and ischemic dementia, and the memory impaired by scopolamine.

[Clinical Applications] (1) Pharyngitis and tonsillitis; (2) biliary infection, bacillary dysentery, and pustuloderma; (2) septicemia and pyemia; (3) post-apoplectic sequelae; (4) hypertension; (5) presenile dementia.

Daochi San **(Redness-removing Powder)**: *Radix Rehmannia* (rehmannia root), *Radix Glycyrrhizae* (licorice root), *Caulis Clematidis* (clematis stem), and *Herba Lophatheri* (lophatherum), mixed at equal amount in weight and ground into powder, 9 g twice daily.

This formula is also made into pills known as ***Daochi Wan*** **(Redness-removing Pill)**.

[Effects] Clears the Heart of fire and induce diuresis.

[Indications] Heat or fire in the Heart Meridian, manifested by ulceration of the mouth or tongue with thirst and desire for cold drinks, flushed face and hot sensation in the chest; or in treating downward transmission of Heart fire with difficult and painful urination or even hematuria.

[Analysis] Rehmannia root clears the Heart of fire and reduces heat from the blood, and also replenishes Kidney *yin*, i.e., water, which checks hyperactivity of fire. Clematis stem, bitter in taste and cold in nature, also clears up the Heart fire. Both are the principal ingredients of the formula. Lophatherum is the adjuvant, which removes heat with urine. Licorice reduces heat, removes toxicity, and moderates the actions of the other ingredients.

[Clinical Applications] Stomatitis and acute urinary tract infection with Heart-fire syndrome.

Qingwei San **(Powder for Clearing Stomach Fire)**: *Rhizoma Coptidis* (goldthread rhizome) 4.5 g, *Radix Angelicae Sinensis* (Chinese angelica root) 6 g, *Radix Rehmanniae* (rehmannia root) 12 g, *Cortex Moutan* (moutan bark) 9 g, and *Rhizoma Cimicifugae* (bugbane rhizome) 3 g, to be made into a decoction.

[Effects] Clears the Stomach of fire and reduces heat in the blood.

[Indications] Accumulation of heat in the Stomach with upward attack of fire manifested by toothache, bleeding and swollen gums, foul breath, reddened tongue with yellow coating, and slippery and rapid pulse.

[Analysis] Goldthread rhizome is the principal ingredient, to clear the Stomach of fire. Bugbane rhizome is also a febrifugal and detoxicant, serving as an adjuvant. Heat usually penetrates blood when it is accumulated in the Stomach. That is why it is necessary to use rehmannia and *moutan* bark to reduce heat in the blood. In this formula, the latter two are auxiliaries.

[Clinical Applications] Stomatitis and periodontitis with the above-mentioned manifestations.

Longdan Xiegan Tang **(Decoction of Gentian to Purge the Liver)**: *Radix Gentianae* (gentian root) 9 g, *Radix Bupleuri* (thorowax root) 6 g, *Rhizoma Alismatis* (alismatis rhizome) 12 g, *Semen Plantaginis* (plantain seed) 9 g, *Caulis Clematidis* (clematis stem) 9 g, *Radix Rehmanniae* (rehmannia root) 9 g, *Radix Angelicae Sinensis*

(Chinese angelica root) 3 g, *Fructus Gardeniae* (cape-jasmine fruit) 9 g, *Radix Scutellariae* (skullcap root) 9 g, and *Radix Glycyrrhizae* (licorice root) 6 g, to be made into a decoction.

The ready-to-use preparation of this formula is ***Longdan Xiegan Wan*** **(Pill of Gentian to Purge the Liver)**.

[Effects] Clears the Liver and the Gallbladder of excess fire and the Lower Energizer of damp-heat.

[Indications] (1) Excess fire of the Liver and the Gallbladder, manifested by dizziness, costal and hypochondriac pain, bitterness in the mouth, restlessness, swollen and painful eyes, and impaired hearing; (2) Damp-heat of the Liver pouring down into the Lower Energizer, manifested by turbid urine, pudendal swelling, vulval pruritus and morbid leukorrhea.

[Analysis] The principal ingredient of the formula is gentian root, which is specifically good for purging fire from the Liver and the Gallbladder. Skullcap root acts on the upper and cape-jasmine fruit on the lower, both being adjuvants and helping gentian root clear up excess fire from the Liver and Gallbladder Meridians. Plantain seed, clematis stem and alismatis rhizome are also adjuvants. They are diuretics, which expel pathogens from the body with urine. Rehmannia root and Chinese angelica root are auxiliaries which nourish the Liver to prevent any damage to the latter either by pathogenic fire or by fire-purging herbs. Thorowax root directs other ingredients to act on the Liver, and licorice moderates their actions.

[Clinical Applications] Conjunctivitis, media otitis, hypertension, icteric hepatitis, cholecystitis, urinary tract infection, pelvic inflammations, and orchitis, all in the acute stage.

Yinchenhao Tang **(Oriental Wormwood Decoction)**: *Herba Artemisiae Scopariae* (oriental wormwood) 30 g, *Fructus Gardeniae* (cape-jasmine fruit) 12 g, and *Radix et Rhizoma Rhei* (rhubarb) 6 g, to be made into a decoction.

[Effects] Clears damp-heat and relieves jaundice.

[Indications] Icterus due to damp-heat, manifested by bright yellow discoration of the skin and sclera accompanied by deep-colored urine, constipation, thirst, abdominal distension, yellow greasy tongue coating, and deep replete or slippery pulse (*yang* jaundice).

[Analysis] Oriental wormwood is the principal ingredient which clears up damp-heat and promotes the secretion and excretion of bile. Cape-jasmine fruit and rhubarb are adjuvants, which remove damp-heat through diuresis and catharsis respectively.

[Clinical Applications] Acute icteric hepatitis and cholecystitits with a damp-heat syndrome as described above.

Gegen Qin Lian Tang **(Decoction of Kudzuvine, Skullcap and Goldthread)**: *Radix Puerariae* (Kudzuvine root, gegen) 15 g, *Radix Scutellariae* (skullcap root) 9 g, *Rhizoma Coptidis* (goldthread rhizome) 9 g, *Radix Glycyrrhizae* (licorice root) 3 g, to be made into a decoction.

[Effects] Clears the interior of heat and relieves the exterior syndrome.

[Indications] Heat entering the interior while the exterior syndrome has not yet been relieved, manifested by chills, fever and diarrhea with mucous discharge, thirst, reddened tongue with yellow coating, and rapid pulse.

[Analysis] In this formula, kudzuvine root is an herb to relieve exterior syndromes, but it also reduces heat and arrests diarrhea; skullcap root and goldthread rhizome clear up damp-heat. Licorice root regulates the Spleen and the Stomach, and moderates drug effects.

[Clinical Applications] Acute gastro-enteritis or dysentery in the initial stage.

Shashen Maidong Tang **(Decoction of Glehnia and Lilyturf)**: *Radix Glehniae* (glehnia root) 9 g, *Rhizoma Polygonati Odorati* (fragrant solomonseal rhizome) 9 g, *Radix Ophiopogonis* (lilyturf root) 9 g, *Radix Trichosanthis* (snakegourd root) 12 g, *Semen Lablab Album* (white lablab seed) 9 g, *Folium Mori* (mulberry leaf) 6 g, and *Radix Glycyrrhizae* (licorice root) 3 g, to be made into a decoction.

[Effects] Relieves dryness of the Lungs and the Stomach.

[Indications] Dryness of the Lungs and the Stomach, manifested by dryness of the mouth, thirst, dry cough, and reddened tongue with scanty coating.

[Analysis] Except for mulberry leaf, which disperses dryness-heat and lablab seed and licorice, which tonify *qi*, all the other ingredients are *yin* tonics for the Lungs and the Stomach.

[Clinical Applications] Bronchitis and other respiratory diseases with dryness of the Lungs.

Qinghao Biejia Tang **(Decoction of Chinghao and Turtle Shell)**: *Herba Artemisiae Chinghao* (sweet wormwood) 6 g, *Carapax Trionycis* (turtle shell) 15 g, *Radix Rehmanniae* (rehmannia root), *Rhizoma Anemarrhenae* (anemarrhena rhizome) 6 g, and *Cortex Moutan* (moutan bark) 9 g, to be made into a decoction.

[Effects] Nourishes *yin* and expels heat.

[Indications] Lingering of pathogenic heat in *yin*, manifested by low-grade fever, aggravated in the evening and alleviated in the morning, with no sweating when the temperature drops; reddened tongue and thready, rapid pulse.

[Analysis] Sweet wormwood and turtle shell are the principal ingredients, which dispel the asthenic heat and nourish *yin,* respectively. Rehmannia root and anemarrhena rhizome nourish *yin* and reduce heat, and *moutan* bark purges fire from *yin*. They are auxiliaries.

[Clinical Applications] Acute febrile diseases at the late stage when the high fever has subsided, or low-grade fever after surgical operation without infection.

FORMULAS FOR CLEARING UP INTERNAL COLD

Lizhong Wan **(Pill for Regulating the Middle Energizer)**: *Radix Ginseng* (ginseng), *Rhizoma Zingiberis* (dried ginger), *Radix Glycyrrhizae* (licorice root), and *Rhizoma Atractylodis Macrocephalae* (white atractylodes rhizome), 9 g each, to be made into a decoction[6].

[Effects] Warms the Middle Energizer, dispels cold and invigorates the Spleen and the Stomach.

[Indications] Deficiency-cold of the Spleen and the Stomach with diarrhea, vomiting, abdominal pain and anorexia.

[Analysis] It is interesting to note that, although ginseng is used and put in the first place in the formula, most authors in the literature agree that dried ginger is the principal ingredient which warms the Middle Energizer and dispels pathogenic cold, while ginseng is an adjuvant which replenishes the Spleen *qi*, and white atractylodes is an auxiliary which invigorates the Spleen and removes dampness. Licorice moderates the actions of other ingredients, and at the same time it reinforces the Spleen and the Stomach to some extent.

[Clinical Applications] Chronic colitis and gastro-intestinal spasms with deficiency-cold syndrome of the Spleen and the Stomach.

***Fuzi Lizhong Wan* (Aconite Pill for Regulating the Middle Energizer)** = *Lizhong Wan* (Pill for Regulating the Middle Energizer) + *Radix Aconiti Lateralis Preparata* (prepared aconite lateral root). The aconite pill is more potent in dispelling cold, not only indicated in the treatment of chronic gastritis, chronic colitis, peptic ulcer, and excessive menstrual bleeding with deficiency-cold syndrome of the Spleen and the Stomach, but also effective for acute gastroenteritis due to direct attack of exogenous cold.

***Xiao Jianzhong Tang* (Mild Decoction for Strengthening the Middle Energizer)**: *Extractum Malti* (malt extract) 24 g, *Radix Paeoniae Alba* (white peony root) 12 g, *Ramulus Cinnamomi* (cinnamon twig) 9 g, *Radix Glycyrrhizae* (licorice root) 9 g, *Rhizoma Zingiberis Recens* (fresh ginger) 9 g, and *Fructus Jujubae* (Chinese date) 12pc, to be made into a decoction.

[Effects] Warms the Spleen and the Stomach, and relieves pain.

[Indications] Deficiency-cold of the Spleen and the Stomach, manifested by epigastric pain alleviated by warmth and pressure, pale complexion, and white tongue coating.

[Analysis] In this formula, deficiency of *yang* is treated in both direct and indirect ways. Cinnamon twig directly warms the Spleen and the Stomach. In addition, another method "reinforcing *yang* by using drugs pungent in flavor and sweet in taste" is applied. Malt extract and Chinese date are sweet, and fresh ginger is pungent. The combined use of these substances promotes the generation of *yang* of the Spleen and the Stomach. Careful analysis of the formula will reveal that it is actually a derivative of Decoction of Cinnamon Twig with minor change of the dosage, but addition of malt extract markedly enhances the warming effect of cinnamon twig, making the formula able to dispel cold from the interior. White peony root is increased in dosage, for it has an antispasmodic action to relieve abdominal pain when it is used together with licorice.

[Clinical Applications] Peptic ulcer, chronic gastritis, and functional disorders of the stomach with deficiency-cold syndrome.

---

[6]Some formulas orginated for making pills or powder are also often used in the form of decoctions for increasing the efficacy or suiting the needs of treatment by modifying certain ingredients. In these cases the formulas still bear the names of pill or powder.

***Huangqi Jianzhong Tang* (Astragalus Decoction for Strengthening the Middle Energizer)** = *Xiao Jianzhong Tang* (Mild Decoction for Strengthening the Middle Energizer) + Radix Astragali (milkvetch root).

With the addition of milkvetch root, the formula has a more tonifying effect than *Xiao Jianzhong Tang*, and is used for treating deficiency-cold of the Spleen and the Stomach if the deficiency state is prominent.

***Shen Fu Tang* (Decoction of Ginseng and Aconite)**: *Radix Ginseng (ginseng)* 12 g, and *Radix Aconiti Lateralis Preparata* (prepared aconite lateral root) 9 g.

[Effects] Restores the vital functions after collapse and shock.

[Indications] Exhaustion of the original *qi* with collapse or shock manifested by cold limbs, cold sweat, faint respiration and scarcely perceptible pulse.

[Analysis] In the formula ginseng is used to reinforce the oringinal *qi* for resuscitation, so ginseng of good quality is preferred, and cannot be replaced by *Radix Codonopsis Pilosulae* (*dangshen*) nor by *Radix Panacis Quinquefolii* (American ginseng). Prepared aconite lateral root warming and tonifying *yang-qi*, helps ginseng to restore the vital functions.

[Modern Pharmacology] (1) Antishock effect: In treating hemorrhagic shock, the decoction elevates the blood pressure slowly but persistently, and markedly lowers the blood lactic acid level and plasma cathepsin activity. (2) Cardiotonic action: The decoction shows a positive inotropic action. It inhibits the ATPase of myocardial cell memebrane, more potently than either of the ingredients alone. (3) Antiarrythmic action: The decoction counteracts various arrythmias induced by pitressin, chloroform or aconitine. (4) Action to dilate the coronary artery: The decoction dilates the coronary artery and protects the heart from ischemia induced by pitressin.

[Clinical Applications] Shock, heart failure, and arrythmias.

FORMULAS FOR ELIMINATING DAMP

Damp in the body is either exogenous or endogenous. According to the severity and the site of the affection, damp can be eliminated by using aromatic damp-resolvants, diuretics and febrifuging diuretics.

Damp affections can be encountered in epidemic diseases, diarrhea, dysentery, edema, morbid leukorrhea, etc. The common manifestations are a heavy sensation in the body, headache as if the head were tightly bound, lassitude, swelling, or lingering fever, accompanied by greasy tongue coating and soft or slippery pulse.

Retention of damp in the Middle Energizer is usually marked by anorexia, nausea, vomiting, diarrhea, and thick greasy tongue coating. Retention of damp in the Lower Energizer is often manifested by oliguria, diarrhea and leukorrhea. Edema or ascites indicates severe retention of damp.

The key points in the composition of damp-expelling formulas are as follows:

1. The drugs should be selected according to the severity of the pathogenic damp.

For example, for mild damp affections or retention of summer damp, fragrant damp-resolving drugs such as *Herba Pogostemonis* (caplin patchouli), *Herba Eupatorii* (eupatorium), and *Fructus Amomi* (spiny amomum fruit) are preferred; for severe damp affections or disturbance of the Spleen by cold-damp, damp-eliminating drugs bitter in taste and warm in property are often used. In case of a severe damp affection with formation of edema, diuretics, such as *Poria* (fuling or poria), *Polyporus* (umbellate polypore), *Rhizome Alismatis*, (water plantain tuber), *Semen Plantaginis* (plantain seed), *Semen Coicis* (coix seed), and *Talcum* (talc) are prescribed. Even without edema, a severe damp affection can be treated with diuretics.

2. Long-term retained damp may be transformed into heat. In some cases, the affection is due to damp-heat from the beginning. In both conditions, drugs to eliminate damp-heat should be added. If the damp-heat is retained in the Bladder, *Herba Dianthi* (lilac pink), *Herba Polygoni Avicularis* (common knotgrass), *Caulis Aristolochiae Manshuriensis* (Manshurian Dutchmans-pipe stem) and other febrifuging diuretics are suitable; if it is in the Large Intestine, damp-eliminating febrifugals such as *Radix Pulsatillae* (pulsatilla root), *Cortex Fraxini* (ash bark), *Radix Scutellariae* (skullcap root), and *Rhizoma Coptidis* (goldthread rhizome) are indicated.

3. Damp and water are the same kind of thing. Both retention of damp and accumulation of water are attributed to functional disorders of the Lungs, the Spleen and the Kidneys. The major part of syndrome differentiation is to determine which *zang*-organ is primarily impaired. If impediment of the Lungs plays the major role, it is necessary to remove the obstructing pathogenic factors from the Lungs in order to expel the damp. If the retention of damp and water is due to disordered Spleen function, invigoration of the Spleen will remove the damp and water. When deficiency of Kidney *yang* causes accumulation of water-damp, the principal treatment is to warm Kidney *yang*, resolve damp and induce diuresis.

4. Damp is apt to impede the flow of *qi*, resulting in distension, and a feeling of stuffiness or fullness. The impeded *qi* flow, in turn, further impairs the movement of water and damp. Therefore, addition of ingredients to promote the flow of *qi* and relieve distension is beneficial to the removal of damp. The drugs commonly used are *Pericarpium Citri Reticulatae* (tangerine peel), *Fructus Aurantii* (bitter orange), *Cortex Magnoliae Officinalis* (officinal magnolia bark), *Radix Aucklandiae* (costus root), *Pericarpium Arecae* (areca peel, and *Semen Arecae* (areca seed).

***Pingwei San* (Stomach-pacifying Powder)**: *Rhizoma Atractylodis* (atractylodes rhizome), *Cortex Magnoliae Officinalis* (officinal magnolia bark), *Pericarpium Citri Reticulatae* (tangerine peel), and *Radix Glycyrrhizae* (licorice root) mixed at a ratio of 3:2:2:1 in weight and ground into powder, 6-9 g each dose. Or to be taken as a decoction with *Rhizoma Atractylodis* (atractylodes rhizome) 9 g, *Cortex Magnoliae Officinalis* (officinal magnolia bark) 6 g, *Pericarpium Citri Reticulatae* (tangerine peel) 6 g, *Radix Glycyrrhizae* (licorice root) 3 g, Rhizoma Zingiberis Recens (fresh ginger) 3 slices, and *Fructus Ziziphi Jujubae* (Chinese date) 3 pieces.

[Effects] Resolves damp and invigorates the Spleen.

[Indications] Disturbance of the Spleen and the Stomach by damp, manifested by anorexia, epigastric and abdominal distension, nausea, vomiting, tastelessness in the mouth, lassitude, loose stools, thick white greasy coating of the tongue.

[Analysis] The principal ingredient of the formula is atractylodes rhizome which eliminates damp and invigorates the Spleen. Officinal magnolia bark removing damp and relieving distension; tangerine peel regulating the flow of *qi* and resolving damp; licorice root, fresh ginger, and Chinese date harmonizing the Spleen and the Stomach, are all adjuvants and auxiliaries.

[Clinical Applications] Chronic gastritis and chronic colitis with the above-mentioned manifestations.

Huoxiang Zhengqi San **(Powder of Patchouli for Restoring Normal *Qi*)**: *Herba Pogostemonis* (cablin patchouli) 9 g, *Folium Perillae* (perilla leaf) 6 g, *Radix Angelicae Dahuricae* (dahurian angelica root) 3 g, *Pericarpium Arecae* (areca peel) 9 g, *Poria* (fuling or poria) 9 g, *Rhizoma Atractylodis* (atractylodes rhizome) or *Rhizoma Atractylodis Macrocephalae* (white atractylodes rhizome) 6 g, *Rhizoma Pinelliae* (processed pinellia tuber) 9 g, *Cortex Magnoliae Officinalis* (officinal magnolia bark) 6 g, *Radix Platycodi* (platycodon root) 4.5 g, and *Radix Glycyrrhizae* (licorice root) 4.5 g, to be made into a decoction as a daily dose, or to be mixed and ground into powder, 6-9 g each dose.

Its ready-to-use preparations include ***Huoxiang Zhengqi Shui*** **(Liquid of Patchouli for Restoring Normal *Qi*)**, and ***Huoxiang Zhengqi Pian*** **(Tablets of Patchouli for Restoring Normal *Qi*)**.

[Effects] Relieves exterior damp syndromes, harmonize the Spleen and the Stomach, and resolves the turbid damp in the interior.

[Indications] Summer-damp affection or exterior syndrome accompanied by retention of damp in the interior, manifested by chills, fever, headache, fullness or distension in the chest and abdomen, anorexia, nausea, vomiting, abdominal pain, diarrhea, tastelessness in the mouth, greasy tongue coating, and soft pulse.

[Analysis] This formula is derived from *Pingwei San* (Stomach-pacifying Powder) or *Erchen Tang* (Decoction of Pinellia Tuber and Tangerine Peel) to resolve damp in combination with drugs to relieve the exterior syndrome. Cablin patchouli, a fragrant substance, is the principal ingredient to resolve turbid damp or summer damp and relieve the exterior syndrome. Perilla leaf dispelling wind-cold, is an adjuvant. Dahurian angelica root dispels wind and platycodon root ventilates the Lungs, both enhancing the action of cablin patchouli. Officinal magnolia bark, and areca peel eliminate damp and relieve distention; medicated leaven and tangerine peel pacify the Stomach for arresting vomiting; atractylodes, poria and licorice resolves damp and invigorate the Spleen, also enhancing the patchouli's action in resolving the turbid damp.

[Modern Pharmacology] (1) Effects on the gastro-intestinal tract: The formula relieves intestinal spasms induced by cholinomimetic agents. The spasmolytic effect is similar as that of atropine, but the action of the formula on the intestinal molitility is bi-directional: inhibitory for a hyperkinetic intestine, and excitatory for a hypokinetic intestine. This may explain the effect of the formula on regulating the gastro-intestinal function. In addition, the formula markedly increases the absorption of glucose and water during diarrhea. (2) Analgesic action: The formula shows an analgesic effect in the laboratory. (3) Effects on bacteria and immune function: The formula exhibits a broad spectrum of bacteriostatic actions. It also enhances the cellular immunity.

[Clinical Applications] Influenza with gastro-intestinal symptoms, and acute gastro-enteritis.

***Wuling San* (Powder of Five Drugs with Poria)**: *Poria* (fuling or poria) 9 g, *Polyporus* (umbellated polypore) 9 g, *Rhizoma Atractylodis Macrocephalae* (white atractylodes rhizome) 9 g, *Rhizoma Alismatis* (water-plantain tuber) 6 g, and *Ramulus Cinnamomi* (cinnamon twig) 3 g; to be made into a decoction.

[Effects] Facilitates urination and induces diuresis.

[Indications] (1) Oliguria and dire thirst with vomiting immediately after drinking in an exterior syndrome after excessive sweating. (2) Retention of water-damp marked by oliguria, edema, lower abdominal distension or diarrhea.

[Analysis] Umbellated polypore, poria and water-plantain tuber are all principal ingredients to induce diuresis. White atractylodes rhizome, invigorating the Spleen for removing the water-damp, is an adjuvant. Cinnamon twig assists the micturition of the Bladder, serving as an auxiliary.

[Modern Pharmacology] (1) The decoction shows diuretic action both in the clinic and in the laboratory. It increases not only the urine output but also the urinary excretion of Na^+, K^+ and Cl^- by inhibiting the reabsorbing function of the renal tubules. (2) Effect on electrolyte metabolism: The formula was originally designed for the treatment of oliguria and dire thirst after excessive sweating (probably dehydration with disordered distribution of water and electrolytes). Modern research has revealed that the decoction has the action to regulate electrolyte metabolism in the condition of great loss of water. It acts on the osmotic receptor and reduces the secretion of antidiuretic hormone.

[Clinical Applications] Nephritic edema, postpartum or postoperative retention of urine, acute gastro-enteritis with diarrhea and vomiting.

***Bazheng San* (Overall Correction Powder)**: *Semen Plantaginis* (plantain seed) 12 g, *Caulis Aristolochiae Manshuriensis* (Manshurian dutchmans-pipe stem) 6 g, *Herba Dianthi* (lilac pink) 15 g, *Herba Polygoni Avicularis* (common knotgrass) 15 g, *Pulvis Talci* (talc) 12 g, *Radix Glycyrrhizae* (licorice root) 3 g, *Fructus Gardeniae* (cape-jasmine fruit) 6 g, *Radix et Rhizoma Rhei Preparata* (prepared rhubarb) 6 g, *and Medulla Junci* (rush pith) 3 g, to be made into a decoction.

[Effects] Clears heat, purges fire, induces diuresis and relieves stranguria.

[Indications] Damp-heat in the Bladder, manifested by urgency of micturition with difficulty, turbid and red urine, urodynia, reddened tongue with yellow coating and rapid pulse.

[Analysis] In this formula manshurian dutchmans-pipe stem, plantain seed, talc and rush pith induce diuresis and at same time quench fire; lilac pink and common knotgrass clear heat and relieve stranguria. They are supplemented with prepared rhubarb and cape-jasmine fruit, which purge the fire, and licorice root, which ward off the side effects of bitter and cold-propertied drugs on the Stomach, and also relieves pain during urination.

[Clinical Applications] Acute urinary tract infection with a damp-heat syndrome,

FORMULAS FOR DISPELLING WIND-DAMP (ANTIRHEUMATIC FORMULAS)

***Duhuo Jisheng Tang* (Decoction of Pubescent Angelica and Mulberry Mistletoe)**: *Radix Angelicae pubescentis* (pubescent angelica root) 6 g, *Ramulus Loranthi* (mulberry mistletoe) 15 g, *Radix Achyranthis Bidentatae* (twotoothed achyranthes root) 9 g, *Cortex Eucommiae* (eucommia bark) 9 g, *Herba Asari* (wild ginger) 1.5 g, *Radix Gentianae Macrophyllae* (large-leaf gentian root) 6 g, *Radix Saposhnikoviae* (saposhnikovia root) 6 g, *Ramulus Cinnamomi* (cinnamon twig) 3 g, *Radix Angelicae Sinensis* (Chinese angelica root) 9 g, *Radix Paeoniae Alba* (white peony root) 9 g, *Radix Rehmanniae Preparata* (prepared rehmannia root) 9 g, *Rhizoma Chuanxiong* (*chuanxiong*) 6 g, *Poria* (fuling or poria) 9 g, *Radix Codonopsis Pilosulae* (dangshen) 9 g, *and Radix Glycyrrhizae* (licorice) 3 g, to be made into a decoction.

The ready-to-use preparation of this formula is called ***Duhuo Jisheng Wan* (Pill of Pubescent Angelica and Mulberry Mistletoe)**.

[Effects] Dispels wind, cold and damp, and tonifies the Liver, Kidneys, *qi* and blood.

[Indications] Chronic wind-cold-damp affections associated with deficiency conditions of the Liver and the Kidneys marked by arthralgia, muscular contracture and lumbago.

[Analysis] In this formula pubescent angelica root, large-leaf gentian root, saposhnikovia root, wild ginger and cinnamon twig dispel wind-damp and warm the meridians to relieve pain; *dangshen*, poria, licorice, Chinese angelica root, *chuanxiong*, rehmannia root, and peony root tonify *qi* and blood, and activate blood circulation; mulberry mistletoe, twotoothed achyranthes root, and eucomia bark replenish the Liver and the Kidneys, and strengthen the tendons and bones. Therefore, this formula removes evil *qi* and at the same time supports normal *qi*.

[Clinical Applications] Rheumatoid arthritis, sciatica, and lumbar muscle strain accompanied by a syndrome of the Liver, Kidneys, *qi* and blood deficiency.

FORMULAS FOR PURGATION

Purgation is not limited to the treatment of constipation. In Chinese medicine, it is an important therapy for eliminating various pathogenic agents such as retained heat, stagnated cold and accumulated fluid by opening the bowels. It is particularly useful when the pathogenic agents are retained in the *fu*-organs, as it is emphasized that the *fu*-organs function well only when they are unobstructed. Since excessive purgation may cause damage to the normal *qi* of the human body, drastic purgative formulas are contraindicated in patients with an exterior syndrome, in the aged with debility, in women in pregnancy or during the menstrual period, and in those with impairment of fluids either due to delivery or due to disease. Even in a patient indicated for drastic purgation, it should be discontinued as soon as the pathogenic agents are removed.

***Da Chengqi Tang* (Drastic Purgative Decoction)**: *Radix et Rhizoma Rhei* (rhubarb) 9 g, *Natrii Sulfas* (sodium sulfate) 15 g, *Fructus Aurantii Immaturus* (immature bitter orange) 9 g, and *Cortex Magnoliae Officinalis* (officinal magnolia bark) 9 g. Add rhubarb when the decoction of immature bitter orange and officinal magnolia bark is nearly done. Then pour the liquid on sodium sulfate.

[Effects] Drastically purges impacted heat.

[Indications] Impaction of heat in the Stomach and Large Intestine, marked by tidal fever in the afternoon, abdominal pain with tenderness, constipation, prickled tongue with brown coating, deep and slippery pulse, and even delirium.

[Analysis] In the formula rhubarb is the principal ingredient which eliminates excessive heat by purgation. Sodium sulfate is the adjuvant, which helps the purgation by softening the fecal masses. Immature bitter orange and magnolia bark are auxilaries which dissipate the accumulation and relieve abdominal distention.

[Modern Pharmacology] (1) Purgative action: The decoction causes purgation by increasing the intestinal motility and the volume of the intestinal contents. Rhubarb stimulates the large intestine and augments the peristalsis; sodium sulfate holds water in the intestines in amounts sufficient to maintain its isotonic concentration; immature bitter orange and officinal magnolia bark also excite the smooth muscle of the intestines. The purgative effect of the decoction is due to direct action on the intestines, for the effect cannot be blocked by atropine. (2) Antibacterial and anti-inflammatory actions: The decoction has a bacteriostatic or even bacteriocidal effect on Staphylococcus aureus both in vitro and in vivo. In experimenal inflammations. the decoction suppresses the capillary permeability, lowers the activity of hyaluronidase, reduces inflammatory exudation and prevents the spreading of the inflammation. (3) Effect on experimental ileus: Clinically, the decoction has a good effect in treating ileus, intussusception and volvulus. Experimentally, injection of the decoction into the intestinal cavity induces total reduction of the retrograde intussusception and artificial volvulus, and promotes the passage of intestinal contents through the partially obstructed intestine. In experimental intestinal obstruction, a large amount of vasoactive internal polypeptide (VIP) is released, which is an important factor in inducing intestinal congestion, edema and exudation. However, after infusion of the decoction into the duodenum the plasma VIP level is greatly lowered and the pathological changes of the intestine are markedly mitigated. (4) Effect on experimental respiratory distress syndrome: Oleic-acid-induced respiratory distress syndrome manifested by cough, dyspnea, and abdominal distension may be taken as a model of “excessive heat in the Lungs and the Large Intestine.” The decoction can elevate the partial pressure of oxygen in arterial blood and reduce the pulmonary lesion.

[Clinical Applications] A variety of recipes have been derived from this formula for treating acute pancreatitis, ileus, and acute pneumonia with constipation.

Xiexin Tang **(Decoction for Purging the Heart of Fire)**: *Radix et Rhizoma Rhei* (rhubarb) 6 g, *Rhizoma Coptidis* (goldthread rhizome) 6 g, and *Radix Scutellariae* (skullcap root) 9 g, to be made into a decoction.

This is a basic combination for forming a variety of fire-quenching and detoxifying formulas indicated in treating syndromes of excess fire, toxic heat, and damp-heat with the heat in preponderance.

Wenpi Tang **(Spleen-warming Decoction)**: *Radix et Rhizoma Rhei* (rhubarb) 6 g, *Radix Aconiti Lateralis Preparata* (prepared aconite lateral root) 9 g, *Rhizoma Zingiberis (dried ginger) 6 g, Radix Codonopsis Pilosulae* (dangshen) 9 g, and *Radix Glycyrrhizae Preparata* (prepared licorice) 3 g.

[Effects] Warms the Spleen and drives away the retained cold.

[Indications] Constipation due to retained cold, or chronic dysentery accompanied by abdominal pain, cold limbs, white and slippery tongue coating, and deep and stringy pulse.

[Analysis] In the formula, ginger and aconite lateral root are warming drugs to disperse cold, *dangshen* and licorice tonify the Spleen and replenish *qi*, and rhubarb is added for purgation. Thus, the main ingredients are warm in nature to invigorate the Spleen function. However, only warming the Spleen may not be enough to remove the retained cold, and purgation alone may further impair the Spleen. So, this is a formula of combined elimination and tonification, with tonification in preponderance.

[Clinical Applications] Chronic dysentery and intestinal obstruction with deficiency-cold syndrome of the Spleen.

Maren Wan **(Laxative Pill with Cannabis Seed)**: *Semen Cannabis* (hemp seed), *Radix et Rhizoma Rhei* (rhubarb), *Fructus Aurantii Immaturus* (immature bitter orange), *Cortex Magnoliae Officinalis* (officinal magnolia bark), *Semen Armeniacae Amarum* (bitter apricot seed), and *Radix Peoniae Alba* (white peony root), mixed at a ratio of 4:2:2:1:1:1 in weight, add equal amount of honey and made into pills, 6-12 g twice a day. The formula may also be used for making a decoction by using appropriate amount of each ingredient. The pill is a mild laxative for treating constipation.

FORMULAS FOR MEDIATION

Formulas for Mediation Between the Exterior and the Interior

Xiao Chaihu Tang **(Minor Bupleurum Decoction)**: *Radix Bupleuri* (thorowax root) 9 g, *Radix Scutellariae* (skullcap root) 9 g, *Rhizoma Pinelliae Preparata* (prepared pinellia tuber) 6 g, *Rhizoma Zingiberis Recens* (fresh ginger) 3 slices, *Fructus Ziziphi Jujubae* (Chinese date) 3 pieces, *Radix Glycyrrhizae* (licorice root) 3 g, and *Radix Codonopsis Pilosulae* (*dangshen*) 6 g.

[Effects] Mediates between the exterior and the interior.

[Indications] Half-exterior half-interior syndrome marked by alternate chills and fever, stuffiness in the chest, anorexia, nausea, vomiting, bitterness in the mouth, dryness of the throat, dizziness, thin white coating of the tongue, and stringy and rapid pulse.

[Analysis] Diaphoresis is good for dispelling the evil in the exterior portion of the body, and purgation for elimination of the evil in the interior, but neither of them is appropriate if the evil exists between the exterior and the interior. Thorowax root disperses the evil from the half-exterior, and skullcap root clears the pathogenic heat from the half-interior. So, the combined use of these two drugs relieves the half-exterior half-interior syndrome. Pinellia tuber and fresh ginger are added for arresting nausea and vomiting. *Dangshen*, Chinese date and licorice are used for strengthening normal *qi*.

[Clinical Applications] Pleurisy, pyelonephritis, cholecystitis, infectious hepatitis, and colds during menstruation with the above-mentioned manifestations.

Da Chaihu Tang **(Major Bupleurum Decoction)**: *Radix Bupleuri* (thorowax root) 9 g, *Radix Scutellariae* (skullcap root) 9 g, *Radix Peoniae Alba* (white peony root) 9 g, *Rhizoma Pinelliae Preparata* (prepared pinellia tuber) 9 g, *Radix et Rhizoma Rhei* (rhubarb) 6 g, *Fructus Aurantii Immaturus* (immature bitter orange) 9 g, *Fructus Ziziphi Jujubae* (Chinese date) 3 pieces, and *Rhizoma Zingiberis Recens* (fresh ginger) 3 slices, to be made into a decoction.

[Effects] Mediates between the exterior and the interior, and purges the impacted heat in the interior.

[Indications] Half-exterior half-interior syndrome combined with interior heat, marked by alternate chills and fever, nausea, vomiting, abdominal pain with distension, constipation, bitterness in the mouth, yellow coating of the tongue, and stringy taut and forceful pulse.

[Analysis] This formula is derived from *Xiao Chaihu Tang* (Minor Bupleurum Decoction) by subtraction of *dangshen* and licorice root, and addition of rhubarb, immature bitter orange and white peony root. So it is a formula of mediation together with purgation.

[Clinical Applications] Acute cholecystitis and acute pancreatitis with the above-mentioned manifestations.

Formulas for Mediation Between the Liver and the Spleen (or Stomach)

Xiaoyao San **(Ease Powder)**: *Radix Bupleuri* (thorowax root) 6 g, *Radix Angelicae Sinensis* (Chinese angelica root) 9 g, *Radix Paeoniae Alba* (white peony root) 9 g, *Rhizoma Atractylodis Macrocephalae* (white atractylodes rhizome) 9 g, *Poria* (fuling or poria) 9 g, and *Radix Glycyrrhizae* (licorice root) 4.5 g for making decoction, or mixed at the ratio of 2:2:2:2:2:1 in weight, respectively, ground into powder, 6-9 g twice daily. It is also made into pills, called ***Xiaoyao Wan*** **(Ease Pill)**.

[Effects] Relieves depression of Liver *qi*, invigorates the Spleen and nourishes blood.

[Indications] Depressed Liver *qi* with dysfunction of the Spleen and blood deficiency, manifested by hypochondriac pain, headache, dizziness, lassitude and anorexia, or menstrual disorders, distension in the breasts, and stringy, thready pulse.

[Analysis] It is a formula based on *Sini San* (Powder for Relieving Stagnation with Cold Limbs) with removal of immature bitter orange and addition of Chinese angelica root to nourish blood and white atractylodes rhizome and poria to invigorate the Spleen.

[Clinical Applications] Irregular menstruation, dysmenorrhea, and chronic liver or gallbladder diseases with the above manifestations.

Dan Zhi Xiaoyao San **(Ease Powder with *Moutan* and Gardenia)**: *Xiaoyao San* (Ease Powder) plus *Cortex Moutan* (tree peony bark) and *Fructus Gardeniae* (Cape-jasmine fruit); to be made into a decoction or powder. Its ready-to-use preparation is called ***Dan Zhi Xiaoyao Wan*** **(Ease Pill with *Moutan* and Gardenia)**.

Its indications and clinical applications are similar to those of *Xiaoyao San* (Ease Powder), if there is endogenous heat (hot sensation in the palms and soles, low fever and night sweating) in addition.

Tongxie Yaofang **(Essential Formula for Diarrhea with Abdominal Pain)**: *Rhizoma Atractylodis Macrocephalae* (white atractylodes rhizome) 9 g, *Radix Paeoniae Alba* (white peony root) 9 g, *Pericarpium Citri Reticulatae* (tangerine peel) 9 g, and *Radix Saposhnikoviae (*saposhnikovia root) 6 g, to be made into a decoction.

[Effects] Soothes the Liver, invigorates the Spleen, relieves abdominal pain and arrests diarrhea.

[Indications] Attack on the Spleen by the hyperactive Liver ("Wood overcomes earth") with diarrhea accompanied by borborygmi and abdominal pain. The diarrhea is usually characterized by its close relationship with emotional changes and the abdominal pain cannot be alleviated by bowel movements. There is no sign indicating the presence of excess heat nor deficiency cold. The pulse is often stringy.

[Analysis] In this formula, white atractylodes rhizome invigorates the Spleen, and white peony root soothes the Liver and arrests pain, both serving as the principal ingredients. Tangerine peel regulates *qi* of the Middle Energizer, and saposhnikovia root dissipates stagnated Liver *qi* and regulates the Spleen function, both being adjuvants.

[Clinical Applications] Chronic colitis and other gastro-intestinal disease with the above-mentioned manifestations.

FORMULAS FOR REGULATING THE FLOW OF *QI*

Disorders of the flow of *qi* chiefly refer to stagnation of *qi* and upward perversion of *qi*. Therefore, there are two categories of formulas for regulating the flow of *qi*: one for promoting the flow of *qi* and the other for sending down the flowing *qi*.

Stagnation of *qi* chiefly involves *qi* of the Spleen and the Stomach (*qi* of the Middle Energizer, or middle *qi* for short) and *qi* of the Liver. Stagnation of the middle *qi* is chiefly manifested by epigastric or abdominal distension, alleviated by belching or passing flatus and accompanied by nausea, anorexia, borborygmi and abnormal bowel movements. Stagnation of the Liver *qi* is marked by distending pain in the lateral pectoral, hypochondriac and/or lower abdominal regions where the Liver Meridian passes, accompanied by irritability or menstrual disorders.

Upward perversion of *qi* involves the Lung and the Stomach, and occasionally the Kidney (referring to its function in receiving air). Formulas for sending down the Lung *qi* are mostly antiasthmatic, and those for sending Stomach *qi* are antiemetic.

Sini San **(Powder for Relieving Stagnation with Cold Limbs)**: *Radix Bupleuri* (thorowax root) 6 g, *Radix Paeoniae Alba* (white peony root) 6 g, *Fructus Aurantii Immaturus* (immature bitter orange) 6 g, and *Radix Glycyrrhizae* (licorice root) 6 g, to be made into a decoction.

[Effects] Harmonizes the Liver and the Spleen, and relieves stagnated heat.

[Indications] Heat in the interior with cold extremities or abdominal pain with diarrhea and stringy pulse.

[Analysis] This formula was originally used for treating abdominal pain and cold limbs due to interior stagnation of *yang-qi* with obstruction of its distribution to the extremities. Since stagnation of *yang-qi* is virtually stagnation of Liver *qi*, now this formula is taken as the basic formula for regulating the flow of Liver *qi*.

In the formula, thorowax root and white peony root are the principal ingredients. The former relieves stagnation of Liver *qi* and transmits *yang-qi* to the exterior, and the latter nourishes the Liver. The action of immature bitter orange is descending in direction while that of thorowax root ascending. Therefore, they are used together to disperse stagnated *qi*. A combination of white peony root and licorice root relieves spasms and pain.

[Clinical Applications] Used as the basic formula for treating chronic hepatitis, cholecytitis, intercostal neuralgia and dysmenorrhea with the above-mentioned manifestations.

Chaihu Shugan San **(Bupleurum Powder for Soothing the Liver)**: *Radix Bupleuri* (thorowax root) 6 g, *Radix Paeoniae Alba* (white peony root) 4.5 g, *Fructus Aurantii Immaturus* (immature bitter orange) 4.5 g, and *Radix Glycyrrhizae* (licorice root) 1.5 g, *Pericarpium Citri Reticulatae* (tangerine peel) 6 g, *Rhizoma Chuanxiong* (*chuanxiong*) 4.5 g and *Rhizoma Cyperi* (cyperus tuber) 4.5 g, to be made into a decoction. It is a derivative of *Sini San* (Powder for Relieving Stagnation with Cold Limbs) by adding tangerine peel, *chuanxiong* and cyperus tuber. All the additional ingredients have the action of regulating the flow of *qi*, but tangerine peel also resolves phlegm, *chuanxiong* promotes blood circulation, and cyperus tuber relieves pain and menstrual disorders. This formula is often used for treating stagnation of Liver *qi* with hypochondriac pain or dysmenorrhea.

Banxia Houpo Tang **(Decoction of Pinellia and Magnolia)**: *Rhizoma Pinelliae* (pinellia tuber) 9 g, *Cortex Magnoliae Officinalis* (officinal magnolia bark) 6 g, *Poria* (fuling or poria) 9 g, *Folium Perillae* (perilla leaf) 3 g, and *Rhizoma Zingiberis Recens* (fresh ginger) 3 slices, to be made into a decoction.

[Effects] Relieves depressed Liver *qi* and resolves phlegm.

[Indications] Retention of depressed *qi* combined with phlegm, marked by the feeling of a lump in the throat which is unable to be spat out or swallowed ("globus hystericus"), accompanied by stuffiness in the chest.

[Analysis] Pinellia tuber resolves phlegm, and officinal magnolia bark promotes the flow of *qi*. Both of them are the principal ingredients in the formula. Perilla leaf assists magnolia bark to remove the depressed *qi*, poria invigorates the Spleen and removes the damp, assisting pinellia tuber to resolve the phlegm, and fresh ginger helps to send down the upward perverted *qi*. All of them are adjunvants and auxiliaries.

[Clinical Applications] Chronic laryngitis, and particularly depression or hysteria with above-mentioned complaints.

Yueju Wan **(Pill for Removing Stagnation)**: *Rhizoma Atractylodis* (atractylodes rhizome), *Rhizoma Cyperi* (cyperus tuber), *Rhizoma Chuanxiong* (*chuanxiong*), *Massa Fermentata Medicinalis* (medicated leaven), and *Fructus Gardeniae* (cape-jasmine fruit), mixed in equal amounts, ground into powder or made into pills. 6-9 g twice daily.

[Effects] Promotes the flow of *qi* and relieves stagnation syndromes.

[Indications] Various kinds of stagnation syndromes (stagnation of *qi*, blood, phlegm, fire, damp and food), particularly stagnation of *qi*, manifested by stuffiness in the chest, epigastric distension and pain, acid regurgitation, vomiting and indigestion.

[Analysis] The principal ingredient in this formula is cyperus tuber, which dissipates the stagnated *qi* to relieve distension and pain in the chest and abdomen. All the rest are adjuvant ingredients: *Chuanxiong* promotes the blood flow to treat stagnation of blood for relieving stabbing pains in the chest. Atractylodes rhizome removes damp and invigorates the Spleen to relieve stagnation of phlegm for treating stuffiness in the chest with expectoration. Cape-jasmine fruit reduces heat and purges the stagnated fire, to relieve vomiting and acid regurgitation. Medicated leaven promotes digestion, to cure epigastric distension and anorexia due to stagnation of food.

[Clinical Applications] Functional disorders of the gastro-intestinal tract, peptic ulcer, chronic gastritis, hepatitis, and cholecystitis with the above-mentioned manifestations.

Dingchuan Tang **(Asthma-relieving Decoction)**: *Herba Ephedrae* (ephedra) 9 g, *Semen Armeniacae Amarum* (bitter apricot seed) 4.5 g, *Cortex Mori* (mulberry bark) 9 g, *Fructus Perillae* (perilla fruit) 6 g, *Semen Ginkgo* (ginkgo seed) 9 g, *Flos Farfarae* (coltsfoot flower) 9 g, *Rhizoma Pinelliae* (pinellia tuber) 9 g, *Radix Scutellariae* (skullcap root) 4.5 g, and *Radix Glycyrrhizae* (licorice root) 3 g, to be made into a decoction.

[Effects] Facilitates the flow of Lung *qi* and resolves phlegm.

[Indications] Asthma due to exterior attack of wind-cold with interior accumulation of phlegm-heat, manifested by difficulty in breathing accompanied by sticky yellow phlegm or chills and fever, yellow greasy tongue coating and slippery, rapid pulse.

[Analysis] The principal ingredient, ephedra, relieves both asthma and exterior syndrome. Bitter apricot seed strengthens the antiasthmatic effect. Mulberry bark and skullcap root relieve coughing and asthma by clearing the Lungs of heat. Perilla fruit, pinellia tuber and coltsfoot flower send down Lung *qi*, arrest coughing and resolves phlegm, further enhancing the antiasthmatic effect of ephedra and bitter apricot seed. Ginkgo seed has three actions: to resolve phlegm, relieve asthma, and minimize the diaphoretic effect of ephedra. Licorice moderates the actions of the other ingredients, and itself is an antitussive and expectorant.

[Clinical Applications] Asthmatic bronchitis with the above-mentioned manifestations.

***Jupi Zhuru Tang* (Decoction of Tangerine Peel and Bamboo Shavings)**: *Pericarpium Citri Reticulatae* (tangerine peel) 9 g, *Caulis Bambusae in Taeniam* (bamboo shavings) 9 g, *Radix Ginseng* (ginseng) 3 g, *Radix Glycyrrhizae* (licorice root) 6 g, *Rhizoma Zingiberis Recens* (fresh ginger) 9 g, and *Fructus Jujubae* (Chinese date) 5pc, to be made into a decoction.

[Effects] Regulates the Stomach *qi* and arrests its upward perversion.

[Indications] Hiccups and vomiting due to weakness of the Stomach with heat marked by reddened tongue and deplete, rapid pulse.

[Analysis] Tangerine peel regulates the flow of Stomach *qi* and relieves vomiting, and bamboo shavings clear the Stomach of heat and arrest hiccups. They are the principal ingredients in the formula. Fresh ginger is an important herb for stopping vomiting, suitable for treating vomiting of the cold type. Together with bamboo shavings, the antiemetic effect of ginger is brought into full play, while its hot nature is neutralized. Ginseng is a tonic for the Stomach, regulating the formula and at the same time replenishing Stomach *qi*. Licorice root and Chinese date harmonize the Stomach function.

[Clinical Applications] Persistent hiccups after surgical operation, vomiting during pregnancy and neurogenic vomiting.

FORMULAS FOR REGULATING BLOOD CONDITIONS

Blood disorders can be divided into five categories: deficiency of blood, heat in blood, cold in blood, stasis of blood and discharge of blood (bleeding). The formulas for treating deficiency, heat and cold of blood are discussed in tonic formulas and formulas for clearing up internal heat and internal cold, respectively.

Formulas for Activating Blood Circulation and Removing Stasis

Blood stasis is usually a complicated condition. A variety of disorders may serve as the origin of blood stasis, such as stagnation of *qi*, deficiency of *qi*, deficiency of blood, heat in blood and cold in blood. In all these cases, corresponding ingredients to treat the fundamental disorders should be added to herbs for activating blood circulation and removing stasis. On the other hand, even without these fundamental disorders, it is preferable to add some ingredients to promote the flow of *qi* for facilitating blood circulation, and to add some tonic ingredients in order to prevent impairment of genuine *qi* by removing blood stasis.

Blood stasis may occur in different locations and cause a great variety of diseases. Therefore, the formulas used to remove blood stasis are large in number and complicated in composition. Here, only a few basic formulas are discussed.

Siwu Tang **(Decoction of Four Ingredients)** is one of the basic formulas. This formula is to be discussed in detail in Tonic Formulas as a blood tonic, but it also has the action of activating blood circulation and removing stasis. It contains four ingredients: *Radix Rehmanniae Preparata* (prepared rehmannia root), *Radix Angelicae Sinensis* (Chinese angelica root), *Rhizoma Chuanxiong* (*chuanxiong*) and *Radix Paeoniae Alba* (white peony root). It has both the effects of nourishing blood and activating blood circulation to remove stasis. When the latter effect is stressed, white peony root is usually replaced by red peony root; if the stagnated blood is related to heat, rehmannia root is used instead of prepared rehmannia root.

Tao Hong Siwu Tang **(Decoction of Four Ingredients with Peach Seed and Safflower)**: *Radix Angelicae Sinensis* (Chinese angelica root), *Rhizoma Chuanxiong* (*chuanxiong*), *Radix Paeoniae Alba* (white peony root), *Radix Rehmanniae* (rehmannia root), *Semen Persicae* (peach seed), and *Flos Carthami* (safflower), to be made into a decoction.

[Effects] Activates blood circulation and regulates menstration.

[Indications] Menstrual disorders due to blood stasis.

[Analysis] The formula is a simple and useful derivative of *Siwu Tang* (decoction of Four Ingredients). In the formula all the ingredients except rehmannia root are herbs to activate blood circulation and remove stasis. Chinese angelica root and rehmannia root have the action of nourishing blood, and *chuanxiong* promotes the flow of *qi*. The dosage of each ingredient is variable in accordance with the patient's condition.

[Clinical Applications] (1) Menstrual disorders, especially delayed menstrual cycle, abdominal pain just before the period, difficulty in menstrual discharge due to blood clots or incessant uterine bleeding due to blood stasis; (2) traumatic injuries or skin diseases with blood stasis.

Xuefu Zhuyu Tang **(Decoction for Removing Blood Stasis in Chest)**: *Semen Persicae* (peach seed) 12 g, *Flos Carthami* (safflower) 9 g, *Radix Angelicae Sinensis* (Chinese angelica root) 9 g, *Rhizoma Chuanxiong* (*chuanxiong*) 4.5 g, *Radix Paeoniae Rubra* (red peony root) 6 g, *Radix Rehmanniae* (rehmannia root) 9 g, *Radix Bupleuri* (thorowax root) 3 g, *Fructus Aurantii* (bitter orange) 6 g, *Radix Platycodi* (platycodon root) 4.5 g, *Radix Cyathulae* (cyathula root) 9 g, and *Radix Glycyrrhizae* (licorice root) 3 g, to be made into a decoction.

[Effects] Activates blood circulation, removes stasis, promotes the flow of *qi* and relieves pain.

[Indications] Blood stasis in the chest marked by pectoral pain with darkened tongue and hesitant pulse.

[Analysis] The formula contains *Tao Hong Siwu Tang* (Decoction of Four Ingredients with Peach Seed and Safflower) plus thorowax root, bitter orange, platycodon root, cyathula root and licorice root. Chinese angelica root, *chuanxiong*, red peony root, peach seed and safflower activate blood circulation and remove stasis, and cyathula root expels obstruction in blood vessels, and removes the stagnated blood by directing it downward. All these ingredients are the primary components of the formula.

Blood circulation depends on the motion of *qi*, especially on the motion of Lung *qi* for even distribution of blood and on the motion of Liver *qi* for smooth flow of blood. Therefore, in the formula, platycodon root and bitter orange are added for promoting the flow of *qi* in the chest, and thorowax root for promoting Liver *qi* flow. Rehmannia root by nourishing blood and reducing heat, together with Chinese angelica root, prevents impairment of blood during the process of eliminating blood stasis. Licorice root moderates the actions of the other ingredients. All the additional ingredients are secondary components of the formula.

[Modern Pharmacology] (1) Actions on the blood and the cardiovascular system: The decoction inhibits ADP-induced platelet aggregation, reduces blood viscosity, and improves various hemorheological indices. It also greatly improves the microcirculatory distubances induced by dextran. It dilates blood vessels, particularly the coronary and cerebral arteries, and increases the blood supply to the myocardium and the brain. It protects the heart from experimental myocardial infaction, and reduces the vascular resistance in cerebral vascular spasms induced by norepinephrine. (2) Effects on chronic inflammation: The decoction suppresses the genesis of DNA in the process of granulation, and hence counteracts the formation of chronic granulomatous lesions. Since the anti-inflammatory effect is accompanied by atrophy of the thymus and hypertrophy of the adrenal, the effect is presumably related to the action of the decoction on the adrenal cortex.

[Clinical Applications] Coronary heart disease, disseminated intravascular coagulation and various kinds of pains (such as headache, chest pain, abdominal pain and lumbago) due to blood stasis.

***Shaofu Zhuyu Tang* (Decoction for Removing Blood Stasis in the Lower Abdomen)**: *Radix Angelicae Sinensis* (Chinese angelica root) 9 g, *Rhizoma Chuanxiong* (*chuanxiong*) 3 g, *Radix Paeoniae Rubra* (red peony root) 6 g, *Pollen Typhae* (cat-tail pollen) 9 g, *Feces Trogopterorum* (trogopterus dung) 6 g, *Myrrha* (myrrh) 6 g, *Rhizoma Corydalis* (corydalis tuber) 3 g, *Fructus Feniculi* (fennel fruit) 7 pieces, *Rhizoma Zingiberis Preparata* (prepared ginger) 0.5g, and *Cortex Cinnamomi* (cinnamon bark) 3 g, to be made into a decoction.

[Effects] Removes blood stasis, warms the meridians in the lower abdomen, and relieves pain.

[Indications] Mass formation in the lower abdomen, pain during the menstrual period, or irregular menstruation with blood clots.

[Analysis] In the formula, Chinese angelica root, red peony root and *chuanxiong* activate blood circulation and remove blood stasis; cat-tail pollen, trogopterus dung, myrrh, and corydalis tuber eliminate blood stasis and relieve pain; fennel fruit, ginger and cinnamon bark warm the meridians, particularly in the lower abdominal region.

[Clinical Applications] Dysmenorrhea, menstrual disorders and chronic pelvic inflammations with blood stasis.

***Buyang Huanwu Tang* (*Yang*-Reinforcing Decoction for Treating Hemiplegia)**[7]: *Radix Astragali* (milkvetch root) 60g, *Radix Angelicae Sinensis* (Chinese angelica root) 6 g, *Radix Paeoniae Rubrum* (red peony root) 6 g, *Lumbricus* (earthworm) 3 g, *Rhizoma Chuanxiong* (*chuanxiong*) 3 g, *Semen Persicae* (peach seed) 3 g, and *Flos Carthami* (safflower) 3 g, to be made into a decoction.

[Effects] Replenishes *qi*, activates blood circulation and removes obstruction for collateral meridians.

[Indications] Postapoplectic hemiplegia.

[Analysis] This is also a derivative of *Tao Hong Siwu Tang* (Decoction of Four Ingredients with Peach Seed and Safflower). Rehmannia root is subtracted, and milkvetch root and earthworm are added. In addition, milkvetch root is used in a very large dose and becomes the principal ingredient of the formula. According to traditional Chinese medicine, paralysis or loss of voluntary motion indicates serious deficiency of *qi* (energy), and so a large dose of *qi*-replenishing herb, milkvetch root, is used. On the other hand, severe deficiency of *qi* is bound to result in blood stasis, and numbness is attributed to obstruction of collateral meridians with stagnated blood flow. That is why all the circulating-activating and stasis-removing ingredients in *Tao Hong Siwu Tang* (Decoction of Four Ingredients with Peach Seed and Safflower) are used with an additional herb to remove obstruction in collateral meridians, namely, earthworm.

[Modern Pharmacology] (1) Effects on the cerebrovascular system: The decoction dilates the cerebral arteries and persistently increases the cerebral blood flow. (2) Effects on the heart: The decoction strengthens the contractibility of the myocardium, but has no influence on the myocardial oxygen consumption, heart rate or blood pressure. (3) Effect on the blood: The decoction markedly inhibits the platelet aggregation induced by adenosine diphosphate, and reduces blood viscosity. (4) Effects on atherosclerosis: The decoction not only reduces the serum cholesterol and triglycerid levels in experimental hyperlipemia, but also removes the atherosclerotic plaques. (5) Repair effects on damage to the nervous system: In the laboratory, the decoction mitigates the degeneration and necrosis of the neurons after traumatic injury and promotes their renovation.

[Clinical Applications] Cerebrovascular diseases (cerebral thrombosis, cerebral embolism, cerebrovascular spasm and postapolectic sequelae, but contraindicated in active cerebral hemorrhage) and other neurological diseases (such as sciatica, peripheral nervous damage and Parkinson's disease).

---

[7]In ancient China, many famous physicians were also literati of great attainments. They often gave herbal formulas elegant names. *Buyang Huanwu Tang* is one example. The meaning of each Chinese character can be expressed as follows: *bu* - to reinforce, *yang* - the opposite of *yin*, *huan* - to restore, *wu* - the number 5, and *tang* - decoction. In the Chinese language, each number has ab extended meaning. For example, one implies “same,” two implies “different,” ten implies “perfect” or “whole,” and “five” refers to “half.” Therefore, the name of the formula means that it is a *yang*-reinforcing prescription to restore the diseased half of the body.

Hemostatic Formulas

Acute hemorrhage is often due to trauma, or due to heat or fire which forces the blood to flow out of the vessel, while chronic bleeding is attributed to failure of the Spleen to control the blood. In addition, stagnated blood is also a common cause of bleeding, though the stagnated blood itself may be the result of bleeding. Therefore, it is emphasized in Chinese medicine when stopping bleeding blood stagnation should be avoided.

Generally, hemorrhagic conditions should be treated in accordance with the cause. For example, if hematuria occurs as a manifestation of Heart fire, *Daochi San* (Powder for Eliminating Redness) is indicated. Prolonged dribbling of menstrual flow due to failure of Spleen *qi* to control blood can be properly treated with *Guipi Wan* (Spleen-Invigorating Pill).

Among the preparations purely for stopping bleeding, the most famous one is *Yunnan Baiyao* (White Drug-Powder of Yunnan). It can be used both topically and orally for treating various kinds of bleeding, including traumatic bleeding. It not only stops bleeding effectively, but also relieves pain and removes blood stasis. Its chief component is *Radix Notoginseng* (notoginseng), but the formula has not been made public.

TONIC FORMULAS

Formulas that replenish and strengthen *qi*, blood, *yin* and *yang* of the *zang-fu* organs are called tonic formulas. They are used to treat deficiency syndromes and can be divided into four categories:

1. *Qi* tonic formulas: for treating deficiency of *qi*.
2. Blood tonic formulas: for treating deficiency of blood.
3. *Yin* tonic formulas: for treating deficiency of *yin*.
4. *Yang* tonic formulas: for treating deficiency of *yang*.

Qi Tonic Formulas

***Sijunzi Tang* (Decoction of Four Noble Ingredients)**: *Radix Ginseng* (ginseng) or *Radix Codonopsis* (dangshen) 12 g, *Rhizoma Atractylodis Macrocephalae* (white atractylodes root) 9 g, *Poria* (fuling or poria) 9 g, and *Radix Glycyrrhizae Preparata* (prepared licorice root) 4.5 g, to be made into a decoction.

Its ready-to-use preparation in pills is called ***Sijunzi Wan* (Pill of Four Noble Ingredients)**.

[Effects] Replenishes *qi* and invigorates the Spleen.

[Indications] *Qi* deficiency of the Spleen and the Stomach marked by poor appetite, loose stools, shortness of breath and lack of strength.

[Analysis] All the four ingredients have the action of invigorating the Spleen and replenishing *qi*. In addition, white atractylodes and poria also remove dampness. Thus, the formula can be taken for a long period of time without side effects.

[Modern Pharmacology] (1) Effects on the gastro-intestinal tract: The decoction inhibits the increased peristalsis of the gastro-intestinal tract induced by reserpine or neostigmine and the tonic contraction induced by acetylcholine. (2) Effects on the immune functions: The decoction strengthens the phagocytosis of macrophages, elevates the lymphocyte transformation rate, and promotes the production of hemolysin antibody. (3) Effects on metabolism and hemopoiesis: The decoction accelerates the formation of red blood cells and increases energy metabolism. (4) Antineoplastic and antimutational actions: In the laboratory, the decoction suppresses the growth of S_{180} sarcoma, and prevents the chromosomal aberration induced by cyclophosphamide.

[Clinical Applications] (1) Chronic gastritis, chronic colitis, peptic ulcer and chronic hepatitis, and chronic fatigue syndrome with deficiency of the Spleen and Stomach *qi*. (2) Used in chemotherapy of cancers for strengthening the latter's antineoplastic effect and minimizing the side effects.

Liujunzi Tang **(Decoction of Six Noble Ingredients)**: Decoction of Four Noble Ingredients plus *Rhizoma Pinelliae* (Pinellia tuber) and *Pericarpium Citri Reticulatae* (tangerine peel).

This is actually a combination of *Sijunzi Tang* (Decoction of Four Nobel Ingredients) and *Erchen Tang* (Decoction of Pinellia Tuber and Tangerine Peel).

The effect of *Sijunzi Tang* (Decoction of Four Nobel Ingredients) is to invigorate the functions of the Spleen and the Stomach, and that of *Erchen Tang* (Decoction of Pinellia Tuber and Tangerine Peel) is to expel damp-phlegm. Therefore, their combination, i.e., *Liujunzi Tang* (Decoction of Six Noble Ingredients), has the action of invigorating the functions of the Spleen and the Stomach and removing damp-phlegm, and is indicated for treating weakness of the Spleen and the Stomach with accumulation of damp-phlegm, manifested by anorexia, loose stools, coughing and profuse frothy sputum (accumulation of phlegm in the Lungs), or epigastric distension, vomiting and acid regurgitation (accumulation of damp-phlegm in the Stomach).

The ready-to-use preparation of the formula is ***Liujunzi Wan*** **(Pill of Six Noble Ingredients)**.

Xiang Sha Liujunzi Tang **(Decoction of Six Noble Ingredients with Costus and Amomum)** is a modification of *Liujunzi Tang* (Decoction of Six Noble Ingredients). It is composed of Decoction of Six Noble Ingredients plus *Radix Aucklandiae* (costus root) and *Fructus Amomi* (amomum fruit). As mentioned in the "Basic combinations" of herbs, costus root and amomum fruit are often used together for regulating the flow of *qi* and removing damp from the Spleen and the Stomach. It has similar indications as Decoction of Six Noble Ingredients but is more effective.

Its ready-to-use preparation is ***Xiang Sha Liujunzi Wan*** **(Pill of Six Noble Ingredients with Costus and Amomum)**.

Shen Ling Baizhu Wan **(Pill of Ginseng, Poria and White Atractylodes)** is another formula derived from *Sijunzi Tang* (Decoction of Four Noble Ingredients). It contains the following ingredients: *Radix Ginseng* (ginseng) or *Radix Codonopsis* (dangshen), *Rhizoma Atractylodis Macrocephalae* (white atractylodes root), *Poria* (fuling or poria), *Radix Glycyrrhizae Preparata* (prepared licorice root), *Rhizoma Dioscoreae* (Chinese yam), *Semen Lablab Album* (white lablab seed), *Semen Coicis* (coix seed), *Semen Nelumbinis* (lotus seed), *Fructus Amomi* (amomum fruit), and *Radix Platycodi* (platycodon root).

Shen Ling Baizhu Wan itself is a ready-to-use preparation, but decoction is also often prescribed according to the composition of the pills.

[Effects] Replenishes *qi*, invigorates the Spleen, removes damp and relieves diarrhea.

[Indications] Deficiency of Spleen and Stomach *qi*, manifested by reduced food intake, epigastric distress after meal, diarrhea, lassitude and lack of strength, emaciation, sallow complexion, pale tongue with white coating, and relaxed pulse.

[Analysis] In this formula, all the ingredients except amomum fruit and platycodon root are tonic herbs for the Spleen. Furthermore, Chinese yam, white lablab seed, coix seed and lotus seed also have the action of removing damp and relieving diarrhea. Amomum fruit is a carminative promoting the flow of *qi*, so that the formula replenishes *qi* but will not cause any stagnation of *qi* thereby. Another interesting point in the composition of this formula is the use of platycodon root. It is a herb acting on the Lungs instead of the Spleen and the Stomach. It acts as a conductant to direct all the tonics upward, so that not only the Spleen and the Stomach, but also the Lungs will be invigorated. Two advantages can be thus obtained. One is the prevention of deficiency of Lung *qi*. As the "son" organ of the Spleen according to the Five Elements Theory, the Lungs are apt to be impaired in protracted weakness of the Spleen. The other is further strengthening of *qi*. Since the Lungs dominate *qi*, invigorating the Lungs will give more replenishment of *qi*.

[Clinical Applications] Chronic bronchitis, chronic diarrhea, indigestion, and menstrual disorders with deficiency syndrome of Spleen and Stomach *qi*.

Buzhong Yiqi Tang **(Decoction for Reinforcing the Middle Energizer and Replenishing *Qi*)**: *Radix Astragali* (milkvetch root) 15-20 g, *Radix Ginseng* (ginseng) 9 g, *Rhizoma Atractylodis Macrocephalae* (white atractylodes rhizome) 9 g, *Radix Glycyrrhizae* (licorice root) 4.5 g, *Radix Angelicae Sinensis* (Chinese angelica root) 9 g, *Pericardium Citri Reticulatae* (tangerine peel) 6 g, *Rhizome Cimicifugae* (bugbane rhizome) 3 g, and *Radix Bupleuri* (thorowax root) 3 g, to be made into decoction.

The ready-to-use preparation of this formula is ***Buzhong Yiqi Wan*** **(Pill for Reinforcing the Middle Energizer and Replenishing *Qi*)**.

[Effects] Tonifies the Spleen and the Stomach, and elevates *qi*.

[Indications] Weakness of the Spleen and Stomach with sinking of *qi*, manifested by chills, fever and headache with sweating, accompanied by anorexia, lack of strength, pale tongue with white coating and feeble pulse; or disorders characterized by ptosis and protracted diarrhea.

[Analysis] From the composition, it can be clearly seen that the formula is related to *Sijunzi Tang* (Decoction of Four Nobel Ingredients), but has a remarkable difference from the latter's other derivative formulas. First of all, the principal ingredient is changed to Radix Astragali (milkvetch root). Second, Poria (fuling or poria) is not used in this formula. Third, bugbane rhizome and thorowax root, two major herbs that elevate *yang qi*, are added.

Since the principal ingredient has been changed, it is usually not taken as a derivative of *Sijunzi Tang* (Decoction of Four Noble Ingredients). Milkvetch root not only replenishes *qi* of the Spleen and the Lungs, it also elevates *yang qi*. Together with bugbane rhizome and thorowax root, this formula has a potent effect of elevating *yang qi*, and is effective for treating sinking syndromes. Sinking syndromes are usually due to protracted deficiency of Spleen *qi*. That is why the "four noble ingredients" except poria are used. Poria is chiefly for removing dampness through diuresis. In deficiency of Spleen *qi*, the Spleen fails to transmit and distribute the essential fluid throughout the body, which results in accumulation of dampness. Whenever Spleen *qi* is invigorated, especially if *yang qi* is elevated, all the accumulated fluid will be transmitted to the Lungs and then redistributed. Therefore, poria is no longer necessary.

[Clinical Applications] (1) Repeated attacks of influenza, persistent fever in influenza or postinfluenzal asthenia with the above-mentioned manifestations; (2) Prolapse of the rectum, prolapse of the uterus, gastroptosis, blepharoptosis as well as protracted diarrhea due to sinking of *qi*.

Shengmai San **(Pulse-activating Powder)**: *Radix Ginseng* 3-9 g, *Radix Ophiopogonis* (lilyturf root) 15 g, and *Fructus Schisandrae* (magnoliavine fruit) 3-9 g, to be made into a decoction.

The ready-to-use preparation of this formula is ***Shenmai Yin*** **(Pulse-activating Drink)**, which is composed of ginseng, lilyturf root and magnoliavine fruit at a ratio of 1:2:1 in weight.

[Effects] Replenishes *qi* and *yin* and arrests sweating.

[Indications] Deficiency of both *qi* and *yin*, manifested by profuse sweating, dryness of the throat and mouth, shortness of breath, thirst, lassitude, and faint pulse.

[Analysis] It is a formula for replenishing both *qi* and *yin*. It is called pulse-activating because it can be used for emergency treatment of exhausted *qi* and *yin* with a scarcely perceptible pulse. More frequently, it is used for deficiency of *qi* and *yin* in various chronic diseases and after acute febrile diseases, manifested by lassitude, thirst, and spontaneous sweating.

In this formula, ginseng strengthens *qi*, lilyturf replenishes *yin*, and magnoliavine fruit consolidates *qi* and *yin*, and also arrests sweating by its astringent action.

[Modern Pharmacology] (1) Effects on the cardiovascular system: The formula shows a prominent positive inotropic action, enhancing the myocardial contractibility and cardiac output, by inhibiting the activity of myocardial Na^+, K^+-ATPase. It markedly increases the coronary blood flow, improves the myocardial blood supply, and adjusts the metabolism of the myocardium to tolerate hypoxia. It counteracts the arrhythmia induced by pitressin, chloroform or aconitine. Its anti-chock effect has been demonstrated in hemorrhagic shock, endotoxic shock, cardiogenic shock and burn shock. In the treatment of shock, it improves the microcirculation and gradually raises the blood pressure, but in acute myocardial infarction with hypertension it lowers the blood pressure. So, its effect on blood pressure is bi-directional. (2) Effects on the immune function: The formula stimulates the reticulo-endothelial system, and increases the peripheral matured T lymphocytes. (3) Effects on the pituitary-adrenocortical system: The formula quickly stimulates the pituitary-adrenocortical function, accelerates the formation and releases of ACTH, and greatly elevates the plasma corticosterone level. The formula increases the plasma corticosterone much more than an equivalent amount of genosides, suggesting that magnoliavine fruit also plays a role in this respect. (4) Effects on the blood: The formula has an anticoagulant effect: It suppresses blood platelet aggregation induced by adenosine diphosphate, prolongs prothrombin time and prothrombin consumption time, and reduces plasma fibrinogen content.

[Clinical Applications] Myocardial infarction with cardiogenic shock, infectious shock, coronary heart disease with angina pectoris, arrythmias in pulmonary heart disease and myocarditis.

Blood Tonic Formulas

Blood deficiency may be generalized or mainly invole a certain *zang*-organ, particularly the Heart or the Liver. In comparison with modern Western concepts, generalized blood deficiency is only partially comparable with anemia, for severe anemia is usually diagnosed as deficiency of *qi* and blood. Therefore, potent blood tonic formulas in Chinese medicine are composed of both blood tonics and *qi* tonics.

Danggui Buxue Tang **(Blood Tonic Decoction with Chinese Angelica)**: *Radix Astragali* (milkvetch root) 30 g, and *Radix Angelicae Sinensis* (Chinese angelica root) 6 g, to be made into a decoction.

[Effects] Replenishes *qi* and generates blood.

[Indications] Deficiency of blood due to blood loss, manifested by sallow complexion, lassitude, lack of strength, low fever, and large but feeble pulse.

[Analysis] The formula only contains two ingredients, namely, milkvetch root, a *qi* tonic, and Chinese angelica root, a blood tonic. It is interesting to note that the *qi* tonic is used in a much larger dose than the blood tonic. According to the traditional theory, it is believed that blood is generated by *qi*. This explains the rationale of using *qi* tonics for the treatment of blood deficiency. However, modern experimental research has shown that milkvetch root itself is an active hemopoietic agent.

In this context, probably another question would be raised: Why not use milkvetch root alone for the treatment of blood deficiency? In fact, milkvetch root can be used alone, and there is a ready-to-use preparation called *Huangqi Gao* (Soft Extract of Milkvetch

Root). This preparation contains only a moderate dose of milkvetch root, and so is mild in action and good for long-term use. If a quicker effect is expected, a larger dose of milkvetch root is necessary. Then the rule of combining ingredients should be followed. Both milkvetch root and Chinese angelica root are tonics; but the former pertains to *yang* and the latter to *yin*. Large doses of milkvetch root may cause dryness, while Chinese angelica root has some moistening effect. Therefore, combined use of these two ingredients not only enhances the effect of generating blood, but also minimizes the side effects. After all, Chinese angelica root has been traditionally taken as the representative drug for treating blood deficiency. That is why the formula is called *Danggui Buxue Tang* (Blood Tonic Decoction with Chinese Angelica), though the principal ingredient of the formula is milkvetch root.

[Clinical Applications] Posthemorrhagic anemia.

Siwu Tang **(Decoction of Four Ingredients)**: *Radix Angelicae Sinensis* (Chinese angelica root) 9 g, *Rhizoma Chuanxiong* (*chuanxiong*) 6 g, *Radix Paeoniae Alba* (white peony root) 9 g, and *Radix Rehmanniae Preparata* (prepared rehmannia root) 15 g; to be made into a decoction.

[Effects] Tonifies blood and regulates menstruation.

[Indications] Menstrual disorders due to deficiency and stagnation of blood.

[Analysis] This formula is chiefly used for treating deficiency of Liver blood, and taken as the basic formula for treating menstrual disorders. Unlike *Danggui Buxue Tang* (Blood Tonic Decoction with Chinese Angelica) in which the dosage, or at least the proportion between the ingredients, is fixed, i.e., the dosage of milkvetch root should be five times that of Chinese angelica root, the dosage of each ingredient in this formula listed above is just an example and can be varied along with the indications. It is also hard to say which one is the principal ingredient. In fact, the principal ingredient can also be varied according to the dosage and indications.

All the four ingredients in the formula are blood tonics, but in addition, each has its own special action. Chinese angelica root activates blood circulation for removing stasis, *chuanxiong* promotes the flow of *qi*, white peony root soothes the Liver, and prepared rehmannia root replenishes Kidney *yin*. Therefore, for replenishing blood, prepared rehmannia root is the principal ingredient; for regulating menstruation, Chinese angelica root should take the first place; for removing blood stasis, Chinese angelica root and *chuanxiong* are more important than the others, and white peony root is usually replaced by red peony root; for treating adverse flow of Liver *qi*, white peony root takes priority.

[Modern Pharmacology] (1) Antianemic effect: The decoction can improve the hemopoietic function of bone marrow in mice with hemorrhagic anemia, accelerating the increase of red blood cells, hemoglobin and reticulocytes. (2) Immune-enhancing effect: The decoction enhances phagocytosis of the reticulo-endothelial cells, and promotes the peripheral lymphocyte transformation and interferon induction. (3) Effect on hypoxia: The decoction counteracts atmospheric hypoxia, myocardial hypoxia caused by isoproterenol, cerebral anoxia caused by ligation of common carotid artery and cytohypoxia by sodium nitrite. (4) Effect on blood platelet aggregation: The decoction inhibits ADP- (adenosine diphosphate-) induced platelet aggregation by increasing the platelet cAMP and ferulic acid contents.

[Clinical Applications] Dysmenorrhea, amenorrhea, and anemia.

There is no ready-to-use preparation of this formula, but many kinds of pills for treating blood deficiency or regulating menstruation are based on it. For example, *Ai Fu Nuangong Wan* (Uterus-warming Pill of Argyi and Cyperus), a commonly used preparation for treating menstrual disorders, is a derivative of the above formula.

***Ai Fu Nuangong Wan* (Uterus-warming Pill of Argyi and Cyperus)**: *Folium Artemisiae Argyi* (argyi leaf), *Rhizoma Cyperi* (cyperus rhizome), *Fructus Evodiae* (evodia fruit), *Cortex Cinnamomi* (cinnamon bark), *Radix Angelicae Sinensis* (Chinese angelica root), *Rhizoma Chuanxiong* (*chuanxiong*), *Radix Paeoniae Alba* (white peony root), *Radix Rehmanniae Preparata* (prepared rehmannia root), *Radix Astragali* (Milkvetch root) and *Radix Dipsaci* (teasel root).

This formula consists of Decoction of Four Ingredients to replenish blood for the Thoroughfare and Conception vessels, cyperus to regulate menstruation and relieve pain, argyi, cinnamon and evodia to warm the uterus and also relieve pain, milkvetch root to replenish *qi* and teasel root to replenish the Liver and Kidneys. Therefore, warming the uterus and regulating menstruation, it is effective for treating menstrual disorders of deficiency-cold type. It should be noted that, although the formula also contains milkvetch root and Chinese angelica root, it is not taken as a derivative of *Danggui Buxue Tang* (Blood Tonic Decoction with Chinese Angelica). This is because whenever we say Blood Tonic Decoction with Chinese Angelica, we always mean that the dosage of milkvetch root is five times or at least much larger than that of Chinese angelica, but in Uterus-warming Pill of Argyi and Cyperus the dosage of milkvetch root is not so large.

Tonic Formulas for Both *Qi* and Blood

***Bazhen Tang* (Decoction of Eight Precious Ingredients)**: *Radix Ginseng* (ginseng) 6 g, *Rhizoma Atractylodis Macrocephalae* (white atractylodes rhizome) 9 g, *Poria* (fuling or poria) 9 g, *Radix Glycyrrhizae* (licorice root) 3 g, *Radix Angelicae Sinensis* (Chinese angelica root) 9 g, *Radix Paeoniae Alba* (white peony root) 9 g, *Rhizoma Chuanxiong* (*chuanxiong*) 9 g, and *Radix Rehmanniae Preparata* (prepared rehmannia root) 9g, to be made into a decoction.

Its ready-to-use preparation is ***Bazhen Wan* (Pill of Eight Precious Ingredients)**

[Effects] Tonifies *qi* and blood.

[Indications] Deficiency of both *qi* and blood manifested by pallor or sallow complexion, dizziness, lack of strength, shortness of breath, palpitations, anorexia, pale tongue with thin white coating, and weak pulse.

[Analysis] Apparently this is a combination of two formulas: *Si Junzi Tang* (Decoction of Four Noble Ingredients), the basic *qi* tonic formula, and *Siwu Tang*

(Decoction of Four Ingredients), the basic blood tonic formula.

[Clinical Applications] Anemia or general debility with the above-mentioned manifestations.

The formula is further developed into more complicated formulas. For example, ***Shiquan Dabu Wan*** **(Pill of Ten Powerful Tonics)** = Pill of Eight Precious Ingredients + *Radix Astragali* (milkvetch root) and *Cortex Cinnamomi* (cinnamon bark). It replenishes both *qi* and blood with warming effect and is more potent than Pill of Eight Precious Ingredients, particularly useful for recuperation.

Guipi Tang **(Spleen-Invigorating Decoction)**: *Radix Astragali* (milkvetch root) 12 g, *Rhizoma Atractylodis Macrocephalae* (white atractylodes rhizome) 9 g, *Poria* (fuling or poria) 9 g, *Arillus Longan* (longan aril) 9 g, *Semen Ziziphi Spinosae* (spiny date seed) 9 g, *Radix Ginseng* (ginseng) 9 g, *Radix Aucklandiae* (costus root) 4.5 g, *Radix Glycyrrhizae* (licorice root) 4.5 g, *Radix Angelicae Sinensis* (Chinese angelica root) 9 g, and *Radix Polygalae* (milkwort root) 9 g, to be made into a decoction.

The ready-to-use preparation of this formula is ***Guipi Wan*** **(Spleen-invigorating Pill)** or ***Renshen Guipi Wan*** **(Spleen-Invigorating Pill with Ginseng)**.

[Effects] Invigorates the Spleen, nourishes the Heart, replenishes *qi* and tonifies blood.

[Indications] Deficiency of both Spleen *qi* and Heart blood, marked by any of the following groups of manifestations: (1) insomnia and palpitations accompanied by sallow complexion, pale tongue and white coating; (2) pallor, lack of strength and reduced food intake due to deficiency of *qi* and blood; (3) various kinds of bleeding due to failure of the Spleen to control blood.

[Analysis] This formula is also a derivative of *Sijunzi Tang* with the addition of milkvetch root to replenish *qi*, Chinese angelica root and longan aril to nourish blood. Spiny date seed induces tranquilization, and milkwort root is a sedative and antidepressant. Costus root regulates the flow of the Spleen *qi*. So this is a formula for replenishing both *qi* and blood, invigorating the Spleen and calming the Heart (mind).

[Clinical Applications] Anxiety states, functional uterine bleeding, and thrombocytopenic purpura with the above-mentioned manifestations.

Yin Tonic Formulas

For practical purposes, deficiency of *yin* in clinical diagnosis only refers to deficiency of vital essence and body fluids. Theoretically, blood pertains to *yin*, but owing to its particular significance, deficiency of blood is separated from deficiency of *yin*. Each *zang-fu* organ has its own essence and fluids, and so there are different patterns of *yin* deficiency, such as deficiency of Heart *yin*, deficiency of Liver *yin*, and so on. General deficiency of *yin* is usually attributed to deficiency of Kidney *yin*, because the Kidneys store essence which comes from all other organs if in excess, and sends essence to other organs if needed. Owing to the particularly important role of the Kidneys in supplying *yin*, many formulas for replenishing *yin* contain *yin* tonics for the Kidneys.

Deficiency of *yin* may produce endogenous heat. Therefore, in formulas for replenishing *yin*, some ingredients to reduce heat are frequently added.

Yin tonics may impair the appetite or cause stagnation of *qi* or retention of fluid. So ingredients to invigorate the Spleen, to regulate the flow of *qi* or to induce diuresis are sometimes added to *yin* tonic formulas.

Liuwei Dihuang Tang **(Decoction of Six Ingredients with Rehmannia)**: *Radix Rehmanniae Preparata* (prepared rehmannia root) 18 g, *Fructus Corni* (dogwood fruit) 9 g, *Rhizoma Dioscoreae* (Chinese yam) 9 g, *Rhizoma Alismatis* (alismatis rhizome) 6 g, *Cortex Moutan* (moutan bark) 6 g, and *Poria* (fuling or poria) 6 g, to be made into a decoction.

Its ready-to-use preparation is ***Liuwei Dihuang Wan*** **(Pill of Six Ingredients with Rehmannia)**. In fact, the pill was first formulated, and the composition of the decoction follows the pill recipe.

[Effects] Replenishes Kidney *yin*.

[Indications] Deficiency of Kidney *yin* manifested by weakness and soreness of loins and knees, dizziness, tinnitus, impaired hearing, night sweating, afternoon fever or feverishness in the palms and soles, dribbling of urine, reddened tongue with scanty coating, and a deep, thready and rapid pulse.

[Analysis] This is the basic formula for replenishing Kidney *yin*. It shows a special pattern of ingredient combination with the following features:

(1) It is a well-recognized formula for replenishing Kidney *yin*, but it also includes tonic ingredients for the Liver and the Spleen. Prepared rehmannia root as the principal ingredient is used in a much larger dosage than all other ingredients. Dogwood fruit is a *yin* tonic for both the Liver and the Kidneys. Because "the Liver and the Kidneys have the same source," replenishing Liver *yin* will increase Kidney *yin*. Rhizoma Dioscoreae (Chinese yam) invigorates the Spleen. "The Spleen provides the material basis of the acquired constitution"; it supplies nutrients to form essence. So, addition of this ingredient is also helpful for replenishing Kidney *yin*.

(2) The whole formula is a combination of three tonics or replenishing ingredients with three reducing or removing ingredients. Besides the above-mentioned tonics which replenish the Kidneys, Liver and Spleen respectively, the formula includes alismatis rhizome, a diuretic which removes excessive water, poria which removes damp, and *moutan* bark which reduces endogenous heat. Damp and excessive water are products of disordered water metabolism in Kidney insufficiency. Endogenous heat is an accompaniment of *yin* deficiency. So, this formula serves as a good example to illustrate a treatment of both the incidental and fundamental aspects of a disease.

(3) The reducing or removing ingredients used in the formula have other functions: alismatis rhizome prevents stagnation caused by prepared rehmannia root, moutan bark corrects the warm nature of dogwood fruit, and poria enhances the Spleen-invigorating effect of Chinese yam by removing damp.

[Modern Pharmacology] (1) Effects on the immune function: The formula shows immunoenhancing effect, including increasing the activity of Fc and C3b receptors of macrophages, promoting the lymphocyte transformation and inducing the production of interferon; (2) Antineoplastic actions: The decoction shows antineoplastic effects in the laboratory. It cannot directly kill tumor cells, but inhibits cancer growth by enhancing the host's immunosurveillance. In addition, it can lessen the toxic and side effects of chemotherapeutic agents (adriamycin, vintristin, cyclophosphamide and 5-FU), and protect the blood, heart, liver and kidney from the damage of chemotherapy. (3) Effects on the liver and lipid metabolism: The decoction prevents liver damage from carbon tetrachloride and thioacetamide. It is interesting to note that when the formula is divided into two decoctions, one only containing the three tonics, and the other, the three reducing ingredients, none of the decoction shows the liver-protecting effect. In experimental hyperlipemia, the formula can reduce serum cholersterol and fat content in the liver. The decoction containing the reducing ingredients shows similar effect as the whole formula. Further analysis of the formula has revealed that the effective ingredients on blood lipids are alismatis rhizome and *moutan* bark. (4) Effects on carbohydrate metabolism: The formula reduces blood sugar and elevates the hepatic content of glycogen. (5) Effects on calcium and phosphorus metabolism. The formula was orginally designed for treating rickets in children. (According to traditional Chinese medical theory, rickets is a morbid condition due to Kidney deficiency, for the Kidneys dominate the bones.) In experimental rickets, the formula maintains the normal Ca and P metabolism, and increases the deposit of Ca and P in the bones. (6) Effects on sexual function: The formula increases the number of sperms and coapulations in animal experiments. (7) Effect on hearing: The formala lessens the impairment of hearing caused by gentamycin in the laboratory.

[Clinical Applications] Diabetes mellitus, hypertension, chronic nephritis, menopausal syndrome with *yin* deficiency of the Liver and the Kidneys.

On basis of this formula a series of rehmannia pills have been developed.

Zhi Bai Dihuang Wan **(Rehmannia Pill with Anemarrhena and Phellodendron)**: *Liuwei Dihuang Wan* (Pill of Six Ingredients with Rehmannia) + *Rhizoma Anemarrhenae* (anemarrhena rhizome) and *Cortex Phellodendri* (phellodendron bark).

It has the action of replenishing *yin* and subduing fire, and is indicated in treating deficiency of *yin* with exuberant fire manifested by consumptive fever, night sweating, soreness of the loins and knees, and dryness of mouth or sore throat.

Qi Ju Dihuang Wan **(Rehmannia Pill with Wolfberry and Chrysanthemum)**: *Liuwei Dihuang Wan* (Pill of Six Ingredients with Rehmannia) + *Fructus Lycii* (wolfberry fruit) and *Flos Chrysanthemi* (chrysanthemum flower).

It is used for treating *yin* deficiency of the Liver and the Kidneys with blurred vision or dryness of and pain in the eyes.

Mai Wei Dihuang Wan **(Rehmannia Pill with Lilyturf and Schisandra)**: *Liuwei Dihuang Wan* (Pill of Six Ingredients with Rehmannia) + *Radix Ophiopogonis* (lilyturf root) and *Fructus Schisandrae* (magnoliavine fruit).

It has the action of replenishing Lung and Kidney *yin*, and is used for treating consumptive diseases with coughing, hemoptysis, afternoon fever and night sweating.

Yiguan Jian **(Ever Effective Decoction)**: *Radix Glehniae* (glehnia root) 9 g, *Radix Ophiopogonis* (lilyturf root) 9 g, *Radix Rehmanniae* (rehmannia root) 18-30 g, *Radix Angelicae Sinensis* (Chinese angelica root) 9 g, *Fructus Lycii* (wolfberry fruit) 9-18 g, and *Fructus Toosendan* (Szechwan chinaberry) 4.5 g, to be made into a decoction.

It is indicated in the treatment of hypochondriac and epigastric pain accompanied by dryness of the throat and mouth due to *yin* deficiency with *qi* stagnation. In this *yin* tonic formula, a small amount of Szechwan chinaberry is added to soothe the flow of *qi*.

Zuogui Yin **(Yin-directing Decoction)**: *Radix Rehmanniae Preparata* (prepared rehmannia root) 15-30 g, *Rhizoma Dioscoreae* (Chinese yam) 6 g, *Fructus Lycii* (wolfberry fruit) 6 g, *Poria* (fuling or poria) 6 g, *Fructus Corni* (dogwood fruit) 4.5 g, and *Radix Glycyrrhizae Preparata* (prepared licorice root) 3 g, to be made into a decoction.

[Effects] Replenishes Kidney *yin*.

[Indications] Deficiency of Kidney *yin* manifested by aching of the loins, nocturnal emission, night sweating, dryness of the mouth and throat, thirst, reddened tongue with no coating, and thready and rapid pulse.

[Analysis] This formula is also derived from *Liuwei Dihuang Wan* (Pill of Six Ingredients with Rehmannia) by subtraction of two "reducing" ingredients, namely alismatis rhizome and moutan bark, and addition of two more tonics, namely, wolfberry fruit for replenishing *yin*, and prepared licorice root for tonifying the Spleen.

[Clinical Applications] Chronic diseases or convalescence after a severe disease with a deficiency syndrome of Kidney *yin*.

Yang Tonic Formulas

Jingui Shenqi Wan **(Kidney-*Qi* Pill of Golden Chamber)** or ***Shenqi Wan*** **(Kidney-*Qi* Pill)** for short: *Radix Rehmanniae Preparata* (prepared rehmannia root), *Fructus Corni* (dogwood fruit), *Rhizoma Dioscoreae* (Chinese yam), *Rhizoma Alismatis* (alismatis rhizome), *Cortex Moutan* (moutan bark), *Poria* (fuling or poria), *Radix Aconiti Lateralis Preparata* (prepared aconite lateral root), and Ramulus Cinnamomi (cinnamon twig), mixed at the ratio of 8:4:4:3:3:3:1:1 in weight, ground into powder and made into pills, 6-9 g twice daily. This formula is often used for making decoctions with appropriate dosage of the ingredients.

[Effects] Reinforces Kidney *yang*.

[Indications] Deficiency of Kidney *yang* marked by aching in the lower back, weakness of the legs, cold sensation in the lower portion of the body and abnormal urination (oliguria or polyuria) accompanied by pale and plump tongue, and weak pulse sinking at the *chi* section.

[Analysis] The formula is composed of *Liuwei Dihuang Wan* (Pill of Six Ingredients with Rehmannia) plus cinnamon twig and prepared aconite lateral root. However, it is not taken as a derivative of Pill of Six Ingredients with Rehmannia. It is called Kidney-*Qi* Pill of the Golden Chamber because it first came into being in the book *Synopsis of Prescriptions of the Golden Chamber* (written in 219), about 900 years earlier than the Pill of Six Ingredients with Rehmannia, first recorded in *Key to Therapeutics of Children's Diseases* (in 1119). Therefore, it is reasonable to say that the latter is a derivative of *Jingui Shenqi Wan* (Kidney-*Qi* Pill of the Golden Chamber). Pill of Six Ingredients with Rehmannia = Kidney-*Qi* Pill − cinnamon twig − aconite lateral root.

An interesting issue worth discussing is its composition. It is a formula for reinforcing Kidney *yang*, but the principal ingredient is prepared rehmannia root, a *yin* tonic. Among the eight ingredients of the formula, only cinnamon and aconite are *yang* drugs, and the other six are related to *yin*, either replenishing or reducing it, as discussed above in the composition of Pill of Six Ingredients with Rehmannia. This can be explained as follows:

(1) According to *yin-yang* theory, *yin* represents the material basis, and *yang* the functional activities. They are interdependent and can be transformed into each other. So it is said that growth of *yang* depends upon normal development of *yin*. This is the main reason why *yin* tonics are used in the formula for reinforcing *yang*, even in larger doses than *yang* tonics.

(2) Kidney *yang* deficiency is always a chronic disease, in which Kidney *yin* deficiency is involved. Therefore, the use of *yin* tonics is necessary.

(3) For treating Kidney *yang* deficiency, long-termed medication is necessary. Because of their warming action, *yang* tonics are apt to impair *yin* fluid, causing dryness. That is why *yin* tonics must be used in combination with *yang* tonics for long-term use.

[Modern Pharmacology] (1) Effects on carbohydrate metabolism: Clinically the formula is effective for treating diabetes mellitus. In the laboratory, the formula shows a hypoglycemic effect in streptozotocin-induced diabetes. The effective ingredient is dogwood fruit, which contains ursolic acid and oleanolic acid as the active principles for diabetes. Since they are fat-soluble, they can hardly be extracted by hot water. This can explain why the pill preparation but not the decoction has been recommended traditionally. (2) Effects on lipid metabolism: The formula prevents the formation of fatty liver and reduces the blood lipids in animals fed with high cholesterol food. (3) Effects on glutathione: The formula markedly increases the glutathione contents in the lens and the testis. So, it can be used for the treatment of cataract and oligospermia. (4) Effects on the neuro-humoral regulation: Clinically, *yang* deficiency of the Kidneys is often associated with hypofunction of the hypothalmic-pituitary-adrenocortical axis. The formula can improve the pituitary-adrenocortical function, increasing the urinary excretion of 17-hydroxycorticosterone and reducing the dosage of cortisone in cortisone-dependent patients. The formula has no testerone-like action, but has some components that may act on the testis, as shown by increasing the combining sites of dihydrotestosterone receptors in the prostate gland.

[Clinical Applications] Chronic nephritis with edema, diabetes mellitus, prostatic hyperplasia, sexual impotence, cataracts and many other diseases associated with deficiency of Kidney *yang*. It is interesting to note that both oliguria and polyuria can be treated with the same formula.

Similar to *Jingui Shenqi Wan* (Kidney-Qi Pill of the Golden Chamber), ***Gui Fu***

***Dihuang Wan* (Rehmannia Pill with Cinnamon and Aconite)**, also called ***Bawei Dihuang Wan* (Pill of Eight Ingredients with Rehmannia)** or ***Gui Fu Bawei Wan* (Pill of Eight Ingredients with Cinnamon and Aconite)**, is often used for reinforcing *yang*. The composition of the latter is the same as that of the former, except that cinnamon twig is replaced by cinnamon bark.

***Jisheng Shenqi Wan* (Revivifying Kidney-*Qi* Pill)**: *Shenqi Wan* (Kidney-*Qi* Pill) plus *Radix Achyranthis Bidentatae* (twotoothed achyranthes root) and *Semen Plantaginis* (plantain seed). It reinforces Kidney *yang* for inducing diuresis, indicated in the treatment of edema and oliguria due to Kidney-*yang* deficiency as seen in nephrotic syndrome.

***Yougui Yin* (*Yang*-directing Decoction)**: *Radix Rehmanniae Preparata* (prepared rehmannia root) 15-30 g, *Fructus Corni* (dogwood fruit) 6 g, *Rhizoma Dioscoreae* (Chinese yam) 6 g, *Fructus Lycii* (wolfberry fruit) 6 g, *Radix Glycyrrhizae Preparata* (prepared licorice root) 4.5 g, *Cortex Eucommiae* (eucommia bark) 6 g, *Radix Aconiti Lateralis Preparata* (prepared aconite lateral root) 6 g, and *Cortex Cinnamomi* (cinnamon bark) 4.5 g, to be made into a decoction.

[Effects] Tonifies Kidney *yang*.

[Indications] Kidney *yang* deficiency manifested by lumbar aching, cold limbs, lassitude, pale tongue with white coating, and deep and thready pulse.

[Analysis] This formula is derived from *Gui Fu Bawei Wan* by subtraction of all the three reducing ingredient, namely, alismatis rhizome, *moutan* bark and poria, and addition of wolfberry fruit and eucommia bark to tonify the Kidneys and the Liver, and prepared licorice to tonify the Spleen.

[Clinical Applications] Chronic diseases with Kidney *yang* deficiency.

***Erxian Tang* (Decoction of Two Elixirs)**: *Rhizoma Curculiginis* (curculigo rhizome) 9 g, *Herba Epimedii* (epimedium) 9 g, *Radix Morindae Officinalis* (morinda root) 9 g, *Radix Angelicae Sinensis* (Chinese angelica root) 9 g, *Cortex Phellodendri* (phellodendron bark) 6 g, *Rhizoma Anemarrhenae* (anemarrhena rhizome) 6 g, to be made into a decoction.

[Effects] Tonifies the Kidneys, purges fire, and regulates the Thoroughfare and Conception vessels.

[Indications] Deficiency of both *yin* and *yang* complicated by exuberant fire.

[Analysis] It is a formula not only for warming Kidney *yang*, but also for replenishing Kidney *yin*, assuaging asthenic Kidney fire, and regulating menstruation. So, it is indicated in the treatment of menopausal syndrome, amenorrhea, hypertension and other chronic diseases with deficiency of both Kidney *yang* and *yin*.

Curculigo rhizome, epimedium and morinda root are Kidney *yang* tonics. Anemarrhena rhizome and phellodendron bark replenish *yin* and assuage fire. Chinese angelica root nourishes blood and regulates menstruation.

[Clinical Applications] Menopausal syndrome, hypertension, and irregular menstruation with the above-mentioned syndrome.

DIGESTANT FORMULAS

Digestants are indicated for indigestion with epigastric and abdominal fullness and distension, fetid belching, acid regurgitation, nausea, vomiting, anorexia, diarrhea or constipation, and thick greasy coating of the tongue.

The key points in the composition of a digestant formula can be described as follows:

1. Digestants are the principal ingredients: *Massa Fermentata Medicinalis* (medicated leaven) and *Fructus Hordei Germinatus* (germinated barley) are good for improving digestion of cereal food, and *Fructus Crataegi* (hawthorn fruit) for meat and fatty food.

2. Retention of undigested food in the stomach often causes disordered flow of Stomach *qi*. If there is upward perverted flow of Stomach *qi* with nausea and vomiting, *Semen Raphani* (radish seed) and *Rhizoma Pinelliae* (pinellia tuber) are often added as anti-emetics. If Stomach *qi* is stagnated, causing epigastric fullness and distension, it is preferable to add *Pericarpium Citri Reticulatae* (tangerine peel), *Radix Aucklandiae* (costus root) and *Fructus Amomi* (spiny amomum fruit), and in severe cases the use of *Fructus Aurantii Immaturus* (immature bitter orange), *Pericarpium Citri Reticulatae Viride* (green tangerine peel) and *Semen Arecae* (areca seed) may be necessary. If the retained food leads to constipation, it is helpful to evacuate the bowels by using *Rhizoma et Radix Rhei* (rhubarb).

3. Prolonged retention of food may induce heat, manifested by yellow tongue coating and thirst. So, some febrifugals such as *Radix Scutellariae* (skullcap root) and *Fructus Forsythiae* (forsythia fruit) are often added in the digestant formulas.

4. It is important to differentiate excess from deficiency in case of indigestion. Indigestion due to eating and drinking too much at one time is usually of the excess type, and can be treated with digestants alone. But if indigestion occurs due to diminished function of the Spleen, the primary treatment should be invigoration of the Spleen, and the use of digestants is auxiliary.

***Baohe Wan* (Lenitive Pill)**: *Fructus Crataegi* (hawthorn fruit), *Massa Pinelliae Fermentata* (medicated leaven), *Semen Raphani* (radish seed), *Poria* (fuling or poria), *Pericarpium Citri Reticulatae* (tangerine peel), Rhizoma Pinelliae (pinellia tuber), and *Fructus Forsythiae* (forsythia fruit), mixed in a ratio of 6:2:1:3:3:3:1 in weight and made into pills, 6-9 g twice daily. The formula may also be used for making a decoction.

[Effects] Promotes digestion and pacifies the Stomach.

[Indications] Indigestion manifested by distension and pain in the epigastrium, anorexia, fetid belching, acid regurgitation, yellow greasy tongue coating, and slippery pulse.

[Analysis] This is a mild formula for treating retention of undigested food. It chiefly contains digestants—hawthorn fruit, medicated leaven and radish seed being the principal ingredients. Since stagnated food is apt to produce damp and heat, the formula contains tangerine peel, poria and pinellia tuber for dispelling damp, and forsythia for clearing heat, all of which are auxiliaries.

[Clinical Applications] Indigestion due to improper diet, but not suitable for diminished Spleen function with retention of food.

Zhi Zhu Wan **(Pill of Bitter Orange and White Atractylodes)**: *Rhizoma Atractylodis Macrocephalae* (white atractylodes rhizome) and *Fructus Aurantii Immaturus* (immature bitter orange), mixed in a ratio of 2:1 in weight and made into pills, 6-9 g twice daily, or made into a decoction with corresponding dosage.

[Effects] Invigorates the Spleen, promotes digestion and removes retained food.

[Indications] Indigestion due to weakened Spleen and Stomach, manifested by epigastric distension, anorexia, or splashing sounds in the stomach.

[Analysis] In this formula, tonification is primary, while elimination is secondary, because the dosage of white atractylodes rhizome is double that of immature bitter orange.

[Clinical Applications] Chronic stomach diseases with the above-mentioned manifestations.

ASTRINGENT FORMULAS

Astringent formulas are used for arresting various kinds of abnormal discharge, such as spontaneous sweating or night sweating, nocturnal emission or spermatorrhea, enuresis or incontinence of urine, protracted diarrhea with fecal incontinence, abnormal uterine bleeding and excessive leukorrhea. It should be noted that many of the above disorders are secondary to deficiency conditions, but most astringent formulas can only give symptomatic relief. Therefore, other formulas for radical treatment are often necessary.

Astringent Formula for Arresting Sweating

Yupingfeng San **(Jade Screen Powder)**: *Radix Astragali* (milkvetch root), *Rhizoma Atractylodis Macrocephalae* (white atractylodes rhizome), and *Radix Saposhnikoviae* (saposhnikovia root), mixed in a ratio of 3:1:1 in weight and ground into powder, 6-9 g twice a day. It is also made into pills, called ***Yupingfeng Wan*** **(Jade Screen Pill)**, and into a solution called ***Yupingfeng Koufuye*** **(Jade Screen Solution)**.

[Effects] Replenishes *qi*, consolidates the superficial defence and arrests sweating.

[Indications] Exterior deficiency syndrome manifested by aversion to wind, spontaneous sweating, pale tongue with white tongue coating, and floating, feeble pulse.

[Analysis] Milkvetch root, the principal ingredient of the formula, replenishes *qi* of the Spleen and the Lungs, particularly the superficial defensive *qi*, and arrests excessive sweating. White atractylodes rhizome invigorating the Spleen and replenishing *qi*, helps milkvetch root to strengthen the superficial defence and arrest sweating. Saposhnikovia root, a herb to dispel pathogenic wind, when used together with *qi* tonics, can dispel pathogens in patients with deficiency of *qi*, causing no adverse effects. So this formula is good for treating spontaneous sweating due to deficiency of superficial defensive *qi* and can also be used for a preventive purpose in those with weak body resistance and vulnerable to exogenous affections.

[Clinical Applications] Prevention of repeated attacks of colds and influenza, particularly in vulnerable individuals.

Astringent Formulas for Arresting Diarrhea

***Sishen Wan* (Pill of Four Miraculous Ingredients)**: *Fructus Psoraleae* (scurfpea fruit), *Fructus Schisandrae* (magnoliavine fruit), *Semen Myristicae* (nutmeg), and *Fructus Evodiae* (evodia fruit), mixed at a ratio of 4:4:2:1 in weight, ground into powder and made into pills, 9-12 g twice daily.

[Effects] Warms the Kidneys and the Spleen, and arrests diarrhea.

[Indications] Deficiency-cold of the Kidneys and the Spleen, manifested by diarrhea daily before dawn, anorexia, lassitude, soreness in the back, cold limbs, pale tongue with thin white coating, and deep, slow and weak pulse.

[Analysis] Scurfpea fruit, pungent in flavor and warm in nature, reinforcing vital fire and dispelling pathogenic cold, is the principal ingredient. Evodia fruit warms the Middle Energizer and dispels cold; nutmeg also warms the Spleen. Both nutmeg and magnoliavine fruit are astringents for arresting diarrhea. Therefore, the action of this formula is to warm the Spleen and the Kidneys, and arrest diarrhea.

[Clinical Applications] Chronic colitis with the above-mentioned manifestations.

Astringent Formula for Arresting Seminal Emission

***Jinsuo Gujing Wan* (Golden Lock Pill for Semen Discharge)**: *Semen Astragali Complanati* (flatstem milkvetch seed), *Semen Euryales* (euryale seed), *Stamen Nelumbinis* (lotus stamen), *Os Draconis Ustum* (calcined dragon's bone), and *Concha Ostreae Usta* (calcined oyster shell), mixed at the ratio of 2:2:2:1:1 in weight, ground into powder and made into pills, 9 g twice daily.

[Effects] Strengthens the Kidneys and arrests seminal discharge.

[Indications] Kidney insufficiency marked by seminal emission and spermatorrhea, lack of strength, soreness in the loins, pale tongue with white coating, and fine, weak pulse.

[Analysis] This is a formula for treating seminal emission and spermatorrhea due to Kidney insufficiency. Flatstem milkvetch seed is the principal ingredient. It reinforces the Kidneys, replenishes vital essence and arrests seminal emission. Euryale seed and lotus stamen are adjuvants which help strengthen the effect of the principal ingredient in arresting seminal discharge. Calcined dragon's bone and oyster shell are also astringents used as auxiliary ingredients in this formula. Therefore, the formula has both the radical effect of reinforcing the Kidneys and the symptomatic effect of arresting seminal discharge, but the latter is the major one.

[Clinical Applications] Seminal emission and spermatorrhea due to Kidney insufficiency. Contraindicated in seminal emission caused by damp-heat in the Lower Energizer.

Astringent Formula for Arresting Abnormal Urination

***Suoquan Wan* (Pill for Reducing Urination)**: *Radix Linderae* (spicebush root), and

Semen Alpiniae Oxyphyllae (sharp-leaf galangal seed), mixed in equal amounts, ground into powder and made into pills.

[Effects] Reinforces the Kidneys and arrests enuresis.

[Indications] Frequent urination in adults and enuresis in children.

[Analysis] Both ingredients are warm in property, reinforce the Kidneys and dispel cold.

Astringent Formula for Arresting Excessive Uterine Bleeding or Leukorrhea

***Guchong Tang* (Decoction for Reinforcing the Thoroughfare Vessel)**: *Rhizoma Atractylodis Macrocephalae* (white atractylodes rhizome) 30 g, *Radix Astragali* (milkvetch root) 18 g, *Os Draconis Ustum* (calcined dragon's bone) 24 g, *Concha Ostreae Usta* (calcined oyster shell) 24 g, *Fructus Corni* (dogwood fruit) 24 g, *Radix Paeoniae Alba* (white peony root) 12 g, *Os Sepiae* (cuttlefish bone) 12 g, *Radix Rubiae* (madder root) 9 g, *Petiolus Trachycarpi Carbonizatus* (carbonized petiole of windmill palm) 6 g, and *Galla Chinensis* (Chinese gall) 1.5 g, to be made into a decoction.

[Effects] Invigorates the Spleen, replenishes *qi*, and arrests bleeding from the Thoroughfare Vessel.

[Indications] Abnormal uterine bleeding and excessive menstrual flow due to failure of the Spleen to control blood.

[Analysis] White atractylodes rhizome and milkvetch root, invigorating the Spleen and replenishing *qi,* are the principal ingredients. Disorders of the Thoroughfare Vessel are often related to insufficiency of the Liver and the Kidneys. So dogwood fruit and white peony root are used to reinforce the Liver and the Kidneys. All the other ingredients are astringents to stop bleeding.

[Clinical Applications] Functional uterine bleeding, excessive bleeding after parturition and peptic ulcer hemorrhage due to deficiency of *qi*.

FORMULAS FOR TRANQUILIZATION

These formulas are used for treating mental restlessness marked by insomnia, fidgetiness or mania. Mental restlessness may be due to various conditions, such as deficiency of Heart blood, exuberance of Heart fire, disturbance of the Heart by phlegm-fire, incoordination of the Heart and the Kidneys, and even dysfunction of the Stomach. To relieve mental restlessness, the primary conditions should be treated correspondingly with addition of proper tranquilizing agents. Tranquilizing agents can chiefly be divided into two categories: those inducing tranquilization by nourishing Heart blood, e.g., *Semen Ziziphi Spinosae* (spiny date seed), *Caulis Polygoni multiflori* (fleece-flower stem), *Radix Polygalae* (milkwort root) and *Semen Biotae* (arborviatae seed); and those inducing tranquilization by their heaviness (minerals or shells), e.g., *Magnetitum* (magnetite), *Margarita* (pearl), *Os Draconis* (dragon's bone) and *Choncha Ostreae* (oyster shell).

***Suanzaoren Tang* (Decoction of Spiny Date Seed)**: *Semen Ziziphi Spinosae* (spiny date seed) 18 g, *Rhizoma Anemarrhenae* (anemarrhena rhizome) 6 g, *Poria* (fuling or poria) 6 g, *Rhizoma Chuanxiong* (chuanxiong) 3 g, and *Radix Glycyrrhizae* (licorice root) 3 g, to be made into a decoction.

The ready-to-use preparation of this formula is ***Suanzaoren Tang Wan*** (**Pill of Spiny Date Seed Decoction**).

[Effects] Nourishes blood, removes heat and induces tranquilization.

[Indications] Insomnia of deficiency type, accompanied by palpitation, night sweating, dizziness, dryness of the throat and mouth, and stringy or thready, rapid pulse.

[Analysis] According to the Five Elements theory, the treatment for an organ in deficiency is by reinforcing its "mother" organ. Fidgetiness and insomnia are symptoms of mental restlessness. Liver, pertaining to wood, is the mother organ of the Heart, which pertains to fire. When Liver blood is insufficient, the blood supply to the Heart (the organ in charge of mental activities) is not adequate, resulting in fidgetiness and insomnia. In addition, deficiency of Liver *yin* is usually accompanied by endogenous heat, which may lead to insomnia by disturbing the normal activities of the Heart, and also to other accompanying symptoms such as dizziness, night sweating, and dryness of the throat and mouth. Spiny date seed is the principal ingredient in the formula. In Chinese, it is called *suanzaoren*, in which *suan* means sour, and *zaoren* is date seed. Sourness pertains to wood, acting on the Liver. Therefore, spiny date seed is primarily considered as a blood tonic of the Liver with a tranquilizing effect.

Poria is an adjuvant to assist spiny date seed in its tranquilizing effect. Anemarrhena rhizome and *chuanxiong* are auxiliary ingredients: the former eliminates endogenous heat, and the latter soothes the Liver and partially corrects the astringent action of spiny date seed. Licorice root moderates the effects of the other ingredients.

[Modern Pharmacology] Modern research has shown the sedative or hypnotic effect of this decoction. The decoction inhibits over-stimulated nerve cells, particularly the cerebral cortex, and spiny date seed plays the principal role. However, there is no modern explanation regarding its effect in nourishing Liver blood.

[Clinical Applications] Insomnia, as described above.

Tianwang Buxin Dan (**Heavenly King's Heart Tonic**): *Radix Rehmanniae* (rehmannia root), *Radix Ginseng* (ginseng) Radix Scrophulariae (figwort root), *Radix Salviae Miltiorrhizae* (red sage root), *Poria* (fuling or poria), *Radix Polygalae* (milkwort root), *Radix Platycodi* (platycodon root), *Fructus Schisandrae* (magnoliavine fruit), *Radix Ophiopogonis* (lilyturf root), *Radix Asparagi* (asparagus root), *Semen Ziziphi Spinosae* (spiny date seed), *Radix Angelicae Sinensis* (Chinese angelica root), *and Semen Biotae* (arborvitae seed), mixed in a ratio of 8:1:1:1:1:1:1:2:2:2:2:2:2 in weight, respectively, and made into pills, 9 g twice daily. The formula may also be used for making decoctions by using the appropriate dosage of each ingredient.

[Effects] Nourishes *yin*-blood of the Heart and the Kidneys, and calms the mind.

[Indications] Deficiency of Heart and Kidney *yin* with exuberance of *yang* marked by insomnia, palpitation, ulceration in the mouth with constipation, reddened tongue with scanty coating, and thready, rapid pulse.

[Analysis] In this formula, rehmannia root and figwort root replenish Kidney *yin* and reduce heat; Chinese angelica root and red sage root nourish Heart blood; lilyturf root and asparagus root replenish Heart *yin*; ginseng and poria tonify Heart *qi*; spiny date seed, arborvitae seed and milkwort root calm the mind; magnoliavine fruit tonifies the Heart by its astringent action; and platycodon root, serving as a conductant, "directs" the effects of other ingredients upward.

[Clinical Applications] Anxiety states with the above-mentioned manifestation.

Guizhi Gancao Longgu Muli Tang **(Decoction of Cinnamon Twig, Licorice Root, Dragon's Bone and Oyster Shell)**: *Ramulus Cinnamomi* (cinnamon twig) 3 g, *Radix Glycyrrhizae* (licorice root) 6 g, *Os Draconis* (dragon's bone) 9 g, and *Concha Ostreae* (oyster shell) 9 g, to be made into a decoction.

[Effects] Warms up the Heart and induces sedation.

[Indications] Deficiency of Heart *yang* with mental flightiness manifested by irritability, palpitation and spontaneous sweating.

[Analysis] Dragon's bone and oyster shell are heavy materials for inducing tranquilization. Cinnamon twig, being warm in nature, reinforces Heart *yang*, and licorice root replenishes Spleen *qi*. Their combined use restores the normal function of the Heart (normal mental activities).

[Clinical Applications] Anxiety states with the above-mentioned manifestations.

WIND-SUBDUING FORMULAS

Here "wind" refers to endogenous wind, which is usually due to exuberance of Liver *yang*. *The Canon of Medicine* states, "Various kinds of (endogenous) wind symptoms such as tremors, convulsions and vertigo are mostly attributed to the Liver." So, endogenous wind is also called "Liver wind." Liver-wind syndromes can generally be classified into three categories: (1) Liver wind due to exuberance of Liver *yang*, either of excess type or of deficiency type (secondary to *yin* deficiency), (2) Liver wind stirred up by extreme heat (high fever), and (3) Liver wind due to deficiency of blood.

Tianma Gouteng Yin **(Decoction of Gastrodia and Uncaria Stem)**: *Rhizoma Gastrodiae* (gastrodia tuber) 6 g, *Ramulus Uncariae* (uncaria stem) 15 g, *Concha Haliotidis* (sea-ear shell), *Ramulus Loranthi* (mulberry mistletoe) 15 g, *Cortex Eucommiae* (eucommia bark) 9 g, Fructus Gardeniae (cape-jasmine fruit) 9 g, Radix Scutellariae (skullcap root) 9 g, *Radix Cyathulae* (cyathula root) 9 g, *Herba Leonuri* (motherwort) 9 g, *Caulis Polygoni Multiflori* (fleece-flower stem) 15 g, *Poria cum Radix Pino* (*fushen*) 12 g, to be made into a decoction.

[Effects] Soothes the Liver, subdues the wind and nourishes *yin*.

[Indications] Liver wind due to deficiency of *yin* with exuberance of *yang* manifested by headache, vertigo, insomnia, reddened tongue, and stringy, rapid pulse.

[Analysis] In this formula, gastrodia tuber, uncaria stem, and sea-ear shell soothe the Liver and subdue Liver wind; cape-jasmine fruit and skullcap root purge fire from the Liver; eucommia bark, mulberry mistletoe and cyathula root nourish Kidney *yin* and Liver blood, and remove obstructions from the collateral meridians; motherwort promotes blood circulation in the collateral meridians; and fleece-flower stem and *fushen* (poria with host wood) are tranquilizers.

[Clinical Applications] Hypertension with Liver wind of deficiency type.

CHAPTER 11

COMMONLY USED PATENT MEDICINES

Traditional Chinese patent medicines are ready-to-use preparations manufactured with traditional Chinese medicinal substances in accordance with the procedures stipulated in formularies. They usually take the forms of pills (including watered pills, honeyed pills, concentrated pills and minute or dropping pills), tablets, capsules, soft extracts, granules and medicinal wine. These have an apparent advantage over decoctions in the convenience of administering the remedy. The number of Chinese patent medicines is also huge. Following are some commonly used ones. Most of them are specified in the current *Pharmacopoeia of the People's Republic of China.*

Medicines for Respiratory Diseases

***Ganmao Qingre Chongji* (Antipyretic Granules for Colds)**

[Ingredients] *Spica Schizonepetae, Herba Menthae, Radix Saposhnikoviae, Radix Bupleuri, Folium Perillae, Radix Puerariae, Radix Platycodi, Semen Armenicae Amarum, Radix Angelicae Dahuricae, Herba Corydalis Bungeanae* and *Rhizoma Phragmitis.*

[Effects] Dispels wind-cold, induces diaphoresis and removes heat.

[Indications] Common cold with headache, fever, chills, general aching, stuffed running nose and cough.

[Usage and Dosage] 12 g, 2 times a day, to be taken with hot water.

***Ganmao Tuire Chongji* (Antipyretic Granules for Flu)**

[Ingredients] *Folium Isatidis, Radix Isatidis, Fructus Forsythiae* and *Rhizoma Bistortae.*

[Effects] Removes toxic heat.

[Indications] Upper respiratory infection, acute tonsillitis, and pharyngitis.

[Usage and Dosage] 18-36 g, 3 times a day, to be taken with hot water.

***Chuanbei Pipa Tangjiang* (Fritillary and Loquat Syrup)**

[Ingredients] *Bulbus Fritillariae Cirrhosae, Folium Eriobotryae, Semen Armeniacae Amarum, Radix Platicodi* and *Mentholum.*

[Effects] Removes heat from the Lungs, resolves phlegm and relieves coughing.

[Indications] Coughing in colds and bronchitis.

[Usage and Dosage] 10 ml, 3 times a day.

***Yin Qiao Jiedu Wan* (Detoxicant Pill of Honeysuckle and Forsythia), *Yin Qiao Jiedu Pian* (Detoxicant Tablet of Honeysuckle and Forsythia)** and ***Yin Qiao Jiedu Chongji* (Detoxicant Granule of Honeysuckle and Forsythia).**

[Ingredients] *Flos Lonicerae, Fructus Forsythiae, Fructus Arctii, Herba Schizonepetae, Herba Menthae, Semen Sojae Preparatum, Radix Platycodi, Radix Glycyrrhizae, Herba Lophatheri* and *Rhizoma Phragmitis.*

[Effects] Relieves exterior syndrome and eliminates toxic heat.

[Indications] Upper respiratory infection with fever, headache, cough, dryness of the mouth and sore throat.

[Usage and Dosage] 1 pill, 4 tablets or 1 pack of granules, 2-3 times a day.

***Yangyin Qingfei Gao* (Extract for Nourishing *Yin* and Clearing the Lungs)**

[Ingredients] *Radix Rehmanniae, Radix Ophiopogonis, Radix Scrophulariae, Bulbus Fritillaria Cirrhosae, Radix Paeoniae Alba, Cortex Moutan, Herba Menthae* and *Radix Glycyrrhizae.*

[Effects] Nourishes *yin*, clears the Lungs of heat, and relieves coughing.

[Indications] Deficiency of Lung *yin* marked by coughing with scanty expectoration, sore throat and dryness of the mouth.

[Usage and Dosage] 10-20 ml, 2-4 times a day.

***Banlangen Chongji* (Isatis-root Granules)**

[Ingredients] *Radix Isatidis.*

[Effects] Removes toxic heat, and reduces swelling.

[Indications] Upper respiratory infection, tonsilitis, mumps; also for prevention and treatment of infectious hepatitis and measles.

[Usage and Dosage] 5 g, 4 times a day.

***Fangfeng Tongsheng Wan* (Miraculous Pill of Saposhnikovia)**

[Ingredients] *Radix Saposhnikoviae, Fructus Forsythiae, Herba Ephedrae, Fructus Gardeniae, Radix et Rhizoma Rhei, Gypsum Fibrosum, Radix Scutellariae, Radix Paeoniae Alba, Rhizoma Chuanxiong*, etc.

[Effects] Dispels wind-heat from both the exterior and interior.

[Indications] Wind-heat affection involving both the exterior and interior marked by headache, sore throat and constipation; urticaria.

[Usage and Dosage] 6 g, 2 times a day.

[Warning] Used with caution in pregnancy.

Medicines for Digestive Diseases

***Huoxiang Zhengqi Shui* (Liquid of Pachouli for Restoring Normal Qi)**

[Ingredients] *Rhizoma Atractylodis, Pericardium Citri Reticulatae, Cortex Magnoliae Officinalis, Radix Angelicae Dahuricae, Pericarpium Arecae, Poria, Rhizoma Pinelliae, Extractum Glycyrrhizae, Oleum Pogostemonis, Oleum Folii Perillae.*

[Effects] Relieves exterior damp syndromes and harmonizes the Spleen and the Stomach.

[Indications] Influenza with gastro-intestinal symptoms, and acute gastro-enteritis.

[Usage and Dosage] 5-10 ml, 2 times a day.

Huoxiang Zhengqi Pian **(Tablet of Pachouli for Restoring Normal *Qi*).**

[Ingredients] *Herba Pogostemonis, Folium Perillae, Radix Angelicae Dahuricae, Pericarpium Arecae, Poria, Rhizoma Atractylodis Macrocephalae, Pericarpium Citri Reticulatae, Rhizoma Pinelliae, Cortex Magnoliae Officinalis, Radix Platycodi* and *Radix Glycyrrhizae.*

[Effects] Relieves exterior damp syndromes and harmonizes the Spleen and the Stomach.

[Indications] Influenza with gastro-intestinal symptoms, and acute gastro-enteritis.

[Usage and Dosage] 6 g, 2 times a day.

Fuzi Lizhong Wan **(Aconite Pill for Regulating the Middle Energizer)**

[Ingredients] *Radix Aconiti Lateralis Preparata, Radix Codonopsis Pilosulate, Rhizoma Zingiberis, Radix Glycyrrhizae* and *Rhizoma Atractylodis Macrocephalae.*

[Effects] Warms and tonifies the Spleen and the Stomach.

[Indications] (1) Chronic gastritis, chronic colitis, peptic ulcer, and excessive menstrual bleeding with deficiency-cold syndrome of the Spleen and the Stomach; (2) Acute gastroenteritis due to direct attack of exogenous cold.

[Usage and Dosage] 6 g of watered-honey pills or 1 big honeyed pill (9 g), 2-3 times a day.

Maren Wan **(Laxative Pill with Cannabis Seed)**

[Ingredients] *Semen Cannabis, Radix et Rhizoma Rhei, Fructus Aurantii Immaturus, Cortex Magnoliae Officinalis, Semen Armeniacae Amarum* and *Radix Peoniae Alba.*

[Effects] Induces laxation.

[Indications] Constipation.

[Usage and Dosage] 6 g of water-honeyed pills or 1 big honeyed pill (9 g), 1-2 times a day.

Yueju Wan **(Pill for Removing Stagnation)**

[Ingredients] *Rhizoma Atractylodis, Rhizoma Cyperi, Rhizoma Chuanxiong, Massa Fermentata Medicinalis* and *Fructus Gardeniae.*

[Effects] Promotes the flow of *qi* and relieves stagnation syndromes.

[Indications] Functional disorders of the gastro-intestinal tract, peptic ulcer, chronic gastritis, hepatitis, cholecystitis with stagnation syndrome marked by stuffiness in the chest, epigastric distension and pain, acid regurgitation, vomiting, and indigestion.

[Usage and Dosage] 6-9 g, 2 times a day.

Xiangsha Yangwei Wan **(Stomachic Pill with Cyperus and Amomum)**

[Ingredients] *Radix Aucklandiae, Fructus Amomi, Rhizoma Atractylodis*

Macrocephalae, Pericarpium Citri Reticulatae, Poria, Rhizoma Pinelliae, Rhizoma Cyperi, Fructus Aurantii Immaturus, Fructus Amomi Rotundus, Cortex Magnoliae Officinalis, Herba Pogostemonis and *Radix Glycyrrhizae.*

[Effects] Regulates the Stomach function.

[Indications] Digestive disorders marked by anorexia, acid regurgitation, epigastric distention and lassitude.

[Usage and Dosage] 9 g, 2 times a day.

Shen Ling Baizhu Wan **(Pill of Ginseng, Poria and White Atractylodes)**

[Ingredients] *Radix Ginseng, Rhizoma Atractylodis Macrocephalae, Poria, Radix Glycyrrhizae Preparata, Rhizoma Dioscoreae, Semen Lablab Album, Semen Coicis, Semen Nelumbinis, Fructus Amomi* and *Radix Platycodi.*

[Effects] Replenishes *qi*, invigorates the Spleen, removes damp and relieves diarrhea.

[Indications] Chronic bronchitis, chronic diarrhea, indigestion, and menstrual disorders with deficiency of Spleen *qi.*

[Usage and Dosage] 6-9 g, 2-3 times a day.

Baohe Wan **(Lenitive Pill)**

[Ingredients] *Fructus Crataegi, Massa Pinelliae Fermentata Semen Raphani, Poria, Pericarpium Citri Reticulatae*, Rhizoma Pinelliae and *Fructus Forsythiae.*

[Effects] Promotes digestion, removes retained food and regulates the Stomach function.

[Indications] Indigestion due to retained food marked by distension and pain in the epigastrium, anorexia, fetid belching, acid regurgitation, yellow greasy tongue coating, and slippery pulse.

[Usage and Dosage] 6-9 g, 2 times a day.

Zhi Zhu Wan **(Pill of Bitter Orange and White Atractylodes)**

[Ingredients] *Rhizoma Atractylodis Macrocephalae* and *Fructus Aurantii Immaturus.*

[Effects] Invigorates the Spleen, promotes digestion and eliminates damp.

[Indications] Indigestion due to weakened Spleen and Stomach marked by epigastric distension, anorexia, or splashing sounds in the stomach.

[Usage and Dosage] 6 g, 2 times a day.

Sishen Wan **(Pill of Four Miraculous Ingredients)**

[Ingredients] *Fructus Psoraleae, Fructus Schisandrae, Semen Myristicae* and *Fructus Evodiae.*

[Effects] Warms the Kidneys and the Spleen, and arrests diarrhea.

[Indications] Chronic colitis with deficiency-cold of the Kidneys and the Spleen, marked by diarrhea daily before dawn, anorexia, lassitude, soreness of the back, cold limbs, pale tongue with thin white coating, and deep, slow and weak pulse.

[Usage and Dosage] 9 g, 1-2 times a day.

Medicines for Cardiovascular Diseases

Fufang Danshen Diwan **(Compound Danshen Dropping Pill)**
[Ingredients] *Radix Salviae Miltiorrhizae, Radix Notoginseng* and *Borneolum.*
[Effects] Removes blood stasis, regulates the flow of *qi*, and relieves pain.
[Indications] Angina pectoris.
[Usage and Dosage] 10 pillets, 3 times a day, to be taken orally or sublingually.
[Warning] Used with caution in pregnancy.

Guanxin Suhe Wan **(Storax Pill for Coronary Heart Disease)**
[Ingredients] *Storax, Borneolum, Olibanum, Lignum Santali Albi* and *Radix Aristolochiae.*
[Effects] Regulates the flow of *qi* in the chest and relieves pain.
[Indications] Angina pectoris.
[Usage and Dosage] 1 pill, 1-3 times a day.
[Warning] Contraindicated in pregnancy.

Shengmai Yin **(Pulse-activating Drink)**
[Ingredients] *Radix Ginseng, Radix Ophiopogonis* and *Fructus Schisandrae.*
[Effects] Replenishes *qi*, nourishes *yin*, and restores normal pulse.
[Indications] Arrhythmias and palpitations due to deficiency of both *qi* and *yin.*
[Usage and Dosage] 10 ml, 3 times a day.

Medicines for Mental Disorders

Suhexiang Wan **(Storax Pill)**
[Ingredients] *Storax, Benzoinum, Borneolum, Pulvis Corni Bubali Concentratus, Moschus, Lignum Santali Album, Lignum Aquilariae Resinatum, Flos Caryophylli, Rhizome Cyperi, Radix Aucklandiae, Olibanum, Fructus Piperis Longi, Rhizoma Atractylodis Macrocephalae, Fructus Chebulae* and *Cinnabairs.*
[Effects] Induces restoration of consciousness as an aromatic stimulant, and promotes the flow of *qi* and relieves pain.
[Indications] Apoplexy with loss of consciousness; angina pectoris.
[Usage and Dosage] 1 pill, 1-2 times a day.
[Warning] Contraindicated in pregnancy.

Angong Niuhuang Wan **(Bezoar Resurrection Pill)**
[Ingredients] *Calculus Bovis, Pulvis Cornus Bubali Concentratus, Moschus, Margarita, Cinnabaris, Realgar, Rhizoma Coptidis, Radix Scutellariae, Fructus Gardeniae, Radix Curcumae, Borneolum Syntheticum.*
[Effects] Removes toxic heat, relieves convulsion, and promotes the restoration of consciousness.
[Indications] Delirium and convulsion due to high fever.
[Usage and Dosage] 1 pill (3 g) at once.

[Warning] Used with caution in pregnancy.

Medicines for Gynecological Diseases

***Ai Fu Nuangong Wan* (Uterus-warming Pill of Argyi and Cyperus)**

[Ingredients] *Folium Artemisiae Argyi, Rhizoma Cyperi, Fructus Evodiae, Cortex Cinnamomi, Radix Angelicae Sinensis, Rhizoma Chuanxiong, Radix Paeoniae Alba, Radix Rehmanniae Preparata, Radix Astragali* and *Radix Dipsaci.*

[Effects] Replenishes *qi*, warms the uterus, and regulates menstruation.

[Indications] Menstrual disorders due to deficiency-cold in the uterus.

[Usage and Dosage] 9 g, 2-3 times a day.

***Xiaoyao San* (Ease Powder)**

[Ingredients] Radix Bupleuri, Radix Angelicae Sinensis, Radix Paeoniae Alba, Rhizoma Atractylodis Macrocephalae, Poria and *Radix Glycyrrhizae.*

[Effects] Soothes the Liver, invigorates the Spleen and nourishes blood.

[Indications] Irregular menstruation, dysmenorrhea, and chronic liver or gallbladder diseases due to depressed Liver *qi* with Spleen dysfunction and blood deficiency.

[Usage and Dosage] 6-9 g, 1-2 times a day.

***Danggui Wan* (Chinese Angelica Pill)**

[Ingredients] *Radix Angelica Sinensis.*

[Effects] Nourishes blood, activates circulation, and regulates menstruation.

[Indications] Menstrual disorders and dysmenorrhea.

[Usage and Dosage] 6 g, 2 times a day.

***Yimucao Gao* (Concentrated Decoction of Motherwort)**

[Ingredients] *Herba Leonuri.*

[Effects] Activates blood circulation and regulates menstruation.

[Indications] Amenorrhea, dysmenorrhea, abdominal pain after parturition due to blood stasis.

[Usage and Dosage] 10 g, 1-2 times a day.

[Warning] Contraindicated in pregnancy.

***Wuji Baifeng Wan* (White Phoenix Pill)**

[Ingredients] *Phoenix, Colla Cornus Cervi, Carapax Trionycis, Concha Ostreae, Otheca Mantidis, Radix Ginseng, Radix Astragali, Radix Angelicae Sinensis, Radix Peoniae Alba, Rhizoma Cyperi, Radix Asparagali, Radix Glycyrrhizae, Radix Rehmanniae, Rhizoma Chuanxiong, Radix Stellariae, Radix Salviae Miltiorrhizae, Rhizoma Dioscoreae, Semen Euryales* and *Cornu Cervi Degelatinatum.*

[Effects] Replenishes *qi* and blood, regulates menstruation, and arrests excessive leukorrhea.

[Indications] Menstrual disorders with abnormal uterine bleeding and excessive leukorrhea due to deficiency of both *qi* and blood.

[Usage and Dosage] 1 big pill (9 g), 2 times a day.

***Gengnian'an Pian* (Menopause-quieting Tablet)**

[Ingredients] *Radix Rehmanniae Preparata, Radix Polygoni Multiflori, Rhizoma Alismatis, Poria, Fructus Schisandrae, Concha Margaritifera Usta, Radix Scrophylariae, Fructus Tritici Levis*, etc.

[Effects] Nourishes *yin*, removes heat and induces tranquilization.

[Indications] Menopausal syndrome marked by afternoon fever, excessive sweating, dizziness, tinnitus, insomnia and unsteady blood pressure.

[Usage and Dosage] 6 tablets, 2-3 times a day.

Medicines for Diseases of the Ear, Nose, Throat and Mouth

***Erlong Zuoci Wan* (Rehmannia Pill for Treating Deafness)**

[Ingredients] *Magnetitum, Radix Rehmanniae, Fructus Corni, Cortex Moutan, Rhizoma Dioscoreae, Poria, Rhizoma Alismatis* and *Radix Bupleuri Marginati.*

[Effects] Replenishes the Kidneys and subdues hyperactive Liver.

[Indications] Tinnitus and impairment of hearing due to *yin* deficiency of the Liver and the Kidneys with exuberance of Liver *yang*.

[Usage and Dosage] 6 g of water-honeyed pills or 9 g of small honeyed pills, 2 times a day.

***Biyan Pian* (Pill for Treating Rhinitis)**

[Ingredients] *Fructus Xanthii, Flos Magnoliae, Radix Saposhnikoviae, Fructus Forsythiae, Flos Chrysanthemi Indici, Fructus Schisandrae, Radix Platycodi, Radix Angelicae Dahuricae, Rhizoma Anemarrhenae, Herba Schizonepetae* and *Radix Glycyrrhizae.*

[Effects] Dispels wind and removes toxic heat from the nose.

[Indications] Acute and chronic rhinitis and sinusitis.

[Usage and Dosage] 3-4 tablets, 3 times a day.

***Daochi Wan* (Redness-removing Pill)**

[Ingredients] *Fructus Forsythiae, Rhizome Coptidis, Fructus Gardeniae, Caulis Aristolochiae Manshuriensis, Radix Scrophulariae, Radix Trichosanthis, Radix Paeoniae Rubra, Radix et Rhizoma Rhei, Radix Scutellariae* and *Talcum.*

[Effects] Removes heat, quenches fire, and relaxes the bowels.

[Indications] Ulcers in the mouth or on the tongue, sore throat, burning sensation during urination, and constipation.

[Usage and Dosage] 3 g, 2 times a day.

***Niuhuang Jiedu Pian* (Bezoar Detoxicant Pill)**

[Ingredients] *Calculus Bovis, Realgar, Gypsum Fibrosum, Radix et Rhizoma Rhei, Radix Scutellariae, Radix Platycodi, Borneolum Syntheticum* and *Radix Glycyrrhizae.*

[Effects] Removes toxic fire.

[Indications] Sore throat, swollen and painful gums, ulcers in the mouth or on the tongue, and inflammation of the eye due to excessive fire.

[Usage and Dosage] 2-4 tablets, 2 times a day.

[Warning] Contraindicated in pregnancy.

Bingpeng San **(Borneolum and Borax Powder)**

[Ingredients] *Borneolum Syntheticum, Borax, Cinnabaris* and *Natrii Sulfas Exsiccatus*.

[Effects] Removes toxic heat, reduces swelling and alleviates pain.

[Indications] Sore throat, painful swelling of the gums, and ulcers in the mouth or on the tongue.

[Usage and Dosage] A small quantity to be insufflated to the afflicted area, several times a day.

Liushen Wan **(Miraculous Pill of Six Ingredients)**

[Ingredients] Calculus Bovis, Moschus, Margarita, Borneolum, Venenum Bufonis and Realgar.

[Effects] Removes toxic heat and relieves pain.

[Indications] Pharyngitis, tonsilitis, stomatitis, periodontitis, mastitis, and boils.

[Usage and Dosage] 8 pillets, 2 times a day; for external use, 10 pellets to be mixed with liquid and applied topically.

Medicines for Rheumatic Conditions

Xiao Huoluo Wan **(Pill for Activating Circulation in Collateral Meridians—Minor Recipe)**

[Ingredients] *Arisaema cum Bile, Radix Aconiti Preparata, Radix Aconiti Kusnezoffii Preparata, Lumbricus, Olibanum* and *Myrrha*.

[Effects] Relieves rheumatic conditions and removes obstructions from the collateral meridians.

[Indications] Rheumatoid arthritis with joint pain, numbness and muscle contracture.

[Usage and Dosage] 3 g, 2 times a day.

[Warning] Contraindicated in pregnancy.

Mugua Wan **(Chaenomeles Fruit Pill)**

[Ingredients] *Fructus Chaenomelis, Radix Angelicae Sinensis, Rhizoma Chuanxiong, Radix Angelicae Dahuricae, Radix Clematidis, Rhizoma Cibotii, Radix Achyranthis Bidentatae, Caulis Spatholobi, Caulis Piperis Futokadsurae, Radix Ginseng, Radix Aconiti Preparata* and *Radix Aconiti Kusnezoffii Preparata*.

[Effects] Dispels wind-cold, removes obstruction from the collateral meridians, and relieves pain.

[Indications] Rheumatic or rheumatoid arthritis with numbness of the limbs, general aching, limpness of the knees and difficulty in walking.

[Usage and Dosage] 30 pills (4.5 g), 2 times a day.

***Guogong Jiu* (Guogong Wine)**

[Ingredients] *Radix Angelicae Sinensis, Rhizoma Chuanxiong, Radix Angelicae Pubescentis, Radix Achyranthis Bidentatae, Fructus Citri Sarcodactylis, Rhizoma Polygonati Odorati*, etc.

[Effects] Relieves rheumatic conditions and muscular contracture.

[Indications] Rheumatoid arthritis with pain in the back and legs, and difficulty in walking.

[Usage and Dosage] 10 ml, 2 times a day.

Medicines for Traumatic Injuries

***Qili San* (Anti-bruises Powder)**

[Ingredients] *Resina Draconis, Olibanum, Myrrha, Flos Carthami, Catechu, Borneolum Syntheticum, Moschus* and *Cinnabaris.*

[Effects] Removes blood stasis, reduces swelling, relieves pain and arrests bleeding.

[Indications] Traumatic injuries with blood stasis, pain and/or bleeding

[Usage and Dosage] 1-1.5 g, 1-3 times a day; for external use, an appropriate quantity to be mixed with liquid and applied topically.

[Warning] Contraindicated in pregnancy.

***Huoxue Zhitong San* (Blood-activating Analgesic Powder)**

[Ingredients] *Radix Angelicae Sinensis, Radix Notoginseng, Olibanum, Borneolum Syntheticum, Eupolyphaga seu Steleophaga* and *Pyritum.*

[Effects] Activates blood circulation, removes stasis, reduces swelling and alleviates pain.

[Indications] Traumatic injury with ecchymosis, swelling and pain.

[Usage and Dosage] 1.5 g, 2 times a day.

[Warning] Contraindicated in pregnancy.

***Yunnan Baiyao* (Yunnan White Drug)**

[Effects] Arrests bleeding, relieves pain and removes blood stasis.

[Indications] Traumatic bleeding, and other hemorrhages.

[Usage and Dosage] 0.2 g, 2-3 times a day.

[Warning] Contraindicated in pregnancy.

Tonic Medicines

***Buzhong Yiqi Wan* (Pill for Reinforcing the Middle Energizer and Replenishing *Qi*)**

[Ingredients] *Radix Astragali, Radix Ginseng, Rhizoma Atractylodis Macrocephalae, Radix Glycyrrhizae, Radix Angelicae Sinensis, Pericarpium Citri Reticulatae, Rhizome Cimicifugae* and *Radix Bupleuri.*

[Effects] Tonifies the Spleen and Stomach, and elevates *qi*.

[Indications] (1) Repeated attacks of influenza, persistent fever in influenza or post-influenza asthenia due to deficiency of *qi*; (2) Prolapse of uterus, gastroptosis, blepharoptosis, protracted diarrhea with prolapse of the rectum, and functional uterine bleeding due to sinking of *qi*.

[Usage and Dosage] 6 g, 3 times a day.

Bazhen Wan **(Pill of Eight Precious Ingredients)**

[Ingredients] *Radix Ginseng, Rhizoma Atractylodis Macrocephalae, Poria, Radix Glycyrrhizae, Radix Angelicae Sinensis, Radix Paeoniae Alba, Rhizoma Chuanxiong* and *Radix Rehmanniae Preparata.*

[Effects] Replenishes *qi* and blood.

[Indications] Deficiency of *qi* and blood with sallow complexion, anorexia, lack of strength and excessive menstruation.

[Usage and Dosage] 6 g or water-honeyed pills or 1 big honeyed pill, 2 times a day.

Shiquan Dabu Wan **(Pill of Ten Powerful Tonics)**

[Ingredients] Ingredients of *Bazhen Wan* + *Radix Astragali* and *Cortex Cinnamomi.*

[Effects] Warms and replenishes *qi* and blood.

[Indications] Deficiency of *qi* and blood with pallor, shortness of breath, palpitations, lack of strength and cold extremities, or excessive menstruation.

[Usage and Dosage] 6 g or water-honeyed pills or 1 big honeyed pill, 2-3 times a day.

Guipi Wan **(Spleen-invigorating Pill)** or ***Renshen Guipi Wan*** **(Spleen-Invigorating Pill with Ginseng)**

[Ingredients] *Radix Astragali, Rhizoma Atractylodis Macrocephalae, Poria, Arillus Longan, Semen Ziziphi Spinosae, Radix Ginseng, Radix Aucklandiae, Radix Glycyrrhizae, Radix Angelicae Sinensis* and *Radix Polygalae.*

[Effects] Invigorates the Spleen, nourishes blood, and induces tranquilization.

[Indications] Deficiency of both the Spleen *qi* and the Heart blood, marked by: (1) Insomnia and palpitations; (2) Pallor, lack of strength and reduced food intake; (3) Various kinds of bleeding such as thrombocytopenic purpura and functional uterine bleeding.

[Usage and Dosage] 6 g of water-honeyed pills or 9 g of small honeyed pills, 3 times a day.

Liuwei Dihuang Wan **(Pill of Six Ingredients with Rehmannia)**

[Ingredients] *Radix Rehmanniae Preparata, Fructus Corni, Rhizoma Dioscoreae, Rhizoma Alismatis, Cortex Moutan* and *Poria.*

[Effects] Replenishes Kidney *yin*.

[Indications] Deficiency of Kidney *yin* marked by dizziness, tinnitus, aching and weakness in the loins and knees, night sweating, seminal emission or diabetes.

[Usage and Dosage] 6 g of water-honeyed pills or 9 g of small honeyed pills, 2 times a day.

***Zhi Bai Dihuang Wan* (Rehmannia Pill with Anemarrhena and Phellodendron)**

[Ingredients] Ingredients of *Liuwei Dihuang Wan* (Pill of Six Ingredients with Rehmannia) + *Rhizoma Anemarrhenae* and *Cortex Phellodendri.*

[Effects] Replenishes *yin* and subdues fire.

[Indications] Deficiency of *yin* with exuberant fire manifested by consumptive fever, night sweating, dryness of mouth or sore throat.

[Usage and Dosage] 6 g of water-honeyed pills or 9 g of small honeyed pills, 2 times a day.

***Qi Ju Dihuang Wan* (Rehmannia Pill with Wolfberry and Chrysanthemum)**

[Ingredients] Ingredients of Liuwei Dihaung Wan (Pill of Six Ingredients with Rehmannia) + *Fructus Lycii* and *Flos Chrysanthemi.*

[Effects] Replenishes Liver and the Kidney *yin.*

[Indications] *yin* deficiency of the Liver and the Kidneys, with blurred vision or dryness and pain in the eyes.

[Usage and Dosage] 6 g of water-honeyed pills or 9 g of small honeyed pills, 2 times a day.

***Mai Wei Dihuang Wan* (Rehmannia Pill with Lilyturf and Schisandra)**

[Ingredients] Ingredients of *Liuwei Dihuang Wan* (Pill of Six Ingredients with Rehmannia) + *Radix Ophiopogonis* and *Fructus Schisandrae.*

[Effects] Replenishes *yin* of the Kidneys and Lungs.

[Indications] *Yin* deficiency of the Kidney and the Lungs marked by coughing, hemoptysis, afternoon fever and night sweating.

[Usage and Dosage] 6 g of water-honeyed pills or 9 g of small honeyed pills, 2 times a day.

***Wuzi Yanzong Wan* (Pill of Five Kinds of Seeds for Offsprings)**

[Ingredients] *Fructus Lycii, Semen Cuscutae, Fructus Rubi, Fructus Schisandrae* and *Semen Plantaginis.*

[Effects] Replenishes Kidney essence.

[Indications] Deficiency of Kidney essence marked by backache, dribbling of urine after micturition, seminal emission, premature ejaculation, impotence and sterility.

[Usage and Dosage] 6 g, 2 times a day.

***Jinsuo Gujing Wan* (Golden Lock Pill for Semen Discharge)**

[Ingredients] *Semen Astragali Complanati, Semen Euryales, Stamen Nelumbinis, Os Draconis Ustum* and *Concha Ostreae Usta.*

[Effects] Strengthens the Kidneys and arrests seminal discharge.

[Indications] Seminal emission and spermatorrhea due to Kidney insufficiency.

[Usage and Dosage] 9 g, 2 times a day.

Guifu Dihuang Wan **(Rehmannia Pill with Cinnamon and Aconite)**

[Ingredients] Ingredients of *Liuwei Dihuang Wan* (Pill of Six Ingredients with Rehmannia) + *Radix Aconiti Lateralis Preparata* and *Cortex Cinnamomi.*

[Effects] Reinforces Kidney *yang*.

[Indications] *Yang* deficiency of the Kidneys marked by cold sensation in the loins and knees, oliguria, edema, or polyuria, as occurring in chronic nephritis with edema, diabetes mellitus, prostatic hyperplasia and sexual impotence.

[Usage and Dosage] 6 g of water-honeyed pills or 9 g of small honeyed pills, 2 times a day.

PART THREE

ACUPUNCTURE AND MOXIBUSTION

INTRODUCTION

In China acupuncture and moxibustion are usually combined as order of *zhen-jiu*, i.e., acupuncture preceding moxibustion. In ancient times, however, they were referred to in the reverse order, as *jiu-ci*, i.e., moxibustion preceding needling, which indicates the earlier application of moxibustion than that of acupuncture.

Both acupuncture and moxibustion were invented by the Chinese as early as in the clan commune period of primitive society about 10,000-4,000 years ago. In the Stone Age, stone needles (called *bian*) were manufactured for therapeutic purposes. From the fifth century B.C., with the introduction and application of iron instruments, stone needles were replaced by metal needles. This greatly promoted acupuncture practice. Cases of successful treatment with acupuncture appeared in the historical records, as did writings on acupuncture and moxibustion.

Initially, acupuncture and moxibustion were applied at the tender points; "pain indicates the point" was the rule to determine the site of treatment. Discovery of the acupoints was a milestone in the progress of this art of healing. After repeated trials, a certain number of points were found to have therapeutic effects. Their locations, actions and indications were defined, and each of them was given a special name. Some of the acupoints were recorded as early as in *The Canon of Medicine*. In the *Zhenjiu Jiayi Jing* (*ABC Classic of Acupunture and Moxibustion*, ca. 259) 349 acupoints were discussed, together with texual research. In the *Zhenjiu Fengyuan* (*Source of Acupuncture and Moxibustion*, 1815) 361 acupoints of the 14 meridians were collected, and this acupoint list is still in use.

Along with the discovery of acupoints, the hypothesis of the meridian system was established, chiefly based on the correlation between the acupoints and internal organs, and the transmission of acupuncture sensation. It provided a theoretical basis for acupuncture and moxibustion, and made them a special branch of Chinese medicine.

CHAPTER 12

THE MERIDIAN SYSTEM

GENERAL CONSIDERATIONS

The meridian system includes meridians and collaterals. These are conduits through which *qi* and blood circulate, and by which the internal organs are related to the superficial organs and tissues, making the body an organic whole. In the Chinese language meridians are *jing* (经), which means the main conduits, and collaterals are *luo* (络), which means the subsidiary conduits. In books on acupuncture written in English, *jing* has frequently been translated as "channel," but according to the Standard Nomenclature of Acupuncture proposed by the World Health Organization, the term "meridian" is recommended. The two translations reflect different concepts. Those who use the word "channel" adhere to the hypothesis that there exists a structure that forms the tube-like passages for *qi* and blood. Since the descriptions of the courses of channels differ greatly from the present knowledge of anatomy, there should be some structure other than the known blood vessels and nerves. Many scientists have engaged in research into the substantial structure of the "channels," but up to now no new structure has been discovered along the "channels." Therefore, the word "meridian" seems to be more appropriate, as it passes through certain points but has no substantial structure.

I. Historical development of the concept of meridian system

One of the puzzling questions about the meridians is whether they are passages for blood. Doubtless, meridians in traditional Chinese medicine include the ducts containing and circulating blood. At the very beginning, both *jing* and *luo* were attributes of *mai* (脉) which means a blood vessel. *Jing* was and still is an abbreviation of *jing-mai*, namely, the main blood vessels running vertically, and *luo*, an abbreviation of *luo-mai*, namely, the subsidiary blood vessels running obliquely and forming a network. At the earliest stage of the development of acupuncture, the treatment was merely to cause bleeding by puncturing the skin at certain points. As *The Canon of Acupuncture* (also called *Miraculous Pivot*, being a part of the *Canon of Medicine*) states, "Acupuncture is completed whenever there is bleeding." At later stages, acupuncture sensation was discovered, and was believed to indicate the movement of *qi*. With repeated practice it was concluded in the *Canon of Acupuncture* that, as the key to acupuncture, therapeutic effect can be achieved only after achieving sensation. Thereafter, *qi* was more closely related to the meridian system than blood.

The development of the hypothesis of the meridian system was not only based on acupuncture. *Qigong* also made contributions to the formation of the hypothesis. During *qigong* exercises, the upward and downward movement of *qi* can be felt. The ancient graphic records of *qi* movement during *qigong* exercise were basically identical to the courses of the meridians. So, in *qigong* and also in acupuncture the meridian system referred more to the passage of *qi* than to the circulation of blood.

If the meridian system were chiefly related to the circulation of blood, the issue would be simplified, and the meridian system could be just taken as the vascular system. The divergence of the traditional description of the meridian system from the modern description of the vascular system could be attributed to the lack of anatomical knowledge in ancient times. However, as *qi* is chiefly involved in the formation of the hypothesis of meridians, the condition would be much more complicated because there is no such concept in modern Western medicine that is exactly equivalent to *qi*. So far as feeling or sensation is concerned, the nervous system probably plays an important role, but neither the course of meridians nor the transmission of acupuncture sensation conforms to the distribution of the nervous system. Therefore, the hypothesis of the meridian system should not be refuted merely by citing the lack of anatomical knowledge of the nervous system.

II. Evidence Indicating the Existence of Meridians in Modern Studies

(1) Transmission of acupuncture sensation along the meridians. Stimulation at an acupoint may give rise to a specific sensation such as soreness, distension or tingling transmitted from the acupoint along the course of the meridian, as described traditionally. This is also called "meridian transmission," and those who can easily feel the meridian transmission are called "meridian-sensitive" persons. In a survey carried out by the China Academy of Traditional Chinese Medicine and others, among 5,906 subjects tested, 65 (1.1%) were found to have meridian transmission along three or more meridians when impulse stimulation with low-frequency electricity was applied to the 12 well points (points located at the ends of the fingers and toes). About 10-20% of the population showed meridian transmission along one or two meridians. The feelings transmitted were described as tingling, fluid-flowing, pulsating, formicating, cooling or heating. The speed of transmission was quite slow, only a few cm per second. Conformity of the meridian transmission to the classical description of meridian courses was observed in 81% of meridian-sensitive persons. On the limbs, the meridian transmission was basically identical to the classical description of meridian courses, while divergence happened occasionally on the trunk, and frequently on the head and face.

(2) Blockade of meridian transmission. It is recorded in monographs on acupuncture written about five hundred years ago that the direction of acupuncture sensation can be changed by pressing the skin with a finger. Modern research has shown that meridian transmission can be blocked by mechanical pressure or cooling. For example, acupuncture at Hegu (LI 4), a point on the dorsum of the hand, between the 1st and 2nd metacarpal bones, and on the radial side of the midpoint of the 2nd metacarpal bone, can produce transmission of acupuncture sensation up to Yingxiang (LI 20) in the nasolabial groove. Pressure at Shousanli (LI 10), a point on the radial side of the dorsal surface of the forearm,

2 *cun* below the cubital crease, blocked the transmission of acupuncture sensation. The sensation disappeared above (proximal to) that point, while it was still there or even augmented below (distal to) that point. Removal of the pressure restored the transmission of acupuncture sensation to Yingxiang (LI 20). This could be repeatedly demonstrated in a short period of time. Similar changes were also demonstrated by local cooling at Shousanli (LI 10) with an ice bag, but it took a longer time to block or restore acupuncture sensation transmission. Examination of the sensory conducting function of the radial nerve showed no change in the incubation period, persistent period and amplitude when pressure was applied to Shousanli (LI 10) during needling at Hegu (LI 4). The above results indicate that blockage of meridian transmission is not due to disturbance of nervous conductivity.

(3) Conformity of linear skin lesions to the meridian courses. It was reported that many patients with linear skin diseases, either congenital (such as nevus verrucosus, pigmented nevus, nevus anemicus, nevus sebaceus and porokeratosis) or acquired (such as neurodermatitis, lichen planus, eczema, and scleroderma), had their lesions distributed in conformity with the meridian courses.

Though the skin lesions differed in morphology in patients with different skin diseases, they were all distributed along the meridian courses, basically identical with the classical descriptions. The linear skin lesions were usually about 1 cm in width. In each patient all the lesions along the same meridian or along several meridians had the same pathological changes; for example, the lesions all occurred in sebaceous glands in patients with nevus sebaceus distributed along the meridian. In some cases, the skin lesion occurred along two or more meridians. These cases provided more evidence to show that conformity of the skin lesions to the meridian courses was not merely a curious coincidence.

(4) Hallucinative meridian transmission in artificial limbs. It has also been reported that phantom limb and meridian transmission can be induced by acupuncture in patients with artificial limbs. This indicates that meridian transmission cannot be taken as evidence to prove the substantial tube-like structure of the meridians. Since the feeling of a phantom limb can be induced by stimulation of the parietal lobe, and eliminated by excision of the postcentral gyrus, indicating the production of a phantom limb feeling in the cerebral cortex, meridian transmission may also be related to the cerebral cortex.

In conclusion, modern studies can confirm only meridian transmission, but not the morphological structure of meridians.

III. The Composition of the Meridian System

The meridian system is composed of (1) twelve regular meridians, (2) twelve divergent meridians, (3) eight extra meridians, (4) fifteen main collaterals, and (5) superficial collaterals and minute collaterals, as shown in the following diagram. In addition, the meridian system also includes the connection of the twelve meridians with the *zang-fu* organs in the interior, and with the muscles, joints, skin zones and acupoints in the exterior (Table XII-1).

1. The twelve regular meridians. The main body of the meridian system is the twelve regular meridians. The nomenclature of the twelve regular meridians is based

on three factors: (1) the hand or foot (on which the meridian courses), (2) the *yin* or *yang* (aspect of the limb along which the meridian runs), and (3) the *zang* or *fu* organ (to which the meridian pertains). The names of the twelve meridians are shown in Table XII-2.

Table XII-1 Composition of the Meridian System

- Twelve Regular Meridians
  - Hand
    - Three *Yin*
      - Lungs (Hand-Taiyin) → Lieque (LU 7)*
      - Pericardium (Hand-Jueyin) → Neiguan (PC 6)*
      - Heart (Hand-Shaoyin) → Tongli (HT 5)*
    - Three *Yang*
      - Large Intestine (Hand-Yangming) → Pianli (LI 6)*
      - Triple Energizer (Hand-Shaoyang) → Waiguan (TE 5)*
      - Small Intestine (Hand-Taiyang) → Zhizen (SI 7)*
  - Foot
    - Three *Yin*
      - Spleen (Foot-Taiyin) → Gongsun (SP 4)*; → Dabao (SP 21)*
      - Liver (Foot-Jueyin) → Ligou (LR 5)*
      - Kidney (Foot-Shaoyin) → Dazhong (KI 5)*
    - Three Yang
      - Stomach (Foot-Yangming) → Fenglong (ST 40)*
      - Gallbladder (Foot-Shaoyang) → Guangming (GB 37)*
      - Bladder (Foot-Taiyang) → Feiyang (BL 58)*
- Eight Extra Meridians
  - Governor Vessel → Collateral of GV → Changqiang (GV 1)*
  - Conception Vessel → Collateral of CV → Jiuwei (CD 15)*
  - Thoroughfare Vessel, Belt Vessel, Yang Heel Vessel, Yin Heel Vessel, Yang Link Vessel, Yin Link Vessel — meet with the above 14 meridians
- Twelve Divergent Meridians
- Twelve Meridian Muscles
- Twelve Cutaneous Zones

(The collaterals listed above for the twelve regular meridians and the Governor and Conception Vessels form the Fifteen Main Collaterals.)

Collaterals: Fifteen Main Collaterals → Superficial Collaterals, Minute Collaterals

* The point from which the main collateral starts.

2. The branches of the twelve meridians. Each regular meridian has its branches going deep into the body, connecting various *zang-fu* organs.

3. The eight extra meridians (vessels). There are eight meridians which do not directly pertain to *zang-fu* organs, nor have their courses on the limbs. They are the Governor Vessel (GV), Conception Vessel (CV), Thoroughfare Vessel (TV), Belt Vessel (BV), *Yang* Heel Vessel (YangHV), *Yin* Heel Vessel (YinHV), *Yang* Link Vessel (YangLV), and *Yin* Link Vessel (YinLV). The Governor Vessel is also called the "sea of *yang* vessels" because it connects with all the six *yang* meridians, and The Conception Vessel called the "sea of *yin* vessels" because it connects with all the six *yin* meridians. The Governor and Conception Vessels have their own acupoints, but all the other extra meridians only have their acupoints attached to the regular meridians. Therefore, it is usually said that the acupoints belong to fourteen meridians (namely, the twelve regular meridians plus the Governor and Conception Vessels).

Table XII-2 Nomenclature of the Twelve Regular Meridians

	Hand (Upper Limb)	Foot (Lower Limb)
Flexor or innter aspect (*yin*)		
Taiyin*	Lungs (LU)	Spleen (SP)
Shaoyin*	Heart (HT)	Kidneys (KI)
Jueyin*	Pericardium (PC)	Liver (LV)
Extensor or outer aspect (*yang*)		
Yangming**	Large Intestine (LI)	Stomach (ST)
Taiyang**	Small Intestine (SI)	Bladder (BL)
Shaoyang**	Triple Energizer (TE)	Gallbladder (GB)

* Taiyin literally means the greater *yin*; it refers to the radial side of the inner (flexor) aspect of the upper limb or the anteromedial side of the lower limb. Shaoyin literally means the lesser *yin*; it refers to the ulnar side of the inner aspect of the upper limb or the medial side of the lower limb. Jueyin literally means reversing *yin*; it refers to the midline of the inner aspect of the upper limb or the posteromedial side of the lower limb.

** Yangming literally means splendid *yang*; it refers to the radial side of the outer (extensor) aspect of the upper limb or the anterolateral side of the lower limb. Taiyang literally means greater *yang*; it refers to the ulnar side of the outer aspect of the upper limb or the posterior side of the lower limb. Shaoyang literally means lesser *yang*; it refers to the midline of the outer aspect of the upper limb or the lateral side of the lower limb.

4. The fifteen main collaterals. Each of the fourteen meridians has a main collateral. Together with the great collateral of the Spleen, there are fifteen in all, which communicate with the exterior and interior of the body.

5. Superficial collaterals and minute collaterals. The collaterals lying just beneath

the skin are called superficial collaterals. Minute collaterals or capillaries are subdivided small branches of the meridians or capillaries. Through these collaterals, *qi* and blood are spread all over the body.

6. The twelve meridian muscle groups. There are twelve groups of muscles along which the meridians travel. These muscles, linking the joints, integrate motion. Disorders of the meridians involving the muscles result in rheumatism, contraction of the limbs, and motion impairment.

7. The twelve cutaneous zones. The cutaneous zones above the courses of the meridians are the superficial areas that reflect pathological conditions of the internal organs, and are also the portals of entry for pathogenic factors.

IV. Distribution of the Meridians

1. The twelve regular meridians

The general rules of the distribution of the regular meridians on the body's surface are: the inner pertains to *yin*, and the outer to *yang*; the abdomen pertains to *yin*, and the back to *yang*; the head is the place where all the *yang* meridians meet, and no superficial part of the *yin* meridians reaches the head. The twelve regular meridians are mainly longitudinally distributed along the limbs, trunk, and head and face, symmetrically on the right and left sides.

The three *yin* meridians of the hand go from the chest (the lungs, heart and pericardium) to the hand, and the three *yin* meridians of the foot from the foot to the abdomen (the spleen, liver and kidneys). On the limbs, they run along the inner aspect, with Taiyin in the anterior, Jueyin in the middle, and Shaoyin in the posterior.

The three *yang* meridians of the hand run from the hand to the head, and the three *yang* meridians of the foot from the head to the foot. On the limbs, they run along the outer aspect, with Yangming in the anterior, Shaoyang in the middle, and Taiyang in the posterior.

The connections of the twelve regular meridians are shown in Table XII-3. The *yin* meridians connect with their interior-exteriorly related *yang* meridians (e.g., the Lung Meridian of Hand Taiyin and the Large Intestine Meridian of Hand Yangming) at the fingers or toes. The *yang* meridians connect with the *yang* meridians of the same name (e.g., the Large Intestine Meridian of Hand Yangming and the Stomach Meridian of Foot Yangming) at the head or face. The *yin* meridians connect with the *yin* meridians in the chest. Thus, the twelve regular meridians form a circle, through which *qi* circulates.

2. The Governor Vessel and Conception Vessel. Both the Governor and Conception Vessels originate in the lower abdomen, and reach the body's surface at the perineum. The Governor Vessel runs along the midline of the back up to the head, and then the face. The Conception vessel runs along the midline of the abdomen and chest up to the chin.

V. Functions of the Meridians

1. Functions in physiology: (1) The meridians link various parts of the body into an organic whole. (2) The meridians are the courses along which *qi* and blood circulate to nourish the body. (3) The meridians protect the body against external pathogenic factors.

2. Functions in pathology: (1) Diseases of the internal organs are often reflected at other sites of the body through the meridians. For example, hypochondriac pain in Liver diseases, supraclavicular pain in Lung diseases, ulceration of the tongue in flaming up of Heart fire, congested eyes in exuberance of Liver fire, impairment of hearing in deficiency of Kidney qi, can all be explained by means of the meridians. (2) Exogenous affection can be transmitted from the exterior to the interior along the meridians. For example, when pathogens attack the body from outside, they stay in the superficial portion first, involving the minute collaterals. If they are not dispelled in time, they will enter the Lungs through the Hand Taiyang Meridian, leading to upper respiratory symptoms. They can be further transmitted to the large intestine from the Hand Taiyang to Foot Yangming Meridians, leading to high fever with constipation.

3. Functions in diagnosis: (1) Diseases of the internal organs may be reflected on the body's surface through the meridians. Inspection and palpation on the course of the meridian may obtain some signs (such as tender points) indicating the impairment of related internal organs. (2) The course of the meridians may give information about differential diagnosis. For example, in the diagnosis of headache, if the headache is located at the vertex, it is related to the Liver Meridian; if it is located at the occipital region involving the nape, it is related to the Bladder Meridian.

4. Functions in treatment. Meridians often serve as the basis of point selection. There are three common ways to select acupoints according to the meridians: (1) Treating the lower part of the body when the symptoms appear in the upper part, e.g., using Taichong (LR 3) on the foot in the treatment of vertical headache. (2) Treating the upper part of the body when the symptoms appear in the lower part, e.g., needling Baihui (GV 20) at the top of the head in the treatment of prolapse of the rectum. (3) Selecting points from the interior-exteriorly related meridians, e.g., using Yanglingquan (GB 34) in the treatment of Liver diseases, and Gongsun (SP 4) in the treatment of Stomach diseases.

THE TWELVE REGULAR MERIDIANS

I. Lung Meridian of Hand-Taiyin (LU) (Fig. XII-1)

Course: The Lung Meridian begins internally in the Middle Energizer, descends to connect with the large intestine, then ascends to the lungs and throat, moves laterally and exits superficially at Zhongfu (LU 1). Then it descends along the lateral side of the arm and forearm, and terminates at Shaoshang (LU 11) on the radial aspect of the thumb, where it connects with the Large Intestine Meridian, with 11 points on either side. It has a branch running from Lieque (LU 7) to the radial side of the tip of the index finger.

Symptomatology: coughing, asthma, shortness of breath, hemoptysis, sore throat, common cold, oppressive feeling in the chest, pain in and numbness of the supraclavicular fossa and dorsal aspect of the forearm, pain and coldness in the shoulder and back.

II. Large Intestine Meridian of Hand-Yangming (LI) (Fig. XII-2)

Course: The Large Intestine Meridian runs from Shangyang (LI 1) on the radial side of the index finger and ascends the dorsal surface of the hand and forearm, the lateral side of the arm, and the dorsal side of the shoulder to Jugu (LI 16) where the meridian enters internally and travels posteriorly to Dazhui (GV 14), and then moves anteriorly to the supraclavicular fossa, where it descends past the diaphragm to connect with the large intestine. The superficial supraclavicular branch ascends the anterior lateral neck and the mandible, connects internally with the lower teeth, encircles the lips and terminates at the opposite Yingxiang (LI 20). There are 20 points on either side.

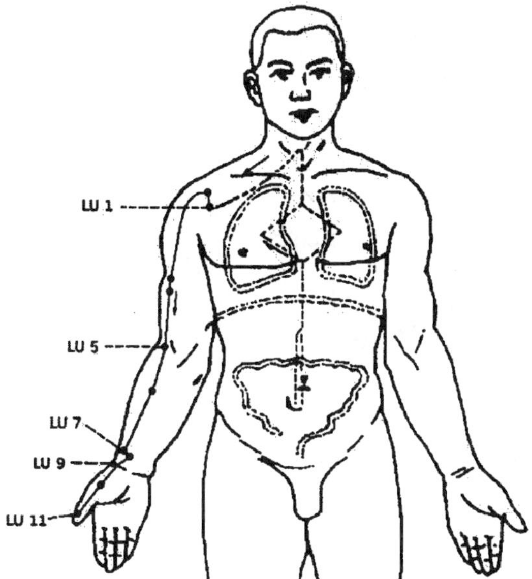

Fig. XII-1 Lung Meridian

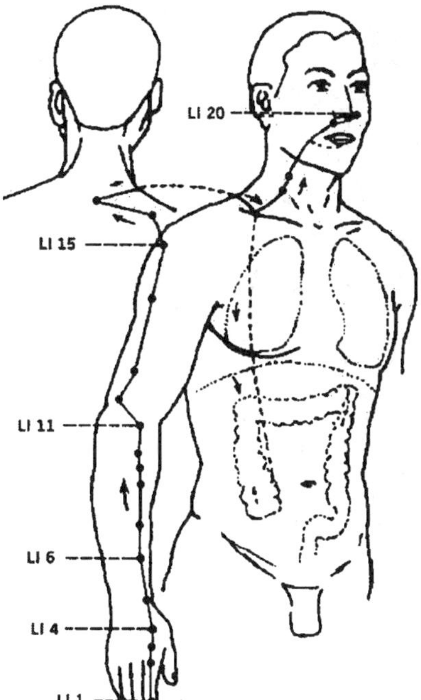

Fig. XII-2 Large Intestine Meridian

Symptomatology: abdominal pain, borborygmi, diarrhea, dysentery, pharyngitis, toothache, rhinorrhea, epistaxis, pain in the shoulder, arm and forefinger, fever and chills.

III. Stomach Meridian of Foot-Yangming (ST) (Fig. XII-3)

Course: The Stomach Meridian originates internally at the lateral edge of the nose, ascends to the medial canthus of the eye, then continues to the first superficial point Chenqi (ST 1) at the inferior border of the orbit, descends to the upper gum, courses around the mouth, and travels up to Touwei (ST 8). From here it continues internally to terminate at Shenting (GV 24). The facial branch descends from Daying (ST 5), turns

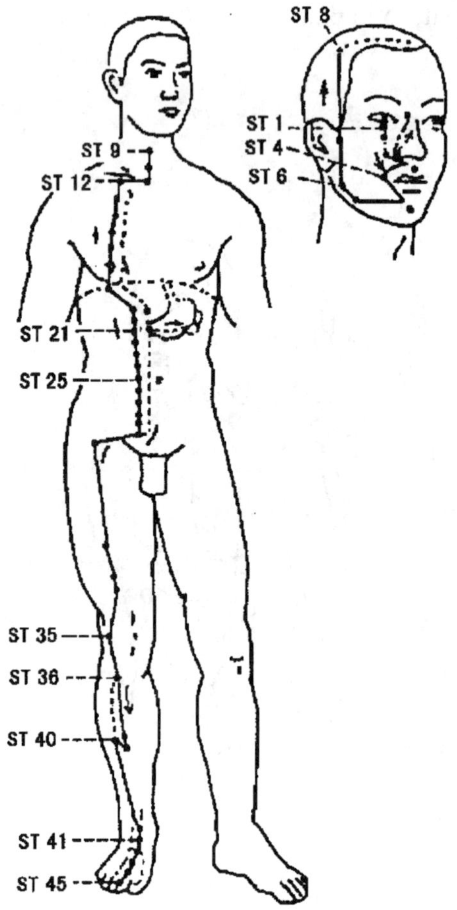

Fig. XII-3 Stomach Meridian

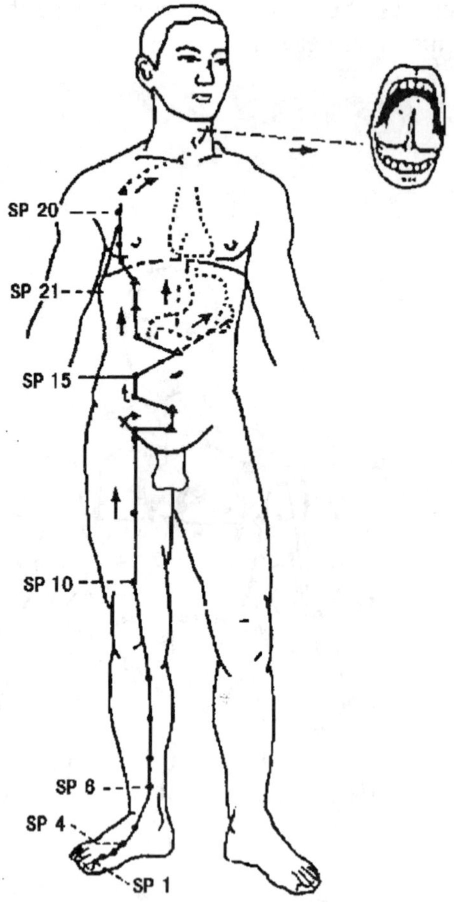

Fig. XII-4 Spleen Meridian

internally and descends past the diaphragm to connect with the stomach and spleen. The supraclavicular fossa branch descends along the midclavicular line to Qichong (ST 30) in the inguinal region, then anteriorly along the lateral margin of the femur to the patella, terminating at Lidui (ST 45) on the lateral side of the tip of the second toe. The gastric branch descends internally past the umbilicus, and terminates at Qichong (ST 30). The tibial branch leaves Zusanli (ST 36) and descends along the fibula, terminating at the lateral side of the tip of the middle toe. The dorsal foot branch leaves Chongyang (ST 42) and descends to the medial side of the big toe at Yingbai (SP 1). There are 45 points on either side.

Symptomatology: borborygmi, abdominal distension, edema, gastralgia, vomiting, epistaxis, facial hemiplegia, sore and swollen throat, and burning sensation in the regions which the meridian passes through the chest, abdomen and lower extremities.

IV. Spleen Meridian of Foot-Taiyin (SP) (Fig. XII-4)

Course: The Spleen Meridian runs from Yingbai (SP 1) on the medial side of the big toe, ascends along the medial side of foot and tibia and antero-medial side of the thigh to the abdomen, entering the abdomen and connecting with the spleen and stomach. The meridian ascends the abdomen at a distance of 4 cun lateral to the Conception Vessel, and terminates superficially at Dabao (SP 21) in the sixth intercostal space on the midaxillary line. The meridian continues internally past the supraclavicular fossa and terminates at the base of the tongue. The gastric branch leaves the stomach and ascends internally past the diaphragm, and connects with the heart. There are 21 points on either side.

Symptomatology: abdominal distension, epigastric pain, nausea and vomiting, diarrhea, eructation jaundice, stiffness of the tongue and pain in the medial aspect of knee.

V. Heart Meridian of Hand-Shaoyin (HT) (Fig. XII-5)

Course: The heart meridian originates in the heart, descends internally past the diaphragm, and connects with the small intestine. The cardiac branch ascends internally paralateral to the esophagus and terminates at the eye. The main branch leaves the heart, traverses the lungs and emerges superficially in the midaxilla at Jiquan (HT 1), and then descends along the ulnar side of the forearm medially, terminating at Shaochong (HT 9) on the radial side of the tip of the little finger, with 9 points on either side.

Symptomatology: cardialgia, thirst, dryness of the throat, jaundice, pain of hypo-chondriac region, pain in the medial aspect of the arm and feverish sensation in the palms.

VI. Small Intestine Meridian of Hand-Taiyang (SI) (Fig. XII-6)

Course: The Small Intestine Meridian runs from Shaoze (SI 1) at the ulnar side of the little finger, ascends the ulnar side of the forearm and the arm, over the scapula to Dazhui (GV 14). The meridian then descends internally to the heart, past the diaphragm to connect with the small intestine. The supraclavicular fossa branch ascends superficially along the lateral side of the neck, past the cheek to the lateral corner of the eye, and terminates at Tinggong (SI 19). The buccal branch leaves the main meridian at the cheek, and ascends to the medial canthus of the eye. There are 19 points on either side.

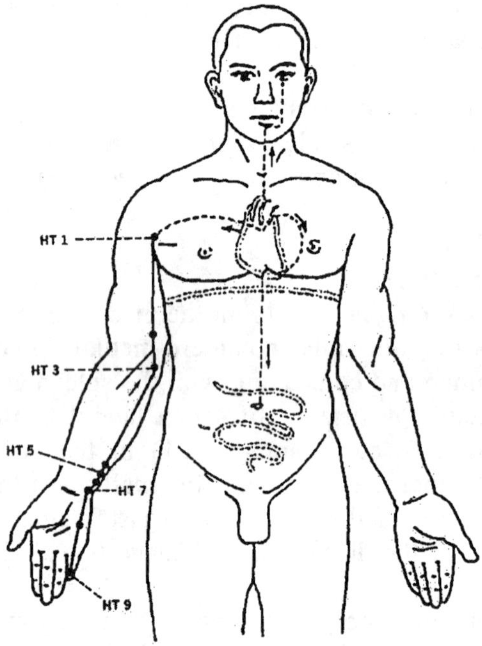

Fig. XII-5 Heart Meridian

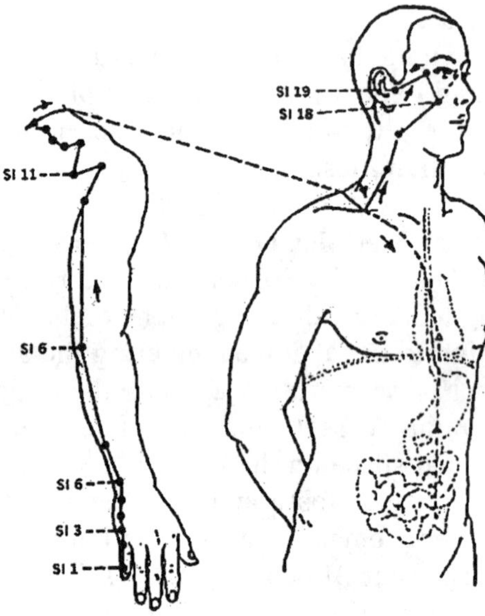

Fig. XII-6 Small Intestine Meridian

Symptomatology: deafness, jaundice, swelling of the neck, sore throat, lower abdominal pain, pain in the shoulder and poster-lateral aspect of the arm.

VII. Bladder Meridian of Foot-Taiyang (BL) (Fig. XII-7)

Course: The Bladder Meridian runs from Jingming (BL 1) at the medial canthus of the eye, ascends the forehead to the vertex, and then enters the brain and exits at the nape of the neck where it divides into two parallel branches: the first branch descends the back at a distance of 1.5 *cun* from the spine. During its course, it connects with the kidneys and urinary bladder, and continues along the posterior side of the thigh to the popliteal fold; the second branch descends the back at a distance of 3 *cun* from the spine, continues along the latero-posterior side of the thigh to popliteal fold where it meets the first branch. The meridian continues to descend along the posterior side of the calf to the lateral malleolus, terminating at Zhiyin (BL 67) on the lateral side of the tip of the little toe. There are 67 points on either side.

Symptomatology: eye disorders, headache, backache, lumbago, leg and foot pain, spasm of calf muscles, dysuria and enuresis.

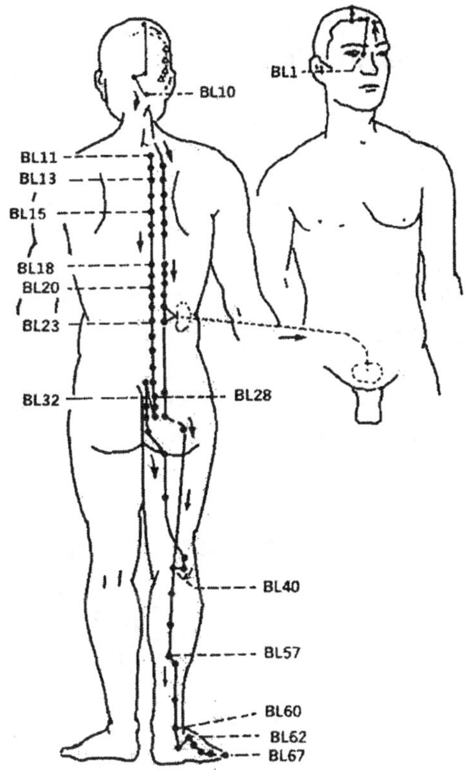

Fig. XII-7 Bladder Meridian

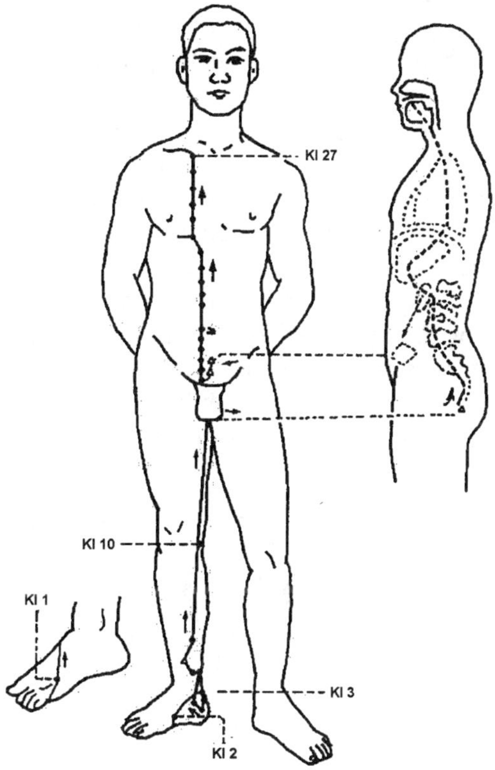

Fig. XII-8 Kidney Meridian

VIII. Kidney Meridian of Foot-Shaoyin (KI) (Fig. XII-8)

Course: The Kidney Meridian begins on the plantar tip of the small toe and travels to Yongquan (KI 1) in the center of the sole, continues along the inner side of the lower limb to the symphysis pubis, turns internally to the kidneys and urinary bladder, and back to the symphysis pubis, descending along the abdomen and chest to Shufu (KI 27) in the depression between the first rib and the lower border of the clavicle, with 27 points on either side. The kidney branch travels through the liver and diaphragm, enters the lungs and follows the trachea and larynx at the base of the tongue.

Symptomatology: enuresis, menoxenia, hemoptysis, dyspnea, dry sensation on the tongue, sore throat, lumbago, edema, diarrhea, pain and atrophy of the postero-medial aspect of the thigh, pain and feverish sensation in the soles.

IX. Pericardium Meridian of Hand-Jueyin (PC) (Fig. XII-9)

Course: The Pericardium Meridian originates in the center of the thorax, connects with the pericardium, and descends to the lower abdomen, linking all three Energizers. The thoracic branch exits superficially at Tianchi (PC 1) near the nipple, and descends along the midline of the anterior side of the arm to Zhongchong (PC 9) at the midpoint of the tip of the middle finger, with 9 points on either side.

Symptomatology: feverish sensation in the palms, spasm of forearm, distension of axilla, fullness in the chest and hypochondriac regions, tachycardia, feverish sensation of face.

X. Triple Energizer Meridian of Hand-Shaoyang (TE) (Fig. XII-10)

Course: The Triple Energizer Meridian runs from Guanchong (TE 1) at the ulnar side of the ring finger, travels along the midline of the posterior side of the arm and through the regions of the shoulder, neck, ear and eye, and terminates at Sizhukong (TE 23) at the lateral canthus, with 23 points on either side. The thoracic branch runs from the supraclavicular fossa to the pericardium and down through the thorax and abdomen, linking the Upper, Middle and Lower Energizers. The auricular branch travels from behind the ear to terminate at the lateral canthus.

Symptomatology: abdominal distension, edema, enuresis, dysuria, headache, deafness, sore throat, eye disorders, and pain in the lateral aspect of the shoulder and arm.

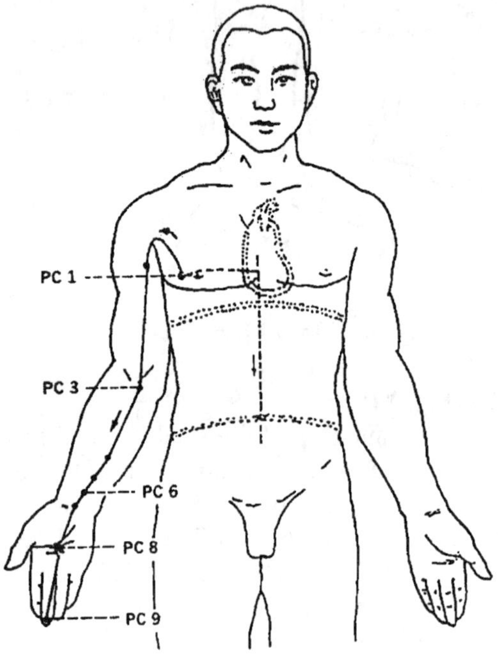

Fig. XII-9 Pericardium Meridian

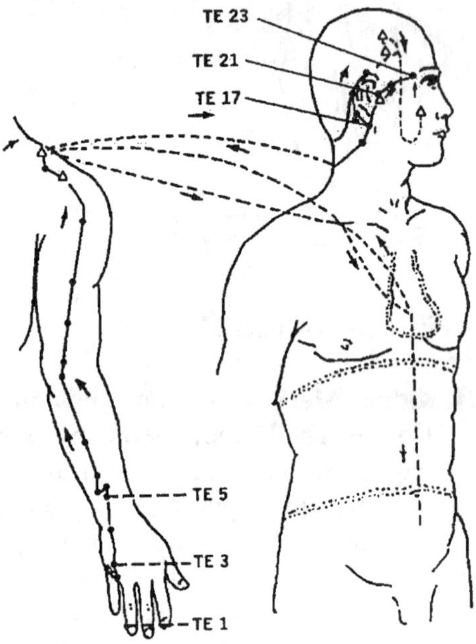

Fig. XII-10 Triple Energizer Meridian

XI. Gallbladder Meridian of Foot-Shaoyang (GB) (Fig. XII-11)

Course: The Gallbladder Meridian runs from Tongziliao (GB 1) at the lateral canthus of the eye, through the regions of the temple, ear, neck, shoulder, flank, and the outer side of the lower limb, terminating at Zuqiaoyin (GB 44) on the lateral side of the tip of the 4th toe, with 44 points on either side. The post-auricular branch travels into the ear and down to the supraclavicular fossa, down into the chest, past the diaphragm, connecting with the gallbladder and liver, and continues down to the lower abdomen into the inguinal groove. The dorsal foot branch leaves the main meridian at Zulinqi (GB 41), terminating at the base of the big toe nail.

Symptomatology: pain of lateral canthus, chest and hypochondriac pain, bitter taste in the mouth, dizziness, malaria, lateral knee pain, and fever.

XII. Liver Meridian of Foot-Jueyin (LR) (Fig. XII-12)

Course: The Liver Meridian runs from Dadun (LR 1) on the big toe just behind the nail, through the inner side of the lower limb, external genitalia and abdomen, to Qimen (LR 14) about 2 *cun* below the nipple, with 14 points on either side. From Qimen (LR 14), the meridian enters the abdomen, crosses the stomach para-laterally to connect with the liver and gallbladder. From the liver, the meridian ascends past the diaphragm along the trachea, larynx and sinus cavity, connecting with the eye, and then ascends to the top of the head, where it meets the Governor Vessel.

Symptomatology: enuresis, dysuria, gynecological pain, lumbago, diarrhea, hernia and mental diseases.

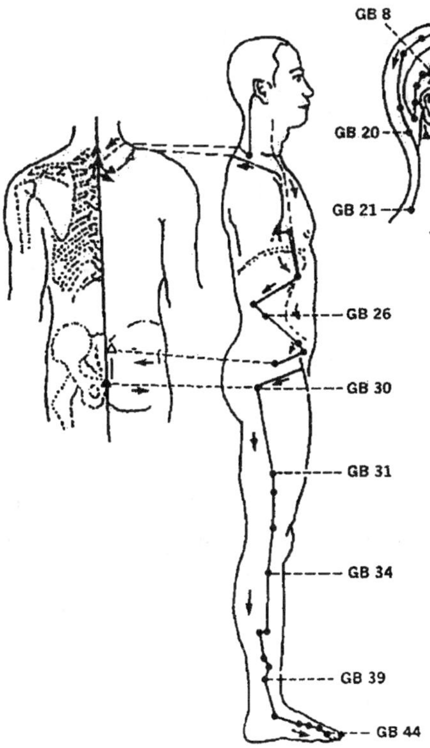

Fig. XII-11 Gallbladder Meridian

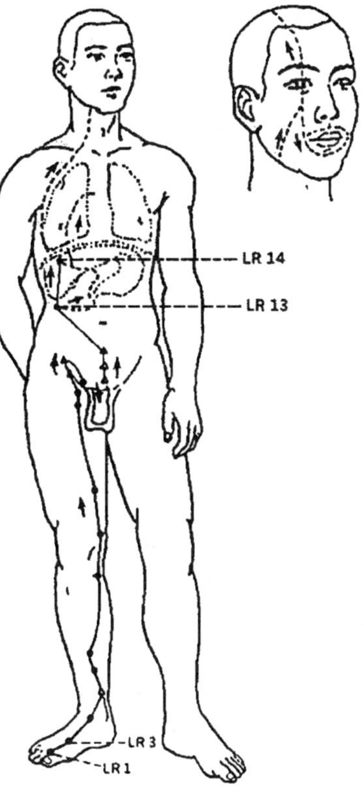

Fig. XII-12 Liver Meridian

THE EIGHT EXTRA MERIDIANS

Governor Vessel (GV) (Fig. XII-13)

Course: The Governor Vessel originates in the lower abdomen, descends and exits at the perineum, and travels from Changqiang (GV 1), a point below the coccyx, along the spinal column to the top of the head, and then descends along the midline of the face down to Yinjiao (GV 28), a point between the upper lip and the upper gum in the labia frenulum, with 28 points.

Symptomatology: syncope, dizziness, headache, lumbago, opisthotonos and diseases of the related internal organs.

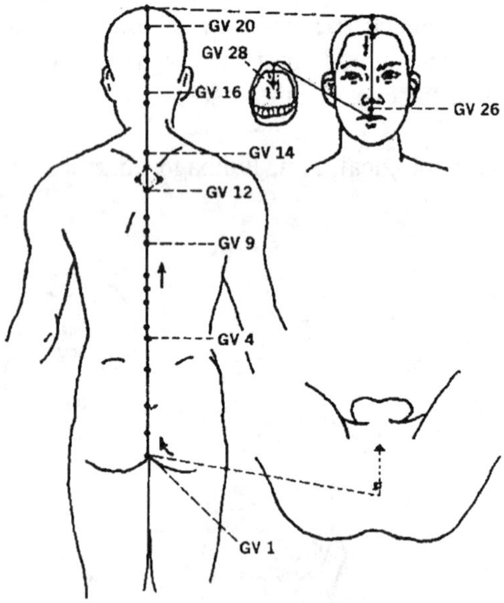

Fig. XII-13 Governor Vessel

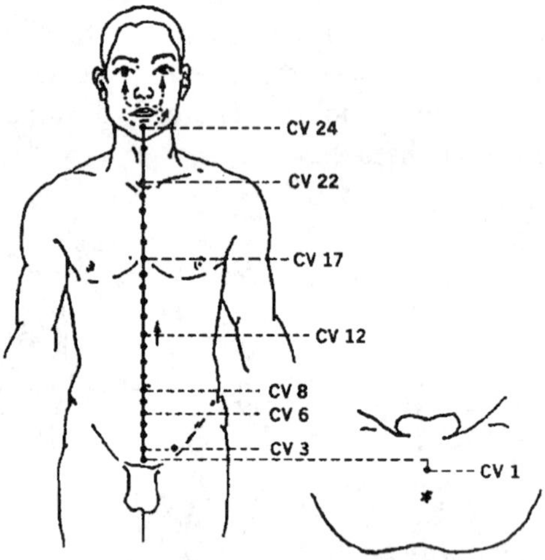

Fig. XII-14 Conception Vessel

Conception Vessel (CV) (Fig. XII-14)

Course: The Conception Vessel originates in the lower abdomen, descends and exits at the perineum, and ascends from Huiyin (CV 1) in the center of the perineum, along the midline of the abdomen and chest to Chengjiang (CV 24), the midpoint of the mentolabial sulcus, with 24 points. The internal portion of this meridian ascends from Chengjiang (CV 24), encircles the mouth and travels to the eyes.

Symptomatology: abdominal pain, retention of urine, enuresis, menstrual disorders, uterine bleeding, hernia, collapse, gastralgia, diarrhea and coughing.

Thoroughfare Vessel (TV)

Course: The Thoroughfare Vessel originates in the lower abdomen (the uterus in the female), comes into confluence with the Kidney Meridian, and then runs upward along both sides of the abdomen to the chest.

Symptomatology: menstrual disorders, abnormal unterine bleeding, abdominal pain and infertility

Belt Vessel (BV)

Course: The Belt Vessel goes round the waist in confluence with a part of the Gallbladder Meridian.

Symptomatology: leukorrhea, prolapse of the uterus, abdominal distension and weakness of the lower back.

***Yang* Heel Vessel (YangHV)**

Course: The *Yang* Heel Vessel originates at Shenmai (BL 62) at the lateral side of the heel, runs upward along the outer side of the lower limb, through the abdomen, chest, shoulder and cheek, and terminates at Fengchi (GB 20) on the nape.

Symptomatology: muscular spasm of the lateral aspect and flaccidity of the medial aspect of the lower extremity, mania and insomnia.

***Yin* Heel Vessel (YinHV)**

Course: The *Yin* Heel Vessel originates at Zhaohai (KI 6) at the inner side of the heel, runs upward along the inner side of the lower limb, through the external genitalia, the abdomen, chest, neck, either side of the nose, and terminates at Jingming (BL 1) at the inner canthus.

Symptomatology: muscular spasm of the medial aspect and flaccidity of the lateral aspect of the lower extremity, sore throat and sleepiness.

***Yang* Link Vessel (YangLV)**

Course: The *Yang* Link Vessel originates at Jinmen (BL 63) below the lateral malleolus, runs upward along the outer side of the lower limb, through the side of the trunk, the shoulder, retroauricular region and forehead, and terminates at Yamen (GV 15).

Symptomatology: chills and fever, dizziness, dyspnea and rheumatalgia.

***Yin* Link Vessel (YinLV)**

Course: The *Yin* Link Vessel originates at Zhubin (KI 9), runs upward along the inner side of the lower limb to the abdomen, where it meets the Spleen, Liver, Kidney, and Stomach Meridians at Fushe (SP 13). It continues up the chest to the throat, where it meets the Conception Vessel at Tiantu (CV 22) and Lianquan (CV 23).

Symptomatology: chest pain, distension of hypochondriac region and swelling of external genitalia.

CHAPTER 13

ACUPOINTS

DEFINITION AND NOMENCLATURE

Acupoints are the sites on the surface of the body to which the *qi* of the organs and meridians flows. Through the physiological connection between the organs and the meridian system, pathological changes of the organs may be reflected at these points. Stimulation of the points by needling, pressure, heat or massage may therefore bring about regulation and treatment of the organs. These sites of stimulation to "clear the meridians, balance *qi* and blood, eliminate pathogenic factors and reinforce the body's resistance" are known as acupoints (needling points) or simply points. There are three categories of points: (1) points of the fourteen meridians, (2) extra-meridian points or simply extra points, and (3) *ashi* (or "ouch") points.[1] *Ashi* points have no fixed location, nor fixed number. They are found by eliciting tenderness or pain at the site of most sensitivity. There are 361 meridian points and dozens of extra-meridian points. All of them have names in Chinese characters, locations and indications.

In 1991, the World Health Organization of the United Nations published a Proposed Standard International Acupuncture Nomenclature, in which an alphanumeric code of the acupoints together with the Chinese phonetic alphabet (*pinyin*) names is recommended. In the alphanumeric code, the alphabetic part is derived from the English translation of the meridian names, while the numbering follows the course of each meridian. For example, Hegu is the fourth point on the Large Intestine Meridian, and so its standard name is Hegu (LI 4), or simply LI 4.

For extra points, 48 were generally recognized. The proposed alphanumeric code consists of a general prefix "EX," denoting "extra points," followed by an alphabetic code indicating the region (HN for head and neck, CA for chest and abdomen, B for back, UE for upper extremity, and LE for lower extremity). Points are numbered from the higher to the lower level for the head, neck and trunk; and from the proximal to the distal for the extremities. For example, Sishencong on the vertex of the head is EX-HN 1, Jingbailao, the lowest extra point on the neck, is EX-HN 15.

---

[1]Ashi (阿是) means "Is it?" Searching for the *ashi* point, the physician asks the patient whether it is the most painful point while pressing with a finger. When the patient answers "yes," the *ashi* point is thus found. This may also be expressed by the patient's exclamation of ouch.

SPECIALLY DESIGNATED POINTS

Specially designated points are points on the 14 meridians that have specific therapeutic effects, and hence are grouped under special names. They are five *shu*-transport points, *yuan*-source points, *luo*-connecting points, front *mu*-curtain points, back *shu*-transport points, influential points, cleft points, crossing points, eight confluence points and lower sea points.

I. Five Shu-Transport Points.

Each of the 12 regular meridians has five specific points distributing distally to the elbows and knees, varying in their condition of the flow of *qi* and blood. They are the *Jing*-well points, *Ying*-spring points, *Shu*-stream points, *Jing*-river points and *He*-sea points. In the names of the five *shu* points, the flow of the meridian *qi* is likened to the flow of water. The well point is the place where the meridian *qi* starts to bubble, the spring point is where the meridian *qi* starts to spout, the stream point is where the flow of the meridian *qi* starts to flourish, the river point is where the meridian *qi* starts to pour, and the sea point signifies the confluence of the rivers. The five *shu* points are listed in Tables XIII-1a and 1b.

Actions of the Five *Shu* Points

1. Well Points (*Jing* Points): Resuscitation for emergency revival.
2. Spring Points (*Ying* Points): Purging fire in cases of febrile diseases.
3. Stream Points (*Shu* Points): Relief of arthralgia. Spring and stream points are used to treat meridian diseases of the exterior portion of the body.
4. River Points (*Jing* Points): Relief of coughing, asthma and disorders of the throat.
5. Sea Points (*He* Points): Treatment of diseases of internal *fu* organs.

Table XIII-1a The Five *Shu*-Transport Points of the *Yin* Meridians

Meridian	Well	Spring	Stream	River	Sea
Hand-Taiyin Lung (LU)	Shaoshang 11	Yuji 10	Taiyuan 9	Jingqu 8	Chize 5
Hand-Jueyin Pericardium (PC)	Zhongchong 9	Laogong 8	Daling 7	Jianshi 5	Quze 3
Hand-Shaoyin Heart (HT)	Shaochong 9	Shaofu 8	Shenmen 7	Lingdao 4	Shaohai 3
Foot-Taiyin Spleen (SP)	Yinbai 1	Dadu 2	Taibai 3	Shangqiu 5	Yinlingquan 9
Foot-Jueyin Liver (LR)	Dadun 1	Xingjian 2	Taichong 3	Zhongfeng 4	Ququan 8
Foot-Shaoyin Kidney (KI)	Yongquan 1	Rangu 2	Taixi 3	Fuliu 7	Yingu 10

Table XIII-1b The Five *Shu*-Transport Points of *Yang* Meridians

Meridian	Well	Spring	Stream	River	Sea
Hand-Yangming	Shangyang	Erjian	Sanjian	Yangxi	Quchi
Large Intestine (LI)	1	2	3	5	11
Hand-Shaoyang	Guanchong	Yemen	Zhongzhu	Zhigou	Tianjing
Triple Energizer(TE)	1	2	3	6	10
Hand-Taiyang Small	Shaoze	Qiangu	Houxi	Yanggu	Xiaohai
Intestine (SI)	1	2	3	5	8
Foot-Yangming	Lidui	Neiting	Xiangu	Jiexi	Zusanli
Stomach (ST)	45	44	43	41	36
Foot-Shaoyang	Zuqiaoyin	Xiaxi	Zulinqi	Yangfu	Yanglingquan
Gallbladder (GB)	44	43	41	38	34
Foot-Taiyang	Zhiyin	Zutonggu	Shugu	Kunlun	Weizhong
Bladder (BL)	67	66	65	60	40

II. Lower Sea Points of the Six *Fu*-Organs

The lower sea points are points on the three *yang* meridians of the foot corresponding to the six *fu*-organs as listed in Table XIII-2. The points are used to treat disorders of the corresponding *fu*-organs. "Stomach" in its broad sense includes the intestines, so the lower sea points of the Large and Small Intestines are on the Stomach Meridian. The Triple Energizer controls water metabolism and eliminates superfluous water through the Bladder, so the lower sea point of the Triple Energizer is on the Bladder Meridian.

Table XIII-2

Acupoint	Corresponding *fu*-organ	Acupoint	Corresponding *fu*-organ
Zusanli (ST 36)	Stomach	Shangjuxu (ST 37)	Large Intestine
Xiajuxu (ST 39)	Small Intestine	Yanglingquan (GB 34)	Gallbladder
Weizhong (BL 40)	Bladder	Weiyang (BL 39)	Triple Energizer

III. Twelve Primary Points (*Yuan* Points)

Each of the twelve regular meridians has a primary point (*yuan* point) where the primary *qi* of the corresponding *zang-fu* organ is retained. Therefore, they are used to treat the disorders of *zang-fu* organs. They are listed in Table XIII-3.

IV. Fifteen Connecting Points (*Luo* Points)

Connecting points are the points for the 14 meridians to connect the interior-exteriorly related *yin* and *yang* meridians as well as the areas supplied by the two meridians. The Spleen Meridian has two, and each of the others has one connecting point, hence 15 in all. The connecting points (listed in Table XIII-4a and 4b) are used to treat disorders involving the two meridians and the corresponding areas.

Table XIII-3 The Twelve Primary Points

Zang-fu organ	Primary Point	*Zang-fu* organ	Primary Point
Three Hand *Yin* Meridians		Three Hand *Yang* Meridians	
Lung	Taiyuan (LU 9)	Large Intestine	Hegu (LI 4)
Pericardium	Daling (PC 7)	Triple Energizer	Yangchi (TE 4)
Heart	Shenmen (HT 7)	Small Intestine	Wangu (SI 4)
Three Foot *Yin* Meridians		Three Foot *Yang* Meridians	
Spleen	Taibai (SP 3)	Stomach	Chongyang (ST 42)
Liver	Taichong (LR 3)	Gallbladder	Qiuxu (GB 40)
Kidney	Taixi (KI 3)	Bladder	Jinggu (BL 64)

Table XIII-4a Connecting Points of the Hand and Foot

Yin Meridian Interior)	Connecting Points		*Yang* Meridian (Exterior)
Hand-Taiyin	Lieque (LU 7)	Pianli (LI 6)	Hand-Yangming
Hand-Jueyin	Neiguan (PC 6)	Waiguan (TE 5)	Hand-Shaoyang
Hand-Shaoyin	Tongli (HT 5)	Zhizheng (SI 7)	Hand-Taiyang
Foot-Taiyin	Gongsun (SP 4)	Fenglong (ST 40)	Foot-Yangming
Foot-Jueyin	Ligou (LR 5)	Guangming (GB 37)	Foot-Shaoyang
Foot-Shaoyin	Dazhong (KI 4)	Feiyang (BL 58)	Foot-Taiyang

Table XIII-4b Connecting Points of the Trunk

Area	Name of Collateral	Point	Collateral
Front of trunk	Collateral of Conception Vessel	Jiuwei (CV 15)	Abdomen
Back of trunk	Collateral of Governor Vessel	Changqiang (GV1)	Head
Side of trunk	Great Collateral of Spleen	Dabao (SP 21)	Hypochondrium

V. Sixteen Cleft Points (Xi Points)

Cleft Points are the points where the meridian *qi* accumulates deeply. Each of the twelve regular meridians, together with *Yin* Heel, *Yang* Heel, *Yin* Link and *Yang* Link Vessels, has a cleft point, hence 16 in all. They are mainly used for treating acute pain and disorders in the area supplied by the pertinent meridian and for examining tenderness (Table XIII-5).

Table XIII-5 Cleft Points

Three Hand *Yin* Meridians		**Three Hand *Yang* Meridians**	
***Zang-fu* organ**	**Cleft Point**	***Zang-fu* organ**	**Cleft Point**
Lung	Kongzui (LU 6)	Large Intestine	Wenliu (LI 7)
Pericardium	Ximen (PC 4)	Triple Energizer	Huizong (TE 7)
Heart	Yinxi (HT 6)	Small Intestine	Yanglao (SI 6)
Three Foot *Yin* Meridians		**Three Foot *Yang* Meridians**	
***Zang-fu* organ**	**Cleft Point**	***Zang-fu* organ**	**Cleft Point**
Spleen	Diji (SP 8)	Stomach	Liangqiu (ST 34)
Liver	Zhongdu (LR 6)	Gallbladder	Waiqiu (GB 36)
Kidney	Shuiquan (KI 5)	Bladder	Jinmen (BL 63)
Extra Meridians			
Vessel	**Point**	**Vessel**	**Point**
Yin Link Vessel	Zhubin (KI 9)	*Yang* Link Vessel	Yangjiao (GB 35)
Yin Heel Vessel	Jiaoxin (KI 8)	*Yang* Heel Vessel	Fuyang (BL 59)

VI. Confluence Points of Eight Vessels

The eight points refer to the points on the limbs where the regular meridians communicate with the eight extra meridians. They are often used in pairs to treat the disorders related to the extra meridians (Table XIII-6).

Table XIII-6 The Confluence Points of the Eight Vessels

Acupoint	Extra Meridian intersected	Indications
Neiguan (PC 6)	→ *Yin* Link Vessel	Disorders of the heart, chest,
Gongsun (SP 4)	→ Thoroughfare Vessel	and stomach
Houxi (SI 3)	→ Governor Vessel	Disorders of the nape, scapula,
Shenmai (BL 62)	→ *Yang* Heel Vessel	ears, and inner canthus
Waiguan (TE 5)	→ Yang Link Vessel	Disorders of the neck, shoulder,
Linqi (GB 41)	→ Belt Vessel	heek, ear and outer canthus
Lieque (LU 7)	→ Conception Vessel	Disorders of the throat and
Zhaohai (KI 6)	→ Yin Heel Vessel	diaphragm

VII. Back-Transport Points (Back-*Shu* Points) and Front-Curtain Points (Front-*Mu* Points)

The specific points on the back where the *qi* of the *zang-fu* organs is infused are called back-transport points (back-*shu* points). They are named in accordance with their corresponding *zang-fu* organs. If a *zang-fu* organ is diseased, its corresponding back-transport point would show abnormal reactions, such as pain on pressure or presence of a nodule. The back-transport points are mainly used to treat disorders of the corresponding *zang-fu* organs or disorders of their related sense organs and tissues.

The specific points on the chest and abdomen where the *qi* of the *zang-fu* organs is concentrated are called front-curtain points (front-*mu* points). They are situated close to the related *zang-fu* organs. Like the back-transport points, the front-curtain points also show abnormal reactions such as tenderness if the corresponding *zang-fu* organs are disordered. The front-curtain points can be used for diagnosis and treating diseases of the corresponding organs. According to the rule of "treating *yin* disease with *yang*, and vice versa," it is customary to treat the disorders of the *zang*-organs with back-transport points and to treat the disorders of the *fu*-organs with front-curtain points.

The back-transport and front-curtain points and their corresponding organs are listed in Table XIII-7.

Table XIII-7 The Back-Transport (Back-*Shu*) and Front-Curtain (Front-*Mu*) Points and Their Corresponding *Zang-fu* Organs

Zang-fu Organ	Back-Transport Point	Front-Curtain Point
Lung	Feishu (BL 13)	Zhongfu (LU 1)
Pericardium	Jueyinshu (BL 14)	Danzhong (CV 17)
Heart	Xinshu (BL 15)	Juque (CV 14)
Liver	Ganshu (BL 18)	Qimen (LR 14)
Gallbladder	Danshu (BL 19)	Riyue (GB 24)
Spleen	Pishu (BL 20)	Zhangmen (LR 13)
Stomach	Weishu (BL 21)	Zhongwan (CV 12)
Triple Energizer	Sanjiaoshu (BL 22)	Shimen (CV 5)
Kidney	Shenshu (BL 23)	Jingmen (GB 25)
Large Intestine	Dachangshu (BL 25)	Tianshu (ST 25)
Small Intestine	Xiaochangshu (BL 27)	Guanyuan (CV 4)
Bladder	Pangguangshu (BL 28)	Zhongji (CV 3)

VIII. The Eight Influential Points

The eight influential points are important acupoints which exert influence on the *zang*, *fu*, *qi*, blood, bones, marrow, tendons and blood vessels, respectively. They are listed in Table XIII-8.

Table XIII-8 Eight Influential Points

Acupoint	Tissue	Acupoint	Tissue
Zhangmen (LR 13)	*Zang*-organs	Zhongwan (CV 12)	*Fu*-organs
Danzhong (CV 17)	*Qi*	Geshu (BL 17)	blood
Yanglingquan(GB 34)	Tendons	Taiyuan (LU 9)	vessels
Dazhu (BL 11)	Bones	Xuanzhong (GB 39)	marrow

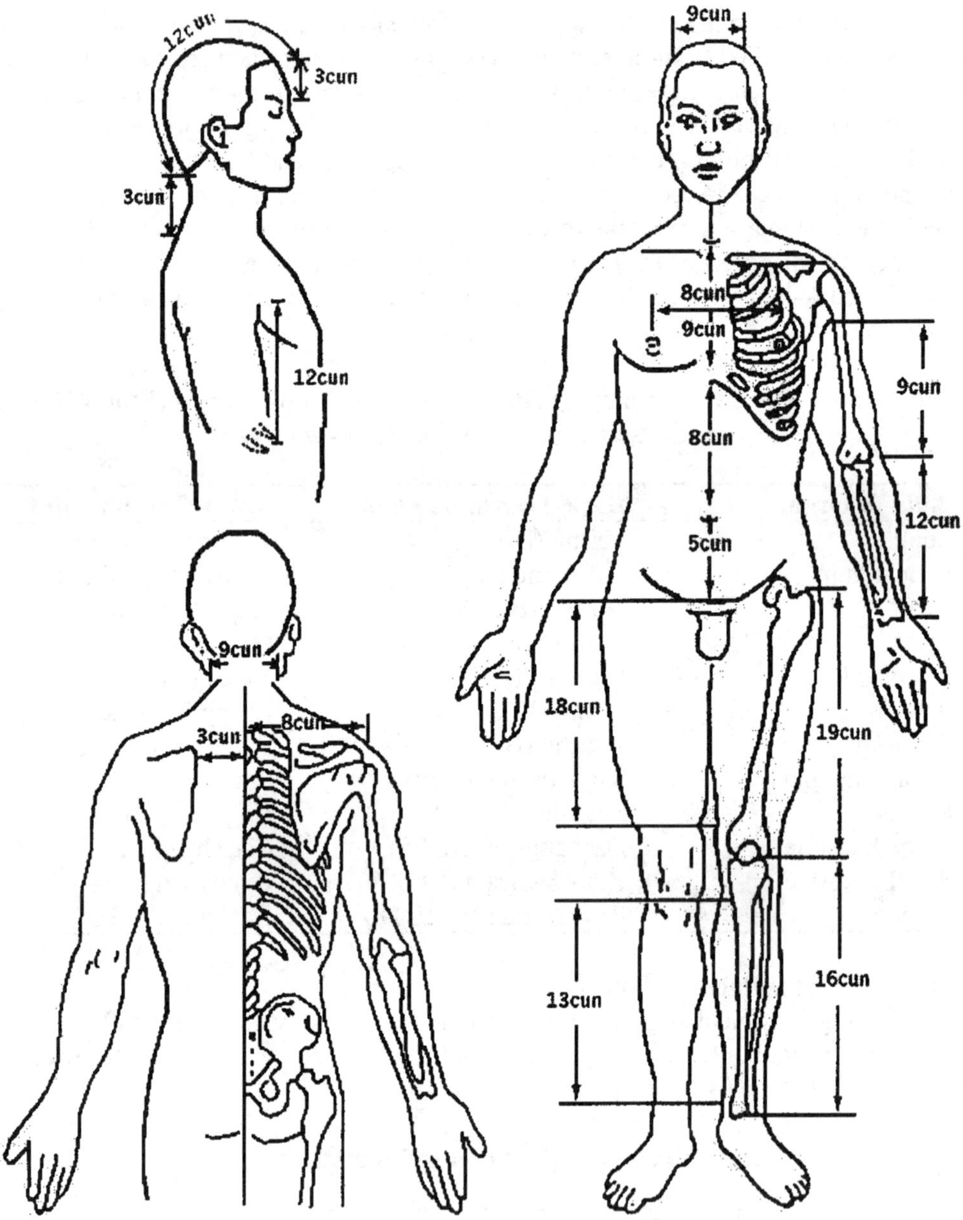

Fig. XIII-1 Proportional measurement

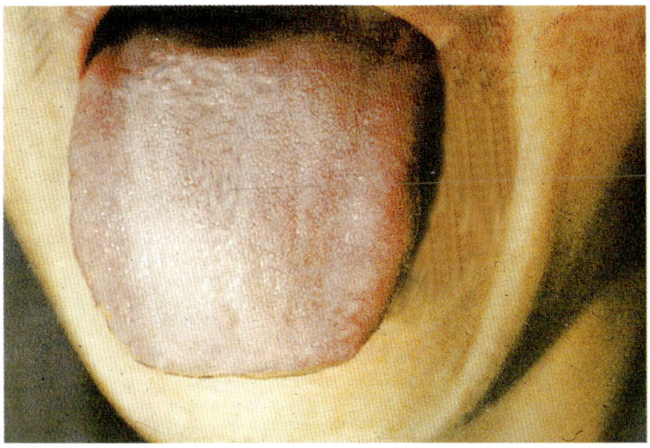

Color Fig. 1 A normal tongue.

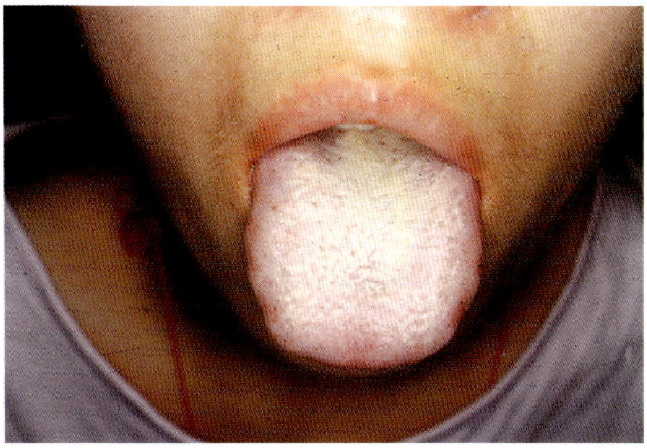

Color Fig. 2 A plump and enlarged tongue with tooth prints on the edges and heavy greasy coating, seen in a patient with chronic pancreatitis, indicating spleen insufficiency with damp accumulation.

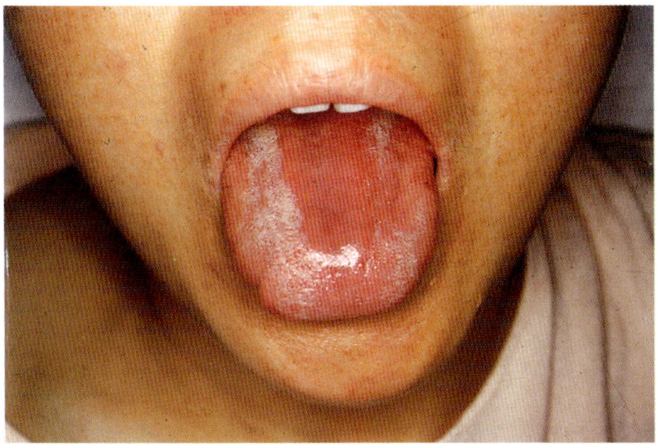

Color Fig. 3 A plump tongue with marked peeling of the coating, seen in a case of chronic pulmonary heart disease with deficiency of *qi* and *yin*.

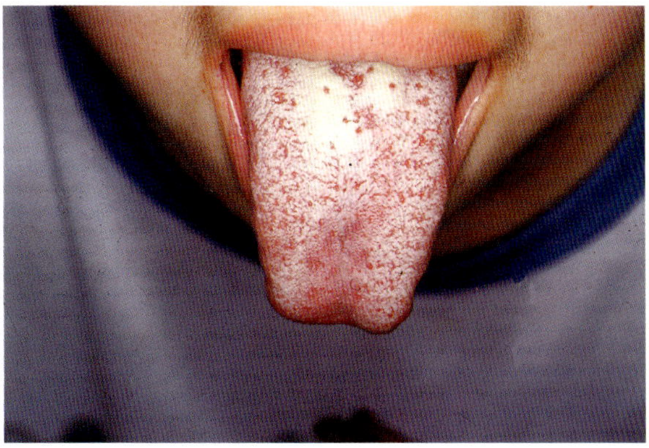

Color Fig. 4 A reddened and prickled tongue with thick coating in a case of Henoch's purpura with kidney involvement, indicating heat in blood.

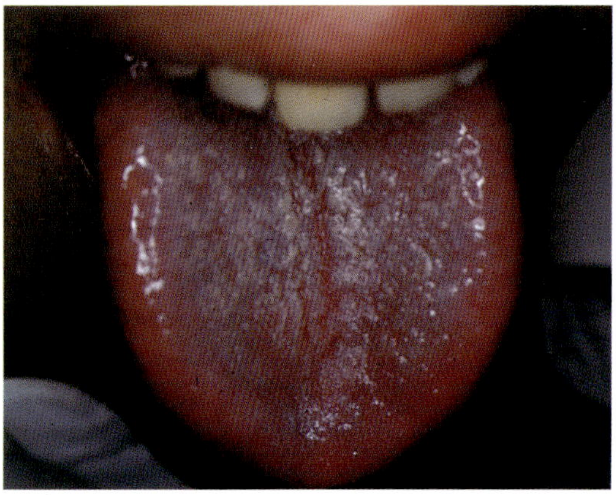

Color Fig. 5 A dark crimson tongue with a longitudinal fissure in the middle, indicating heat in the *ying*-blood system.

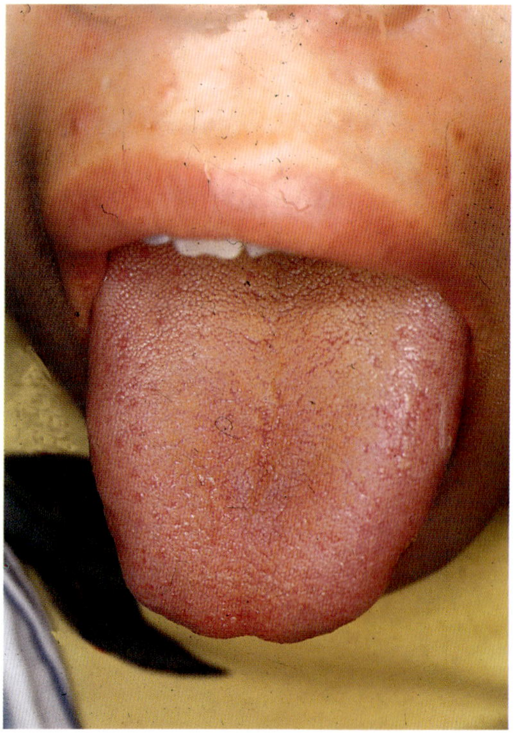

Color Fig. 6 A tongue with a reddened tip and thin yellowish coating in a patient with upper respiratory infection diagnosed as wind-heat affection in Chinese medicine.

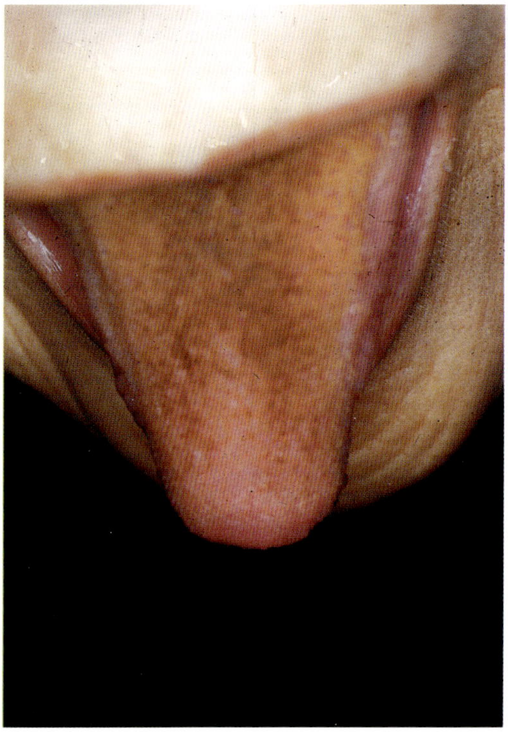

Color Fig.7 A reddened tongue with dry, yellow and brown-grey coating, indicating intense heat with impairment of *yin*, seen in a patient with diadetes mellitus and renal insufficiency.

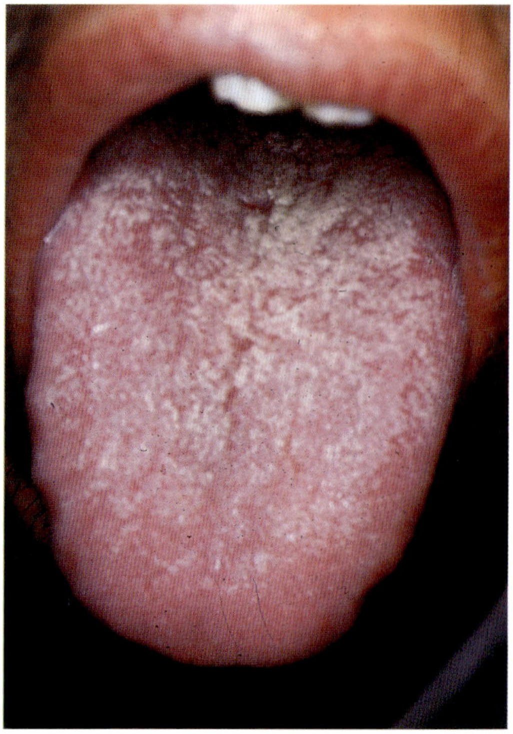

Color Fig. 8 A purple tongue with white greasy coating seen in a patient with coronary heart disease diagnosed as blood stasis due to cold-phlegm in Chinese medicine.

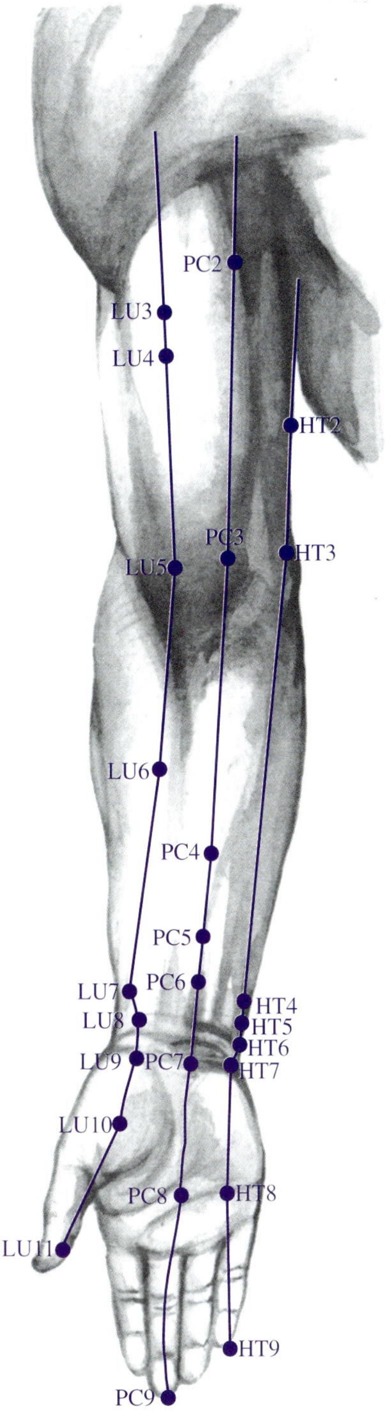

Color Fig. 9 Points of Lung (LU), Pericardium (PC) and Heart (HT) Meridians on the upper extremity

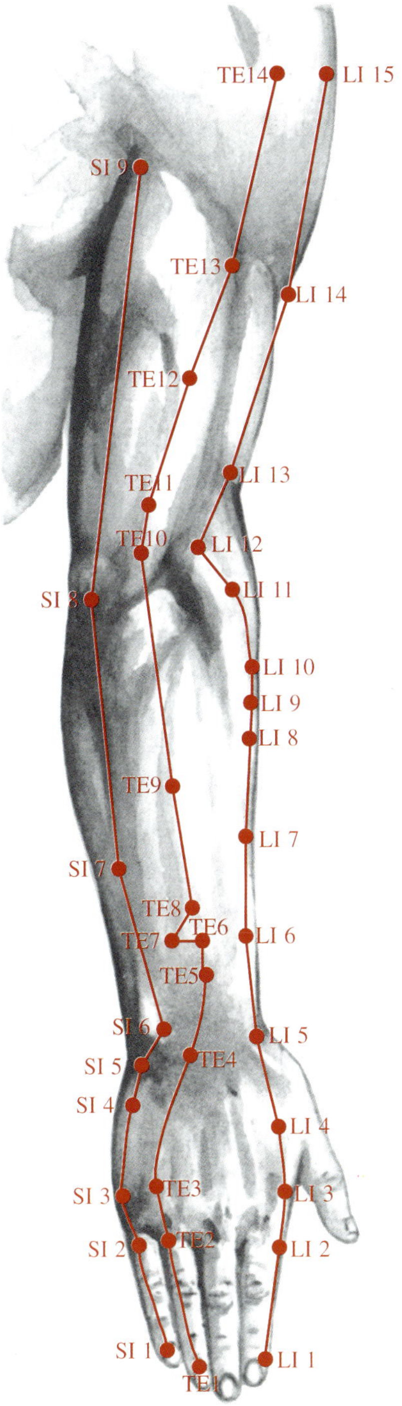

Color Fig. 10 Points of Large Intestine (LI), Triple Energizer (TE) and Small Intestine (SI) Meridians on the upper extremity

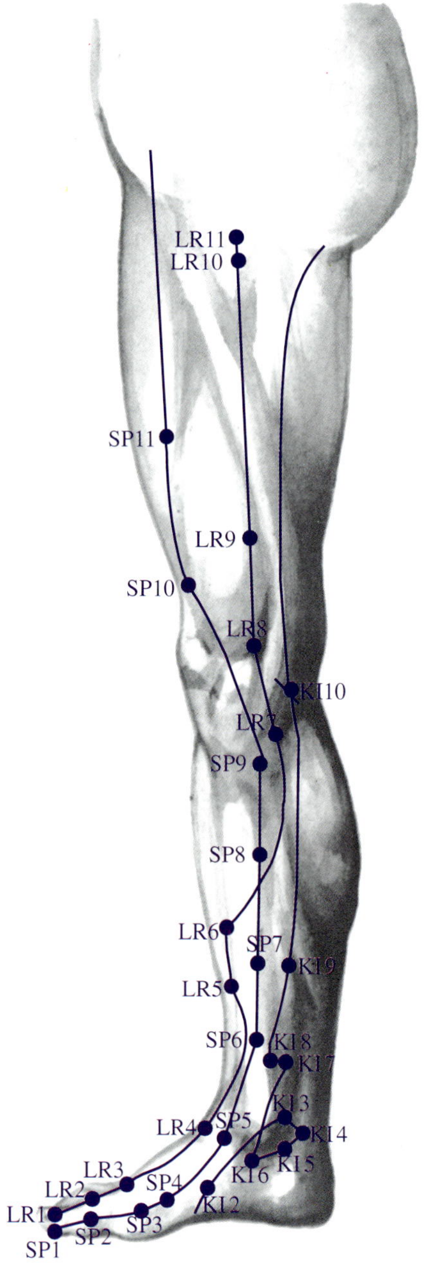

Color Fig. 11 Points of Spleen (SP), Kidney (KI) and Liver (LR) Meridians on the lower extremity

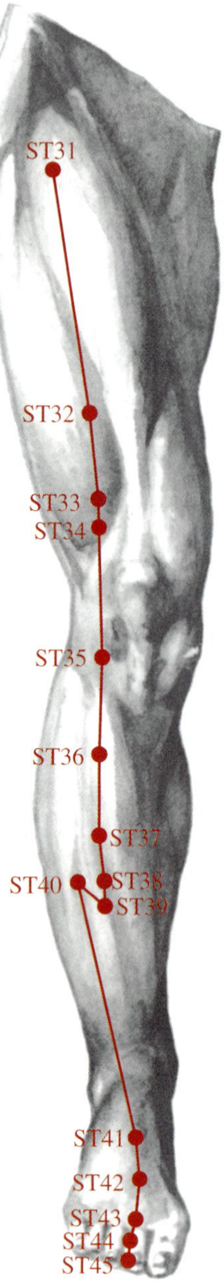

Color Fig. 12 Points of Stomach (ST) Meridian on the lower extremity

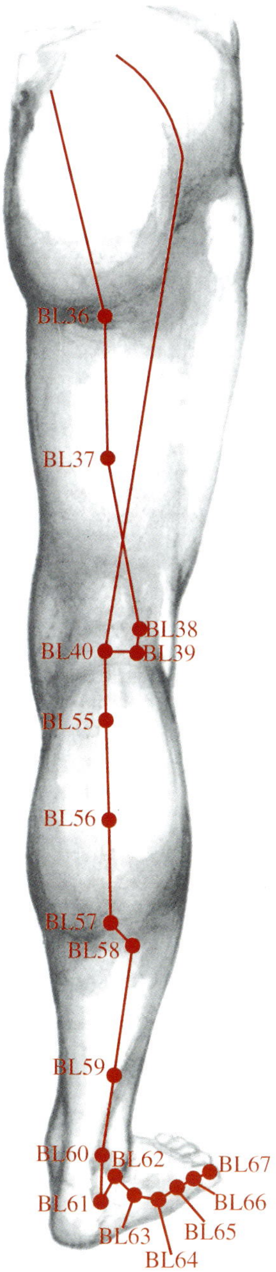

Color Fig. 13 Points of Bladder (BL)
Meridian on the lower extremity

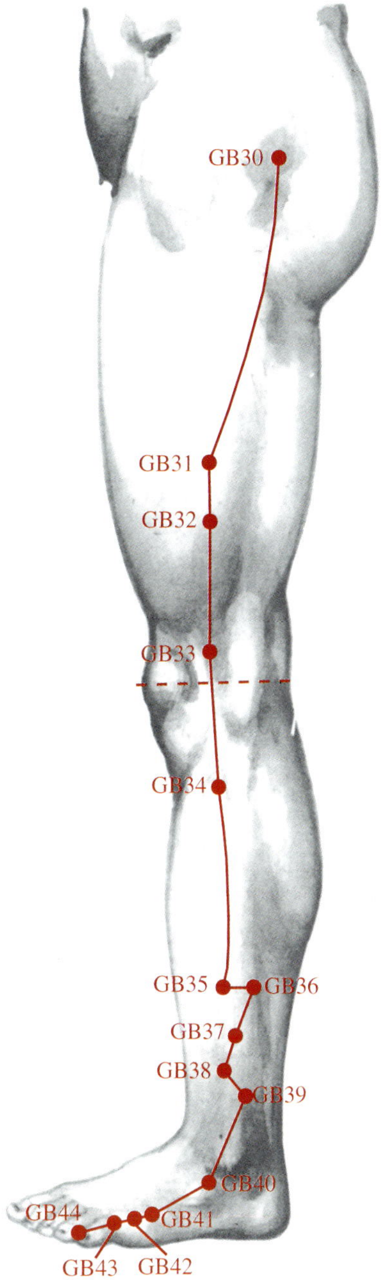

Color Fig. 14 Points of Gallbladder (GB)
Meridian on the lower extremity

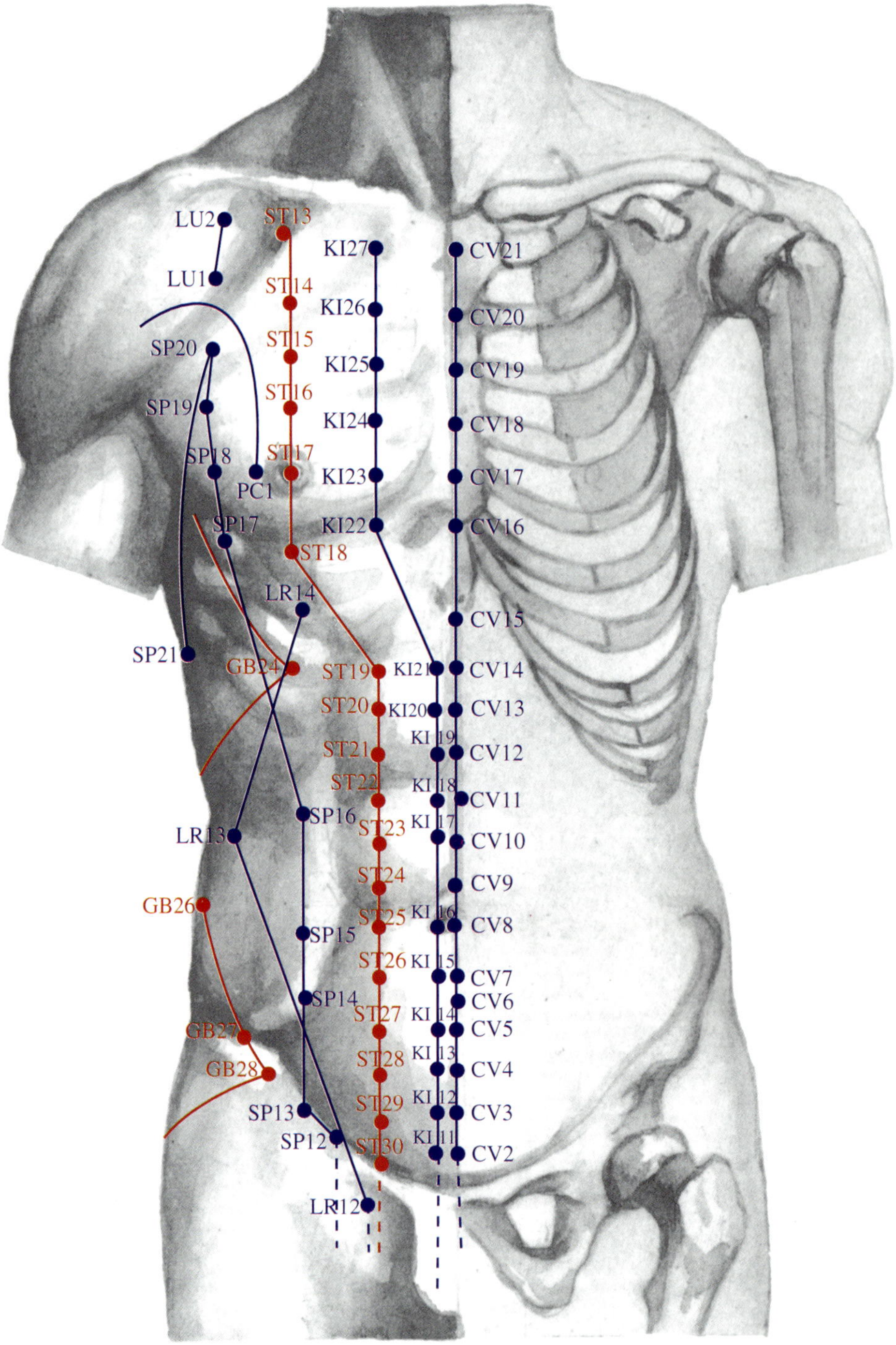

Color Fig. 15 Points of Conception Vessel (CV), Kidney (KI), Stomach (ST), Spleen (SP), Liver (LR), Gallbladder (GB), Pericardium (PC) and Lung (LU) Meridians on the chest and abdomen

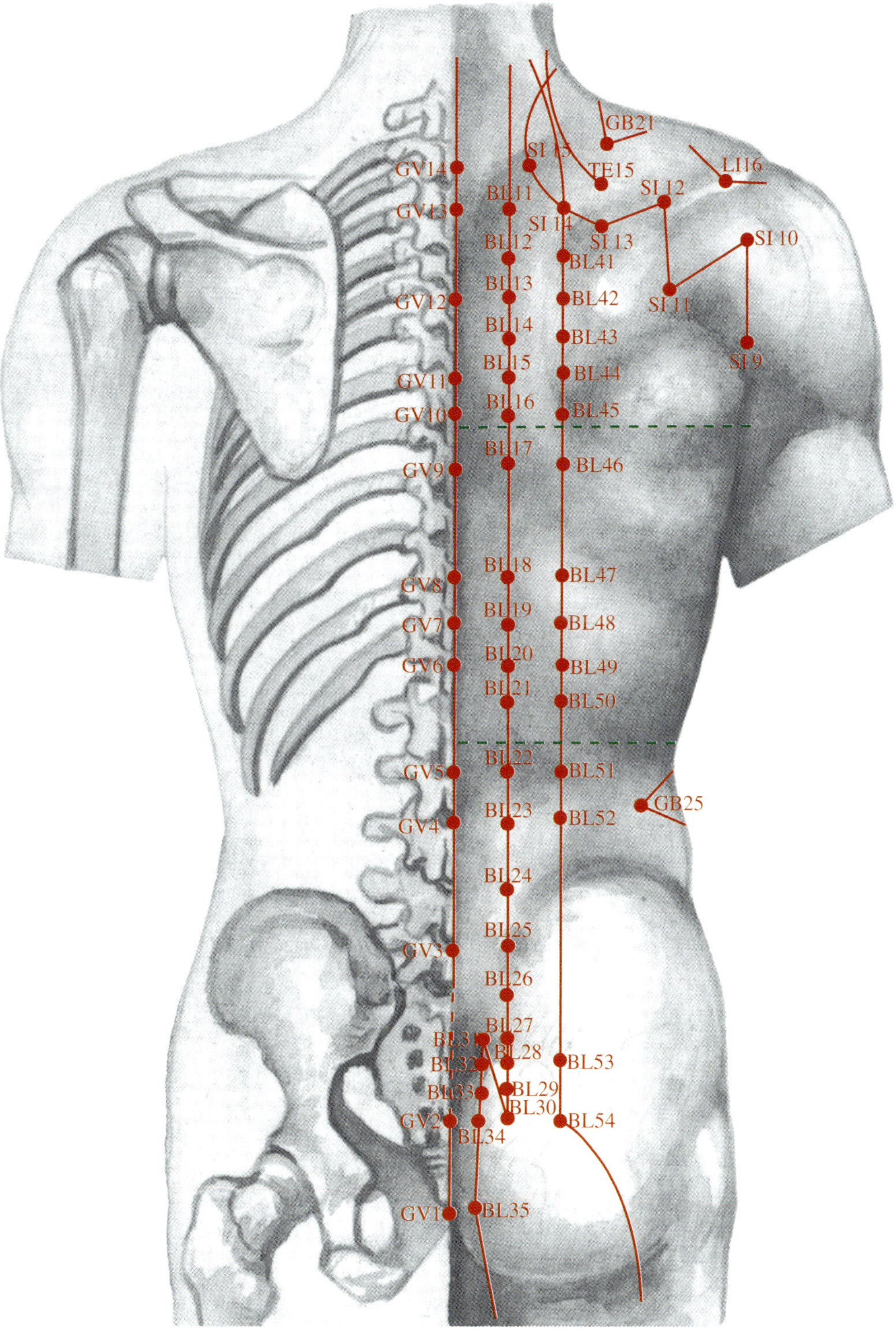

Color Fig. 16 Points of Governor Vessel (GV), Bladder (BL), Gallbladder (GB), Triple Energizer (TE), Small Intestine (SI) and Large Intestine (LI) Meridians on the back

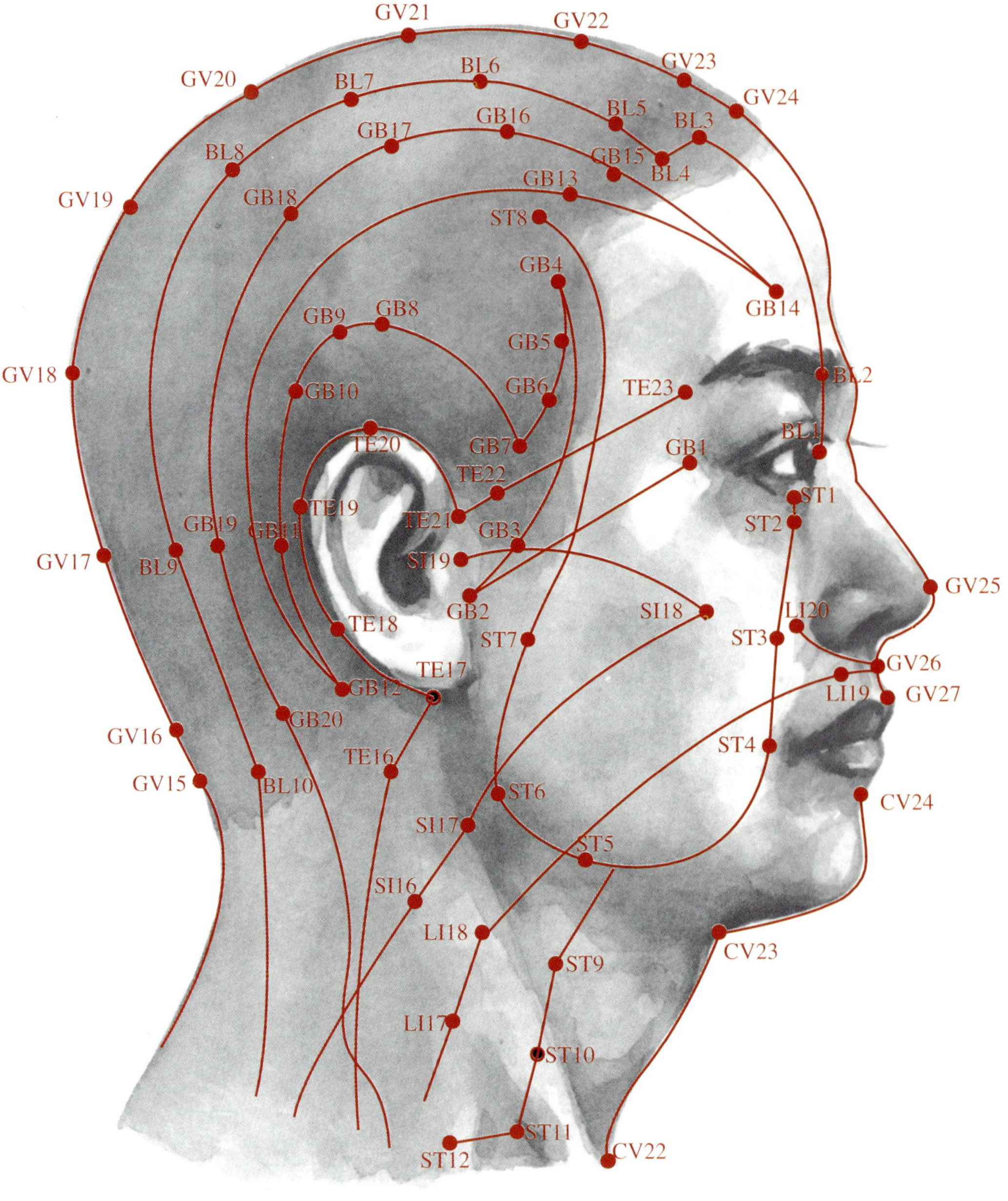

Color Fig. 17 Points on the head

IX. Crossing Points

The crossing points are the points where two or more meridians intersect. They can be used to treat disorders of the pertinent meridians and the intersected meridians. For example, Sanyinjiao (SP 6), a crossing point of the three foot *yin* meridians, is effective for treating disorders of the Liver, Spleen and Kidneys. There are more than 90 crossing points.

Methods of Locating Acupoints

I. Anatomical Landmarks

Anatomical landmarks on the body's surface are the basis for locating acupoints.

1. Fixed landmarks. Fixed landmarks are those that do not change with body movement. They include:

(1) Prominences and depressions of bones, such as medial malleolus, lateral malleolus, tuberosity of the navicular bone, medial condyle of the tibia, lateral epicondyle of the humerus, and acromial extremity of clavicle;

(2) Sense organs: eyes, nose, mouth, ears;

(3) Hair, particularly hairlines;

(4) Nails;

(5) Umbilicus; and

(6) In the majority of cases, nipples.

2. Moving landmarks. Moving landmarks are those that only appear when a body part maintains a specific position, e.g., cubital crease when the arm is flexed, and transverse palmar crease when a fist is made.

II. Proportional Measurement (Fig. XIII-1)

The width or length of various portions of the human body are divided into a certain number of equal units as the standards for proportional measurement. The unit is the *cun*, a Chinese unit of length which literally means an inch, but the proportional *cun* has no definite length; it varies with the size of the body, and so is applicable to patients with different body sizes.

III. Finger Measurement (Table XIII-9, Fig. XIII-2)

The length and width of a patient's finger(s) are taken as a standard for locating the acupoints. The following methods are commonly used:

1. Middle finger measurement: The distance between the two medial ends of the creases of the interphalangeal joints counts as one *cun* when the patient's middle finger is flexed.

2. Thumb measurement: The width of the interphalangeal joint of the patient's thumb counts as one *cun*.

3. Four-finger measurement: The width of four fingers (index, middle, ring and little) close together at the level of the dorsal skin crease of the proximal interphalangeal joint counts as three *cun*.

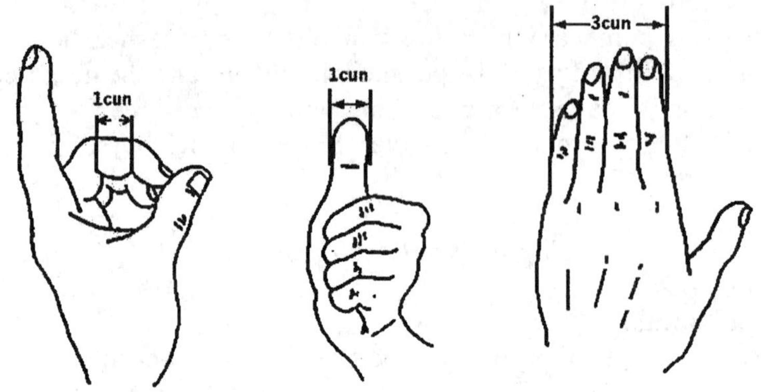

Fig. XIII-2 Middle finger *cun* Thumb *cun* Four-finger measurement

Table XIII-9 Finger Measurement

Body Part	Distance	Proportional Measurement
Head	From anterior hairline to posterior hairline	12 *cun* (longitudinal)
	Between two mastoid processes	9 *cun* (transverse)
Chest & Bdomen	From sternocostal angle to center of umbilicus	8 *cun* (longitudinal)
	Between center of umbilicus and upper border of symphysis pubis	5 *cun* (longitudinal)
	Between the nipples	8 *cun* (transverse)
Back	Between medial border of scapula and posterior midline	3 *cun* (transverse)
Lateral side of chest	From end of axillary fold on lateral side of chest to tip of 11th rib	12 *cun* (longitudinal)
Upper extremities	Between end of axillary fold and transverse cubital crease	9 *cun* (longitudinal)
	Between transverse cubital crease and transverse wrist crease	12 *cun* (longitudinal)
Lower extremities	From upper border of symphysis pubis to medial epicondyle of femur	18 *cun* (longitudinal)
	From lower border of medial condyle of tibia to tip of medial malleolus	13 *cun* (longitudinal)
	From prominence of great trochanter to middle of patella	19 *cun* (longitudinal)
	Between center of patella and tip of lateral malleolus	16 *cun* (longitudinal)
	From tip of lateral malleolus to heel	3 *cun* (longitudinal)

The Acupoints of the 14 Meridians
Points of Lung Meridian of Hand-Taiyin (LU)
(Color Figs. 9 and 15)

1. Zhongfu (LU 1) (Front-Curtain Point of the Lungs) (crossing SP)

[Location] In the anterior thoracic wall, on the level of the 1st intercostal space, 6 *cun* lateral to the anterior midline.

[Effects] Facilitates the flow of Lung *qi* and purges away evil heat from the chest.

[Indications] Coughing, asthma, and pain in the chest, shoulder and back, as occurring in bronchitis, pneumonia, pulmonary tuberculosis and angina pectoris.

[Manipulation] Puncture obliquely 0.5-0.8 *cun* towards the lateral aspect of the chest. Never puncture deeply towards the medial aspect to avoid injuring the lung.

2. Yunmen (LU 2)

[Location] In the anterior thoracic wall, in the depression of the infraclavicular fossa, 6 *cun* lateral to the anterior midline.

[Effects] Facilitates the flow of Lung *qi* and purges away evil heat from the arm.

[Indications] Coughing, asthma, and pain in the chest, shoulder and arm, as occurring in bronchitis, and periarthritis of the shoulder.

[Manipulation] Puncture obliquely 0.5-1.0 *cun* towards the lateral aspect of the chest. Never puncture deeply towards the medial aspect to avoid injuring the lung.

3. Tianfu (LU 3)

[Location] On the medial side of upper arm, 3 *cun* below the anterior end of axillary fold.

[Effects] Facilitates the flow of Lung *qi* and arrests nose bleeding.

[Indications] Coughing, asthma, epistaxis, and pain in the medial aspect of the upper arm.

[Manipulation] Puncture perpendicularly 0.5-1.0 *cun*.

4. Xiabai (LU 4)

[Location] On the medial side of the upper arm, 4 *cun* below the anterior end of axillary fold.

[Effects] Facilitates the flow of Lung *qi* and calms the Heart.

[Indications] Cough in bronchitis, tachycardia, pain in the medial aspect of the upper arm.

[Manipulation] Puncture perpendicularly 0.5-1.0 *cun*.

5. Chize (LU 5) (*He*-Sea Point)

[Location] In the cubital crease, in the depression of the radial side of tendon of biceps muscle.

[Effects] Facilitates the flow of Lung *qi* and purges away fire.

[Indications] Coughing, asthma, hemoptysis, sore throat, afternoon fever, hypertension.

[Manipulation] Puncture perpendicularly 0.5-1.0 *cun*.

6. Kongzui (LU 6) (Cleft Point)

[Location] On the radial side of the palmar surface of forearm, 7 *cun* above the crease of the wrist.

[Effects] Clears up heat, induces diaphoresis, and soothes the throat.

[Indications] Coughing, asthma, pain in the chest, hemoptysis, sore throat, pain in the elbow and arm.

[Manipulation] Puncture perpendicularly 0.5-1.0 *cun*.

7. Lieque (LU 7) (Connecting Point, Confluence Point of the Conception Vessel)

[Location] Superior to the styloid process of the radius, 1.5 *cun* above the transverse crease of the wrist.

[Effects] Facilitates the flow of Lung *qi*, relieves cough, promotes micturition and removes wind from the collateral meridians.

[Indications] Fever and coughing in colds, acute retention of urine, soft tissue injury of the wrist, pain and stiffness in the neck and nape.

[Manipulation] Puncture 0.3-0.5 *cun* obliquely upward.

8. Jingqu (LU 8) (*Jing*-River Point)

[Location] 1 *cun* above the transverse crease of the wrist in the depression on the lateral side of the radial artery.

[Effects] Facilitates the flow of Lung *qi*, soothes the throat, and restores normal pulse.

[Indications] Coughing, asthma, sore throat, chest pain, pain in the wrist, pulseless disease (Takayasu disease).

[Manipulation] Puncture perpendicularly 0.3-0.5 *cun*. Avoid puncturing the radial artery and vein.

9. Taiyuan (LU 9) (*Shu*-Stream Point, Primary Point, Influential Point of Vessels)

[Location] At the radial end of the transverse crease of the wrist, in the depression on the lateral side of the radial artery.

[Effects] Facilitates the flow of Lung *qi*, soothes the throat, and restores normal pulse.

[Indications] Coughing, asthma, hemoptysis, sore throat, palpitations, pulseless disease (Takayasu disease).

[Manipulation] Puncture perpendicularly 0.3-0.5 *cun*. Avoid puncturing the radial artery and vein.

10. Yuji (LU 10) (*Ying*-Spring Point)

[Location] On the radial side of the midpoint of the 1st metacarpal bone, and on the dorso-ventral boundary of the hand.

[Effects] Clears the Lung of heat, arrests cough, and relieves sore throat.

[Indications] Coughing, hemoptysis and acute tonsillitis.

[Manipulation] Puncture slightly obliquely 0.3-0.8 *cun* towards the center of the palm.

11. Shaoshang (LU 11) (*Jing*-Well Point)

[Location] On the radial side of the thumb, 0.1 *cun* proximal to the corner of nail.

[Effects] Induces resuscitation, clears up heat, and relieves sore throat.

[Indications] High fever, loss of consciousness, acute respiratory infection.

[Manipulation] Puncture 0.1 *cun*, or prick to cause bleeding.

Points of Large Intestine Meridian of Hand-Yangming (LI)

(Color Figs. 10, 16, 17 and Fig. XIII-3)

1. Shangyang (LI 1) (*Jing*-Well Point)

[Location] On the radial side of the index finger, 0.1 *cun* proximal to the corner of the nail.

[Effects] Purges away heat, induces resuscitation, and relieves sore throat.

[Indications] Loss of consciousness in cases of stroke or high fever, febrile disease with anhidrosis, sore throat, toothache and swelling of the submandibular region.

[Manipulation] Puncture 0.1 *cun* or prick to cause bleeding.

2. Erjian (LI 2) (*Ying*-Spring Point)

[Location] In the depression of the radial side of the index finger, distal to the metacarpal-phalangeal joint, on the dorso-ventral boundary.

[Effects] Clears up heat, soothes the throat, and improves the vision.

[Indications] Blurred vision, epistaxis, toothache, sore throat, fever.

[Manipulation] Puncture 0.2-0.3 *cun* when the patient's index finger is bent.

3. Sanjian (LI 3) (*Shu*-Stream Point)

[Location] In the depression of the radial side of the index finger, proximal to the metacarpal-phalangeal joint.

[Effects] Purges heat and soothes the throat.

[Indications] Toothache, sore throat, metacarpophalangeal arthritis.

[Manipulation] Puncture 0.5-1.0 *cun* when the patient makes a loose fist.

4. Hegu (LI 4) (Primary Point)

[Location] On the dorsum of the hand, between the 1st and 2nd metacarpal bones, and on the radial side of the midpoint of the 2nd metacarpal bone.

[Effects] Disperses pathogenic wind, purges the Lung of heat, harmonizes the Stomach and Intestines, causes resuscitation, regulates menstruation and induces labor.

[Indications] Fever with anhidrosis or hidrosis, loss of consciousness in stroke, shock, facial paralysis or spasm, trismus, headache, sore throat, constipation, dysentery, amenorrhea, delayed labor, urticaria, pain and motor impairment of the upper limb.

[Manipulation] Puncture perpendicularly 0.5-1.0 *cun*. Avoid injuring the local blood vessels.

[Warning] Contraindicated in pregnancy.

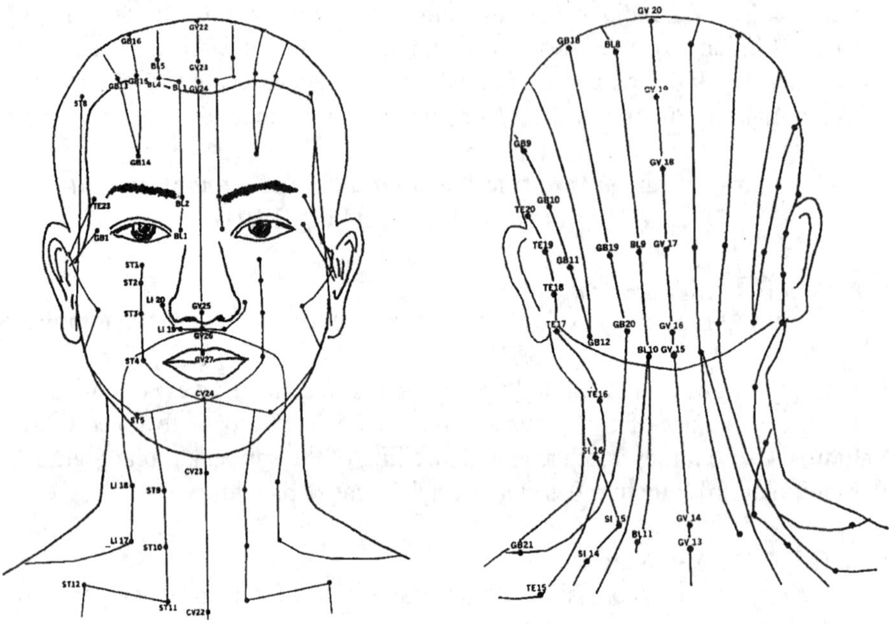

Fig. XIII-3 Points on the head

5. Yangxi (LI 5) (*Jing*-River Point)

[Location] At the radial end of the wrist crease, in the depression between the tendons of the short and long extensor muscles of the thumb.

[Effects] Dispels wind and purges away fire.

[Indications] Headache, inflammation of the eye, toothache, sore throat, pain in the wrist.

[Manipulation] Puncture perpendicularly 0.3-0.5 *cun*. Avoid injuring the local blood vessels.

6. Pianli (LI 6) (Connecting Point)

[Location] On the radial side of the dorsal surface of the forearm, 3 *cun* above the crease of the wrist.

[Effects] Clears the Lung, regulates the water course, and removes obstruction from the collateral meridians.

[Indications] Epistaxis, sore throat, facial paralysis, oliguria with edema, pain in the forearm.

[Manipulation] Puncture 0.5-0.8 *cun* obliquely upward or downward.

7. Wenliu (LI 7) (Cleft Point)

[Location] On the radial side of the dorsal surface of the forearm, 5 *cun* above the crease of the wrist.

[Effects] Removes evil heat, and regulates the gastrointestinal function.

[Indications] Frontal headache, sore throat, stomatitis, borborygmi, abdominal distention, pain in the arm and shoulder.

[Manipulation] Puncture perpendicularly 0.3-0.5 *cun*.

8. Xialian (LI 8)

[Location] On the radial side of the dorsal surface of the forearm, 4 *cun* below the cubital crease.

[Effects] Purges heat from the Yangming Meridian.

[Indications] Abdominal pain, borborygmi, pain in the elbow and arm, motor impairment of the upper limb.

[Manipulation] Puncture perpendicularly 0.5-1.0 *cun*.

9. Shanglian (LI 9)

[Location] On the radial side of the dorsal surface of the forearm, 3 *cun* below the cubital crease.

[Effects] Purges away heat from the Yangming Meridian.

[Indications] Abdominal pain, borborygmi, pain in the arm and shoulder, numbness of the hand and arm, motor impairment of the upper limb.

[Manipulation] Puncture perpendicularly 0.5-1.0 *cun*.

10. Shousanli (LI 10)

[Location] On the radial side of the dorsal surface of the forearm, 2 *cun* below the cubital crease.

[Effects] Regulates the gastrointestinal function.

[Indications] Abdominal pain, diarrhea, toothache, motor impairment of the upper limb, pain in the shoulder and back.

[Manipulation] Puncture perpendicularly 0.8-1.5 *cun*.

11. Quchi (LI 11) (*He*-Sea Point)

[Location] At the lateral end of the cubital crease with the elbow flexed.

[Effects] Disperses heat, soothes the joints, and regulates *qi* and blood.

[Indications] Fever, sore throat, toothache, inflammation of the eye, abdominal pain, constipation, diarrhea, menstrual disorders, urticaria, pain of the elbow and arm, motor impairment of the upper limb.

[Manipulation] Puncture perpendicularly 1.0-1.5 *cun*.

12. Zhouliao (LI 12)

[Location] On the lateral side of the upper arm, superior to the lateral epicondyle of the humerus when the elbow is flexed, 1 *cun* superior and lateral to Quchi (LI 11).

[Indications] Pain in the elbow (external humeral epicondylitis).

[Manipulation] Puncture perpendicularly 0.5-1.0 *cun*.

13. Shouwuli (LI 13)

[Location] On the lateral side of the upper arm, on the line joining Quchi (LI 11) and Jianyu (LI 15), 3 *cun* above Quchi.

[Indications] Pain in the elbow and arm.

[Manipulation] Puncture perpendicularly 0.5-1.0 *cun*.

14. Binao (LI 14)

[Location] On the lateral side of the arm, on the line joining Quchi (LI 11) and Jianyu (LI 15), 7 *cun* above Quchi.

[Indications] Pain in the shoulder and arm, rigidity of the neck.

[Manipulation] Puncture perpendicularly or obliquely upward 0.5-1.0 *cun*.

15. Jianyu (LI 15) (crossing YangHV)

[Location] On the shoulder, in the depression anterior and inferior to the acromion when the arm is abducted.

[Effects] Dispels wind-damp from the meridians, soothes the joints, and reduces heat.

[Indications] Pain in the shoulder and arm (periarthritis of the shoulder), motor impairment of the upper limb, urticaria, hypertension.

[Manipulation] Puncture perpendicularly or obliquely 0.8-1.5 *cun*.

16. Jugu (LI 16) (crossing YangHV)

[Location] On the shoulder, in the depression between the acromial extremity of the clavicle and scapular spine.

[Indications] Pain and motor impairment of the upper limb, pain in the shoulder and back.

[Manipulation] Puncture perpendicularly 0.5-0.8 *cun*. Avoid deep insertion.

17. Tianding (LI 17)

[Location] On the lateral side of the neck, 1 *cun* below Futu (LI 18), on the posterior border of the sterno-cleido-mastoid muscle.

[Effects] Soothes the throat.

[Indications] Sudden loss of voice, sore throat, goiter, numbness of the upper limb.

[Manipulation] Puncture perpendicularly 0.3-0.5 *cun*. Avoid deep insertion.

18. Futu (LI 18)

[Location] On the lateral side of the neck, beside the laryngeal protuberance, between the sternal head and clavicular head of the sternocleidomastoid muscle.

[Effects] Facilitates the flow of Lung *qi*, soothes the throat, and resolves nodulation.

[Indications] Coughing, asthma, sore throat, sudden loss of voice, goiter.

[Manipulation] Puncture perpendicularly 0.3-0.5 *cun*.

19. Kouheliao (LI 19)

[Location] On the upper lip, 0.5 *cun* lateral to Shuigou (GV 26).

[Effects] Removes obstruction from the nose.

[Indications] Rhinitis, facial paralysis.

[Manipulation] Puncture obliquely 0.2-0.3 *cun*.

20. Yingxiang (LI 20) (crossing ST)

[Location] In the nasolabial groove, beside the midpoint of the lateral border of ala nasi.

[Effects] Removes obstruction from the nose, disperses wind and clears up fire.

[Indications] Rhinitis, sinusitis, hyposmia, epistaxis, facial paralysis.

[Manipulation] Puncture obliquely or subcutaneously 0.3-0.5 *cun*.

Points of Stomach Meridian of Foot-Yangming (ST)

(Color Figs.12, 15, 17 and Fig. III-3)

1. Chengqi (ST 1) (crossing CV, YangHV)

[Location] On the face, directly below the pupil when the eyes look straight forward, between the eyeball and the infraorbital ridge.

[Effects] Dispels wind and fire, and improves vision.

[Indications] Inflammation of the eye, night blindness, lacrimation, twitching of the eyelid, facial paralysis.

[Manipulation] Push the eyeball upward with the left thumb and insert the needle along the inferior wall of the orbit 0.3-0.5 *cun*. Lifting-thrusting the needle is prohibited.

2. Sibai (ST 2)

[Location] On the face, directly below the pupil in the depression at the infraorbital foramen.

[Effects] Dispels wind and fire, and improves vision.

[Indications] Inflammation of the eye, blurred vision, twitching of the eyelid, facial paralysis, pain in the face (trigeminal neuralgia).

[Manipulation] Puncture perpendicularly or obliquely 0.3-0.5 *cun*.

3. Juliao (ST 3) (crossing YangHV)

[Location] On the face, directly below the pupil, at the level of the lower border of ala nasi.

[Effects] Dispels wind, and removes obstruction from the nose.

[Indications] Facial paralysis, twitching of the eyelid, pain in the face (trigeminal neuralgia), rhinitis, epistaxis.

[Manipulation] Puncture 0.3-0.5 *cun* perpendicularly or obliquely upward.

4. Dicang (ST 4) (crossing LI, YangHV)

[Location] On the face, directly below the pupil, lateral to the corner of the mouth.

[Indications] Facial paralysis, twitching of the eyelid, salivation.

[Manipulation] Puncture 1.0-1.5 *cun* subcutaneously towards Jiache (ST 6).

5. Daying (ST 5)

[Location] Anterior to the mandibular angle, on the anterior border of masseter muscle, in the groove-like depression appearing when the cheek bulges.

[Indications] Facial paralysis, trismus, pain in the face, toothache.

[Manipulation] Avoid puncturing the artery. Puncture obliquely 0.3-0.5 *cun*.

6. Jiache (ST 6)

[Location] On the cheek, one finger breadth anterior and superior to the mandibular angle, at the prominence of the masseter muscle when the jaw is clenched.

[Indications] Facial paralysis, toothache, swelling of the cheek and face, trismus.

[Manipulation] Puncture 0.3-0.5 *cun* perpendicularly or 1.0-1.5 *cun* subcutaneously towards Dicang (ST 4).

7. Xiaguan (ST 7) (crossing GB)

[Location] On the face, anterior to the ear, in the depression between the zygomatic arch and mandibular notch.

[Effects] Dispels wind, and improves hearing.

[Indications] Impaired hearing, tinnitus, toothache, facial paralysis, pain of the face, motor impairment of the jaw (disorder of temporomandibular joint).

[Manipulation] Puncture perpendicularly 0.3-0.5 *cun*.

8. Touwei (ST 8) (crossing GB, YangLV)

[Location] On the lateral side of the head, 0.5 *cun* above the anterior hairline at the corner of the forehead.

[Effects] Dispels wind from the head, and improves vision.

[Indications] Frontal headache, migraine, blurring of vision, pain in the eye, lacrimation.

[Manipulation] Puncture 0.5-1.0 *cun* subcutaneously with the tip of the needle directed suproposteriorly or inferolaterally.

9. Renying (ST 9)

[Location] On the neck, beside the laryngeal protuberance, and on the anterior border of sternocleidomastoid muscle where the pulsation of the common carotid artery is palpable.

[Effects] Checks upward perversion of *qi*.

[Indications] Coughing, asthma, sore throat, goiter, hypertension, hypotension.

[Manipulation] Avoid puncturing the common carotid artery. Puncture perpendicularly 0.3-0.5 *cun* when the patient is lying supine.

10. Shuitu (ST 10)

[Location] On the anterior border of the sternocleidomastoid muscle, at the midpoint of the line connecting Renying (ST 9) and Qishe (ST 11).

[Effects] Checks upward perversion of *qi*.

[Indications] Coughing, asthma, sore throat, hiccups, goiter.

[Manipulation] Avoid puncturing the artery. Puncture perpendicularly 0.3-0.5 *cun* with no retention of the needle.

11. Qishe (ST 11)

[Location] On the upper border of the medial end of the clavicle, between the sternal head and clavicular head of the sternocleidomastoid muscle.

[Effects] Soothes the throat and disperses goiter.

[Indications] Sore throat, asthma, hiccups, goiter.

[Manipulation] Puncture perpendicularly 0.3-0.5 *cun*.

12. Quepen (ST 12)

[Location] At the center of the supraclavicular fossa, 4 *cun* lateral to the anterior midline.

[Effects] Purges heat from the chest.

[Indications] Coughing, asthma, sore throat, pain in the supraclavicular fossa.

[Manipulation] Avoid puncturing the artery. Puncture perpendicularly 0.3-0.5 *cun*. Deep puncture is prohibited.

13. Qihu (ST 13)

[Location] On the chest, below the midpoint of the lower border of the clavicle, 4 *cun* lateral to the anterior midline.

[Effects] Facilitates the flow of Lung *qi*.

[Indications] Fullness in the chest, cough, asthma, hiccups, pain in the chest and hypochondrium.

[Manipulation] Puncture obliquely 0.3-0.5 *cun*, or subcutaneously 0.5-0.8 *cun*.

14. Kufang (ST 14)

[Location] On the chest, in the 1st intercostal space, 4 *cun* lateral to the anterior midline.

[Effects] Facilitates the flow of Lung *qi*.

[Indications] Fullness and pain in the chest, coughing.

[Manipulation] Puncture obliquely 0.3-0.5 *cun*, or subcutaneously 0.5-0.8 *cun*.

15. Wuyi (ST 15)

[Location] On the chest, in the 2nd intercostal space, 4 *cun* lateral to the anterior midline.

[Effects] Facilitate the flow of Lung *qi*.

[Indications] Fullness and pain in the chest, coughing, asthma, mastitis.

[Manipulation] Puncture obliquely 0.3-0.5 *cun*, or subcutaneously 0.5-0.8 *cun*.

16. Yingchuang (ST 16)

[Location] On the chest, in the 3rd intercostal space, 4 *cun* lateral to the anterior midline.

[Effects] Regulates the flow of *qi*, and promotes lactation.

[Indications] Fullness and pain in the chest, coughing, asthma, mastitis, hyperplasia of mammary glands.

[Manipulation] Puncture obliquely 0.3-0.5 *cun*, or subcutaneously 0.5-0.8 *cun*.

17. Ruzhong (ST 17)

[Location] At the center of the nipple.

[Effects] Serves only as a landmark for locating acupoints on the chest. Puncture and moxibustion are prohibited.

18. Rugen (ST 18)

[Location] On the chest, in the 5th intercostal space, 4 *cun* lateral to the anterior midline.

[Effects] Regulates the flow of *qi*, and promotes lactation.

[Indications] Fullness and pain in the chest, coughing, asthma, insufficient lactation, mastitis, hyperplasia of the mammary glands.

[Manipulation] Puncture obliquely 0.3-0.5 *cun*.

19. Burong (ST 19)

[Location] On the upper abdomen, 6 *cun* above the center of the umbilicus and 2 *cun* lateral to the anterior midline.

[Effects] Harmonizes the Stomach and arrests vomiting.

[Indications] Abdominal distention, vomiting, gastric pain and anorexia.

[Manipulation] Puncture obliquely 0.5-0.8 *cun*.

20. Chengman (ST 20)

[Location] On the upper abdomen, 5 *cun* above the center of the umbilicus and 2 *cun* lateral to the anterior midline.

[Effects] Harmonizes the Stomach and arrests vomiting.

[Indications] Abdominal distention, vomiting, gastric pain and anorexia.

[Manipulation] Puncture perpendicularly or obliquely 0.5-0.8 *cun*.

21. Liangmen (ST 21)

[Location] On the upper abdomen, 4 *cun* above the center of the umbilicus and 2 *cun* lateral to the anterior midline.

[Effects] Harmonizes the Stomach and Intestines, and promotes digestion.

[Indications] Gastric pain, vomiting, anorexia, abdominal distention, diarrhea.

[Manipulation] Puncture perpendicularly or obliquely 0.5-1.0 *cun*.

22. Guanmen (ST 22)

[Location] On the upper abdomen, 3 *cun* above the center of the umbilicus and 2 *cun* lateral to the anterior midline.

[Effects] Regulates the Spleen and Stomach *qi*, and promotes digestion.

[Indications] Abdominal distention and pain, anorexia, borborygmi, diarrhea, and edema.

[Manipulation] Puncture perpendicularly or obliquely 0.5-1.0 *cun*.

23. Taiyi (ST 23)

[Location] On the upper abdomen, 2 *cun* above the center of the umbilicus and 2 *cun* lateral to the anterior midline.

[Indications] Gastralgia, restlessness.

[Manipulation] Puncture perpendicularly or obliquely 0.5-1.0 *cun*.

24. Huaroumen (ST 24)

[Location] On the upper abdomen, 1 *cun* above the center of the umbilicus and 2 *cun* lateral to the anterior midline.

[Indications] Gastralgia, vomiting, and restlessness.

[Manipulation] Puncture perpendicularly or obliquely 0.5-1.0 *cun*.

25. Tianshu (ST 25) (Front-Curtain Point of the Large Intestine)

[Location] On the middle abdomen, 2 *cun* lateral to the center of the umbilicus.

[Effects] Strengthens the Spleen, harmonizes the Intestines, resolves damp, promotes digestion, and regulates menstruation.

[Indications] Abdominal pain (around the umbilicus), borborygmi, constipation, diarrhea, dysentery, irregular menstruation, and edema.

[Manipulation] Puncture perpendicularly or obliquely 0.8-1.2 *cun*.

26. Wailing (ST 26)

[Location] On the lower abdomen, 1 *cun* below the center of the umbilicus and 2 *cun* lateral to the anterior midline.

[Effects] Harmonizes the Intestines, and smoothes the flow of *qi*.

[Indications] Abdominal pain, and dysmenorrhea.

[Manipulation] Puncture perpendicularly or obliquely 0.8-1.2 *cun*.

27. Daju (ST 27)

[Location] On the lower abdomen, 2 *cun* below the center of umbilicus and 2 *cun* lateral to the anterior midline.

[Indications] Lower abdominal distension, dysuria, hernia, seminal emission, premature ejaculation.

[Manipulation] Puncture perpendicularly or obliquely 0.8-1.2 *cun*.

28. Shuidao (ST 28)

[Location] On the lower abdomen, 3 *cun* below the center of the umbilicus and 2 *cun* lateral to the anterior midline.

[Effects] Induces micturition, relieves distention, and regulates menstruation.

[Indications] Lower abdominal distention, retention of urine, edema, and dysmenorrhea.

[Manipulation] Puncture perpendicularly or obliquely 0.8-1.2 *cun*.

29. Guilai (ST 29)

[Location] On the lower abdomen, 4 *cun* below the center of umbilicus and 2 *cun* lateral to the anterior midline.

[Effects] Regulates *qi*, and lifts the uterus.

[Indications] Abdominal pain, and hernia,

[Manipulation] Puncture perpendicularly or obliquely 0.8-1.2 *cun*.

30. Qichong (ST 30)

[Location] Slightly above the inguinal groove, 5 *cun* below the center of the umbilicus and 2 *cun* lateral to the anterior midline.

[Indications] Abdominal pain, borborygmi, hernia, diseases of the male and female genital organs.

[Manipulation] Avoid puncturing the artery. Puncture perpendicularly 0.5-1.0 *cun*.

31. Biguan (ST 31)

[Location] On the anterior side of the upper thigh, at the level of the inferior border of the symphysis pubis, in the depression lateral to the sartorius muscle.

[Effects] Dispels wind, removes obstruction from the collateral meridians, and soothes the lower back and knees.

[Indications] Pain in the thigh, muscular atrophy, numbness, pain or paralysis of the lower limb.

[Manipulation] Puncture perpendicularly 1.0-1.5 *cun*.

32. Futu (ST 32)

[Location] On the anterior side of the thigh, on the line connecting the anterior superior iliac spine and lateral border of the patella, 6 *cun* above the superolateral corner of the patella.

[Effects] Dispels cold-damp, and soothes the lower back and knees.

[Indications] Pain in the lumbar and iliac region, coldness of the knee, paralysis or motor impairment and pain of the lower limbs.

[Manipulation] Puncture perpendicularly 1.0-1.5 *cun*.

33. Yinshi (ST 33)

[Location] On the anterior side of the thigh, on the line connecting the anterior superior iliac spine and lateral border of the patella, 3 *cun* above the superolateral corner of the patella.

[Effects] Dispels cold-damp, and soothes the knees.

[Indications] Pain, numbness and motor impairment of the leg and knee, paralysis of the lower limbs.

[Manipulation] Puncture perpendicularly 0.5-1.0 *cun*.

34. Liangqiu (ST 34) (Cleft Point)

[Location] On the anterior side of the thigh, on the line connecting the anterior superior iliac spine and lateral border of the patella, 2 *cun* above the superolateral corner of the patella, when the knee is flexed.

[Effects] Harmonizes the Stomach, and dispels wind-damp.

[Indications] Pain and numbness of the knee, gastric pain, mastitis, motor impairment of the lower limbs.

[Manipulation] Puncture perpendicularly 0.5-1.0 *cun*.

35. Dubi (ST 35)

[Location] On the knee, in the depression lateral to the patella and its ligament when the knee is flexed.

[Effects] Dispels wind-damp, and soothes the knee.

[Indications] Diseases of the knee joint and soft tissue diseases around the knee joint.

[Manipulation] Puncture perpendicularly 0.5-1.0 *cun*.

36. Zusanli (ST 36) (*He*-Sea Point)

[Location] On the anterolateral side of the leg, 3 *cun* below Dubi (ST 35), one finger breadth from the anterior crest of the tibia.

[Effects] Regulates the Spleen and Stomach, harmonizes the Intestines, checks the upward perversion of *qi*, and strengthens the body resistance.

[Indications] Gastric pain, vomiting, hiccups, abdominal distention, borborygmi, diarrhea, constipation, indigestion, coughing, asthma, edema, emaciation, general weakness, hypotension, hypertension, allergic diseases, anemia, and leucopenia.

[Manipulation] Puncture perpendicularly 1.0-1.5 *cun*.

37. Shangjuxu (ST 37) (Lower Sea Point of the Large Intestine)

[Location] On the anterolateral side of the leg, 6 *cun* below Dubi (ST 35), one finger breadth from the anterior crest of tibia.

[Effects] Regulates the Spleen and Stomach, harmonizes the Intestines.

[Indications] Abdominal pain and distention, borborygmi, diarrhea, constipation, paralysis of the lower limbs.

[Manipulation] Puncture perpendicularly 1.0-1.5 *cun*.

38. Tiaokou (ST 38)

[Location] On the anterolateral side of the leg, 8 *cun* below Dubi (ST 35), one finger breadth from the anterior crest of the tibia.

[Effects] Harmonizes the Stomach and Intestines.

[Indications] Abdominal pain, pain and numbness of the knee and leg, weakness and motor impairment of the foot, pain and motor impairment of the shoulders.

[Manipulation] Puncture perpendicularly 0.5-1.0 *cun*.

39. Xiajuxu (ST 39) (Lower Sea Point of the Small Intestine)

[Location] On the anterolateral side of the leg, 9 *cun* below Dubi (ST 35), one finger breadth from the anterior crest of the tibia.

[Effects] Harmonizes the Intestines, and promotes lactation.

[Indications] Lower abdominal pain, backache referring to the testis, mastitis, numbness and paralysis of the lower limbs.

[Manipulation] Puncture perpendicularly 0.5-1.0 *cun*.

40. Fenglong (ST 40) (Connecting Point)

[Location] On the anterolateral side of the leg, 8 *cun* above the tip of the external malleolus, one finger breadth lateral to Tiaokou (ST 38) or two finger breadths from the anterior crest of the tibia.

[Effects] Harmonizes the Stomach, resolves damp-phlegm, and restores normal mental activity.

[Indications] Headache, dizziness, coughing, asthma, excessive expectoration, vomiting, mania, epilepsy, muscular atrophy, paralysis of the lower limbs.

[Manipulation] Puncture perpendicularly 0.5-1.0 *cun*.

41. Jiexi (ST 41) (*Jing*-River Point)

[Location] On the dorsum of the foot, at the midpoint of the transverse crease between the instep and the leg, in the depression between the tendons of the long extensor muscles of the big toe and of the other toes.

[Effects] Regulates the Spleen, and resolves damp.

[Indications] Pain of the ankle joint, pain and paralysis of the lower limbs, headache, dizziness, abdominal distention, and constipation.

[Manipulation] Puncture perpendicularly 0.3-0.5 *cun*.

42. Chongyang (ST 42) (Primary Point)

[Location] At the prominence of the instep, in the depression between the tendons of the long extensor muscles of the big toe and of the other toes, where the pulsation of the dorsal artery of the foot is palpable.

[Effects] Harmonizes the Stomach, and calms the mind.

[Indications] Pain in the upper teeth, epigastric pain, mania, redness and swelling of the dorsum of the foot, facial paralysis, muscular atrophy and motor impairment of the foot.

[Manipulation] Avoid puncturing the artery. Puncture perpendicularly 0.3-0.5

cun.

43. Xiangu (ST 43) (*Shu*-Stream Point)

[Location] On the instep in the depression distal to the commissure of the 2nd and 3rd metatarsal bones.

[Effects] Induces diuresis, and promotes the flow of *qi*.

[Indications] Facial or general edema, abdominal pain, borborygmi, swelling and pain of the dorsum of the foot.

[Manipulation] Puncture perpendicularly 0.3-0.5 *cun*.

44. Neiting (ST 44) (*Ying*-Spring Point)

[Location] On the instep, at the proximal end of the skin crease of the web between the 2nd and 3rd toes.

[Effects] Clears the Stomach of heat, and promotes digestion.

[Indications] Toothache, pain in the face (trigeminal neuralgia), facial paralysis, fever, sore throat, foul breath, distress in the stomach, abdominal distention, diarrhea, constipation, swelling and pain of the dorsum of the foot.

[Manipulation] Puncture perpendicularly 0.3-0.5 *cun*, or obliquely 0.5-1.0 *cun* with the tip of the needle directed proximally.

45. Lidui (ST 45) (*Jing*-Well Point)

[Location] On the lateral side of the 2nd toe, 0.1 *cun* proximal to the corner of the toenail.

[Effects] Induces resuscitation, and clears the Stomach of heat.

[Indications] Syncope, deviation of the mouth, trismus, fever, toothache, sore throat, dream-disturbed sleep, and mania.

[Manipulation] Puncture 0.1 *cun*, or prick to cause bleeding.

The Points of the Spleen Meridian of Foot-Taiyin (SP)

(Color Figs 11, 15)

1. Yinbai (SP 1) (*Jing*-Well Point)

[Location] On the medial side of the big toe, 0.1 *cun* proximal to the corner of the toenail.

[Effects] Regulates the Spleen, calms the mind, and induces resuscitation.

[Indications] Abdominal distention, hematochezia, menorrhagia, mental disorders, and syncope.

[Manipulation] Puncture 0.1 *cun*, or prick to cause bleeding.

2. Dadu (SP 2) (*Ying*-Spring Point)

[Location] On the medial border of the foot, in the depression just distal to the metatarsophalangeal joint, at the dorso-ventral boundary.

[Effects] Invigorates the Spleen, and resolves dampness.

[Indications] Gastric pain, abdominal distention, diarrhea, constipation, fever with anhidrosis.

[Manipulation] Puncture perpendicularly 0.1-0.3 *cun*.

3. Taibai (SP 3) (*Shu*-Stream Point and Primary Point)

[Location] On the medial border of the foot, in the depression on the medial side of the distal end of the 1st metatarsal, at the dorso-ventral boundary.

[Effects] Supports the Spleen, and promotes digestion.

[Indications] Gastric pain, vomiting, abdominal distention, constipation, diarrhea, and borborygmi.

[Manipulation] Puncture perpendicularly 0.3-0.5 *cun*.

4. Gongsun (SP 4) (Connecting Point, Confluence Point of the Thoroughfare Vessel)

[Location] On the medial border of the foot, anterior and inferior to the proximal end of the 1st metatarsal.

[Effects] Harmonizes the Spleen and Stomach, and regulates the Thoroughfare Vessel.

[Indications] Gastric pain, vomiting, abdominal pain and distention, diarrhea, borborygmi, dysmenorrhea, and retention of placenta.

[Manipulation] Puncture perpendicularly 0.5-0.8 *cun*.

5. Shangqiu (SP 5) (*Jing*-River Point)

[Location] On the medial side of the ankle, in the depression anterior and inferior to the medial malleolus, midway between the tuberosity of the navicular bone and the tip of the medial malleolus.

[Effects] Invigorates the Spleen, and resolves dampness.

[Indications] Abdominal distention, constipation, diarrhea, borborygmi, edema of the lower extremities.

[Manipulation] Puncture perpendicularly 0.2-0.3 *cun*.

6. Sanyinjiao (SP 6) (crossing LR, KI)

[Location] On the medial side of the leg, 3 *cun* above the tip of the medial malleolus, just posterior to the tibia.

[Effects] Promotes the Spleen function, harmonizes the Lower Energizer, regulates the uterus, and dispels wind-damp.

[Indications] Abdominal pain and distention, borborygmi, diarrhea, amenorrhea, irregular menstruation, uterine bleeding, morbid leukorrhea, prolapse of the uterus, prolonged labor, infertility, nocturnal emission, impotence, enuresis, dysuria, edema, hernia, pain in the external genitalia, arthritis of the lower limb with pain and motor impairment, hypertension, insomnia, eczema, and urticaria.

[Manipulation] Puncture perpendicularly 0.5-1.0 *cun*.

[Warning] Contraindicated in pregnancy.

7. Lougu (SP 7)

[Location] On the medial side of the leg, 6 *cun* above the tip of the medial malleolus, just posterior to the tibia.

[Effects] Invigorates the Spleen, and resolves dampness.

[Indications] Abdominal distention, borborygmi, coldness and numbness of the knee and leg, and damp arthralgia.

[Manipulation] Puncture perpendicularly 0.5-1.0 *cun*.

8. Diji (SP 8) (Cleft Point)

[Location] On the medial side of the leg and on the line connecting Yinlingquan (SP 9) and the tip of the medial malleolus, 3 *cun* below Yinlingquan (SP 9).

[Effects] Harmonizes the Spleen, and regulates the Lower Energizer.

[Indications] Abdominal pain and distention, diarrhea, edema, dysuria, nocturnal emission, irregular menstruation, and dysmenorrhea.

[Manipulation] Puncture perpendicularly 0.5-1.0 *cun*.

9. Yinlingquan (SP 9) (*He*-Sea Point)

[Location] On the medial side of the leg, in the depression posterior and inferior to the medial condyle of the tibia.

[Effects] Invigorates the Spleen, resolves dampness, and induces diuresis.

[Indications] Abdominal pain and distention, diarrhea, edema, ascites, jaundice, dysuria, retention of urine, enuresis, incontinence of urine, pain in the external genitalia, dysmenorrhea, and pain in the knee.

[Manipulation] Puncture perpendicularly 0.5-1.0 *cun*.

10. Xuehai (SP 10)

[Location] On the medial side of the thigh, 2 *cun* above the superior medial corner of the patella, on the prominence of the medial head of the quadriceps muscle.

[Effects] Regulates blood, and harmonizes the Lower Energizer.

[Indications] Irregular menstruation, dysmenorrhea, uterine bleeding, amenorrhea, urticaria, eczema, anemia, and pain in the medial aspect of the thigh.

[Manipulation] Puncture perpendicularly 0.5-1.5 *cun*.

11. Jimen (SP 11)

[Location] On the medial side of the thigh, on the line connecting Xuehai (SP 10) and Chongmen (SP 12), 6 *cun* above Xuehai (SP 10).

[Effects] Harmonizes the Lower Energizer, and induces diuresis.

[Indications] Anuria, dysuria, enuresis, pain in the inguinal region, pain and paralysis of the lower limb.

[Manipulation] Puncture perpendicularly 0.5-1.0 *cun*.

12. Chongmen (SP 12) (crossing LR)

[Location] In the inguinal region, 3.5 *cun* lateral to the midpoint of the upper border of the symphysis pubis, lateral to the pulsating external iliac artery.

[Indications] Abdominal pain, hernia, uterine bleeding.

[Manipulation] Avoid puncturing the artery. Puncture perpendicularly 0.5-1.0 *cun*.

13. Fushe (SP 13) (crossing LR, YinLV)

[Location] On the lower abdomen, at the level of 4 *cun* below the center of the umbilicus, 0.7 *cun* laterosuperior to Chongmen (SP 12), and 4 *cun* lateral to the anterior midline.

[Effects] Regulates the Lower Energizer, and disperses the accumulated mass.

[Indications] Lower abdominal pain, and hernia.

[Manipulation] Puncture perpendicularly 0.5-1.0 *cun*.

14. Fujie (SP 14)

[Location] On the lower abdomen, 1.3 *cun* below Daheng (SP 15), and 4 *cun* lateral to the anterior midline.

[Effects] Regulates the Intestines.

[Indications] Pain around the umbilicus, abdominal distention, hernia, diarrhea, and constipation.

[Manipulation] Puncture perpendicularly 0.5-1.0 *cun*.

15. Daheng (SP 15) (crossing YinLV)

[Location] On the middle abdomen, 4 *cun* lateral to the center of the umbilicus.

[Effects] Regulates the Intestines.

[Indications] Abdominal pain and distention, diarrhea, and constipation.

[Manipulation] Puncture perpendicularly or obliquely 0.8-1.2 *cun*.

16. Fu'ai (SP 16) (crossing YinLV)

[Location] On the upper abdomen, 3 *cun* above Daheng (SP 15), and 4 *cun* lateral to the anterior midline.

[Effects] Warms the Middle Energizer, and regulates the Intestines.

[Indications] Abdominal pain, indigestion, diarrhea, and constipation.

[Manipulation] Puncture perpendicularly or obliquely 0.8-1.2 *cun*.

17. Shidou (SP 17)

[Location] On the lateral side of the chest, in the 5th intercostal space, 6 *cun* lateral to the anterior midline.

[Effects] Soothes the chest.

[Indications] Fullness and pain in the chest and costal region.

[Manipulation] Puncture 0.3-0.5 *cun* transversely along the intercostal space.

18. Tianxi (SP 18)

[Location] On the lateral side of the chest, in the 4th intercostal space, 6 *cun* lateral to the anterior midline.

[Effects] Soothes the chest and promotes lactation.

[Indications] Fullness and pain in the chest and costal region, coughing, hiccups, mastitis, insufficient lactation.

[Manipulation] Puncture 0.3-0.5 *cun* transversely along the intercostal space.

19. Xiongxiang (SP 19)

[Location] On the lateral side of the chest, in the 3rd intercostal space, 6 *cun* lateral to the anterior midline.

[Effects] Soothes the chest.

[Indications] Fullness and pain in the chest and costal region.

[Manipulation] Puncture 0.3-0.5 *cun* transversely along the intercostal space.

20. Zhourong (SP 20)

[Location] On the lateral side of the chest, in the 2nd intercostal space, 6 *cun* lateral to the anterior midline.

[Effects] Soothes the chest, and promotes the flow of *qi*.

[Indications] Fullness and pain in the chest and costal region, coughing, and hiccups.

[Manipulation] Puncture 0.3-0.5 *cun* transversely along the intercostal space.

21. Dabao (SP 21) (Connecting Point)

[Location] On the lateral side of the chest, in the 6th intercostal space and on the middle axillary line.

[Effects] Soothes the chest and costal region.

[Indications] Pain in the chest and costal region, asthma, and general aching.

[Manipulation] Puncture 0.3-0.5 *cun* transversely along the intercostal space.

The Points of the Heart Meridian of Hand-Shaoyin (HT)

(Color Fig. 9)

1. Jiquan (HT 1)

[Location] At the apex of the axillary fossa, where the pulsation of the axillary artery is palpable.

[Indications] Pain in the costal and cardiac regions, cold pain in the elbow and arm.

[Manipulation] Avoid puncturing the axillary artery. Puncture perpendicularly 0.5-1.0 *cun*.

2. Qingling (HT 2)

[Location] On the medial side of the arm, 3 *cun* above the cubital crease, in the groove medial to the biceps muscle.

[Indications] Pain in the cardiac and costal regions, shoulder and arm.

[Manipulation] Puncture perpendicularly 0.3-0.5 *cun*.

3. Shaohai (HT 3) (He-Sea Point)

[Location] At the midpoint of the line connecting the medial end of the cubital crease and the medial epicondyle of the humerus when the elbow is flexed.

[Indications] Cardiac pain, pain and numbness of the hand and arm, tremor of the hand, and pain in the axilla and costal region.

[Manipulation] Puncture 0.5-1.0 *cun* perpendicularly or obliquely with the tip of the needle directing distally.

4. Lingdao (HT 4) (*Jing*-River Point)

[Location] On the palmar side of the forearm and on the radial side of the tendon of the ulnar flexor muscle of the wrist, 1.5 *cun* proximal to the crease of the wrist.

[Indications] Cardiac pain, pain of the elbow and arm, and sudden loss of voice.

[Manipulation] Puncture perpendicularly 0.3-0.5 *cun*.

5. Tongli (HT 5) (Connecting Point)

[Location] On the palmar side of the forearm and on the radial side of the tendon of the ulnar flexor muscle of the wrist, 1 *cun* proximal to the crease of the wrist.

[Effects] Quiets the Heart, and calms the mind.

[Indications] Palpitations, dizziness, sore throat, sudden loss of voice, aphasia with stiffness of the tongue, and pain in the wrist and elbow.

[Manipulation] Puncture perpendicularly 0.3-0.5 *cun*.

6. Yinxi (HT 6) (Cleft Point)

[Location] On the palmar side of the forearm and on the radial side of the tendon of the ulnar flexor muscle of the wrist, 0.5 *cun* proximal to the crease of wrist.

[Effects] Clears the Heart of fire, calms the mind, and secures the superficies.

[Indications] Cardiac pain, hysteria, night sweating, epistaxis, and sudden loss of voice.

[Manipulation] Puncture perpendicularly 0.3-0.5 *cun*.

7. Shenmen (HT 7) (*Shu*-Stream Point, Primary Point)

[Location] On the wrist, in the depression of the radial side of the tendon of ulnar flexor muscle of the wrist.

[Effects] Calms the mind, clears the Heart of heat, and quenches fire.

[Indications] Cardiac pain, irritability, palpitations, insomnia, hysteria, mania, epilepsy, pain in the costal region, feverish sensation in the palm, and jaundice.

[Manipulation] Puncture perpendicularly 0.3-0.5 *cun*.

8. Shaofu (HT 8) (*Ying*-Spring Point)

[Location] On the palm, between the 4th and 5th metacarpal bones, at the part of the palm touching the tip of the little finger when the fist is clenched.

[Effects] Clears the Heart of fire.

[Indications] Palpitations (including arrhythmia), pain in the chest, pain in the little finger, feverish sensation in the palm, enuresis, dysuria, and pruritus of the external genitalia.

[Manipulation] Puncture perpendicularly 0.3-0.5 *cun*.

9. Shaochong (HT 9) (*Jing*-Well Point)

[Location] On the radial side of the little finger, 0.1 *cun* proximal to the corner of the nail.

[Effects] Induces resuscitations, and purges away heat.

[Indications] Palpitations, pain in the chest and costal regions, mania, fever, loss of consciousness.

[Manipulation] Puncture 0.1 *cun*, or prick to cause bleeding.

The Points of the Small Intestine Meridian of Hand-Taiyang (SI)

(Color Figs 10, 16, 17 and Fig. XIII-3)

1. Shaoze (SI 1) (*Jing*-Well Point)

[Location] On the ulnar side of the little finger, 0.1 *cun* proximal to the corner of the nail.

[Effects] Clears heat, soothes the throat, and promotes lactation.

[Indications] Fever, loss of consciousness, insufficient lactation, and sore throat.

[Manipulation] Puncture 0.1 *cun*, or prick to cause bleeding.

2. Qiangu (SI 2) (*Ying*-Spring Point)

[Location] At the intersection of the dorso-ventral boundary of the hand and the ulnar end of the crease of the 5th metacarpophalangeal joint.

[Effects] Clears up heat, and soothes the tendons.

[Indications] Fever, tinnitus, headache, numbness and itching of the fingers.

[Manipulation] Puncture perpendicularly 0.3-0.5 *cun*.

3. Houxi (SI 3) (*Shu*-Stream Point, Confluence Point of the Governor Vessel)

[Location] At the intersection of the dorso-ventral boundary of the hand and the ulnar end of the distal palmar crease.

[Effects] Clears heat, soothes the tendons, secures the superficies, and communicates with the Governor Vessel.

[Indications] Pain and rigidity of the neck, tinnitus, impaired hearing, sore throat, mania, fever (including fever in malaria), acute lumbar sprain, night sweating, contracture and numbness of the fingers, and pain in the shoulder and elbow.

[Manipulation] Puncture 0.5-0.8 *cun* perpendicularly towards Hegu (LI 4).

4. Wangu (SI 4) (Primary Point)

[Location] On the ulnar border of the hand, in the depression between the proximal end of the 5th metacarpal bone and hamate bone.

[Effects] Disperses the pathogenic factors from the Small Intestine Meridian, and clears damp-heat.

[Indications] Fever with anhidrosis, headache, rigidity of the neck, contracture of the fingers, pain in the wrist, and jaundice.

[Manipulation] Puncture perpendicularly 0.3-0.5 *cun*.

5. Yanggu (SI 5) (*Jing*-River Point)

[Location] On the ulnar border of the wrist, in the depression between the styloid process of the ulna and triangular bone.

[Effects] Clears heat, and soothes the tendons.

[Indications] Fever, pain of the hand and wrist.

[Manipulation] Puncture perpendicularly 0.3-0.5 *cun*.

6. Yanglao (SI 6) (Cleft Point)

[Location] On the ulnar side of the posterior surface of the forearm, in the depression proximal to and on the radial side of the head of the ulna.

[Effects] Soothes the tendons.

[Indications] Pain in the shoulder, elbow and arm, and stiff neck.

[Manipulation] Puncture perpendicularly 0.3-0.5 *cun*.

7. Zhizheng (SI 7) (Connecting Point)

[Location] On the ulnar side of the posterior surface of the forearm and on the line connecting Yanggu (SI 5) and Xiaohai (SI 8), 5 *cun* proximal to Yanggu (SI 5).

[Effects] Restores normal mental activity, and relieves fever from the superficies.

[Indications] Headache, dizziness, pain in the elbow and fingers, fever, and mania.

[Manipulation] Puncture perpendicularly 0.5-0.8 *cun*.

8. Xiaohai (SI 8) (*He*-Sea Point)

[Location] On the medial side of the elbow, in the depression between the olecranon of the ulna and the medial epicondyle of the humerus.

[Effects] Removes obstruction from the Small Intestine Meridian, dispels wind, and restores normal mental activity.

[Indications] Headache, swelling of the cheek, pain in the nape, shoulder, arm and elbow, epilepsy, and mania.

[Manipulation] Puncture 0.5-0.8 *cun* obliquely with the tip of the needle directed distally.

9. Jianzhen (SI 9)

[Location] Posterior and inferior to the shoulder joint, 1 *cun* above the posterior end of the axillary fold when the arm is adducted.

[Indications] Pain in the scapular region, and motor impairment of the hand and arm.

[Manipulation] Puncture perpendicularly 0.5-1.0 *cun*.

10. Naoshu (SI 10) (crossing YangLV, YangHV)

[Location] On the shoulder, above the posterior end of the axillary fold, in the depression below the lower border of the scapular spine.

[Indications] Pain and swelling of the shoulder.

[Manipulation] Puncture perpendicularly 0.5-1.0 *cun*.

11. Tianzong (SI 11)

[Location] On the scapula, in the depression of the center of the subscapular fossa, at the level of the 4th thoracic vertebra.

[Effects] Dispels wind-damp, and promotes lactation.

[Indications] Shoulder pain with difficulty in lifting the arm (periarthritis of the shoulder), stiff neck, mastitis, hyperplasia of mammary glands, insufficient lactation.

[Manipulation] Puncture perpendicularly or obliquely 0.5-1.0 *cun*.

12. Bingfeng (SI 12) (crossing GB, TE, LI)

[Location] On the scapula, at the center of the suprascapular fossa, directly above Tianzong (SI 11), in the depression found when the arm is raised.

[Effects] Disperses wind, and soothes the nape and shoulder.

[Indications] Pain in the scapular region with rigid nape, numbness and aching of the arm (cervical spondylosis).

[Manipulation] Puncture perpendicularly or obliquely 0.5-0.8 *cun*.

13. Quyuan (SI 13)

[Location] On the scapula, at the medial end of the suprascapular fossa, at the midpoint of the line connecting Naoshu (SI 10) and the spinous process of the 2nd thoracic vertebra.

[Effects] Disperses wind, and soothes the shoulder and back.

[Indications] Pain in the shoulder and scapular region (periarthritis of the shoulder and cervical spondylosis).

[Manipulation] Puncture perpendicularly 0.3-0.5 cum or obliquely 0.5-0.8 *cun*.

14. Jianwaishu (SI 14)

[Location] On the back, 3 *cun* lateral to the midpoint between the spinous processes of the 1st and 2nd thoracic vertebrae.

[Effects] Disperses wind, and soothes the shoulder and back.

[Indications] Pain in the shoulder and back, and stiff neck.

[Manipulation] Puncture obliquely 0.3-0.8 *cun*.

[Warning] Deeper puncture may cause pneumothorax, and so is prohibited.

15. Jianzhongshu (SI 15)

[Location] On the back, 2 *cun* lateral to the midpoint between the spinous processes of the 7th cervical and 1st thoracic vertebrae.

[Effects] Facilitates the flow of Lung *qi*, and checks its upward perversion.

[Indications] Coughing, asthma, pain in the shoulder and back.

[Manipulation] Puncture obliquely 0.3-0.8 *cun*.

[Warning] Deeper puncture may cause pneumothorax, and so is prohibited.

16. Tianchuang (SI 16)

[Location] On the lateral side of the neck, at the posterior border of the sternocleidomastoid muscle, and at the level of the laryngeal protuberance.

[Effects] Soothes the throat, and induces subsidence of swelling.

[Indications] Sore throat, sudden loss of voice, impaired hearing, tinnitus, stiffness and pain in the neck.

[Manipulation] Puncture Perpendicularly 0.3-0.8 *cun*.

17. Tianrong (SI 17)

[Location] On the lateral side of the neck, posterior to the mandibular angle, in the depression of the anterior border of the sternocleidomastoid muscle.

[Effects] Soothes the throat, and induces subsidence of swelling.

[Indications] Sore throat, sudden loss of voice, impaired hearing, tinnitus, stiffness and pain in the neck.

[Manipulation] Avoid puncturing the artery. Puncture perpendicularly 0.5-0.8 *cun*.

18. Quanliao (SI 18) (crossing TE)

[Location] On the face, directly below the outer canthus, in the depression below the zygomatic bone.

[Effects] Dispels wind, and soothes the face and cheek.

[Indications] Facial paralysis, twitching of eyelids, pain in the face, toothache, swelling of the cheek.

[Manipulation] Puncture perpendicularly 0.5-0.8 *cun*.

19. Tinggong (SI 19) (crossing GB, TE)

[Location] On the face, anterior to the tragus and posterior to the mandibular condyloid process, in the depression found when the mouth is open.

[Effects] Improves hearing, and calms the mind.

[Indications] Impaired hearing, tinnitus, vertigo, otorrhea, disorders of temporomandibular joint, toothache.

[Manipulation] Puncture perpendicularly 0.5-1.0 *cun* when the mouth is open.

The Points of the Bladder Meridian of Foot-Taiyang (BL)
(Color Figs. 13, 16, 17 and Fig. XIII-3)

1. Jingming (BL 1) (crossing SI, ST)

[Location] On the face, in the depression about 0.1 *cun* superior to the inner canthus.

[Effects] Disperses wind, and improves vision.

[Indications] Various eye diseases (conjunctivitis, keratitis, dacryoadenitis, optic neuritis, optic atrophy, night blindness, myopia, etc.)

[Manipulation] Gently push the eye-ball to the side and slowly insert the needle 0.5-0.8 *cun* perpendicularly along the medial orbital wall. Twisting or lift-thrusting the needle is prohibited. Press the puncture site for one or two minutes to stem bleeding.

2. Cuanzhu (BL 2)

[Location] On the face, in the depression of the medial end of the eyebrow, at the supraorbital notch.

[Effects] Dispels wind, purges away heat, and improves vision.

[Indications] Frontal headache, eye diseases (conjunctivitis, keratitis, dacryoadenitis, optic neuritis, optic atrophy, myopia, etc.), facial paralysis, and insomnia.

[Manipulation] Puncture 0.3-0.5 *cun* obliquely or subcutaneously along the eyebrow arch.

3. Meichong (BL 3)

[Location] On the head, directly above Cuanzhu (BL 2), 0.5 *cun* above the anterior hairline.

[Effects] Dispels wind, removes obstruction from the nose, and induces tranquilization.

[Indications] Headache, stuffed-up nose, vertigo, and epilepsy.

[Manipulation] Puncture subcutaneously 0.3-0.5 *cun*.

4. Qucha (BL 4)

[Location] On the head, 0.5 *cun* above the anterior hairline and 1.5 *cun* lateral to Shenting (GV 24).

[Effects] Dispels wind and removes obstruction from the nose.

[Indications] Headache, nasal obstruction, and epistaxis.

[Manipulation] Puncture subcutaneously 0.3-0.5 *cun*.

5. Wuchu (BL 5)

[Location] On the head, 1 *cun* above the anterior hairline and 1.5 *cun* lateral to the midline.

[Effects] Dispels wind, purges away heat, and removes obstruction from the nose.

[Indications] Headache, blurring of vision, epilepsy, and convulsion.

[Manipulation] Puncture subcutaneously 0.3-0.5 *cun*.

6. Chengguang (BL 6)

[Location] On the head, 2.5 *cun* above the anterior hairline and 1.5 *cun* lateral to the midline.

[Effects] Dispels wind and removes obstruction from the nose.

[Indications] Headache, and stuffed-up nose.

[Manipulation] Puncture subcutaneously 0.3-0.5 *cun*.

7. Tongtian (BL 7)

[Location] On the head, 4 *cun* above the anterior hairline and 1.5 *cun* lateral to the midline.

[Effects] Dispels wind and removes obstruction from the nose.

[Indications] Headache, dizziness, stuffed-up and runny nose, and epistaxis.

[Manipulation] Puncture subcutaneously 0.3-0.5 *cun*.

8. Luoque (BL 8)

[Location] On the head, 5.5 *cun* above the anterior hairline and 1.5 *cun* lateral to the midline.

[Effects] Dispels wind, removes obstruction from the nose, and calms the mind.

[Indications] Headache, dizziness, stuffed and runny nose (rhinitis, sinusitis), hypertension, and mania.

[Manipulation] Puncture subcutaneously 0.3-0.5 *cun*.

9. Yuzhen (BL 9)

[Location] On the occiput, 2.5 *cun* above the posterior hairline and 1.3 *cun* lateral to the midline, in the depression at the level of the upper border of the external occipital protuberance.

[Effects] Dispels wind, improves vision, and removes obstruction from the nose.

[Indications] Headache, dizziness, ophthalmalgia, myopia, stuffed-up nose and loss of the sense of smell.

[Manipulation] Puncture subcutaneously 0.3-0.5 *cun*.

10. Tianzhu (BL 10)

[Location] On the nape, in the depression of the lateral border of the trapezius muscle and 1.3 *cun* lateral to the midpoint of the posterior hairline.

[Effects] Dispels wind, clears heat, and removes obstruction from the nose.

[Indications] Headache, stuffed-up nose, sore throat, stiff neck, and pain in the shoulder and back.

[Manipulation] Puncture perpendicularly 0.5-0.8 *cun*.

11. Dazhu (BL 11) (Influential Point of Bones) (crossing SI)

[Location] On the back, 1.5 *cun* lateral to the midpoint between the spinous processes of the 1st and 2nd thoracic vertebrae.

[Effects] Dispels wind, and clears heat.

[Indications] Headache, pain in the back and scapular region, stiff neck, and fever with anhidrosis.

[Manipulation] Puncture 0.5-0.8 *cun* obliquely downward or laterally. Avoid deep insertion that may puncture a lung.

12. Fengmen (BL 12) (crossing GV)

[Location] On the back, 1.5 *cun* lateral to the midpoint between the spinous processes of the 2nd and 3rd thoracic vertebrae.

[Effects] Dispels wind, and facilitates the flow of *qi*.

[Indications] Common cold with fever, headache and coughing, and backache.

[Manipulation] Puncture 0.5-0.8 *cun* obliquely downward or laterally. Avoid deep insertion that may puncture a lung.

13. Feishu (BL 13) (Back-Transport Point of the Lungs)

[Location] On the back, 1.5 *cun* lateral to the midpoint between the spinous processes of the 3rd and 4th thoracic vertebrae.

[Effects] Regulates the flow of Lung *qi*, tonifies the Lungs, and clears heat.

[Indications] Coughing, asthma, chest pain, hemoptysis, afternoon fever, and night sweating.

[Manipulation] Puncture 0.5-0.8 *cun* obliquely downward or laterally. Avoid deep insertion that may puncture a lung.

14. Jueyinshu (BL 14) (Back-Transport Point of the Pericardium)

[Location] On the back, 1.5 *cun* lateral to the midpoint between the spinous processes of the 4th and 5th thoracic vertebrae.

[Effects] Soothes the chest, and calms the mind.

[Indications] Cardiac pain, palpitations, stuffiness in the chest.

[Manipulation] Puncture 0.5-0.8 *cun* obliquely downward or laterally. Avoid deep insertion that may puncture a lung.

15. Xinshu (BL 15) (Back-Transport Point of the Heart)

[Location] On the back, 1.5 *cun* lateral to the midpoint between the spinous processes of the 5th and 6th thoracic vertebrae.

[Effects] Calms the mind, and purges away heat.

[Indications] Cardiac pain, palpitations, forgetfulness, nocturnal emission, night sweating, mania, and epilepsy.

[Manipulation] Puncture 0.5-0.8 *cun* obliquely downward or laterally. Avoid deep insertion that may puncture a lung.

16. Dushu (BL 16)

[Location] On the back, 1.5 *cun* lateral to the midpoint between the spinous processes of the 6th and 7th thoracic vertebrae.

[Effects] Soothes the chest, and checks upward perversion of *qi*.

[Indications] Cardiac pain, hiccups, and borborygmi.

[Manipulation] Puncture 0.5-0.8 *cun* obliquely downward or laterally. Avoid deep insertion that may puncture a lung.

17. Geshu (BL 17) (Influential Point of Blood)

[Location] On the back, 1.5 *cun* lateral to the midpoint between the spinous processes of the 7th and 8th thoracic vertebrae.

[Effects] Soothes the chest and diaphragm, and clears heat from blood.

[Indications] Hiccups, belching, vomiting, difficulty in swallowing, asthma, coughing, hemoptysis, afternoon fever, and night sweating.

[Manipulation] Puncture 0.5-0.8 *cun* obliquely downward or laterally. Avoid deep insertion that may puncture a lung.

18. Ganshu (BL 18) (Back-Transport Point of the Liver)

[Location] On the back, 1.5 *cun* lateral to the midpoint between the spinous processes of the 9th and 10th thoracic vertebrae.

[Effects] Soothes the Liver and the hypochondrium, removes damp-heat, and improves vision.

[Indications] Jaundice, pain in the hypochondriac region, bloodshot eyes, blurring of vision, night blindness, mental disorders, epilepsy, backache, hemoptysis, and epistaxis.

[Manipulation] Puncture 0.5-0.8 *cun* obliquely downward or laterally. Avoid deep insertion that may puncture a lung.

19. Danshu (BL 19) (Back-Transport Point of the Gallbladder)

[Location] On the back, 1.5 *cun* lateral to the midpoint between the spinous processes of the 10th and 11th thoracic vertebrae.

[Effects] Regulates the Liver and Gallbladder, and soothes the chest and hypochondrium.

[Indications] Jaundice, bitter taste of the mouth, pain in the chest and hypochondriac region.

[Manipulation] Puncture 0.5-0.8 *cun* obliquely downward or laterally. Avoid deep insertion that may puncture a lung.

20. Pishu (BL 20) (Back-Transport Point of the Spleen)

[Location] On the back, 1.5 *cun* lateral to the midpoint between the spinous processes of the 11th and 12th thoracic vertebrae.

[Effects] Invigorates the Spleen, nourishes blood, and resolves dampness.

[Indications] Epigastric pain, abdominal distention, jaundice, vomiting, diarrhea, profuse menstruation, edema, anorexia, and backache.

[Manipulation] Puncture 0.5-0.8 *cun* obliquely downward or laterally. Avoid deep insertion that may puncture a lung.

21. Weishu (BL 21) (Back-Transport Point of the Stomach)

[Location] On the back, 1.5 *cun* lateral to the midpoint between the spinous processes of the 12th thoracic and 1st lumbar vertebrae.

[Effects] Invigorates the Spleen and Stomach, and removes undigested food.

[Indications] Epigastric pain, anorexia, abdominal distention, borborygmi, diarrhea, nausea, and vomiting.

[Manipulation] Puncture 0.5-0.8 *cun* obliquely downward or laterally.

22. Sanjiaoshu (BL 22) (Back-Transport Point of the Triple Energizer)

[Location] At the lower back, 1.5 *cun* lateral to the midpoint between the spinous processes of the 1st and 2nd lumbar vertebrae.

[Effects] Regulates the Triple Energizer, and induces diuresis.

[Indications] Borborygmi, abdominal distention, indigestion, vomiting, diarrhea, edema, pain and stiffness of the lower back.

[Manipulation] Puncture perpendicularly or obliquely 0.5-1.0 *cun*.

23. Shenshu (BL 23) (Back-Transport Point of the Kidney)

[Location] At the lower back, 1.5 *cun* lateral to the midpoint between the spinous processes of the 2nd and 3rd lumbar vertebrae.

[Effects] Tonifies the Kidneys, soothes the back, and improves hearing and vision.

[Indications] Impotence, nocturnal emission, enuresis, irregular menstruation, excessive leukorrhea, low back pain, weakness of the knees, blurred vision, dizziness, tinnitus, impaired hearing, edema, asthma, and diarrhea.

[Manipulation] Puncture perpendicularly or obliquely 1.0-1.5 *cun*.

24. Qihaishu (BL 24)

[Location] At the lower back, 1.5 *cun* lateral to the midpoint between the spinous processes of the 3rd and 4th lumbar vertebrae.

[Effects] Regulates the Lower Energizer, and strengthens the back and knees.

[Indications] Low back pain, irregular menstruation, dysmenorrhea, and asthma.

[Manipulation] Puncture perpendicularly or obliquely 0.5-1.5 *cun*.

25. Dachangshu (BL 25) (Back-Transport Point of the Large Intestine)

[Location] At the lower back, 1.5 *cun* lateral to the midpoint between the spinous processes of the 4th and 5th lumbar vertebrae.

[Effects] Regulates the Large Intestine, and soothes the lower back and legs.

[Indications] Low back pain, borborygmi, abdominal distention, diarrhea, constipation, pain and motor impairment of the lower limb, sciatica.

[Manipulation] Puncture perpendicularly or obliquely 1.0-1.5 *cun*.

26. Guanyuanshu (BL 26)

[Location] At the lower back, 1.5 *cun* lateral to the midpoint between the spinous processes of the 5th lumbar and 1st sacral vertebrae.

[Effects] Tonifies the Kidneys, and strengthens the lower back.

[Indications] Low back pain, abdominal distention, diarrhea, enuresis, frequent urination, and sciatica.

[Manipulation] Puncture perpendicularly or obliquely 1.0-1.5 *cun*.

27. Xiaochangshu (BL 27) (Back-Transport Point of the Small Intestine)

[Location] On the sacrum, at the level of the 1st posterior sacral foramen, 1.5 *cun* lateral to the median sacral crest.

[Effects] Regulates the Small Intestine, and removes damp-heat.

[Indications] Lower abdominal pain and distention, dysentery, morbid leukorrhea, enuresis, hematuria, nocturnal emission, low back pain, and sciatica.

[Manipulation] Puncture perpendicularly or obliquely 0.5-1.5 *cun*.

28. Pangguangshu (BL 28) (Back-Transport Point of the Bladder)

[Location] On the sacrum, at the level of the 2nd posterior sacral foramen, 1.5 *cun* lateral to the median sacral crest.

[Effects] Regulates the Bladder, and strengthens the lower back.

[Indications] Retention of urine, enuresis, frequent urination, diarrhea, constipation, and pain and stiffness in the lower back.

[Manipulation] Puncture perpendicularly 1.0-1.5 *cun*.

29. Zhonglüshu (BL 29)

[Location] On the sacrum, at the level of the 3rd posterior sacral foramen, 1.5 *cun* lateral to the median sacral crest.

[Effects] Strengthens the lower back, and arrests diarrhea.

[Indications] Diarrhea, pain and stiffness in the lower back.

[Manipulation] Puncture perpendicularly 1.0-1.5 *cun*.

30. Baihuanshu (BL 30)

[Location] On the sacrum, at the level of the 4th posterior sacral foramen, 1.5 *cun* lateral to the median sacral crest.

[Effects] Removes damp-heat, and strengthens the lower back and legs.

[Indications] Enuresis, dysuria, morbid leukorrhea, irregular menstruation, pain and cold sensation of the lower back, paralysis of the leg, constipation tenesmus, and prolapse of the rectum.

[Manipulation] Puncture perpendicularly 1.0-1.5 *cun*.

31. Shangliao (BL 31)

[Location] on the sacrum, at the midpoint between the posterosuperior iliac spine and the posterior midline, at the 1st posterior sacral foramen.

[Effects] Regulates the Lower Energizer, and strengthens the lower back and legs.

[Indications] Low back pain, dysuria, constipation, irregular menstruation, morbid leukorrhea, and prolapse of the uterus.

[Manipulation] Puncture perpendicularly 1.0-1.2 *cun*.

32. Ciliao (BL 32)

[Location] On the sacrum, medial and inferior to the posterosuperior iliac spine, just at the 2nd posterior sacral foramen.

[Effects] Regulates the Lower Energizer, and strengthens the lower back and legs.

[Indications] Low back pain, hernia, irregular menstruation, dysmenorrhea, morbid leukorrhea, impotence, nocturnal emission, enuresis, dysuria, pain and motor impairment of the lower limb.

[Manipulation] Puncture perpendicularly 1.0-1.2 *cun*.

33. Zhongliao (BL 33)

[Location] On the sacrum, medial and inferior to Ciliao (BL 32), at the 3rd posterior sacral foramen.

[Effects] Regulates the Lower Energizer, and strengthens the lower back and legs.

[Indications] Low back pain, dysuria, constipation, diarrhea, irregular menstruation, and morbid leukorrhea.

[Manipulation] Puncture perpendicularly 1.0-1.2 *cun*.

34. Xialiao (BL 34)

[Location] On the sacrum, medial and inferior to Zhongliao (BL 33), at the 4th posterior sacral foramen.

[Effects] Regulates the Lower Energizer, and strengthens the lower back and egs.

[Indications] Low back pain, lower abdominal pain, dysuria, constipation, and morbid leukorrhea.

[Manipulation] Puncture perpendicularly 1.0-1.2 *cun*.

35. Huiyang (BL 35)

[Location] On the sacrum, 0.5 *cun* lateral to the tip of the coccyx.

[Effects] Regulates the Lower Energizer.

[Indications] Diarrhea, constipation, retention of urine, incontinence of urine, hemorrhoids.

[Manipulation] Puncture perpendicularly 0.5-1.0 *cun*.

36. Chengfu (BL 36)

[Location] On the posterior side of the thigh, at the midpoint of the inferior gluteal crease.

[Effects] Strengthens the lower back and legs.

[Indications] Pain in the lower back and gluteal region, pain and motor impairment of the leg.

[Manipulation] Puncture perpendicularly 1.0-2.0 *cun*.

37. Yinmen (BL 37)

[Location] On the posterior side of the thigh and on the line connecting Chengfu (BL 36) and Weizhong (BL 40), 6 *cun* below Chengfu (BL 36).

[Effects] Strengthens the lower back and legs.

[Indications] Pain in the lower back, pain and motor impairment of the leg.

[Manipulation] Puncture perpendicularly 1.0-2.0 *cun*.

38. Fuxi (BL 38)

[Location] At the lateral end of the popliteal crease, 1 *cun* above Weiyang (BL 39), medial to the tendon of the biceps muscle of the thigh.

[Effects] Soothes the tendons.

[Indications] Numbness of the gluteal and femoral regions, contracture of the tendons in the popliteal fossa.

[Manipulation] Puncture perpendicularly 0.5-1.0 *cun*.

39. Weiyang (BL 39) (Lower Sea Point of the Triple Energizer)

[Location] At the lateral end of the popliteal crease, medial to the tendon of the biceps muscle of the thigh.

[Effects] Soothes the tendons, and regulates the Lower Energizer.

[Indications] Stiffness and pain of the lower back, distention and fullness of the lower abdomen, edema, dysuria, and cramp in the leg.

[Manipulation] Puncture perpendicularly 0.5-1.0 *cun*.

40. Weizhong (BL 40) (*He*-Sea Point)

[Location] At the midpoint of the popliteal crease, between the tendon of the biceps muscle of the thigh and the semitendinous muscle.

[Effects] Purges heat, soothes the tendons, and strengthens the lower back and legs.

[Indications] Low back pain, motor impairment of the hip joint, muscle contracture in the popliteal fossa, pain and motor impairment of the lower limb, abdominal pain, vomiting, diarrhea, erysipelas, and eczema.

[Manipulation] Avoid puncturing the popliteal artery. Puncture perpendicularly 0.3-1.0 *cun* or prick superficially to cause bleeding.

41. Fufen (BL 41) (crossing SI)

[Location] On the back, 3 *cun* lateral to the midpoint between the spinous processes of the 2nd and 3rd thoracic vertebrae.

[Indications] Stiffness and pain in the shoulder, back and neck.

[Manipulation] Puncture perpendicularly 0.3-0.5 *cun*.

42. Pohu (BL 42)

[Location] On the back, 3 *cun* lateral to the midpoint between the spinous processes of the 3rd and 4th thoracic vertebrae.

[Effects] Regulates and tonifies the Lungs.

[Indications] Pulmonary tuberculosis, hemoptysis, cough, asthma, stiff neck, and pain in the shoulder and back.

[Manipulation] Puncture perpendicularly 0.3-0.5 *cun*.

43. Gaohuang (BL 43)

[Location] On the back, 3 *cun* lateral to the midpoint between the spinous processes of the 4th and 5th thoracic vertebrae.

[Effects] Warms and tonifies the Lungs.

[Indications] Pulmonary tuberculosis, coughing, asthma, hemoptysis, and night sweating.

[Manipulation] Puncture perpendicularly 0.3-0.5 *cun*.

44. Shentang (BL 44)

[Location] On the back, 3 *cun* lateral to the midpoint between the spinous processes of the 5th and 6th thoracic vertebrae.

[Effects] Soothes the chest, and calms the mind.

[Indications] Asthma, cardiac pain, palpitations, stuffiness in the chest, stiffness and pain in the back.

[Manipulation] Puncture obliquely 0.3-0.5 *cun*.

45. Yixi (BL 45)

[Location] On the back, 3 *cun* lateral to the midpoint between the spinous processes of the 6th and 7th thoracic vertebrae.

[Effects] Soothes the chest.

[Indications] Coughing, asthma, and pain in the shoulder and back.

[Manipulation] Puncture obliquely 0.3-0.5 *cun*.

46. Geguan (BL 46)

[Location] On the back, 3 *cun* lateral to the midpoint between the spinous processes of the 7th and 8th thoracic vertebrae.

[Effects] Checks upward perversion of *qi*.

[Indications] Dysphagia, hiccups, vomiting, belching, and pain and stiffness of the back.

[Manipulation] Puncture obliquely 0.3-0.5 *cun*.

47. Hunmen (BL 47)

[Location] On the back, 3 *cun* lateral to the midpoint between the spinous processes of the 9th and 10th thoracic vertebrae.

[Effects] Soothe the Liver, and harmonizes the Middle Energizer.

[Indications] Pain in the chest and hypochondriac region, back pain, vomiting, and diarrhea.

[Manipulation] Puncture obliquely 0.3-0.5 *cun*.

48. Yanggang (BL 48)

[Location] On the back, 3 *cun* lateral to the midpoint between the spinous processes of the 10th and 11th thoracic vertebrae.

[Effects] Soothes the Liver, and harmonizes the Middle Energizer.

[Indications] Borborygmi, abdominal pain, diarrhea, pain in the hypochondriac region, and jaundice.

[Manipulation] Puncture obliquely 0.3-0.5 *cun*.

49. Yishe (BL 49)

[Location] On the back, 3 *cun* lateral to the midpoint between the spinous processes of the 11th and 12th thoracic vertebrae.

[Effects] Invigorates the Spleen, relieves distention, and removes damp-heat.

[Indications] Abdominal distention, borborygmi, vomiting, diarrhea, and difficulty in swallowing.

[Manipulation] Puncture obliquely 0.3-0.5 *cun*.

50. Weicang (BL 50)

[Location] On the back, 3 *cun* lateral to the midpoint between the spinous processes of the 12th thoracic and 1st lumbar vertebrae.

[Effects] Invigorates the Spleen and Stomach, and relieves distention.

[Indications] Abdominal distention, pain in the epigastric region and back, and infantile indigestion.

[Manipulation] Puncture obliquely 0.3-0.5 *cun*.

51. Huangmen (BL 51)

[Location] At the lower back, 3 *cun* lateral to the midpoint between the spinous processes of the 1st and 2nd lumbar vertebrae.

[Effects] Regulates the Middle Energizer.

[Indications] Abdominal pain, constipation, and abdominal mass (splenomegaly).

[Manipulation] Puncture obliquely 0.3-0.5 *cun*.

52. Zhishi (BL 52)

[Location] At the lower back, 3 *cun* lateral to the midpoint between the spinous processes of the 2nd and 3rd lumbar vertebrae.

[Effects] Tonifies the Kidneys, and strengthens the lower back.

[Indications] Impotence, nocturnal emission, enuresis, frequent urination, dysuria, irregular menstruation, pain in the back and knees, and edema.

[Manipulation] Puncture perpendicularly or obliquely sideward 0.5-1.0 *cun*.

53. Baohuang (BL 53)

[Location] On the buttock and at the level of the 2nd posterior sacral foramen, 3 *cun* lateral to the median sacral crest.

[Effects] Regulates the Middle Energizer, and promotes micturition.

[Indications] Borborygmi, abdominal distention, pain in the lower back, and retention of urine.

[Manipulation] Puncture perpendicularly 1.0-1.5 *cun*.

54. Zhibian (BL 54)

[Location] On the buttock and at the level of the 4th posterior sacral foramen, 3 *cun* lateral to the median sacral crest.

[Effects] Strengthens the lower back and legs, and regulates the Lower Energizer.

[Indications] Pain in the lumbosacral region, motor impairment of the leg, dysuria, swelling around the external genitalia, hemorrhoids, and constipation.

[Manipulation] Puncture perpendicularly 1.5-2.0 *cun*.

55. Heyang (BL 55)

[Location] On the posterior side of the leg, 2 *cun* below Weizhong (BL 40).

[Effects] Strengthens the lower back and legs.

[Indications] Pain in the lower back, pain and paralysis in the lower limbs.

[Manipulation] Puncture perpendicularly 1.0-1.5 *cun*.

56. Chengjin (BL 56)

[Location] On the posterior side of the leg and on the line connecting Weizhong (BL 40) and Chengshan (BL 57), at the center of the gastrocnemius muscle belly, 5 *cun* below Weizhong (BL 40).

[Effects] Soothes and strengthens the lower back and legs.

[Indications] Spasm of the gastrocnemius, and acute pain in the lower back.

[Manipulation] Puncture perpendicularly 1.0-1.5 *cun*.

57. Chengshan (BL 57)

[Location] On the posterior midline of the leg, between Weizhong (BL 40) and Kunlun (BL 60), 8 *cun* below Weizhong (BL 40), in the depression formed below the gastrocnemius muscle belly when the leg is stretched.

[Effects] Soothes and strengthens the lower back and legs.

[Indications] Low back pain, spasm of the gastrocnemius, hemorrhoids, and constipation.

[Manipulation] Puncture perpendicularly 1.0-1.5 *cun*.

58. Feiyang (BL 58) (Connecting Point)

[Location] On the posterior side of the leg, 7 *cun* directly above Kunlun (BL 60) and 1 *cun* lateral and inferior to Chengshan (BL 57).

[Effects] Clears the head and eyes, and strengthens the lower back and legs.

[Indications] Headache, blurred vision, nasal obstruction, epistaxis, pain in the back, weakness of the leg.

[Manipulation] Puncture perpendicularly 1.0-1.5 *cun*.

59. Fuyang (BL 59) (Cleft Point of the *Yang* Heel Vessel) (crossing Yang LV, Yang HV)

[Location] On the posterior side of the leg, posterior to the lateral malleolus, 3 *cun* directly above Kunlun (BL 60).

[Effects] Clears up the head and eyes, and strengthens the lower back and legs.

[Indications] Heavy sensation in the head, headache, low back pain, and paralysis of the lower limbs.

[Manipulation] Puncture perpendicularly 0.5-1.0 *cun*.

60. Kunlun (BL 60) (*Jing*-River Point)

[Location] Posterior to the lateral malleolus, in the depression between the tip of the external malleolus and the Achilles tendon.

[Effects] Dispels wind-heat, regulates the uterus, and soothes the lower back and legs.

[Indications] Headache, blurred vision, epistaxis, stiff neck, pain in the shoulder, back and arm, acute low back pain (lumbar sprain), sciatica, abnormal fetal position, prolonged labor, and retention of placenta.

[Manipulation] Puncture perpendicularly 0.5-1.0 *cun*.

61. Pucan (BL 61) (crossing YangLV, YangHV)

[Location] On the lateral side of the foot, in the depression posterior and inferior to the external malleolus, 1.5 *cun* directly below Kunlun (BL 60).

[Indications] Muscular atrophy and weakness of the lower limb, and pain in the heels.

[Manipulation] Puncture perpendicularly 0.3-0.5 *cun*.

62. Shenmai (BL 62) (Confluence Point of the *Yang* Heel Vessel) (crossing YangLV, YangHV)

[Location] On the lateral side of the foot, in the depression directly below the external malleolus.

[Effects] Clears the head, and strengthens the lower back and legs.

[Indications] Headache, dizziness, insomnia, epilepsy, mania, backache, and aching of the legs.

[Manipulation] Puncture perpendicularly 0.3-0.5 *cun*.

63. Jinmen (BL 63) (Cleft Point) (crossing YangLV, YangHV)

[Location] On the lateral side of the foot, directly below the anterior border of the external malleolus, in the depression lateral to the cuboid bone.

[Effects] Clears the mind, and soothes the tendons.

[Indications] Mania, epilepsy, backache, pain in the external malleolus, motor impairment and pain in the lower limbs.

[Manipulation] Puncture perpendicularly 0.3-0.5 *cun*.

64. Jinggu (BL 64) (Primary Point)

[Location] On the lateral side of the foot, in the depression below the 5th metatarsal bone, at the dorso-ventral boundary.

[Effects] Clears the head, and strengthens the lower back and legs.

[Indications] Headache, stiff neck, epilepsy, and pain in the lower back and thigh.

[Manipulation] Puncture perpendicularly 0.3-0.5 *cun*.

65. Shugu (BL 65) (*Shu*-Stream Point)

[Location] On the lateral side of the foot, in the depression posterior to the 5th metatarsophalangeal joint, at the dorso-ventral boundary.

[Effects] Dispels wind-heat, and soothes the back.

[Indications] Headache, stiff neck, mania, backache, and pain in the lower limb.

[Manipulation] Puncture perpendicularly 0.3-0.5 *cun*.

66. Zutonggu (BL 66) (*Ying*-Spring Point)

[Location] On the lateral side of the foot, in the depression anterior to the 5th metatarsophalangeal joint.

[Effects] Dispels heat, and clears the head.

[Indications] Headache, stiff neck, blurred vision, epistaxis, and mania.

[Manipulation] Puncture perpendicularly 0.2-0.3 *cun*.

67. Zhiyin (BL 67) (*Jing*-Well Point)

[Location] On the lateral side of the little toe, 0.1 *cun* proximal to the corner of toenail.

[Effects] Dispels wind-heat, and facilitates delivery.

[Indications] Headache, nasal obstruction, epistaxis, abnormal fetal position, prolonged labor, and retention of placenta.

[Manipulation] Puncture 0.1 *cun*, or prick to cause bleeding.

The Points of the Kidney Meridian of Foot-Shaoyin (KI)

(Color Figs. 11 and 15)

1. Yongquan (KI 1) (*Jing*-Well Point)

[Location] On the sole, in the depression when the foot is in plantar flexion, approximately at the junction of the anterior third and posterior two thirds of the sole.

[Effects] Purges away heat, and induces resuscitation.

[Indications] Headache, dizziness, sore throat, loss of voice, feverish sensation in the sole, and loss of consciousness.

[Manipulation] Puncture perpendicularly 0.3-0.5 *cun*.

2. Rangu (KI 2) (*Ying*-Spring Point)

[Location] On the medial border of the foot, in the depression below the tuberosity of navicular bone.

[Effects] Purges heat, and induces subsidence of swelling.

[Indications] Sore throat, dysuria, swelling and pain of the dorsum of foot.

[Manipulation] Puncture perpendicularly 0.3-0.5 *cun*.

3. Taixi (KI 3) (*Shu*-Stream Point, Primary Point)

[Location] On the medial side of the foot, posterior to the medial malleolus, in the depression between the tip of the medial malleolus and the Achilles tendon.

[Effects] Tonifies the Kidneys, and bears down fire.

[Indications] Sore throat, toothache, impaired hearing, tinnitus, dizziness, hemoptysis, asthma, insomnia, nocturnal emission, impotence, frequent urination, and pain in the lower back.

[Manipulation] Puncture perpendicularly 0.3-0.5 *cun*.

4. Dazhong (KI 4) (Connecting Point)

[Location] On the medial side of the foot, posterior and inferior to the medial malleolus, in the depression medial to the attachment of the Achilles tendon.

[Effects] Tonifies the Kidneys, and clears up heat.

[Indications] Hemoptysis, asthma, stiffness and pain in the lower back, dysuria, and pain in the heels.

[Manipulation] Puncture perpendicularly 0.3-0.5 *cun*.

5. Shuiquan (KI 5) (Cleft Point)

[Location] On the medial side of the foot, 1 *cun* directly below Taixi (KI 3), in the depression of the medial side of the tuberosity of the calcaneum.

[Effects] Regulates menstruation and tonifies the Kidneys

[Indications] Amenorrhea, irregular menstruation, dysmenorrhea, dysuria.

[Manipulation] Puncture perpendicularly 0.3-0.5 *cun*.

6. Zhaohai (KI 6) (Confluence Point of the *Yin* Heel Vessel) (crossing YinHV)

[Location] On the medial side of the foot, in the depression 1 *cun* below the medial malleolus.

[Effects] Tonifies the Kidneys, calms the mind, and soothes the throat.

[Indications] Irregular menstruation, morbid leukorrhea, prolapse of the uterus, pruritus vulvae, frequent micturition, retention of urine, constipation, epilepsy, insomnia, sore throat, and asthma.

[Manipulation] Puncture perpendicularly 0.3-0.5 *cun*.

7. Fuliu (KI 7) (*Jing*-River Point)

[Location] On the medial side of the leg, 2 *cun* directly above Taixi (KI 3), on the anterior border of the Achilles tendon.

[Effects] Regulates the Intestines, tonifies the Kidneys, induces diuresis, and arrests sweating.

[Indications] Edema, abdominal distention, diarrhea, borborygmi, night sweating, spontaneous sweating, low back pain, lumbar sprain, and pain in the heel.

[Manipulation] Puncture perpendicularly 0.5-0.8 *cun*.

8. Jiaoxin (KI 8) (Cleft Point of the *Yin* Heel Vessel) (crossing YinHV)

[Location] On the medial side of the leg, 2 *cun* above Taixi (KI 3) and 0.5 *cun* anterior to Fuliu (KI 7), posterior to the medial border of the tibia.

[Effects] Regulates menstruation and the Lower Energizer.

[Indications] Irregular menstruation, dysmenorrhea, uterine bleeding, prolapse of the uterus, diarrhea, constipation, pain and swelling of the testis.

[Manipulation] Puncture perpendicularly 0.5-0.8 *cun*.

9. Zhubin (KI 9) (Cleft Point of the *Yin* Link Vessel) (crossing YinLV)

[Location] On the medial side of the leg and on the line connecting Taixi (KI 3) and Yingu (KI 10), 5 *cun* above Taixi (KI 3).

[Effects] Regulates the Lower Energizer, and calms the mind.

[Indications] Pain due to hernia, pain in the foot and lower leg, and mental disorders.

[Manipulation] Puncture perpendicularly 0.5-0.8 *cun*.

10. Yingu (KI 10) (*He*-Sea Point)

[Location] On the medial side of the popliteal fossa, between the tendons of the semitendinous and semimembranous muscles when the knee is flexed.

[Effects] Regulates the Lower Energizer, and calms the mind.

[Indications] Impotence, uterine bleeding, dysuria, pain due to hernia, pain in the knee and popliteal fossa, and mental disorders.

[Manipulation] Puncture perpendicularly 0.5-1.0 *cun*.

11. Henggu (KI 11) (crossing BV)

[Location] On the lower abdomen, 5 *cun* below the center of the umbilicus and 0.5 *cun* lateral to the anterior midline.

[Effects] Regulates the Lower Energizer, and tonifies the Kidneys.

[Indications] Fullness and pain of the lower abdomen, dysuria, enuresis, impotence, nocturnal emission, and pain in the external genitalia.

[Manipulation] Puncture perpendicularly 0.5-1.0 *cun*.

12. Dahe (KI 12) (crossing TV)

[Location] On the lower abdomen, 4 *cun* below the center of the umbilicus and 0.5 *cun* lateral to the anterior midline.

[Effects] Regulates the Lower Energizer, and tonifies the Kidneys.

[Indications] Impotence, nocturnal emission, morbid leukorrhea, pain in the external genitalia, and prolapse of the uterus.

[Manipulation] Puncture perpendicularly 0.5-1.0 *cun*.

13. Qixue (KI 13) (crossing TV)

[Location] On the lower abdomen, 3 *cun* below the center of the umbilicus and 0.5

cun lateral to the anterior midline.

[Effects] Regulates menstruation, and arrests diarrhea.

[Indications] Irregular menstruation, dysmenorrhea, dysuria, abdominal pain, and diarrhea.

[Manipulation] Puncture perpendicularly 0.5-1.0 *cun*.

14. Siman (KI 14) (crossing TV)

[Location] On the lower abdomen, 2 *cun* below the center of the umbilicus and 0.5 *cun* lateral to the anterior midline.

[Effects] Regulates menstruation, and relieves distention.

[Indications] Abdominal pain and distention, diarrhea, irregular menstruation, dysmenorrhea, and postpartum abdominal pain.

[Manipulation] Puncture perpendicularly 0.5-1.0 *cun*.

15. Zhongzhu (KI 15) (crossing TV)

[Location] On the lower abdomen, 1 *cun* below the center of the umbilicus and 0.5 *cun* lateral to the anterior midline.

[Effects] Regulates the Lower Energizer, and opens the bowels.

[Indications] Irregular menstruation, abdominal pain, and constipation.

[Manipulation] Puncture perpendicularly 0.5-1.0 *cun*.

16. Huangshu (KI 16) (crossing TV)

[Location] On the middle abdomen, 0.5 *cun* lateral to the center of the umbilicus.

[Effects] Regulates the Intestines.

[Indications] Abdominal pain and distention, constipation, and diarrhea.

[Manipulation] Puncture perpendicularly 0.5-1 *cun*.

17. Shangqu (KI 17) (crossing TV)

[Location] On the upper abdomen, 2 *cun* above the center of the umbilicus and 0.5 *cun* lateral to the anterior midline.

[Effects] Regulates the Intestines.

[Indications] Abdominal pain, diarrhea, and constipation.

[Manipulation] Puncture perpendicularly 0.5-1.0 *cun*.

18. Shiguan (KI 18) (crossing TV)

[Location] On the upper abdomen, 3 *cun* above the center of the umbilicus and 0.5 *cun* lateral to the anterior midline.

[Effects] Regulates the Stomach, Intestines and Uterus.

[Indications] Vomiting, abdominal pain, constipation, postpartum abdominal pain, and infertility.

[Manipulation] Puncture perpendicularly 0.5-1.0 *cun*.

19. Yindu (KI 19) (crossing TV)

[Location] On the upper abdomen, 4 *cun* above the center of the umbilicus and 0.5 *cun* lateral to the anterior midline.

[Effects] Regulates the Stomach and Intestines.

[Indications] Abdominal pain, borborygmi, epigastric pain, constipation, and vomiting.

[Manipulation] Puncture perpendicularly 0.5-1.0 *cun*.

20. Futonggu (KI 20) (crossing TV)

[Location] On the upper abdomen, 5 *cun* above the center of the umbilicus and 0.5 *cun* lateral to the anterior midline.

[Effects] Regulates the Stomach and intestines.

[Indications] Abdominal pain and distension, vomiting, and indigestion.

[Manipulation] Puncture perpendicularly 0.5-1.0 *cun*.

21. Youmen (KI 21) (crossing TV)

[Location] On the upper abdomen, 6 *cun* above the center of the umbilicus and 0.5 *cun* lateral to the anterior midline.

[Effects] Regulates the Stomach, and checks upward perversion of *qi*.

[Indications] Epigastric pain, indigestion, nausea, vomiting, and morning sickness.

[Manipulation] Puncture perpendicularly 0.3-0.8 *cun*.

[Warning] Deep puncture may injure the liver.

22. Bulang (KI 22)

[Location] On the chest, in the 5th intercostal space, 2 *cun* lateral to the anterior midline.

[Effects] Soothes the chest, and checks upward perversion of *qi*.

[Indications] Coughing, asthma, fullness in the chest and costal region, vomiting, and anorexia.

[Manipulation] Puncture obliquely 0.3-0.8 *cun*.

[Warning] Deep puncture may injure the heart.

23. Shenfeng (KI 23)

[Location] On the chest, in the 4th intercostal space, 2 *cun* lateral to the anterior midline.

[Effects] Facilitates the flow of *qi*, and promotes lactation.

[Indications] Coughing, asthma, fullness in the chest and costal region, and mastitis.

[Manipulation] Puncture obliquely 0.3-0.8 *cun*.

24. Lingxu (KI 24)

[Location] On the chest, in the 3rd intercostal space, 2 *cun* lateral to the anterior midline.

[Effects] Soothes the chest, and facilitates the flow of *qi*.

[Indications] Coughing, asthma, and fullness in the chest and costal region.
[Manipulation] Puncture obliquely 0.3-0.8 *cun*.

25. Shencang (KI 25)

[Location] On the chest, in the 2nd intercostal space, 2 *cun* lateral to the anterior midline.
[Effects] Soothes the chest, and facilitates the flow of *qi*.
[Indications] Coughing, asthma, and chest pain.
[Manipulation] Puncture obliquely 0.3-0.8 *cun*.

26. Yuzhong (KI 26)

[Location] On the chest, in the 1st intercostal space, 2 *cun* lateral to the anterior midline.
[Effects] Facilitates the flow of *qi*, and relieves asthma.
[Indications] Coughing, asthma, and fullness in the chest and costal region.
[Manipulation] Puncture obliquely 0.3-0.8 *cun*.

27. Shufu (KI 27)

[Location] On the chest, below the lower border of the clavicle, 2 *cun* lateral to the midline.
[Effects] Facilitates the flow of *qi*, and relieves asthma.
[Indications] Coughing, asthma, and chest pain.
[Manipulation] Puncture obliquely 0.3-0.8 *cun*.

The Points of the Pericardium Meridian of Hand-Jueyin (PC)

(Color Figs. 9 and 15)

1. Tianchi (PC 1) (crossing GB)

[Location] On the chest, in the 4th intercostal space, 1 *cun* lateral to the nipple and 5 *cun* lateral to the anterior midline.
[Effects] Soothes the chest, and induces subsidence of swelling.
[Indications] Suffocating sensation in the chest, cardiac pain (angina pectoris), pain in the costal region (intercostal neuralgia), swelling and pain of the axillary region.
[Manipulation] Puncture obliquely 0.3-0.8 *cun*.
[Warning] Deep puncture may cause pneumothorax.

2. Tianquan (PC 2)

[Location] On the medial side of the arm, 2 *cun* below the anterior end of the axillary fold, between the long and short heads of the biceps muscle of the arm.
[Effects] Soothes the Heart and the chest.
[Indications] Cardiac pain, palpitation, sensation of fullness in the costal region, pain in the chest, back and the medial aspect of the arm.
[Manipulation] Puncture perpendicularly 0.5-0.8 *cun*.

3. Quze (PC 3) (*He*-Sea Point)

[Location] At the midpoint of the cubital crease, on the ulnar side of the tendon of the biceps muscle of the arm.

[Effects] Soothes the Heart, purges away heat, and induces sedation.

[Indications] Cardiac pain, palpitations, fever, irritability, stomachache, vomiting, pain in the elbow and arm, and tremor of the hand and arm.

[Manipulation] Puncture perpendicularly 0.5-0.8 *cun*.

4. Ximen (PC 4) (Cleft Point)

[Location] On the palmar side of the forearm and on the line connecting Quze (PC 3) and Daling (PC 7), 5 *cun* above the crease of the wrist.

[Effects] Soothes the Heart, purges away heat, and induces sedation.

[Indications] Cardiac pain, palpitation, epistaxis, hematemesis, hemoptysis, chest pain, and epilepsy.

[Manipulation] Puncture perpendicularly 0.5-1.0 *cun*.

5. Jianshi (PC 5) (*Jing*-River Point)

[Location] On the palmar side of the forearm, 3 *cun* above the crease of the wrist, between the tendons of the long palmar muscle and radial flexor muscle of the wrist.

[Effects] Soothes the Heart and the chest, calms the mind, harmonizes the Stomach, and cures malaria.

[Indications] Cardiac pain, palpitation, stomachache, vomiting, fever, irritability, malaria, mental disorders, epilepsy, swelling of the axilla, and contracture of the elbow and arm.

[Manipulation] Puncture perpendicularly 0.5-1.0 *cun*.

6. Neiguan (PC 6) (Connecting Point, Confluence Point of the *Yin* Link Vessel)

[Location] On the palmar side of the forearm, 2 *cun* above the crease of the wrist, between the tendons of the long palmar muscle and radial flexor muscle of the wrist.

[Effects] Soothes the Heart and the chest, calms the mind, harmonizes the Stomach, checks upward perversion of *qi*, and cures malaria.

[Indications] Cardiac pain, palpitations, stuffy feeling in the chest, pain in the costal region, stomachache, nausea, vomiting, hiccups, mental disorders, epilepsy, insomnia, fever, irritability, malaria, contracture and pain in the elbow and arm.

[Manipulation] Puncture perpendicularly 0.5-1.0 *cun*.

7. Daling (PC 7) (*Shu*-Stream Point, Primary Point)

[Location] At the midpoint of the crease of the wrist, between the tendons of the long palmar muscle and radial flexor muscle of the wrist.

[Effects] Soothes the Heart, and calms the mind.

[Indications] Cardiac pain, palpitations, stomachache, vomiting, mental disorders, epilepsy, stuffy feeling in the chest, pain in the costal region, insomnia, and irritability.

[Manipulation] Puncture perpendicularly 0.3-0.5 *cun*.

8. Laogong (PC 8) (*Ying*-Spring Point)

[Location] At the center of the palm, between the 2nd and 3rd metacarpal bones, and in the part touching the tip of the middle finger when a fist is made.

[Effects] Purges the Heart of fire, and calms the mind.

[Indications] Cardiac pain, mental disorders, epilepsy, and foul breath.

[Manipulation] Puncture perpendicularly 0.3-0.5 *cun*.

9. Zhongchong (PC 9) (*Jing*-Well Point)

[Location] At the center of the tip of the middle finger.

[Effects] Clears up heat, and induces resuscitation.

[Indications] Cardiac pain, palpitations, loss of consciousness, aphasia, fever, heat stroke, and convulsion.

[Manipulation] Puncture 0.1 *cun*, or prick to cause bleeding.

The Points of the Triple Energizer Meridian of Hand-Shaoyang (TE)

(Color Figs. 10, 16, 17 and Fig. XIII-3)

1. Guanchong (TE 1) (*Jing*-Well Point)

[Location] On the ulnar side of the ring finger, 0.1 *cun* proximal to the corner of the nail.

[Effects] Purges heat, and soothes the throat and tongue.

[Indications] Headache, redness of the eye, sore throat, stiffness of the tongue, fever, and irritability.

[Manipulation] Puncture 0.1 *cun*, or prick to cause bleeding.

2. Yemen (TE 2) (*Ying*-Spring Point)

[Location] On the dorsum of the hand, between the ring and little fingers, 0.5 *cun* proximal to the margin of the web.

[Effects] Purges heat, and improves hearing.

[Indications] Headache, redness of the eye, sudden deafness, sore throat, and pain in the arm.

[Manipulation] Puncture obliquely 0.3-0.5 *cun*.

3. Zhongzhu (TE 3) (*Shu*-Stream Point)

[Location] On the dorsum of the hand, proximal to the 4th metacarpophalangeal joint, in the depression between the 4th and 5th metacarpals.

[Effects] Purges away heat, and improves hearing.

[Indications] Headache, redness of the eye, deafness, tinnitus, sore throat, fever, pain in the elbow and arm, and motor impairment of the fingers.

[Manipulation] Puncture perpendicularly or obliquely 0.3-0.5 *cun*.

4. Yangchi (TE 4) (Primary Point)

[Location] At the midpoint of the dorsal crease of the wrist, in the depression on the ulnar side of the tendon of the common extensor muscle of the fingers.

[Effects] Regulates the primary *qi* of the Triple Energizer.

[Indications] Pain in the wrist, arm and shoulder, and impaired hearing.

[Manipulation] Puncture perpendicularly 0.3-0.5 *cun*.

5. Waiguan (TE 5) (Connecting Point, Confluence Point of *Yang* Link Vessel)

[Location] On the dorsal side of the forearm, 2 *cun* proximal to the dorsal crease of the wrist, between the radius and ulna.

[Effects] Disperses wind, and clears heat.

[Indications] Fever, headache, pain in the cheek, impaired hearing, tinnitus, motor impairment of the elbow and arm, pain of the fingers, and tremor of the hand.

[Manipulation] Puncture perpendicularly 0.5-1.0 *cun*.

6. Zhigou (TE 6) (*Jing*-River Point)

[Location] On the dorsal side of the forearm, 3 *cun* proximal to the dorsal crease of the wrist, between the radius and ulna.

[Effects] Clears heat, and opens the bowels.

[Indications] Tinnitus, impaired hearing, fever, constipation, sudden hoarseness, aching and heavy sensation of the shoulder and back.

[Manipulation] Puncture perpendicularly 0.5-1.0 *cun*.

7. Huizong (TE 7) (Cleft Point)

[Location] On the dorsal side of the forearm, 3 *cun* proximal to the dorsal crease of the wrist, on the ulnar side of Zhigou (TE 6) and on the radial border of the ulna.

[Effects] Clears the mind, and improves hearing.

[Indications] Deafness, pain in the ear, epilepsy, and pain of the arm.

[Manipulation] Puncture perpendicularly 0.5-1.0 *cun*.

8. Sanyangluo (TE 8)

[Location] On the dorsal side of the forearm, 4 *cun* proximal to the dorsal crease of the wrist, between the radius and ulna.

[Effects] Improves hearing.

[Indications] Deafness, sudden hoarseness, pain in the chest and costal region, pain in the hand and arm, and toothache.

[Manipulation] Puncture perpendicularly 0.5-1.0 *cun*.

9. Sidu (TE 9)

[Location] On the dorsal side of the forearm, 5 *cun* distal to the tip of the olecranon, between the radius and ulna.

[Effects] Improves hearing, and soothes the throat.

[Indications] Deafness, toothache, migraine, sudden hoarseness, and pain in the forearm.

[Manipulation] Puncture perpendicularly 0.5-1.0 *cun*.

10. Tianjing (TE 10) (*He*-Sea Point)

[Location] On the lateral side of the upper arm, in the depression 1 *cun* proximal to the tip of the olecranon.

[Effects] Disperses wind, clears up heat, and resolves nodulation.

[Indications] Migraine, pain in the neck, shoulder and arm, epilepsy, scrofula, and goiter.

[Manipulation] Puncture perpendicularly 0.3-0.5 *cun*.

11. Qinglengyuan (TE 11)

[Location] On the lateral side of the upper arm, 2 *cun* above the tip of the olecranon and 1 *cun* above Tianjing (TE 10).

[Effects] Removes damp-heat.

[Indications] Pain and motor impairment of the shoulder and arm, migraine, and jaundice.

[Manipulation] Puncture perpendicularly 0.3-0.5 *cun*.

12. Xiaoluo (TE 12)

[Location] On the lateral side of the upper arm, at the midpoint of the line connecting Qinglengyuan (TE 11) and Naohui (TE 13).

[Indications] Headache, stiff neck, and motor impairment and pain of the arm.

[Manipulation] Puncture perpendicularly 0.5-0.8 *cun*.

13. Naohui (TE 13)

[Location] On the lateral side of the upper arm and on the line connecting the tip of the olecranon and Jianliao (TE 14), 3 *cun* below Jianliao (TE 14), and on the postero-inferior border of the deltoid muscle.

[Effects] Resolves nodulation.

[Indications] Goiter, and pain in the shoulder and arm.

[Manipulation] Puncture perpendicularly 0.5-0.8 *cun*.

14. Jianliao (TE 14)

[Location] On the shoulder, posterior to Jianyu (LI 15), in the depression inferior and posterior to the acromion when the arm is abducted.

[Indications] Pain and motor impairment of the shoulder and upper arm.

[Manipulation] Puncture perpendicularly or obliquely downward 0.8-1.2 *cun*.

15. Tianliao (TE 15)

[Location] On the scapula, at the midpoint between Jianjing (GB 21) and Quyuan (SI 13), at the superior angle of the scapula.

[Indications] Pain in the shoulder and elbow, and stiffness of the neck.

[Manipulation] Puncture perpendicularly 0.3-0.5 *cun*.

16. Tianyou (TE 16)

[Location] On the lateral side of the neck, directly below the posterior border of the mastoid process, on the level of the mandibular angle, and on the posterior border of the sternocleidomastoid muscle.

[Effects] Clears the head of wind, and improves vision and hearing.

[Indications] Headache, stiff neck, facial swelling, blurring of vision, and sudden deafness.

[Manipulation] Puncture perpendicularly 0.3-0.5 *cun*.

17. Yifeng (TE 17) (crossing GB)

[Location] Posterior to the ear lobe, in the depression between the mastoid process and mandibular angle.

[Effects] Soothes the cheek, and improves hearing.

[Indications] Deafness, tinnitus, otorrhea, facial paralysis, toothache, swelling of the cheek, scrofula, and trismus.

[Manipulation] Puncture perpendicularly 0.5-1.0 *cun*.

18. Chimai (TE 18)

[Location] On the head, at the center of the mastoid process, and at the junction of the middle third and lower third of the line connecting Jiaosun (TE 20) and Yifeng (TE 17) along the curve of the ear helix.

[Effects] Improves hearing, and induces sedation.

[Indications] Headache, tinnitus, deafness, and infantile convulsion.

[Manipulation] Puncture obliquely 0.3-0.5 *cun*, or prick to cause bleeding.

19. Luxi (TE 19)

[Location] On the head, at the junction of the upper and middle third of the line connecting Jiaosun (TE 20) and Yifeng (TE 17) along the curve of the ear helix.

[Effects] Improves hearing, and induces sedation.

[Indications] Headache, tinnitus, deafness, pain in the ear, and infantile convulsion.

[Manipulation] Puncture obliquely 0.3-0.5 *cun*, or prick to cause bleeding.

20. Jiaosun (TE 20) (crossing GB, LI)

[Location] On the head, directly above the ear apex just within the hairline.

[Effects] Clears the head and eye of heat, and improves hearing.

[Indications] Tinnitus, inflammation of the eye, swelling of the gum, toothache, and parotitis.

[Manipulation] Puncture subcutaneously 0.3-0.5 *cun*.

21. Ermen (TE 21)

[Location] On the face, anterior to the supratragic notch, in the depression behind the posterior border of the condyloid process of the mandible.

[Effects] Clears the head and eye of heat, and improves hearing.

[Indications] Headache, inflammation of the eye, blurring of vision, twitching of the eyelid, toothache, and facial paralysis.

[Manipulation] Puncture perpendicularly 0.3-0.5 *cun*.

22. Erheliao (TE 22) (crossing SI, GB)

[Location] On the posterior margin of the temples, anterior to the root of the ear auricle at the hairline and posterior to the superficial temporal artery.

[Effects] Improves hearing.

[Indications] Migraine, and tinnitus.

[Manipulation] Avoid puncture the superficial temporal artery. Puncture obliquely 0.1-0.3 *cun*.

23. Sizhukong (TE 23)

[Location] On the face, in the depression of the lateral end of the eyebrow.

[Effects] Disperses wind, and improves vision.

[Indications] Headache, inflammation of the eye, blurring of vision, twitching of the eyelid, toothache, and facial paralysis.

[Manipulation] Puncture perpendicularly 0.3-0.5 *cun*.

The Points of the Gallbladder of Foot-Shaoyang (GB)

(Color Figs. 14, 15, 16, 17 and Fig. XIII-3)

1. Tongziliao (GB 1) (crossing SI, TE)

[Location] On the face, 0.5 *cun* lateral to the outer canthus, on the lateral border of the orbit.

[Effects] Disperses wind-heat, and improves vision.

[Indications] Headache, inflammation of the eye (keratitis, retinitis), failing of vision (optic atrophy), lacrimation, and facial paralysis.

[Manipulation] Puncture subcutaneously 0.3-0.5 *cun* towards Taiyang (EX-HN 5).

2. Tinghui (GB 2)

[Location] On the face, anterior to the intertragic notch, in the depression posterior to the condyloid process of the mandible when the mouth is open.

[Effects] Dispels wind, and improves hearing.

[Indications] Deafness, tinnitus, toothache, disorder of the temporomandibular joint, and facial paralysis.

[Manipulation] Puncture perpendicularly 0.5-0.8 *cun*.

3. Shangguan (GB 3) (crossing TE, ST)

[Location] Anterior to the ear, directly above Xiaguan (ST 7), in the depression above the upper border of the zygomatic arch.

[Effects] Dispels wind, and improves hearing.

[Indications] Headache, deafness, tinnitus, facial paralysis, and toothache.

[Manipulation] Puncture perpendicularly 0.3-0.5 *cun* when the mouth is slightly open.

4. Hanyan (GB 4) (crossing TE, ST)

[Location] Within the hairline of the temporal region, at the junction of the upper fourth and lower three-fourths of the curved line connecting Touwei (ST 8) and Qubin (GB 7).

[Effects] Dispels wind, and induces sedation.

[Indications] Migraine, vertigo, tinnitus, toothache, convulsion, and epilepsy.

[Manipulation] Puncture subcutaneously 0.3-0.5 *cun*.

5. Xuanlu (GB 5)

[Location] Within the hairline of the temporal region, at the midpoint of the curved line connecting Touwei (ST 8) and Qubin (GB 7).

[Indications] Migraine, and facial swelling.

[Manipulation] Puncture subcutaneously 0.3-0.5 *cun*.

6. Xuanli (GB 6) (crossing BL)

[Location] Within the hairline of the temporal region, at the junction of the upper three-fourths and lower fourth of the curved line connecting Touwei (ST 8) and Qubin (GB 7).

[Effects] Dispels wind, and induces sedation.

[Indications] Migraine, tinnitus, and frequent sneezing.

[Manipulation] Puncture subcutaneously 0.3-0.5 *cun*.

7. Qubin (GB 7) (crossing BL)

[Location] On the head, at the crossing point of the vertical posterior hairline of the temple and horizontal line through the ear apex.

[Effects] Dispels wind, and induces sedation.

[Indications] Headache, swelling of the cheek, trismus, pain in the temporal region, and infantile convulsion.

[Manipulation] Puncture subcutaneously 0.3-0.5 *cun*.

8. Shuaigu (GB 8) (crossing BL)

[Location] On the head, directly above the ear apex, 1.5 *cun* within the hairline.

[Effects] Dispels wind-heat, and induces sedation.

[Indications] Migraine, vertigo, vomiting, and infantile convulsion.

[Manipulation] Puncture subcutaneously 0.3-0.5 *cun*.

9. Tianchong (GB 9)

[Location] On the head, directly above the posterior border of the ear root, 2 *cun* above the hairline and 0.5 *cun* posterior to Shuaigu (GB 8).

[Effects] Dispels wind, and induces sedation.

[Indications] Headache, epilepsy, and convulsion.

[Manipulation] Puncture subcutaneously 0.3-0.5 *cun*.

10. Fubai (GB 10) (crossing BL)

[Location] On the head, posterior and superior to the mastoid process, at the junction of the middle third and upper third of the curved line connecting Tianchong (GB 9) and Wangu (GB 12)

[Indications] Headache, tinnitus, and deafness.

[Manipulation] Puncture subcutaneously 0.3-0.5 *cun*.

11. Touqiaoyin (GB 11) (crossing BL)

[Location] On the head, posterior and superior to the mastoid process, at the junction of the middle third and lower third of the curved line connecting Tianchong (GB 9) and Wangu (GB 12)

[Indications] Headache, tinnitus, and deafness.

[Manipulation] Puncture subcutaneously 0.3-0.5 *cun*.

12. Wangu (GB 12) (crossing BL)

[Location] On the head, in the depression posterior and inferior to the mastoid process.

[Effects] Dispels wind, clears up heat, and calms the mind.

[Indications] Headache, insomnia, swelling of the cheek, retroauricular pain, facial paralysis, and toothache.

[Manipulation] Puncture obliquely 0.3-0.5 *cun*.

13. Benshen (GB 13) (crossing YangLV)

[Location] On the head, 0.5 *cun* above the anterior hairline, 3 *cun* lateral to Shenting (GV 24).

[Effects] Dispels wind, and induces sedation.

[Indications] Headache, insomnia, dizziness, and epilepsy.

[Manipulation] Puncture subcutaneously 0.3-0.5 *cun*.

14. Yangbai (GB 14) (crossing YangLV)

[Location] On the forehead, directly above the pupil, 1 *cun* above the eyebrow.

[Effects] Dispels wind from the head and eyes.

[Indications] Frontal headache, pain of the orbital ridge, dizziness, twitching of the eyelids, ptosis of the eyelids, and lacrimation.

[Manipulation] Puncture subcutaneously 0.3-0.5 *cun*.

15. Toulinqi (GB 15) (crossing BL, YangLV)

[Location] On the head, directly above the pupil and 0.5 *cun* above the anterior hairline, midway between Shenting (GV 24) and Touwei (ST 8).

[Effects] Dispels wind from the head and nose.

[Indications] Headache, dizziness, lacrimation, rhinorrhea, and nasal obstruction.

[Manipulation] Puncture subcutaneously 0.3-0.5 *cun*.

16. Muchuang (GB 16) (crossing YangLV)

[Location] On the head, 1.5 *cun* above the anterior hairline and on the line joining Toulinqi (GB 15) and Fengchi (GB 20).

[Effects] Clears the head and eye of heat.

[Indications] Headache, dizziness, inflammation of the eye, and nasal obstruction.

[Manipulation] Puncture subcutaneously 0.3-0.5 *cun*.

17. Zhengying (GB 17) (crossing YangLV)

[Location] On the head, 2.5 *cun* above the anterior hairline and on the line joining Toulinqi (GB 15) and Fengchi (GB 20).

[Indications] Migraine, and dizziness.

[Manipulation] Puncture subcutaneously 0.3-0.5 *cun*.

18. Chengling (GB 18) (crossing YangLV)

[Location] On the head, 4 *cun* above the anterior hairline and on the line joining Toulinqi (GB 15) and Fengchi (GB 20).

[Effects] Dispels wind, and removes nasal obstruction.

[Indications] Headache, dizziness, epistaxis, and stuffed-up nose.

[Manipulation] Puncture subcutaneously 0.3-0.5 *cun*.

19. Naokong (GB 19) (crossing YangLV)

[Location] On the head, directly above Fengchi (GB 20) and at the level of the upper border of the external occipital protuberance.

[Effects] Dispels wind, and induces sedation.

[Indications] Headache, dizziness, stiff neck, and epilepsy.

[Manipulation] Puncture subcutaneously 0.3-0.5 *cun*.

20. Fengchi (GB 20) (crossing YangLV)

[Location] On the nape, below the occipital bone, at the level of Fengfu (GV 16), in the depression between the upper ends of the sternocleidomastoid and trapezius muscles.

[Effects] Dispels wind, induces diuresis, and clears the head and eyes.

[Indications] Headache, dizziness, insomnia, pain and stiffness of the neck, blurred vision, inflammation of the eye, tinnitus, convulsion, epilepsy, infantile convulsion, fever with anhidrosis, nasal obstruction and rhinorrhea.

[Manipulation] Puncture 0.5-0.8 *cun* towards the tip of the nose.

[Warning] Deep puncture towards the contralateral auricle is dangerous, for the needle may enter the cranial cavity and injure the brain.

21. Jianjing (GB 21) (crossing YangLV)

[Location] On the shoulder, midway between Dazhui (GV 14) and the acromion.

[Effects] Soothes the shoulder and back, and promotes lactation.

[Indications] Pain and stiffness of the neck, pain in the shoulder and back, motor impairment of the arm, insufficient lactation, and mastitis.

[Manipulation] Puncture perpendicularly 0.3-0.5 *cun*.

22. Yuanye (GB 22)

[Location] On the mid-axillary line when the arm is raised, 3 *cun* below the axilla, in the 4th intercostal space.

[Indications] Fullness of the chest, swelling of the axillary region, pain in the costal region, pain and motor impairment of the arm.

[Manipulation] Puncture 0.3-0.5 *cun* transversely along the intercostal space.

23. Zhejin (GB 23)

[Location] On the lateral side of the chest, 1 *cun* anterior to Yuanye (GB 22), in the 4th intercostal space.

[Indications] Fullness of the chest, and pain in the costal region.

[Manipulation] Puncture 0.3-0.5 *cun* subcutaneously along the intercostal space.

24. Riyue (GB 24) (Front-Curtain Point of the Gallbladder) (crossing SP)

[Location] In the 7th intercostal space, 4 *cun* lateral to the anterior midline.

[Effects] Checks upward perversion of *qi*, and promotes bile secretion and lactation.

[Indications] Pain in the hypochondriac region, acid regurgitation, hiccups, vomiting, jaundice, and mastitis.

[Manipulation] Puncture obliquely 0.3-0.5 *cun*.

25. Jingmen (GB 25) (Front-Curtain Point of the Kidney)

[Location] On the lateral side of the waist, just below the free end of the 12th rib.

[Effects] Relieves distention, and strengthens the lower back.

[Indications] Abdominal distention, borborygmi, diarrhea, and pain in the hypochondriac region and lower back.

[Manipulation] Puncture perpendicularly 0.3-0.5 *cun* or obliquely 0.5-1.0 *cun*.

26. Daimai (GB 26) (crossing BV)

[Location] On the lateral side of the abdomen, at the crossing point of a vertical line through the free end of the 11th rib and a horizontal line through the umbilicus.

[Effects] Regulates the Belt Vessel, and strengthens the lower back.

[Indications] Irregular menstruation, amenorrhea, morbid leukorrhea, hernia, and pain in the hypochondriac region and lower back.

[Manipulation] Puncture obliquely 0.5-1.0 *cun*.

27. Wushu (GB 27) (crossing BV)

[Location] On the lateral side of the abdomen, anterior to the anterosuperior iliac spine, 3 *cun* below the level of the umbilicus.

[Effects] Regulates the Belt Vessel and the Lower Energizer.

[Indications] Morbid leukorrhea, lower abdominal pain, constipation, hernia, and pain of the lower back.

[Manipulation] Puncture perpendicularly 0.5-1.0 *cun*.

28. Weidao (GB 28) (crossing BV)

[Location] On the lateral side of the abdomen, anterior and inferior to the anterosuperior iliac spine, 0.5 *cun* anterior and inferior to Wushu (GB 27)

[Effects] Regulates the Belt Vessel and the Lower Energizer.

[Indications] Morbid leukorrhea, lower abdominal pain, hernia, and prolapse of uterus.

[Manipulation] Puncture perpendicularly 0.5-1.0 *cun*.

29. Juliao (GB 29) (crossing YangHV)

[Location] On the hip, at the midpoint of the line connecting the anterosuperior iliac spine and the prominence of the great trochanter.

[Effects] Soothes the lower back and hip, and dispels wind-damp.

[Indications] Pain and numbness in the thigh and lumbar region, and paralysis of the lower limb.

[Manipulation] Puncture perpendicularly 0.5-1.0 *cun*.

30. Huantiao (GB 30) (crossing BL)

[Location] At the junction of the middle third and lateral third of the line connecting the prominence of the great trochanter and the sacral hiatus when the patient is in a lateral recumbent position with the thigh flexed.

[Effects] Soothes the lower back and legs, and dispels wind-damp.

[Indications] Pain of the lumbar region and thigh, and paralysis of the lower limb.

[Manipulation] Puncture perpendicularly 1.5-2.5 *cun*.

31. Fengshi (GB 31)

[Location] On the lateral midline of the thigh, 7 *cun* above the popliteal crease, or at the place touching the tip of the middle finger when the patient stands erect with the arms hanging down.

[Effects] Dispels wind-damp, and soothes the leg and foot.

[Indications] Pain in the thigh and lumbar region, paralysis of the lower limb, and general pruritus.

[Manipulation] Puncture perpendicularly 1.0-1.5 *cun*.

32. Zhongdu (GB 32)

[Location] On the lateral side of the thigh, 2 *cun* below Fengshi (GB 31).

[Effects] Dispels wind-damp, and soothes the leg and foot.

[Indications] Pain of the thigh and knee, and paralysis of the lower limbs.

[Manipulation] Puncture perpendicularly 1.0-1.5 *cun*.

33. Xiyangguan (GB 33)

[Location] On the lateral side of the knee, 3 *cun* above Yanglingquan (GB 34), in the depression above the external epicondyle of the femur.

[Indications] Swelling and pain of the knee, and numbness of the leg.

[Manipulation] Puncture perpendicularly 0.5-1.0 *cun*.

34. Yanglingquan (GB 34) (*He*-Sea Point, Influential Point of Tendons)

[Location] On the lateral side of the leg, in the depression anterior and inferior to the head of the fibula.

[Effects] Purges the Liver and Gallbladder of damp-heat, and soothes the knees.

[Indications] Paralysis of the lower limb, swelling and pain of the knee, jaundice with hypochondriac pain, and bitter taste in the mouth and vomiting.

[Manipulation] Puncture perpendicularly 1.0-1.5 *cun*.

35. Yangjiao (GB 35) (Cleft Point of the *Yang* Link Vessel)

[Location] On the lateral side of the leg, 7 *cun* above the tip of the external malleolus, on the posterior border of the fibula.

[Indications] Paralysis of the leg.

[Manipulation] Puncture perpendicularly 0.5-1.0 *cun*.

36. Waiqiu (GB 36) (Cleft Point)

[Location] On the lateral side of the leg, 7 *cun* above the tip of the external malleolus, on the anterior border of the fibula.

[Indications] Pain in the neck, chest, hypochondrium and thigh.

[Manipulation] Puncture perpendicularly 0.5-1.0 *cun*.

37. Guangming (GB 37) (Connecting Point)

[Location] On the lateral side of the leg, 5 *cun* above the tip of the external malleolus, on the anterior border of the fibula.

[Effects] Removes obstruction from the collateral meridians, and improves vision.

[Indications] Pain in the knee, pain and paralysis of the lower limb, blurring of vision, night blindness, and distending pain in the breast.

[Manipulation] Puncture perpendicularly 0.5-1.0 *cun*.

38. Yangfu (GB 38) (*Jing*-River Point)

[Location] On the lateral side of the leg, 4 *cun* above the tip of the external malleolus, slightly anterior to the anterior border of the fibula.

[Effects] Purges the Gallbladder of fire.

[Indications] Migraine, pain in the chest, axillary and hypochondriac regions and lateral aspect of the leg,

[Manipulation] Puncture perpendicularly 0.5-1.0 *cun*.

39. Xuanzhong (GB 39) (Influential Point of the Marrow)

[Location] On the lateral side of the leg, 3 *cun* above the tip of the external malleolus, on the anterior border of the fibula.

[Effects] Purges the Gallbladder of fire.

[Indications] Apoplexy with hemiplegia, pain in the hypochondriac region, spastic pain in the leg.

[Manipulation] Puncture perpendicularly 0.3-0.5 *cun*.

40. Qiuxu (GB 40) (Primary Point)

[Location] Anterior and inferior to the external malleolus, in the depression lateral to the tendon of the long extensor muscle of the toes.

[Effects] Purges the Gallbladder of fire.

[Indications] Pain in the hypochondriac region with vomiting (cholecystitis, cholelithiasis), paralysis of the lower limb, pain and swelling of the external malleolus.

[Manipulation] Puncture perpendicularly 0.5-1.0 *cun*.

41. Zulinqi (GB 41) (*Shu*-Stream Point, Confluence Point of the Belt Vessel)

[Location] On the lateral side of the instep, proximal to the 4th metatarsophalangeal joint, in the depression lateral to the tendon of the extensor muscle of the little toe.

[Effects] Clears the head, soothes the thoracic and hypochondriac regions, and purges away fire.

[Indications] Headache, dizziness, scrofula, pain in the hypochondriac region, distending pain of the breast, irregular menstruation, pain and swelling of the dorsum of foot, and spastic pain in the foot and toe.

[Manipulation] Puncture perpendicularly 0.3-0.5 *cun*.

42. Diwuhui (GB 42)

[Location] On the lateral side of the instep, proximal to the 4th metatarsophalangeal joint, in the depression between the 4th and 5th metatarsals, medial to the tendon of the extensor muscle of the little toe.

[Effects] Soothes the thoracic region.

[Indications] Distending pain of the breast, swelling and pain of the dorsum of foot.

[Manipulation] Puncture perpendicularly 0.3-0.5 *cun*.

43. Xiaxi (GB 43) (*Ying*-Spring Point)

[Location] On the lateral side of the instep, between the 4th and little toes, proximal to the margin of the web.

[Effects] Clears the head, and soothes the thoracic and hypochondriac regions.

[Indications] Headache, vertigo, tinnitus, impaired hearing, swelling of the cheek, fullness in the chest, pain in the hypochondriac region, distending pain in the breast, fever.

[Manipulation] Puncture perpendicularly 0.3-0.5 *cun*.

44. Zuqiaoyin (GB 44) (*Jing*-Well Point)

[Location] On the lateral side of the 4th toe, 0.1 *cun* proximal to the corner of toenail.

[Effects] Purges away heat, improves hearing, and soothes the hypochondriac region.

[Indications] Migraine, impaired hearing, tinnitus, dream-disturbed sleep, hypochondriac pain, and fever.

[Manipulation] Puncture superficially 0.1-0.2 *cun*.

The Points of the Liver Meridian of Foot-Jueyin (LR)

(Color Figs. 11 and 15)

1. Dadun (LR 1) (*Jing*-Well Point)

[Location] On the lateral side of the big toe, 0.1 *cun* proximal to the corner of the toenail.

[Effects] Soothes the liver, and regulates blood.

[Indications] Hernia, enuresis, uterine bleeding, prolapse of the uterus, and prolonged labor.

[Manipulation] Puncture superficially 0.1-0.2 *cun*, or prick to cause bleeding.

2. Xingjian (LR 2) (*Ying*-Spring Point)

[Location] On the instep between the 1st and 2nd toes, proximal to the margin of the web.

[Effects] Clears the Liver and the eyes of heat, and induces sedation.

[Indications] Hypochondriac pain, abdominal distention, headache, dizziness, vertigo, inflammation of the eye, deviation of the mouth, hernia, painful urination, retention of urine, irregular menstruation, epilepsy, insomnia, and convulsion.

[Manipulation] Puncture obliquely 0.3-0.5 *cun*.

3. Taichong (LR 3) (*Shu*-Stream Point, Primary Point)

[Location] On the instep, in the depression of the proximal end of the 1st interosseous metatarsal space.

[Effects] Clears the Liver and the eye of heat, and induces sedation.

[Indications] Headache, dizziness, vertigo, inflammation of the eye, depression, convulsion, epilepsy, deviation of the mouth, hypochondriac pain, uterine bleeding, hernia, enuresis, retention of urine, and pain in the anterior aspect of the medial malleolus.

[Manipulation] Puncture perpendicularly 0.3-0.5 *cun*.

4. Zhongfeng (LR 4) (*Jing*-River Point)

[Location] On the instep, 1 *cun* anterior to the medial malleolus, midway between Shangqiu (SP 5) and Jiexi (ST 41), in the depression medial to the tendon of the anterior tibial muscle.

[Effects] Soothes the Liver, and clears the Lower Energizer of heat.

[Indications] Hernia, pain in the external genitalia, retention of urine, and distending pain in the hypochondrium.

[Manipulation] Puncture perpendicularly 0.3-0.5 *cun*.

5. Ligou (LR 5) (Connecting Point)

[Location] On the medial side of the leg, 5 *cun* above the tip of the medial malleolus, on the medial border of the tibia.

[Effects] Regulates the Lower Energizer and menstruation.

[Indications] Retention of urine, enuresis, hernia, irregular menstruation, morbid leukorrhea, pruritus vulvae, and weakness of the leg.

[Manipulation] Puncture perpendicularly 0.3-0.5 *cun*.

6. Zhongdu (LR 6) (Cleft Point)

[Location] On the medial side of the leg, 7 *cun* above the tip of the medial malleolus, on the medial border of the tibia.

[Effects] Soothes the Liver, and regulates the Lower Energizer and menstruation.

[Indications] Abdominal and hypochondriac pain, diarrhea, hernia, uterine bleeding, and prolonged lochia.

[Manipulation] Puncture perpendicularly 0.5-0.8 *cun*.

7. Xiguan (LR 7)

[Location] On the medial side of the leg, posterior and inferior to the medial epicondyle of tibia, 1 *cun* posterior to Yinlingquan (SP 9), at the upper end of the medial head of the gastrocnemius muscle.

[Indications] Pain in the knee.

[Manipulation] Puncture perpendicularly 0.5-1.0 *cun*.

8. Ququan (LR 8) (*He*-Sea Point)

[Location] On the medial side of the knee, at the medial end of the popliteal crease when the knee is flexed, posterior to the medial epicondyle of the tibia, in the depression of the anterior border of the insertions of the semimembranous and semitendinous muscles.

[Effects] Clears the Liver of fire and damp-heat.

[Indications] Prolapse of the uterus, lower abdominal pain, retention of urine, pain in the external genitalia, pruritus vulvae, and pain in the medial aspect of the knee and thigh.

[Manipulation] Avoid puncturing the popliteal artery. Puncture perpendicularly 0.5-1.0 *cun* when the knee is bent.

9. Yinbao (LR 9)

[Location] On the medial side of the thigh, 4 *cun* above the medial epicondyle of the femur, between the medial vastus muscle and sartorius muscle.

[Effects] Regulates urination and menstruation.

[Indications] Pain in the lumbosacral region, lower abdominal pain, enuresis, retention of urine, and irregular menstruation.

[Manipulation] Puncture perpendicularly 0.5-1.0 *cun*.

10. Zuwuli (LR 10)

[Location] On the medial side of the thigh, 3 *cun* directly below Qichong (ST 30), on the lateral border of the long abductor muscle of the thigh.

[Effects] Facilitates micturition.

[Indications] Lower abdominal distention and fullness, and retention of urine.

[Manipulation] Puncture perpendicularly 0.5-1.0 *cun*.

11. Yinlian (LR 11)

[Location] On the medial side of the thigh, 2 *cun* directly below Qichong (ST 30), on the lateral border of the long abductor muscle of the thigh.

[Effects] Regulates menstruation.

[Indications] Irregular menstruation, morbid leukorrhea, lower abdominal pain, and pain in the thigh and leg.

[Manipulation] Puncture perpendicularly 0.5-1.0 *cun*.

12. Jimai (LR 12)

[Location] In the inguinal groove, lateral and inferior to Qichong (ST 30), 2.5 *cun* lateral to the anterior midline.

[Effects] Regulates the Lower Energizer.

[Indications] Lower abdominal pain, hernia, and pain in the external genitalia.

[Manipulation] Avoid puncturing the artery. Puncture perpendicularly 0.3-0.5 *cun*.

13. Zhangmen (LR 13) (Front-Curtain Point of the Spleen, Influential Point of *Zang*-organs)

[Location] On the lateral side of the abdomen, below the free end of the 11th rib and at the level of the umbilicus.

[Effects] Soothes the Liver, invigorates the Spleen, and promotes digestion.

[Indications] Abdominal distention, borborygmi, hypochondriac pain, vomiting diarrhea, and indigestion.

[Manipulation] Puncture perpendicularly 0.3-0.5 or obliquely 0.5-1.0 *cun*.

[Warning] Deep perpendicular puncture is dangerous; it may injure the liver on the right side and the spleen on the left side.

14. Qimen (LR 14) (Front-Curtain Point of the Liver)

[Location] On the chest, directly below the nipple, in the 6th intercostal space, 4 *cun* lateral to the anterior midline.

[Effects] Soothes the Liver, and relieves stagnation and depression of *qi*.

[Indications] Hypochondriac pain, abdominal distention, hiccups, acid regurgitation, mastitis, and depression.

[Manipulation] Puncture obliquely 0.3-0.5 *cun*.

The Points of the Governor Vessel (GV)

(Color Figs. 16, 17 and Fig. XIII-3)

1. Changqiang (GV 1) (Connecting Point) (crossing KI)

[Location] At the midpoint of the line connecting the tip of the coccyx and anus.

[Effects] Lifts the anus, regulates bowel movements, and induces sedation.

[Indications] Prolapse of the rectum, constipation, diarrhea, bloody stools, hemorrhoids, pain in the lower back, and epilepsy.

[Manipulation] Puncture perpendicularly 0.5-1.0 *cun*.

2. Yaoshu (GV 2)

[Location] In the hiatus of the sacrum.

[Effects] Regulates blood, and soothes the lumbosacral region.

[Indications] Irregular menstruation, pain and stiffness of the lower back, hemorrhoids, and weakness of the lower limbs.

[Manipulation] Puncture obliquely upward 0.5-1.0 *cun*.

3. Yaoyangguan (GV 3)

[Location] On the midline of the lower back, in the depression below the spinous process of the 4th lumbar vertebra.

[Effects] Soothes the lower back and leg, and warms the Kidney.

[Indications] Irregular menstruation, impotence, pain in the lumbosacral region, pain, numbness and motor impairment of the lower limb.

[Manipulation] Puncture perpendicularly 0.5-1.0 *cun*.

4. Mingmen (GV 4)

[Location] On the midline of the back, in the depression below the spinous process of the 2nd lumbar vertebra.

[Effects] Soothes the back, warms the Kidney, and regulates menstruation.

[Indications] Pain and stiffness of the lower back, impotence, irregular menstruation, diarrhea, indigestion, and morbid leukorrhea.

[Manipulation] Puncture perpendicularly 0.5-1.0 *cun*.

5. Xuanshu (GV 5)

[Location] On the midline of the back, in the depression below the spinous process of the 1st lumbar vertebra.

[Effects] Soothes the back, and promotes digestion.

[Indications] Pain and stiffness of the lower back, diarrhea, and indigestion.

[Manipulation] Puncture perpendicularly 0.5-1.0 *cun*.

6. Jizhong (GV 6)

[Location] On the midline of the back, in the depression below the spinous process of the 11th thoracic vertebra.

[Effects] Invigorates the Spleen, and resolves damp.

[Indications] Epigastric pain, diarrhea, jaundice, stiffness and pain in the back.

[Manipulation] Puncture perpendicularly 0.5-1.0 *cun*.

7. Zhongshu (GV 7)

[Location] On the midline of the back, in the depression below the spinous process of the 10th thoracic vertebra.

[Indications] Epigastric pain, and pain and stiffness of the back.

[Manipulation] Puncture perpendicularly 0.5-1.0 *cun*.

8. Jinsuo (GV 8)

[Location] On the midline of the back, in the depression below the spinous process of the 9th thoracic vertebra.

[Effects] Induces sedation.

[Indications] Epilepsy, stiffness of the back, and epigastric pain.

[Manipulation] Puncture perpendicularly 0.5-1.0 *cun*.

9. Zhiyang (GV 9)

[Location] On the midline of the back, in the depression below the spinous process of the 7th thoracic vertebra.

[Effects] Clears the Liver and Gallbladder of heat, and soothes the chest.

[Indications] Jaundice, coughing, asthma, stiffness of the back, and pain in the chest and back.

[Manipulation] Puncture obliquely upward 0.5-1.0 *cun*.

10. Lingtai (GV 10)

[Location] On the midline of the back, in the depression below the spinous process of the 6th thoracic vertebra.

[Effects] Clears the chest of heat.

[Indications] Coughing, asthma, backache, and stiff neck.

[Manipulation] Puncture obliquely upward 0.5-1.0 *cun*.

11. Shendao (GV 11)

[Location] On the midline of the back, in the depression below the spinous process of the 5th thoracic vertebra.

[Effects] Soothes the Heart, and calms the mind.

[Indications] Cardiac pain, palpitations, anxiety, pain and stiffness of the back.

[Manipulation] Puncture obliquely upward 0.5-1.0 *cun*.

12. Shenzhu (GV 12)

[Location] On the midline of the back, in the depression below the spinous process of the 3rd thoracic vertebra.

[Effects] Facilitates the flow of Lung *qi*, and induces sedation.

[Indications] Coughing, asthma, epilepsy, and pain and stiffness of the back.

[Manipulation] Puncture obliquely upward 0.5-1.0 *cun*.

13. Taodao (GV 13) (crossing BL)

[Location] On the midline of the back, in the depression below the spinous process of the 1st thoracic vertebra.

[Effects] Disperses wind, and purges away heat.

[Indications] Headache, fever, malaria, and stiffness of the back.

[Manipulation] Puncture obliquely upward 0.5-1.0 *cun*.

14. Dazhui (GV 14) (crossing BL, GB, ST)

[Location] On the posterior midline, in the depression below the 7th cervical vertebra.

[Effects] Replenishes *qi*, and relieves fever.

[Indications] Fever, malaria, coughing, asthma, and stiffness of the neck and back.

[Manipulation] Puncture obliquely upward 0.5-1.0 *cun*.

15. Yamen (GV 15) (crossing YangLV)

[Location] On the nape, 0.5 *cun* directly above the midpoint of the posterior hairline, in the depression below the 1st cervical vertebra.

[Effects] Clears the mind, and facilitates the movement of the tongue.

[Indications] Mental disorders, epilepsy, deafness and mute, sudden hoarseness of voice, aphasia with stiffness of the tongue, occipital headache, and stiff neck.

[Manipulation] Puncture perpendicularly 0.5-0.8 *cun*.

[Warning] Upward oblique or deep puncture is strictly prohibited, for it may cause subarachnoid hemorrhage or injure the medullary bulb.

16. Fengfu (GV 16) (crossing YangLV)

[Location] On the nape, 1 *cun* directly above the midpoint of the posterior hairline, directly below the external occipital protuberance.

[Effects] Dispels wind, clears the mind, and facilitates the movement of the tongue.

[Indications] Headache, stiff neck, blurring of vision, epistaxis, sore throat, post-apoplectic aphasia, and mental disorders.

[Manipulation] Puncture perpendicularly 0.5-0.8 *cun*.

[Warning] Deep puncture is strictly prohibited, for it may cause subarachnoid hemorrhage or injure the medullary bulb.

17. Naohu (GV 17) (crossing BL)

[Location] On the midline of the head, 2.5 *cun* above the posterior hairline and 1.5

cun above Fengfu (GV 16), in the depression on the upper border of the external occipital protuberance.

[Effects] Dispels wind, and induces sedation.

[Indications] Headache, dizziness, pain and stiffness of the neck, and epilepsy.

[Manipulation] Puncture subcutaneously 0.3-0.5 *cun*.

18. Qiangjian (GV 18)

[Location] On the midline of the head, 1.5 *cun* directly above Naohu (GV 17), midway between Fengfu (GV 16) and Baihui (GV 20).

[Effects] Dispels wind, and clears the head and eyes.

[Indications] Headache, stiff neck, blurring of vision, mania.

[Manipulation] Puncture subcutaneously 0.3-0.5 *cun*.

19. Houding (GV 19)

[Location] On the midline of the head, 3 *cun* above Naohu (GV 17).

[Effects] Dispels wind, and induces sedation.

[Indications] Headache, vertigo, mania, and epilepsy.

[Manipulation] Puncture subcutaneously 0.3-0.5 *cun*.

20. Baihui (GV 20) (crossing BL)

[Location] On the midline of the head, 7 *cun* above the posterior hairline, at the midpoint of the line connecting the apexes of both ears.

[Effects] Extinguishes the Liver wind, calms the mind, induces resuscitation, and elevates *qi*.

[Indications] Headache, vertigo, tinnitus, nasal obstruction, apoplectic aphasia, loss of consciousness, mental disorders, and prolapse of the rectum and the uterus.

[Manipulation] Puncture subcutaneously 0.3-0.5 *cun*.

21. Qianding (GV 21)

[Location] On the midline of the head, 1.5 *cun* anterior to Baihui (GV 20).

[Effects] Dispels wind, and improves vision.

[Indications] Vertical headache, dizziness, and blurring of vision.

[Manipulation] Puncture subcutaneously 0.3-0.5 *cun*.

22. Xinhui (GV 22)

[Location] On the midline of the head, 2 *cun* posterior to the anterior hairline, 3 *cun* anterior to Baihui (GV 20)

[Effects] Dispels wind, and improves vision.

[Indications] Headache, dizziness, and blurring of vision.

[Manipulation] Puncture subcutaneously 0.3-0.5 *cun*.

[Warning] Puncture at this point is prohibited in infants with metopism.

23. Shangxing (GV 23)

[Location] On the midline of the head, 1 *cun* above the anterior hairline.

[Effects] Clears the head, calms the mind, and removes obstruction from the nose.

[Indications] Headache, epistaxis, rhinorrhea, and mental disorders.

[Manipulation] Puncture subcutaneously 0.3-0.5 *cun*.

[Warning] Puncture at this point is prohibited in infants with metopism.

24. Shenting (GV 24) (crossing BL, ST)

[Location] On the midline of the head, 0.5 *cun* above the anterior hairline.

[Effects] Calms the mind, dispels wind, and removes obstruction from the nose.

[Indications] Epilepsy, anxiety, palpitations, insomnia, headache, dizziness, and rhinorrhea.

[Manipulation] Puncture subcutaneously 0.3-0.5 *cun*, or prick to cause bleeding.

25. Suliao (GV 25)

[Location] On the tip of the nose.

[Effects] Induces resuscitation, and removes obstruction from the nose.

[Indications] Loss of consciousness, nasal obstruction, rhinorrhea, epistaxis, rosacea.

[Manipulation] Puncture perpendicularly 0.2-0.3 *cun*, or prick to cause bleeding.

26. Shuigou (GV 26) (crossing ST, LI)

[Location] On the face, at the junction of the upper third and middle third of the philtrum.

[Effects] Induces resuscitation, clears the mind, and soothes the lower back.

[Indications] Mental disorders, epilepsy, hysteria, infantile convulsion, fainting, loss of consciousness, trismus, deviation of the mouth, pain and stiffness of the lower back.

[Manipulation] Puncture obliquely upward 0.3-0.5 *cun*.

27. Duiduan (GV 27)

[Location] On the face, on the median tubercle of the upper lip, at the junction of the skin and upper lip.

[Effects] Clears the mind, and purges away heat.

[Indications] Mental disorders, twitching of the lip, pain and swelling of the gums.

[Manipulation] Puncture obliquely upward 0.2-0.3 *cun*.

28. Yinjiao (GV 28)

[Location] On the inside of the upper lip, at the junction of the labial frenulum and upper gum.

[Effects] Clears the mind, and purges away heat.

[Indications] Mental disorders, pain and swelling of the gums, and rhinorrhea.

[Manipulation] Prick to cause bleeding.

The Points of the Conception Vessel (CV)

(Color Figs. 15, 17 and Fig. XIII-3)

1. Huiyin (CV 1) (crossing TV)

[Location] On the perineum, at the midpoint between the posterior border of the scrotum and anus in the male, and between the posterior commissure of the large labia and anus in the female.

[Effects] Lifts the anus, and induces resuscitation.

[Indications] Prolapse of the rectum, hemorrhoids, retention of urine, enuresis, and loss of consciousness.

[Manipulation] Puncture perpendicularly 0.5-1.0 *cun*.

2. Qugu (CV 2) (crossing LR)

[Location] On the midline of the lower abdomen, at the midpoint of the upper border of the pubic symphysis.

[Effects] Facilitates micturition, secures essence, and checks vaginal discharge.

[Indications] Retention and dribbling of urine, enuresis, impotence, nocturnal emission, morbid leukorrhea, irregular menstruation, dysmenorrhea, and hernia.

[Manipulation] Puncture perpendicularly 0.5-1.0 *cun*.

3. Zhongji (CV 3) (Front-Curtain Point of the Bladder) (crossing SP, LR, KI)

[Location] On the midline of the lower abdomen, 4 *cun* below the center of the umbilicus.

[Effects] Facilitates micturition, secures essence, and regulates menstruation.

[Indications] Frequent urination, enuresis, retention of urine, impotence, nocturnal emission, uterine bleeding, irregular menstruation, dysmenorrhea, morbid leukorrhea, and prolapse of the uterus.

[Manipulation] Puncture perpendicularly 0.5-1.0 *cun*.

4. Guanyuan (CV 4) (Front-Curtain Point of the Small Intestine) (crossing SP, LR, KI)

[Location] On the midline of the lower abdomen, 3 *cun* below the center of the umbilicus.

[Effects] Tonifies the Kidneys, and regulates the Lower Energizer.

[Indications] Enuresis, retention of urine, frequent urination, irregular menstruation, dysmenorrhea, uterine bleeding, postpartum hemorrhage, morbid leukorrhea, lower abdominal pain, diarrhea, and prolapse of the uterus.

[Manipulation] Puncture perpendicularly 0.5-1.0 *cun*.

5. Shimen (CV 5) (Front-Curtain Point of the Triple Energizer)

[Location] On the midline of the lower abdomen, 2 *cun* below the center of the umbilicus.

[Effects] Regulates the Lower Energizer.

[Indications] Abdominal pain, diarrhea, edema, anuria, enuresis, amenorrhea, uterine bleeding, postpartum hemorrhage, and morbid leukorrhea.

[Manipulation] Puncture perpendicularly 0.5-1.0 *cun*.

6. Qihai (CV 6)

[Location] On the midline of the lower abdomen, 1.5 *cun* below the center of the umbilicus.

[Effects] Replenishes and regulates *qi*.

[Indications] Abdominal pain, diarrhea, constipation, hernia, edema, enuresis, impotence, irregular menstruation, dysmenorrhea, amenorrhea, postpartum hemorrhage, morbid leukorrhea, and asthma.

[Manipulation] Puncture perpendicularly 0.8-1.2 *cun*.

7. Yinjiao (CV 7) (crossing TV)

[Location] On the midline of the lower abdomen, 1 *cun* below the center of the umbilicus.

[Effects] Induces diuresis, and regulates menstruation.

[Indications] Abdominal distention, edema, hernia, irregular menstruation, uterine bleeding, postpartum hemorrhage, morbid leukorrhea, pruritus vulvae, and abdominal pain around the umbilicus.

[Manipulation] Puncture perpendicularly 0.8-1.2 *cun*.

8. Shenque (CV 8)

[Location] At the center of the umbilicus.

[Effects] Warms the Middle Energizer, and checks diarrhea.

[Indications] Abdominal pain, borborygmi, and diarrhea.

[Manipulation] Puncture is prohibited.

9. Shuifen (CV 9)

[Location] On the midline of the upper abdomen, 1 *cun* above the center of the umbilicus.

[Effects] Induces diuresis, and relieves spasm.

[Indications] Abdominal pain, borborygmi, diarrhea, edema, and retention of urine.

[Manipulation] Puncture perpendicularly 0.5-1.0 *cun*.

10. Xiawan (CV 10) (crossing SP)

[Location] On the midline of the upper abdomen, 2 *cun* above the center of the umbilicus.

[Effects] Regulates the Middle Energizer.

[Indications] Epigastric and abdominal pain, borborygmi, indigestion, vomiting, and diarrhea.

[Manipulation] Puncture perpendicularly 0.5-1.2 *cun*.

11. Jianli (CV 11)

[Location] On the midline of the upper abdomen, 3 *cun* above the center of the umbilicus.

[Effects] Regulates the Middle Energizer.

[Indications] Epigastric pain, abdominal distention, borborygmi, and anorexia.

[Manipulation] Puncture perpendicularly 0.5-1.2 *cun*.

12. Zhongwan (CV 12) (Front-Curtain Point of the Stomach, Influential Point of *Fu*-organs) (crossing ST, SI, TE)

[Location] On the midline of the upper abdomen, 4 *cun* above the center of the umbilicus.

[Effects] Regulates the Middle Energizer.

[Indications] Epigastric pain, acid regurgitation, nausea vomiting, abdominal distention, borborygmi, diarrhea, indigestion, and insomnia.

[Manipulation] Puncture perpendicularly 0.5-1.2 *cun*.

13. Shangwan (CV 13) (crossing ST, SI)

[Location] On the midline of the upper abdomen, 5 *cun* above the center of the umbilicus.

[Effects] Regulates the Middle Energizer.

[Indications] Epigastric pain, nausea vomiting, abdominal distention, and insomnia.

[Manipulation] Puncture perpendicularly 0.5-1.2 *cun*.

14. Juque (CV 14) (Front-Curtain Point of the Heart)

[Location] On the midline of the upper abdomen, 6 *cun* above the center of the umbilicus.

[Effects] Soothes the Heart, calms the mind, and harmonizes the Stomach.

[Indications] Precordial and epigastric pain, difficulty in swallowing, nausea, vomiting, acid regurgitation, mental disorders, and palpitations.

[Manipulation] Puncture perpendicularly 0.3-0.5 *cun* or obliquely downward 0.5-0.8 *cun*.

15. Jiuwei (CV 15) (Connecting Point)

[Location] On the midline of the upper abdomen, 7 *cun* above the center of the umbilicus, in the depression below the xiphoid process.

[Effects] Soothes the Heart, and clears the mind.

[Indications] Precordial pain, mental disorders, and epilepsy.

[Manipulation] Puncture obliquely downward 0.3-0.5 *cun*.

16. Zhongting (CV 16)

[Location] On the anterior midline of the chest, at the level of the 5th intercostal space.

[Effects] Soothes the chest, and checks upward perversion of *qi*.

[Indications] Distention and fullness in the chest and costal region, hiccups, nausea.

[Manipulation] Puncture subcutaneously 0.3-0.5 *cun*.

17. Danzhong (CV 17) (Front-Curtain Point of the Pericardium, Influential Point of *Qi*)

[Location] On the anterior midline of the chest, at the level of the 4th intercostal space.

[Effects] Facilitates the flow of *qi*, soothes the chest, and promotes lactation.

[Indications] Asthma, pain and fullness in the chest, palpitations, difficulty in swallowing, hiccups, and insufficient lactation.

[Manipulation] Puncture subcutaneously 0.3-0.5 *cun*.

18. Yutang (CV 18)

[Location] On the anterior midline of the chest, at the level of the 3rd intercostal space.

[Effects] Soothes the chest, and checks upward perversion of *qi*.

[Indications] Pain in the chest, cough, asthma, and vomiting.

[Manipulation] Puncture subcutaneously 0.3-0.5 *cun*.

19. Zigong (CV 19)

[Location] On the anterior midline of the chest, at the level of the 2nd intercostal space.

[Effects] Soothes the chest, and checks upward perversion of *qi*.

[Indications] Pain in the chest, coughing, and asthma.

[Manipulation] Puncture subcutaneously 0.3-0.5 *cun*.

20. Huagai (CV 20)

[Location] On the anterior midline of the chest, at the level of the 1st intercostal space.

[Effects] Soothes the chest, and checks upward perversion of *qi*.

[Indications] Pain in the chest and costal region, coughing, and asthma.

[Manipulation] Puncture subcutaneously 0.3-0.5 *cun*.

21. Xuanji (CV 21)

[Location] On the anterior midline, at the center of the sternal manubrium, 1 *cun* below Tiantu (CV 22).

[Effects] Soothes the chest, and checks perversion of *qi*.

[Indications] Pain and fullness in chest, cough, asthma, and difficulty in swallowing (esophageal and cardiac spasm)

[Manipulation] Puncture subcutaneously 0.3-0.5 *cun*.

22. Tiantu (CV 22) (crossing YinLV)

[Location] On the anterior midline of the neck, at the center of the suprasternal fossa.

[Effects] Facilitates the flow of *qi*, and soothes the throat.

[Indications] Asthma, cough, sore throat, sudden hoarseness of voice, hiccups, difficulty in swallowing, and goiter.

[Manipulation] First puncture perpendicularly 0.1-0.2 *cun*, and then insert the needle downward along the posterior aspect of the sternum 0.5-1.0 *cun*. Avoid puncturing the trachea.

23. Lianquan (CV 23) (crossing YinLV)

[Location] On the anterior midline of the neck, above the laryngeal protuberance, in the depression above the upper border of the hyoid bone.

[Effects] Restores the normal function of the tongue and throat.

[Indications] Aphasia with stiffness of the tongue in apoplexy, sudden hoarseness of voice, and difficultly in swallowing.

[Manipulation] Puncture obliquely 0.5-1.0 *cun* toward the tongue root.

24. Chengjiang (CV 24) (crossing ST)

[Location] On the face, in the depression at the midpoint of the mentolabial sulcus.

[Effects] Disperses wind, and soothes the mouth and teeth.

[Indications] Swelling of the gums, toothache, salivation, mental disorders, and deviation of the eye and mouth.

[Manipulation] Puncture obliquely upward 0.2-0.3 *cun*.

EXTRA POINTS (EX)

The Points of the Head and Neck (HN) (Fig. XIII-4)

1. Sishencong (EX-HN 1)

[Location] Four points on the vertex of the head, 1 *cun* anterior, posterior and lateral to Baihui (GV 20).

[Indications] Headache, vertigo, insomnia, forgetfulness, and epilepsy.

[Manipulation] Puncture subcutaneously 0.5-1.0 *cun*.

2. Dangyang (EX-HN 2)

[Location] At the frontal part of the head, directly above the pupil, 1 *cun* above the anterior hairline.

[Indications] Headache, dizziness, and inflammation of the eye.

[Manipulation] Puncture subcutaneously 0.5-1.0 *cun*.

3. Yintang (EX-HN 3)

[Location] On the forehead, at the midpoint between the eyebrows.
[Indications] Frontal headache, rhinorrhea, epistaxis, and insomnia.
[Manipulation] Puncture subcutaneously 0.3-0.5 *cun*.

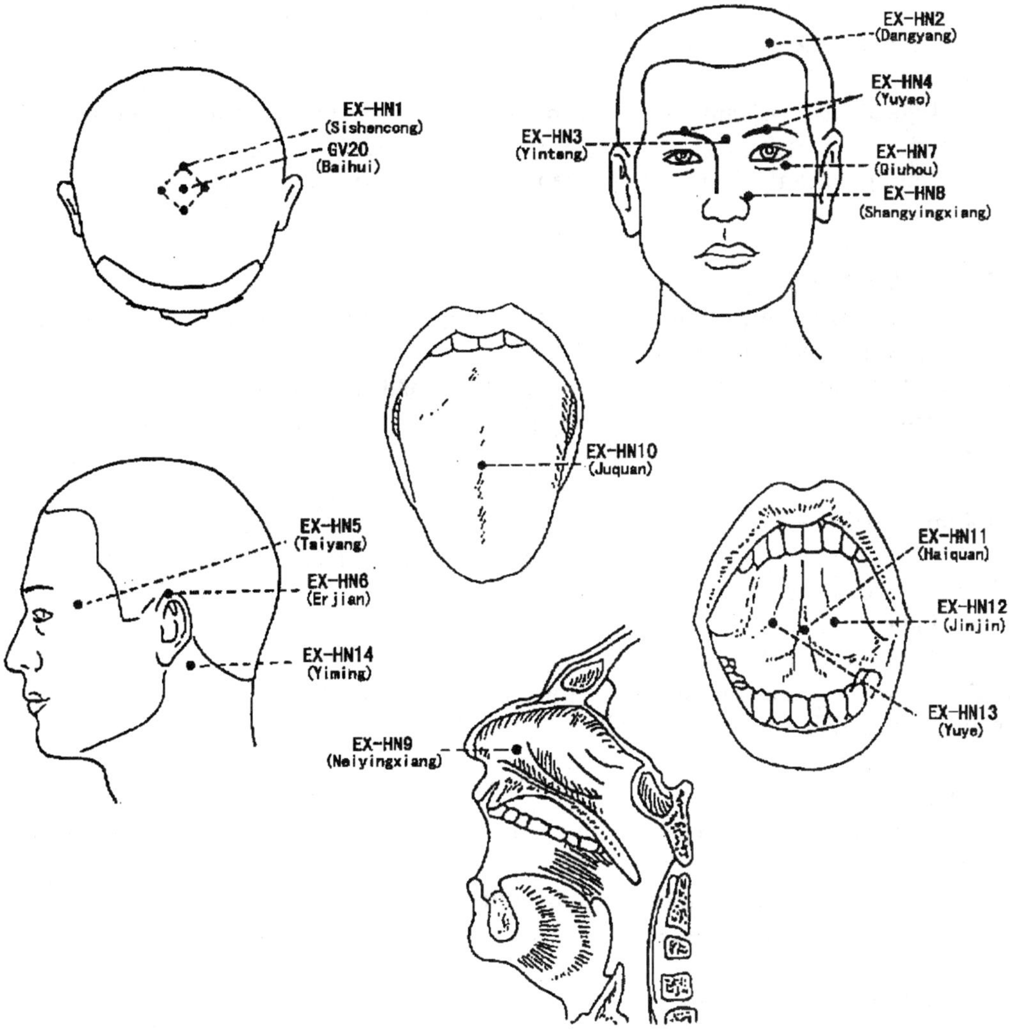

Fig. XIII-4 Extra points of the head and neck

4. Yuyao (EX-HN 4)

[Location] On the forehead, directly above the pupil, in the eyebrow.

[Indications] Pain in the supraorbital region, twitching of the eyelid, ptosis, cloudiness of the cornea, and inflammation of the eye.

[Manipulation] Puncture subcutaneously 0.3-0.5 *cun*.

5. Taiyang (EX-HN 5)

[Location] On the temporal part of the head, in the depression one finger breadth behind the midpoint between the lateral end of the eyebrow and the outer canthus.

[Indications] Migraine, temporal headache, eye diseases, and deviation of the eye and mouth.

[Manipulation] Puncture perpendicularly 0.3-0.5 *cun*, or prick to cause bleeding.

6. Erjian (EX-HN 6)

[Location] On the temporal part of the head, where the tip of the auricle touches when the ear is folded forward.

[Indications] Inflammation of the eye, nebula, and fever.

[Manipulation] Puncture perpendicularly 0.1-0.2 *cun*, or prick to cause bleeding.

7. Qiuhou (EX-HN 7)

[Location] On the face, at the junction of the lateral fourth and medial three-fourths of the infraorbital margin.

[Indications] Eye diseases.

[Manipulation] Push the eyeball upward gently, and then puncture perpendicularly 0.5-1.0 *cun* along the infraorbital margin slowly without lifting, thrusting, twisting or rotating the needle.

8. Shangyingxiang (EX-HN 8)

[Location] On the face, at the junction of the alar cartilage of the nose and the nasal concha, near the upper end of the nasolabial groove.

[Indications] Allergic, atrophic or hypertrophic rhinitis.

[Manipulation] Puncture subcutaneously upward about 0.5 *cun*.

9. Neiyingxiang (EX-HN 9)

[Location] In the nostril, at the junction between the mucosa of the alar cartilage of the nose and the nasal concha.

[Indications] Inflammation of the eye, sunstroke, and syncope.

[Manipulation] Prick to cause bleeding.

10. Juquan (EX-HN 10)

[Location] In the mouth, at the midpoint of the dorsal midline of the tongue.

[Indications] Aphasia with stiffness of the tongue in apoplexy, and protrusion of the tongue.

[Manipulation] Prick to cause bleeding.

11. Haiquan (EX-HN 11)

[Location] In the mouth, at the midpoint of the frenulum of the tongue.

[Indications] Swelling or protrusion of the tongue, and hiccups.

[Manipulation] Prick to cause bleeding.

12. Jinjin (EX-HN 12)

[Location] In the mouth, on the vein in the left side of the frenulum of the tongue.

[Indications] Swelling of the tongue, vomiting, and aphasia with stiffness of the tongue.

[Manipulation] Prick to cause bleeding.

13. Yuye (EX-HN 13)

[Location] In the mouth, on the vein on the right side of the frenulum of the tongue.

[Indications] Swelling of the tongue, vomiting, and aphasia with stiffness of the tongue.

[Manipulation] Prick to cause bleeding.

14. Yiming (EX-HN 14)

[Location] On the nape, 1 *cun* posterior to Yifeng (TE 17).

[Indications] Eye diseases, tinnitus, dizziness, headache, and insomnia.

[Manipulation] Puncture perpendicularly 0.5-0.8 *cun*.

15. Jingbailao (EX-HN 15)

[Location] On the nape, 2 *cun* directly above Dazhui (GV 14) and 1 *cun* lateral to the posterior midline.

[Indications] Scrofula, cough, asthma, and stiff neck.

[Manipulation] Puncture perpendicularly 0.3-0.5 *cun*.

The Points of the Chest and Abdomen (CA) (Fig. XIII-5)

Zigong (EX-CA 1)

[Location] On the lower abdomen, at the level of 4 *cun* below the center of the umbilicus and 3 *cun* lateral to the midline.

[Indications] Prolapse of the uterus, and irregular menstruation.

[Manipulation] Puncture perpendicularly 0.8-1.2 *cun*.

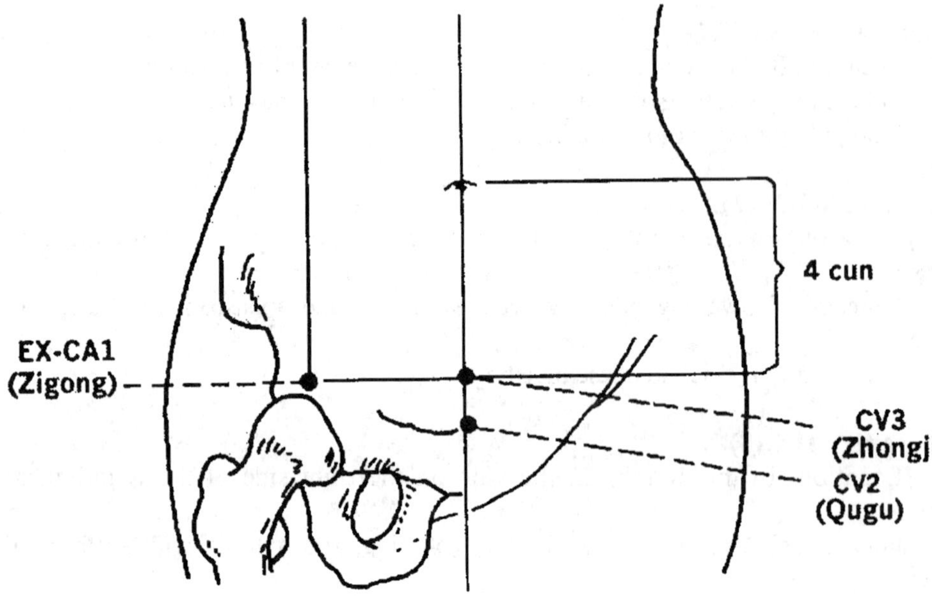

Fig. XIII-5 Extra points of the abdomen

The Points of the Back (B) (Fig. XIII-6)

1. Dingchuan (EX-B 1)

[Location] On the back, below the spinous process of the 7th cervical vertebra, 0.5 *cun* lateral to the posterior midline.

[Indications] Asthma, cough, urticaria, and stiff neck.

[Manipulation] Puncture perpendicularly 0.5-0.8 *cun*.

2. Jiaji (EX-B 2)

[Location] 17 points on each side of the back, below the spinous processes from the 1st thoracic to the 5th lumbar vertebrae, 0.5 *cun* lateral to the posterior midline.

[Indications] Points at the level of the upper thoracic vertebrae for diseases of the upper limbs, heart and lung; points at the level of the lower thoracic vertebrae for diseases of the stomach and intestines; and points at the level of lumbar vertebrae for diseases of the abdomen and lower limbs.

[Manipulation] Puncture perpendicularly 0.5-1.0 *cun* in the cervical and thoracic regions, and 1.0-1.5 *cun* in the lumbar region.

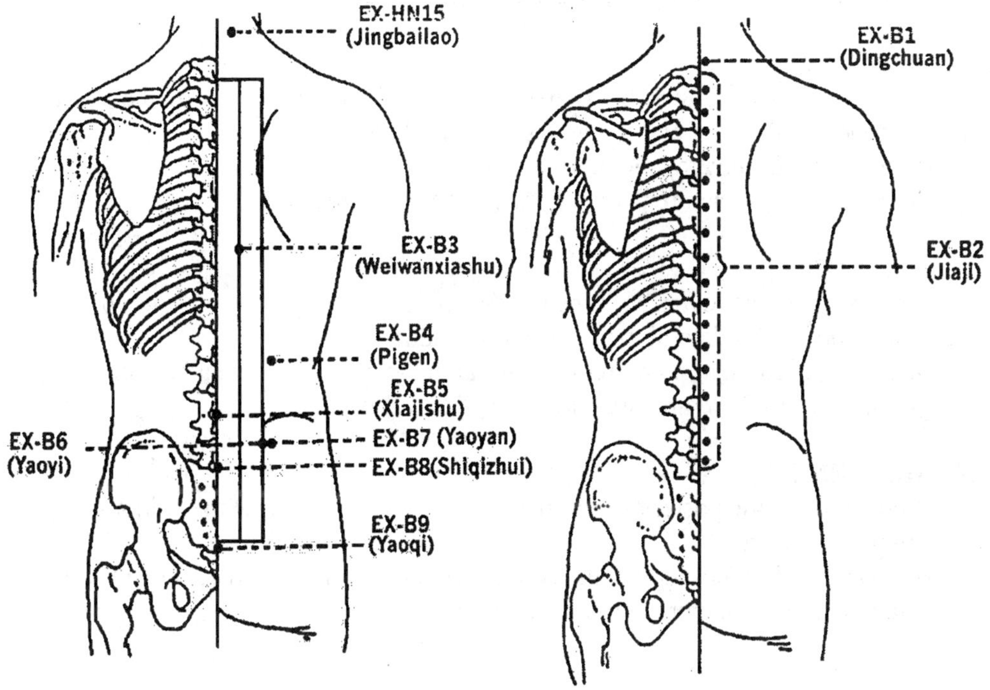

Fig. XIII-6 Extra points of the back

3. Weiwanxiashu (EX-B 3)

[Location] On the back, below the spinous process of the 8th thoracic vertebra, 1.5 *cun* lateral to the posterior midline.

[Indications] Epigastric and abdominal pain, pain in the chest and hypochondriac region, and vomiting.

[Manipulation] Puncture obliquely 0.5-0.8 *cun.*

4. Pigen (EX-B 4)

[Location] On the back, below the spinous process of the 1st lumbar vertebra, 3.5 *cun* lateral to the posterior midline.

[Indications] Hepatosplenomegaly, and lumbago.

[Manipulation] Puncture perpendicularly 0.5-0.8 *cun.*

5. Xiajishu (EX-B 5)

[Location] On the midline of the lower back, below the spinous process of the 3rd lumbar vertebra.

[Indications] Lumbago, abdominal pain, hernial pain, diarrhea, and enuresis.

[Manipulation] Puncture perpendicularly 0.5-1.0 *cun*.

6. Yaoyi (EX-B 6)

[Location] On the lower back, between the spinous processes of the 4th and 5th lumbar vertebrae, 3.0 *cun* lateral to the posterior midline.

[Indications] Lumbago, and uterine bleeding.

[Manipulation] Puncture perpendicularly 0.5-1.0 *cun*.

7. Yaoyan (EX-B 7)

[Location] On the lower back, below the spinous process of the 4th lumbar vertebra, in the depression 3.5 *cun* lateral to the posterior midline.

[Indications] Lumbar pain, frequent urination, and irregular menstruation.

[Manipulation] Puncture perpendicularly 0.8-1.2 *cun*.

8. Shiqizhui (EX-B 8)

[Location] On the posterior midline of the lower back, below the spinous process of the 5th lumbar vertebra.

[Indications] Lumbosacral pain, dysmenorrhea, uterine bleeding, and enuresis.

[Manipulation] Puncture perpendicularly 0.8-1.2 *cun*.

9. Yaoqi (EX-B 9)

[Location] On the posterior midline, 2 *cun* directly above the tip of the coccyx.

[Indications] Headache, insomnia, and epilepsy.

[Manipulation] Puncture subcutaneously upward 1.0-2.0 *cun*.

The Points of the Upper Extremities (UE) (Fig. XIII-7)

1. Zhoujian (EX-UE 1)

[Location] On the posterior side of the elbow, at the tip of the olecranon when the elbow is flexed.

[Indications] Scrofula.

[Manipulation] Apply moxibustion only.

2. Erbai (EX-UE 2)

[Location] Two points on the palmar side of each forearm, 4 *cun* proximal to the crease of the wrist, on each side of the tendon of the radial flexor muscle of the wrist.

[Indications] Hemorrhoids, and prolapse of the rectum.

[Manipulation] Puncture perpendicularly 0.5-1.0 *cun*.

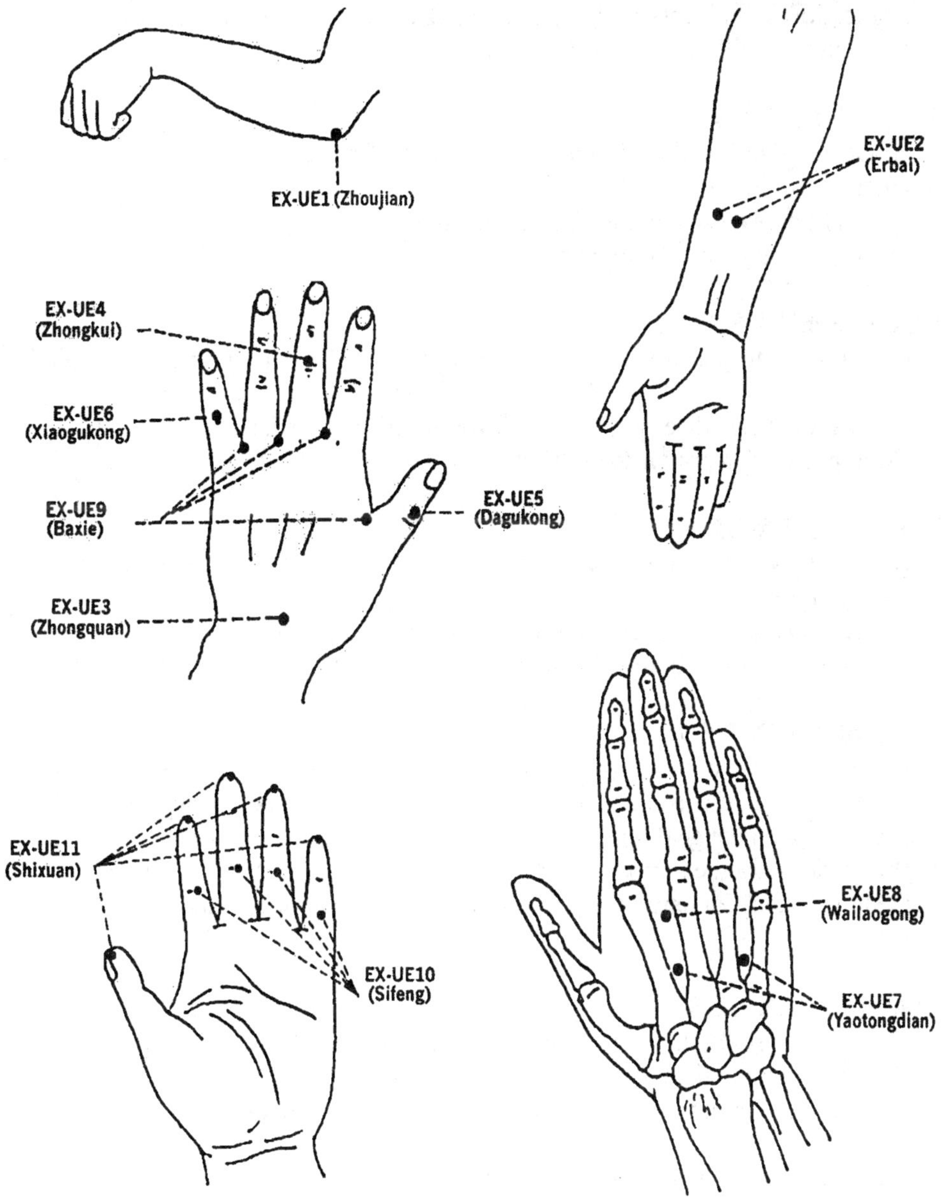

Fig. XIII-7 Extra points of the upper extremities

3. Zhongquan (EX-UE 3)

[Location] On the dorsal crease of the wrist, in the depression on the radial side of the tendon of the common extensor muscle of the fingers.

[Indications] Stuffiness in the chest, epigastric pain, and heat sensation in the palm.

[Manipulation] Puncture perpendicularly 0.3-0.5 *cun*.

4. Zhongkui (EX-UE 4)

[Location] On the dorsal side of the middle finger, at the center of the proximal interphalangeal joint.

[Indications] Nausea, vomiting, and hiccups.

[Manipulation] Apply moxibustion.

5. Dagukong (EX-UE 5)

[Location] On the dorsal side of the thumb, at the center of the interphalangeal joint.

[Indications] Eye diseases, epistaxis, vomiting and diarrhea.

[Manipulation] Apply moxibustion.

6. Xiaogukong (EX-UE 6)

[Location] On the dorsal side of the little finger, at the center of the proximal interphalangeal joint.

[Indications] Eye diseases, sore throat, and pain of the finger.

[Manipulation] Apply moxibustion.

7. Yaotongdian (EX-UE 7)

[Location] Two points on the dorsum of each hand, between the 2nd and 3rd and between the 4th and 5th metacarpal bones, midway between the dorsal crease of the wrist and the metacarpophalangeal joint.

[Indications] Acute lumbar sprain.

[Manipulation] Puncture 0.3-0.5 *cun* perpendicularly or obliquely toward the center of the palm.

8. Wailaogong (EX-UE 8)

[Location] On the dorsum of the hand, between the 2nd and 3rd metacarpal bones, and 0.5 *cun* proximal to the metacarpophalangeal joint.

[Indications] Numbness and contracture of the fingers, indigestion, and stiff neck.

[Manipulation] Puncture obliquely 0.5-1.0 *cun*.

9. Baxie (EX-UE 9)

[Location] Four points on the dorsum of each hand, in the web between each of the fingers.

[Indications] Fever, numbness and contracture of the finger, and redness and swelling of the dorsum of the hand.

[Manipulation] Puncture obliquely 0.3-0.5 *cun*, or prick to cause bleeding.

10. Sifeng (EX-UE 10)

[Location] Four points on each hand, on the palmar side of the index, middle, ring and little fingers and at the center of the proximal interphalangeal joints.

[Indications] Indigestion and malnutrition in children.

[Manipulation] Prick to cause bleeding.

11. Shixuan (EX-UE 11)

[Location] Ten points on both hands, at the tips of the ten fingers, 0.1 *cun* from the free margin of the nails.

[Indications] Loss of consciousness, fainting, high fever, heat stroke, and infantile convulsions.

[Manipulation] Puncture superficially 0.1-0.2 *cun*, or prick to cause bleeding.

The Points of the Lower Extremities (LE) (Fig. XIII-8)

1. Kuangu (EX-LE 1)

[Location] Two points on each thigh, in the lower part of the anterior surface of the thigh, 1.5 *cun* lateral and medial to Liangqiu (ST 34).

[Indications] Knee pain, pain and paralysis of the leg.

[Manipulation] Puncture perpendicularly 0.5-1.0 *cun*.

2. Heding (EX-LE 2)

[Location] Above the knee, in the depression of the midpoint of the upper border of the patella.

[Indications] Pain in the knee, weakness and motor impairment of the leg.

[Manipulation] Puncture perpendicularly 0.3-0.5 *cun*.

3. Baichongwo (EX-LE 3)

[Location] On the medial side of the thigh, 3 *cun* above the superior medial corner of the patella when the knee is flexed, i.e., 1 *cun* above Xuehai (SP 10).

[Indications] Urticaria, eczema, and intestinal parasitosis.

[Manipulation] Puncture perpendicularly 1.0-1.2 *cun*.

4. Neixiyan (EX-LE 4)

[Location] In the depression medial to the patellar ligament when the knee is flexed.

[Effects] Knee pain, weakness of the leg.

[Indications] Knee pain, and weakness of the leg.

[Manipulation] Puncture perpendicularly 0.5-1.0 *cun*.

5. Xiyan (EX-LE 5)

[Location] In the depression on the lateral side of the patellar ligament when the knee is flexed.

[Indications] Knee pain, and weakness of the leg.

[Manipulation] Puncture perpendicularly 0.5-1.0 *cun.*

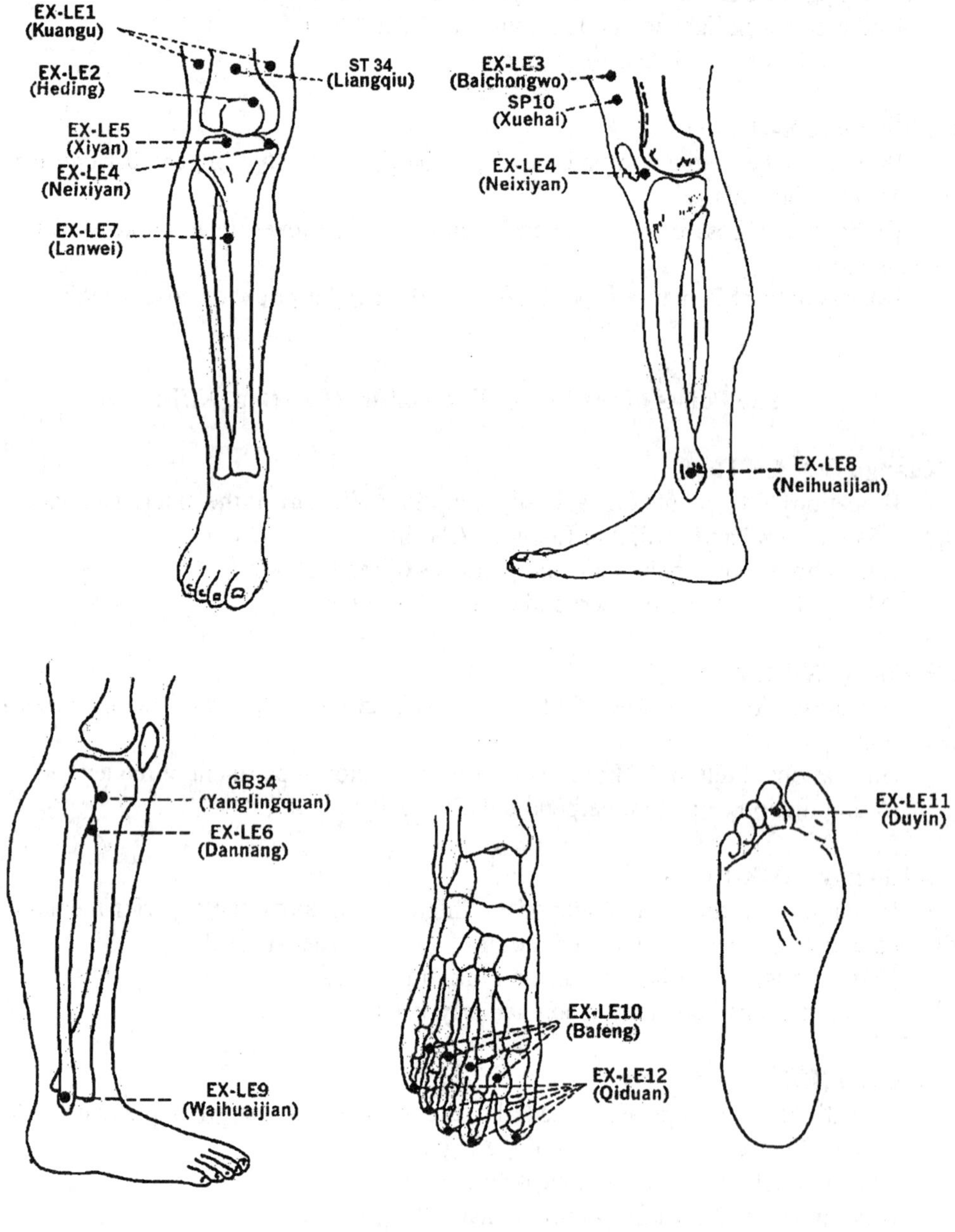

Fig. XIII-8 Extra points of the lower extremities

6. Dannang (EX-LE 6)

[Location] At the upper part of the lateral surface of the leg, 2 *cun* directly below the depression anterior and inferior to the head of the fibula.

[Indications] Acute and chronic cholecystitis, cholelithiasis, biliary ascariasis, and weakness and numbness of the lower limb.

[Manipulation] Puncture perpendicularly 1.0-1.5 *cun*.

7. Lanwei (EX-LE 7)

[Location] At the upper part of the anterior surface of the leg, 5 *cun* below Dubi (ST 35), one finger breadth lateral to the anterior crest of the tibia.

[Indications] Acute and chronic appendicitis, and paralysis of the lower limb.

[Manipulation] Puncture perpendicularly 1.0-1.5 *cun*.

8. Neihuaijian (EX-LE 8)

[Location] On the medial side of the foot, at the tip of the medial malleolus.

[Indications] Toothache, tonsillitis, and systremma.

[Manipulation] Only used for moxibustion.

9. Waihuaijian (EX-LE 9)

[Location] On the lateral side of the foot, at the tip of the lateral malleolus.

[Indications] Toothache, tonsillitis, and systremma.

[Manipulation] Prick to cause bleeding.

10. Bafeng (EX-LE 10)

[Location] Eight points on the insteps of both feet, 0.5 *cun* proximal to the web margin between each two neighboring toes.

[Indications] Pain in the toes, and redness and swelling of the dorsum of the foot.

[Manipulation] Puncture obliquely 0.5-0.8 *cun*.

11. Duyin (EX-LE 11)

[Location] On the plantar side of the 2nd toe, at the center of the distal interphalangeal joint.

[Indications] Abdominal pain, vomiting, retained placenta, and menoxenia.

[Manipulation] Puncture perpendicularly 0.1-0.2 *cun*.

12. Qiduan (EX-LE 12)

[Location] Ten points at the tips of the toes of both feet, 0.1 *cun* from the free margin of each toenail.

[Indications] Syncope, numbness of the toes.

[Manipulation] Puncture perpendicularly 0.1-0.2 *cun*, or prick to cause bleeding.

CHAPTER 14

TECHNIQUES OF ACUPUNCTURE AND MOXIBUSTION

ACUPUNCTURE

Needles. Filiform needles are the mostly commonly used acupuncture needles. They are made of stainless steel, with length ranging from 0.5 (13 mm) to 5 *cun* (125 mm), and caliber ranging from gauge 26 (0.45 mm in diameter) to gauge 33 (0.26 mm in diameter). A filiform needle contains the following parts: tip, body, root and handle as shown in Fig. XIV-1. Use of disposable needles and guiding tubes is recommended.

Operation. The process of acupuncture operation includes insertion, manipulation, retention and withdrawal of the needle.

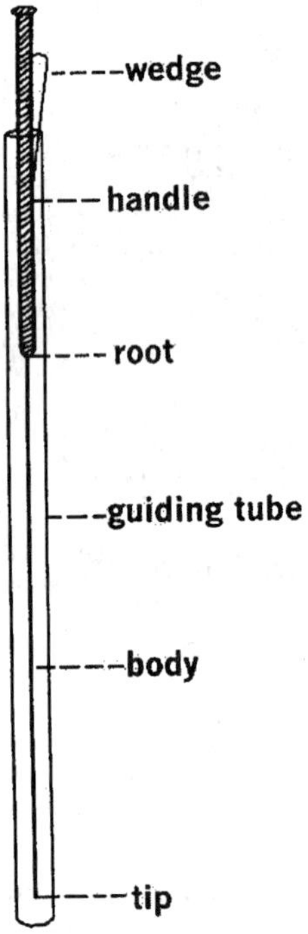

Fig. XIV-1

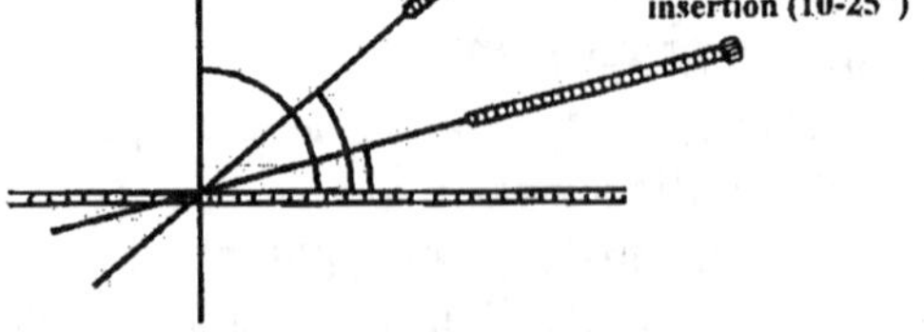

Fig. XIV-2 Direction of needle insertion

1. Insertion of the needle

(1) Method of needle insertion

It is preferable to use acupuncture needles with guiding tubes, sterilized and sealed. Take out the wedge that fixes the needle in the guiding tube, and place the tube with the tip of the needle lightly touching the acupuncture point. Hold the tube with the fingers of one hand, and flick or tap the upper end of the handle of the needle with the index or middle finger of the other hand. The needle will be rapidly inserted through the skin without causing pain. Remove the guiding tube and further insert the needle to the required depth.

(2) Direction of the needle insertion (Fig. XIV-2). Generally, one of the following three directions is used for inserting the needle: perpendicular insertion, oblique insertion and transverse insertion.

In perpendicular insertion, the needle is inserted perpendicularly, forming a 90° angle with the surface of the skin. Most points of the body can be punctured perpendicularly.

In oblique insertion, the needle is inserted obliquely to form an angle of approximately 45° with the surface of the skin. This is indicated for points located where the muscle is thin or close to internal organs.

In transverse insertion, the needle is inserted almost horizontally to form a 15°-25° angle with the surface of the skin. This is preferred for points on the face and head where the muscle is thin.

(3) Depth of needle insertion. The depth of puncturing differs at different points. A deeper puncture is preferred in the treatment of patients with strong constitutions and when a strong stimulation is required. Deeper insertion of the needle is strictly prohibited if a large blood vessel or an important internal organ is located beneath the acupoint.

2. Manipulations of the needle after insertion

A special sensation such as soreness, tingling, distension or heaviness may be experienced by the patient after the needle is inserted to a certain depth. This is called *deqi* (getting the acupuncture sensation). In most instances, manipulation of the needle is necessary to get the acupuncture sensation. As *The Canon of Medicine* states, "The key to an effective acupuncture treatment is to get the sensation."

There are different ways of manipulating the needle after insertion to get the sensation and to produce the desired effect. The basic manipulations are lifting-thrusting and twirling the needle. By using different levels of force and speed, a reinforcement or reduction effect can be achieved.

If no acupuncture sensation appears after the insertion, lift-thrust the needle gently or twirl the needle with the thumb and index finger in one direction with an amplitude of 360° or more, and repeat the manipulation if necessary.

When lifting-thrusting manipulation is applied, after the acupuncture sensation is achieved, reinforcement can be attained by rapid, heavy thrusting and slow, gentle lifting of the needle; reduction can be attained by slow, gentle thrusting and rapid, heavy lifting. Reinforcing manipulation is indicated in cases of deficiency, and reducing manipulation is indicated in cases of excessiveness.

When whirling manipulation is performed, after the acupuncture sensation is achieved, the differentiation of reinforcement and reduction is based on the degree of twirling and the strength with which the needle is twirled. For reduction, the degree of twirling should exceed 360°, with heavy manipulation or with high frequency. For reinforcement, the degree of twirling should be less than 180°, with gentle manipulation or with low frequency.

Besides reinforcement and reduction, manipulation to induce "uniform reinforcement-reduction" is often used. This is a form of needle manipulation, in which the needle is lifted, thrust and twirled evenly with a proper amplitude and favorable angle, indicated when the case is not distinctly excessive or deficient.

3. Retention of the needle

After getting the acupuncture sensation, the needle is usually left in position for 20 minutes. During this period, the manipulation of the needle may be repeated. For relieving severe pain, it is preferable to leave the needle in position longer, with repeated manipulation.

4. Withdrawal of the needle

After twirling the needle back and forth gently, withdraw it and press the puncture site with a sterilized cotton ball to prevent bleeding.

5. Prevention and treatment of adverse reactions

Acupuncture may be compared to a subcutaneous or intramuscular injection. Although there is a potential risk of transmitting infection from one patient to another or of introducing pathogenic organisms, acupuncture is generally a safe procedure if high standards of cleanliness and sterilization are maintained, and aseptic technique is performed.

For avoidance of infection in acupuncture, attention should be paid to the following points: (1) A clean working environment free from dirt and dust, and with adequate light and ventilation is necessary. (2) The practitioner should carefully wash his (her) hands immediately before the acupuncture treatment. If the practitioner wants to palpate the acupuncture point after the needling site has been prepared, his (her) fingertips should be again cleaned with an alcohol swab. (3) The needling sites should be clean and free from wounds or infections. The point should be swabbed with 70% alcohol from the center to the surrounding area with a rotary scrubbing motion. (4) The needle shaft should be maintained in a sterile state, and the practitioner's fingers should not touch the shaft. When inserting a long needle, the shaft may be held in place with a sterile cotton ball. (5) On withdrawing the needle, the insertion site should be pressed with a sterile cotton ball. Once used, needles and cotton balls should be discarded in special containers for infectious waste.

Besides infection, some other risks need to be prevented. They include broken needles, fainting, pain, and inadvertent injury to important organs.

In order to avoid breaking needles, each needle should be carefully checked before use. Defective needles with eroded shafts, or hooked or blunt tips, should be discarded. The patient should adopt a comfortable posture and be requested to remain still and not to change position abruptly during acupuncture.

An untoward reaction that occasionally occurs during acupuncture is fainting. For those who receive acupuncture for the first, treatment in a lying position with gentle manipulation is preferred. If there are symptoms of impending faintness, such as feeling unwell, giddiness, oppressive feeling in the chest, or the complexion turning pale, the needles should be immediately removed and the patient should lie flat with the head down and the legs raised, as the symptoms are probably due to a transient, insufficient blood supply to the brain. Warm drinks are also helpful. The symptoms usually disappear in a few minutes. In severe cases, the following treatment may be applied: (1) press Shuigou (GV 26) with the fingernail; (2) apply moxibustion to Baihui (GV 20) and/or Guanyuan (CV 4) and Qihai (CV 6). If the symptoms are still unrelieved, emergency medical assistance is necessary.

For prevention of fainting, acupuncture should not be performed when the patient is in a state of extreme fatigue, or excessive hunger or excitement.

Pain during needle insertion is usually due to clumsy technique, or to blunt or hooked needles. The "flicking-in" technique with the guiding tube usually causes no pain. The acupuncture sensation of soreness, tingling, distension and heaviness indicating the arrival of *qi* at the point should not be mistaken as a painful reaction.

Pain occurring when the needle is inserted deep into the tissues may be due to contact with the pain receptor nerve fibers. In this case, lift the needle to the superficial portion and carefully insert it again in another direction.

Pain occurring after withdrawal of the needle is often due to excessive stimulation. Pressing and massaging the affected area may relieve the pain.

Stuck needle. After insertion, the needle may become difficult to twirl, lift or thrust, or even to withdraw. This is caused by a muscle spasm or tangling of the muscle fibers around the shaft due to twirling the needle with too wide an amplitude, or rotation in only one direction, or due to movement of the patient.

If the needle is stuck due to excessive rotation, gently rotate the needle in the opposite direction. If it is caused by a muscle spasm, leave it for a while, and then withdraw it by rotating or massaging around the point. Sometimes, it is necessary to insert another needle nearby to divert the patient's attention. If the stuck needle is due to movement of the patient, the original position should be resumed.

Broken needle. Breaks may arise from too forceful manipulation, poor quality of the needle, erosion between the shaft and the handle, strong muscle spasm or a sudden movement of the patient.

Never try to insert a needle if it becomes bent. Too much force should not be used when manipulating needles. The junction between the shaft and the handle is the part that is apt to break. Therefore, one quarter to one third of the shaft should always be kept outside the skin.

If a needle breaks, advise the patient not to move, so as to prevent the broken part of the needle from going deeper into the tissue. If the broken needle protrudes outside the skin, remove it with forceps. If not, press around the site gently until the broken needle is exposed, then remove it with forceps. If the break is due to movement of the patient, ask the patient to resume the original position, and the end of the broken needle will often be exposed. If the above measures fail, surgery is called for.

Injury to important organs. Acupuncture should not cause injury to any organ. In order to avoid injury to the organs, certain areas should not be punctured, for example, the fontanel in babies, the external genitalia, the nipples, the umbilicus and the eyeball. Precautions should be taken when points in proximity to vital organs are punctured. When points on the chest, back and abdomen are punctured, attention should be paid to the depth and direction of needle insertion. Improper manipulation at these points may cause traumatic pneumothorax by injury to the lungs, bleeding due to puncture of the liver or spleen, or hematuria by injury to the kidneys. Inappropriate manipulation at points between or beside the upper cervical vertebrae such as Yamen (GV 15) and Fengfu (GV 16) is even more dangerous. It may cause injury to the medulla oblongata.

Many other points close to the eyeball, trachea and arteries are potentially dangerous, and require special skill and experience. Care should be taken in order to avoid risks as described in the previous chapter under the heading of each point.

6. Contraindications

The following conditions are contraindicated for acupuncture, though most of them are not absolute contraindications:

(1) Pregnancy. It is contraindicated to puncture points on the lower abdomen and lumbosacral region during pregnancy under three months. After three months of pregnancy, points of the upper abdomen and those causing strong sensation such as Hegu (LI 4), Sanyinjiao (SP 6), Kunlun (UB 60) and Zhiyin (UB 67) should also be avoided. Puncture at these points may cause strong uterine contractions, and induce abortion. However, this may be of use in pregnancy for inducing labor or expediting delivery.

(2) Coagulation disorders. Great care should be taken when acupuncture is performed in patients with coagulation disorders. Hemophilia is absolutely contraindicated for puncturing.

(3) Malignant tumors. Puncture of a malignant tumor itself is strictly prohibited, nor should acupuncture be used as the sole treatment for malignant tumors. However, acupuncture can be applied as a complementary measure in combination with other treatments for the relief of pain or other symptoms, and to alleviate side-effects of chemotherapy and radiotherapy.

MOXIBUSTION

Moxibustion is a kind of preventive and therapeutic measure involving the application of heat to certain points of the human body. The material used is mainly moxa wool in form of moxa cones or sticks. Stimulation of the points by heat from the ignited moxa cone or stick warms the relevant meridian, expels cold and damp, induces the smooth flow of *qi* and blood, strengthens *yang*, and treats and prevents diseases.

Various moxibustion techniques are used clinically. They are listed in Table XIV-1.

Table XIV-1 Commonly-used Moxiibustion Techniques

- Moxibustion
  - Moxa cones
    - Direct moxibustion
      - Scarring moxibustion
      - Non-scarring moxibustion
    - Indirect moxibustion
      - Ginger insulation
      - Salt insulation
      - Garlic insulation
      - Medicinal cake insulation
  - Moxa sticks
  - Warming needle

1. Moxibustion with moxa cones

Knead and shape a small amount of moxa wool into a cone the size of a wheat grain (small cone) or half a date stone (big cone). When direct moxibustion is performed, place a moxa cone directly on the skin and ignite it. Indirect moxibustion involves placing a moxa cone with some medical substance (ginger slice, salt, garlic slice or medicinal cake) insulating from the skin. Different names are given to indirect moxibustion with different insulators; for example, when a slice of ginger is used as the insulator, it is called moxibustion with ginger, or simply ginger moxibustion. One moxa cone used at one point is called one unit.

Direct moxibustion can be further divided into scarring moxibustion and non-scarring moxibustion. Scarring moxibustion is also called suppurative moxibustion. When performing the moxibustion, apply some vaseline to the site where the cone is to adhere, then place a big moxa cone on the site, ignite it and let it completely burn out. (Preferably use a slender stick of burning incense to ignite the moxa cone). When the cone is burnt to its base and the patient feels a burning sensation, tap the area around the site to alleviate the pain. Generally, 5-7 units are applied. Since this procedure leads to a local burn, blister, suppuration and scar after healing, at present its use is highly limited. It is only indicated in treating some stubborn chronic diseases, such as bronchial asthma, with the patient's consent.

Non-scarring moxibustion is also called non-suppurative moxibustion. After applying vaseline to the site, place a smaller moxa cone and ignite it. When the cone has burnt halfway down and the patient feels a mild burning pain, remove the cone immediately. This will only cause local redness but no burn, and hence no suppuration or scar. This procedure is often used for treating deficiency of *qi* and blood.

Indirect moxibustion does not cause any burns. Ginger and garlic are cut into slices and the medicinal powder (e.g., pinellia tuber) is made into cakes, all 3 mm thick. The burning of the moxa cones only induces local redness, but no blister. Clinically, ginger moxibustion is often used for treating abdominal pain, diarrhea and vomiting due to cold; garlic moxibustion for treating insect bites and subcutaneous infection at the early stage; and moxibustion with medicinal cake for treating chronic arthritis. Salt-insulated moxibustion is often applied to the umbilicus for general weakness.

2. Moxibustion with moxa sticks

Moxa sticks are made by rolling moxa wool into the shape of a cigar, wrapped with paper made of mulberry bark. When moxibustion is performed, apply an ignited moxa stick over the selected point. It is much more convenient to use moxa sticks than moxa cones, and it is easy to control heat and time during the moxibustion with moxa sticks.

Two methods are often used in moxibustion with moxa sticks: one is warm moxibustion, and the other "sparrow-pecking" moxibustion (Fig. XIV-3). In warm moxibustion, an ignited moxa stick is applied over the point to bring a warmth to the local area for 5 to 10 minutes, with redness of the skin. The heat can be adjusted by varying the distance between the ignited stick and the body's surface to keep the local redness of the skin. In sparrow-pecking moxibustion, the ignited moxa stick is rapidly dabbed above the point. The heat can be adjusted by varying the distance between the ignited stick and the body's surface, as well as by the frequency of dabbing. In both procedures, care should be taken not to cause burns, particularly by the dropping of sparks from a loosely rolled stick. The quality of the moxa stick should be carefully examined before use. Clinically, moxibustion with moxa sticks is often used for treating arthritis cold in property and also for correction of abnormal fetal position.

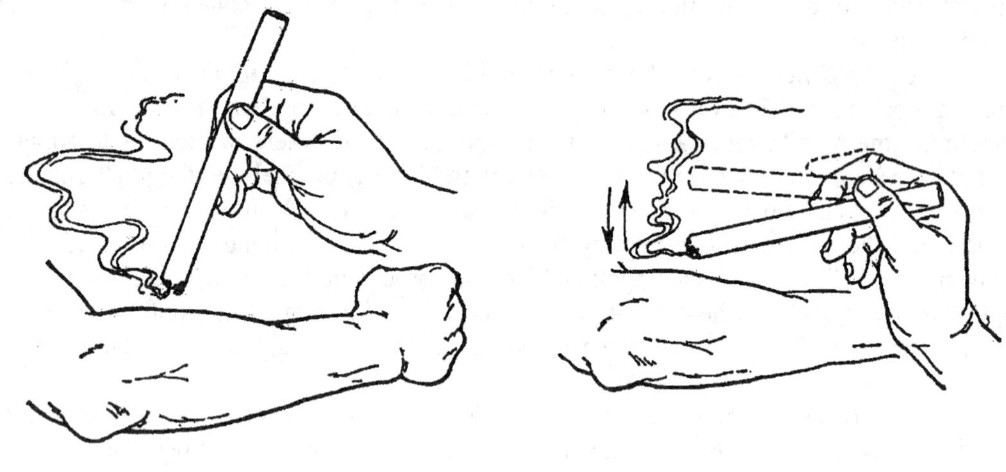

Warm moxibustion "Sparrow-pecking"moxibustion

Fig. XIV-3 Moxibustion with moxa sticks

3. Moxibustion with warming needles

Moxibustion with warming needles is a procedure of acupuncture combined with moxibustion. During acupuncture, when the *qi* has arrived and the needle is retained, an ignited segment of moxa stick 1-2 cm in length is placed on the top of the needle, with the handle of the needle inserted into the moxa wool. One to three segments may be used for each session of treatment. Clinically, this procedure is often used for cold-damp arthralgia or gastrointestinal diseases of the deficiency-cold type.

ELECTROACUPUNCTURE

Electroacupuncture is a modified form of acupuncture therapy, which combines needling and electrical stimulation.

Procedures: One to three pairs of acupoints are selected. After the *qi* is roused by needling, the needles are connected to an electric stimulator. Select the appropriate wave pattern and frequency, and switch on the current at the lowest output. Gradually increase the output as far as the patient can tolerate it or local muscle contractions appear. The electric stimulation usually lasts for 5-20 minutes, but for analgesic purposes a longer period of strong stimulation is needed. When the treatment is completed, switch off the stimulator, disconnect the needles from it, and then remove the needles.

Indications: Electroacupuncture is indicated in a great variety of disorders, particularly for the treatment of pains, rheumatic conditions, and paralysis due to trauma.

Precautions: (1) The stimulator should be carefully examined before use. The output current should only be increased gradually. Sudden increase of the current is strictly prohibited, for it may cause violent muscle contraction with bending or breaking of the needle, or it may not be tolerated by the patient, with subsequent fainting. (2) Electroacupuncture is contraindicated in patients with severe heart disease or in pregnancy.

HYDROACUPUNCTURE

Hydroacupuncture is a kind of therapy in which a drug is injected directly into acupuncture points, and so is also called point injection. The therapeutic effect is based on the combination of mechanical stimulation and pharmacological action at the injection points. Drugs commonly used for this purpose include herbal injections (such as *Radix Angelicae Sinensis, Radix Astragali, Flos Carthami, Radix Salviae Miltiorrhizae* or *Radix Bupleuri*), vitamins (Vitamin B1, B6 or B12), Procain hydrochloride, Atropine, and Adenosine triphosphate.

Procedures: Select acupoints, drug, syringe and needle. After the local skin is sterilized, hold the syringe and insert the needle at the acupoint into the subcutaneous tissue until the arrival of *qi*. If no blood flows into the syringe on suction, inject the drug solution slowly 1-2 ml at each point, or 2-5 ml at sites with thick musculature.

Indications: Hydroacupuncture has a broad spectrum of indications for neurological, respiratory, digestive, locomotive and reproductive disorders. Clinically, it is often used for treating sciatica, trigeminal neuralgia, chronic bronchitis, bronchial asthma, chronic gastritis, chronic colitis, traumatic injuries, fasciomyalgia, impotence and chronic pelvic inflammation.

Precautions: (1) Aseptic technique is strictly required to avoid infection. (2) Deep injections should be avoided when the points on the back are used, in order to avoid injury to internal organs. (3) When the injection is close to a nerve trunk, the needle should be kept away from the nerve trunk. If the tip of the needle touches the nerve trunk and the patient complains of a sensation similar to an electric shock, immediately withdraw the needle and insert it again in another direction. (4) No drug should be injected into an articular cavity, spinal subarachnoid space or blood vessel. (5) Point injection in the lumbosacral region is contraindicated in pregnancy.

CHAPTER 15

BASIC PRINCIPLES OF ACUPUNCTURE TREATMENT

Successful acupuncture treatment depends upon the following factors: (1) appropriate selection of cases, with correct diagnosis, (2) proper selection of acupoints with suitable combinations, and (3) correct selection of manipulations, session intervals and therapeutic courses.

INDICATIONS AND DIAGNOSIS

It is difficult to list the indications of acupuncture treatment. In old textbooks on acupuncture in the Oriental countries, this therapeutic method could be used in the treatment of almost all kinds of diseases. Because of the regulatory mechanism of acupuncture, the broad-spectrum usage of acupuncture was reasonable in ancient times. At present, even for a disease that has effective, specific treatment, acupuncture is still of some use, either as an auxiliary therapy or for symptomatic relief. For example, in cancer patients acupuncture is not indicated for treating the cancer itself, and puncturing the cancer directly is absolutely prohibited; but it may be used for alleviating pain caused by the tumor, and for reducing the side effects of chemotherapy or radiotherapy (such as vomiting and leukopenia).

Classically, acupuncture should be applied in accordance with the traditional Chinese diagnosis, particularly the diagnosis of deficiency versus excess, and cold versus heat. As stated in the *Classic of Acupuncture*, "Reduction is indicated for excess, and reinforcement for deficiency; swiftness for heat, and retentiveness for cold." Reduction means the use of acupoints that have the action of eliminating pathogenic factors, for example, the 12 well points and Quchi (LI 11) for high fever, Shixuan (EX-UE 11) for sunstroke, and Weizhong (BL 40) for severe lumbago; it also means the use of reduction manipulation. Reinforcement means the use of acupoints that have reinforcing actions, such as the back-transport points, Qihai (CV 6), Guanyuan (CV 4) and Zusanli (ST 36); it also means the use of reinforcing manipulation. Swiftness means inserting and thrusting the needle without retention. This is used when Shixuan (EX-UE 11) and the well points are punctured in the treatment of high fever and sunstroke. A longer retention of the needle is necessary for the treatment of cold syndromes. For example, in the treatment of kidney *yang* deficiency with cold sensation in the lower abdomen, puncturing at Guanyuan (CV 4) for a short period of time may not be effective, but a longer retention and then manipulation of the needle often causes warmth.

In addition, if there is no marked manifestation of excess or deficiency, selection of the acupoint is usually in accordance with the meridian involved in the ailment. For example, for digestive disorders points of the Spleen and Stomach Meridians are often used, for respiratory disorders points of the Lung and Large Intestine Meridians are preferred.

SELECTION OF ACUPOINTS

Successful acupuncture treatment, first of all, depends upon proper selection of acupoints. Acupoints can be selected in the following ways:

1. Selection of local or adjacent acupoints

Local or adjacent acupoints are often used for treating diseases of the limbs and superficial parts of the body, for example, acupoints around the eye for eye diseases, acupoints in the auricular region for ear diseases, and Xiyan (EX-LE 5) for knee pain. All these are selections of local acupoints. However, if there is local inflammatory lesion, adjacent points are preferable to local points involved in the inflammation. For example, for arthritis of the elbow, Shousanli (LI 10) is often used instead of Quchi (LI 11) or Chize (LU 5).

Table XV-1 Selection of Remote Acupoints According to the Meridians

Meridians & Acupoints of Choice	Indications
***Yin* meridians of the hand**	**Disorders of the chest**
LU Taiyuan (LU 9), Chize (LU 5)	Respiratory disorders
PC Neiguan (PC 6), Daling (PC 7)	Cardiovascular and mental disorders
HT Shenmen (HT 7), Shaohai (HT 3)	Cardiovascular and mental disorders
***Yang* meridians of the hand**	**Motory and sensory disorders of the upper limb**
LI Hegu (LI 4) Quchi (LI 11)	Diseases of the head, eye, nose, mouth, and throat
TE Zhongzhu (TE 3) Waiguan (TE 5)	Diseases of the head, ear, and neck
SI Houxi (SI 3) Yanglao (SI 6)	Diseases of the occipitus, nape and temporal
***Yin* meridians of the foot**	**Disorders of the abdomen**
SP Gongsun (SP 4), Sanyinjiao (SP 6)	Digestive diseases, bleeding disorders
LR Taichong (LR 3)	Disorders of the liver, gallbladder and genitalia
KI Taixi (KI 3)	Uro-genital disorders
***Yang* meridians of the foot**	**Motory and sensory disorders of the lower limb**
ST Zusanli (ST 36)	Digestive disorders, general weakness
GB Yanglingquan (GB 34)	Disorders of the liver and gallbladder
BL Weizhong (BL 40)	Disorders of the back

2. Selection of remote acupoints

Acupoints on the limbs below the elbow and the knee are usually selected for treating diseases of the head, trunk and internal organs. For instance, Zusanli (ST 36) is used for treating abdominal diseases, Hegu (LI 4) for diseases of the face, Houxi (SI 3) for neck pain. Traditionally, the remote acupoints are selected according to the theory of meridians. Generally, this can be shown in Table XV-1.

3. Selection of points for symptomatic relief

Some acupoints have been found to be specifically effective for relieving certain symptoms, as shown in Table XV-2. Therefore, they are often selected whenever there are such symptoms. However, it should be noted that puncturing at these acupoints may only give symptomatic relief, and the use of other acupoints or other treatment is still necessary.

Table XV-2 Acupoints for relieving common symptoms

Symptoms	Acupoints
Fever	Dazhui (GV 14), Quchi (LI 11), Hegu (LI 4)
Fainting	Shuigou (GV 26), Shixuan (EX-UE 11)
Insomnia	Shenmen (HT 7), Sanyinjiao (SP 6)
Dream-disturbed sleep	Xinshu (BL 15), Shenmen (HT 7)
Palpitations	Neiguan (PC 6), Ximen (PC 4)
Precordial pain	Danzhong (CV 17), Neiguan (PC 6)
Coughing	Tiantu (CV 22), Lieque (LU 7)
Oppression in the chest	Zhongwan (CV 12), Neiguan (PC 6)
Nausea, vomiting	Neiguan (PC 6), Zusanli (ST 36)
Hiccups	Geshu (BL 17), Neiguan (PC 6)
Constipation	Tianshu (ST 25), Zhigou (TE 6)
Abdominal distension	Tianshu (ST 25), Qihai (CV 6), Zusanli (ST 36)
Retention of urine	Sanyinjiao (SP 6), Yinlingquan (SP 9)
Incontinence of urine	Sanyinjiao (SP 6), Qugu (CV 2)
Systremma	Chengshan (BL 57)
Skin itching	Xuehai (SP 10), Sanyinjiao (SP 6)

COMBINATION OF ACUPOINTS

One single acupoint may be enough for a treatment. However, in most instances several acupoints are used in combinations, so as to achieve a better therapeutic effect. Acupoints may be combined in the following ways.

1. Combination of the Back-Transport (Back-Shu) and Front-Curtain (Front-Mu) points.

The disease of an internal organ is often reflected at the back-transport and front-curtain points. They can be selected in combination to achieve a better effect, for example, combined use of Weishu (BL 21) and Zhongwan (CV 12) for gastric disorders, Pangguangshu (BL 28) and Zhongji (CV 3) for dysuria.

2. Combination of the acupoints of the upper and the lower limbs.

One of the common combinations is the use of an acupoint of the upper limb together with another acupoint of the lower limb, for example, combined use of Neiguan (PC 6) and Zusanli (ST 36) for gastric disorders, Hegu (LI 4) and Neiting (ST 44) for sore throat or toothache.

Table XV-3 Examples of combined use of local, adjacent and remote points.

Diseased Area	Local or Adjacent Points	Remote Points
Forehead	Yintang (EX-HN 3), Baihui (GV 20)	Hegu (LI 4), Neiting (ST 44)
Temperol	Taiyang (EX-HN 5), Shuaigu (GB 8)	Zhongzhu (TE 3), Zulinqi (GB 41)
Occipitus	Fengchi (GB 20), Tianzhu (BL 10)	Houxi (SI 3), Kunlun (BL 60)
Vertex	Baihui (GV 20)	Taichong (LR 3)
Eyes	Jingming (BL 1), Chengqi (ST 1)	Hegu (LI 4), Guangming (GB 37)
Nose	Yingxiang (LI 20), Yintang (EX-HN 3)	Hegu (LI 4)
Mouth & teeth	Xiaguan (ST 7), Jiache (ST 6), Dicang (ST 4)	Hegu (LI 4), Neiting (ST 44)
Ears	Yifeng (TE 17), Tinggong (SI 19), Tinghui (GB 2)	Zhongzhu (TE 3), Waiguan (TE 5)
Throat	Tianrong (SI 17)	Hegu (LI 4), Shangyang (LI 1)
Trachea	Tiantu (CV 22)	Lieque (LU 7), Zhaohai (KI 6)
Lungs	Feishu (BL 13), Danzhong (CV 17)	Lieque (LU 7), Chize (LU 5)
Heart	Xinshu (BL 15), Danzhong (CV 17)	Neiguan (PC 6), Shenmen (HT 7)
Stomach	Weishu (BL 21), Zhongwan (CV 12)	Neiguan (PC 6), Zusanli (ST 36)
Liver	Ganshu (BL 18)	Taichong (LR 3), Xingjian (LR 2), Dannang (EX-LE 6)
Gallbladder	Danshu (BL 19)	Yanglingquan (GB 34)
Intestines	Dachangshu (BL 25), Tianshu (ST 25)	Shangjuxu (ST 37), Zusanli (ST 36)
Kidneys	Shenshu (BL 23)	Taixi (KI 3), Fuliu (KI 7)
Bladder	Ciliao (BL 32), Zhongji (CV 3)	Sanyinjiao (SP 6), Yinlingquan (SP 9)
Uterus	Zhongji (CV 3), Guanyuan (CV 4)	Sanyinjiao (SP 6)
Genitalia	Zhongji (CV 3), Qugu (CV 2)	Sanyinjiao (SP 6)
Anus	Changqiang (GV 1), Zhibian (BL 54)	Chengshan (BL 57)
Prostate	Changqiang (GV 1), Guanyuan (CV 4)	Sanyinjiao (SP 6)

3. Combination of acupoints of the right and left sides.

The points of the twelve regular meridians are distributed on both sides of the body symmetrically. They are often used bilaterally for gaining a better result. Without special indication, the acupoints listed in a formula usually refer to those of both sides.

4. Combination of acupoints of the exterior and the interior.

The exterior refers to *yang* meridians, and the interior to *yin* meridians. It is believed that combined use of the points of exterio-interiorly related meridians may show a synergetic effect. For example, for relieving cough, Hegu (LI 4) of Taiyin Meridian (interior) is often used in combination with Taiyuan (LU 9) of Yangming Meridian (exterior).

5. Combination of remote and adjacent or local acupoints.

Examples are shown in Table XV-3.

PART FOUR

COMMON DISEASES

CHAPTER 16
RESPIRATORY DISEASES

COMMON COLD AND INFLUENZA

The common cold and influenza are acute respiratory viral infections. The common cold usually begins with rhinorrhea and sneezing, accompanied by nasal congestion. In most cases, sore throat is frequently present, and there are systemic symptoms such as malaise, headache and mild fever, but in some cases the fever may be high and the general symptoms severe. Severity varies widely within an outbreak, and is presumably dependent on the degree of immunity of the individual. Although rhinoviruses are the most frequently recognized cause of the common cold, enteroviruses may also cause acute respiratory illnesses with rhinitis, sore throat and fever. Respiratory infections caused by enteroviruses often occur in the summer months, and are described as "summer grippe." Influenza in most cases is characterized by the abrupt onset of systemic symptoms, such as headache, feverishness, chilliness, myalgia, or malaise, accompanied by respiratory tract signs, particularly coughing and sore throat. However, a wide spectrum of clinical presentations may occur. In some cases, influenza is just a mild respiratory illness, similar to the common cold. Therefore, it is convenient to discuss these illnesses under the same category. This is particularly true from the perspective of traditional Chinese medicine.

Traditional Chinese medicine holds that attacks of pathogenic wind cause the common cold. The proper expression in the Chinese language for the common cold is "catching wind," and when it occurs in epidemic outbreaks, it is believed to be caused by seasonal pathogens and is called "seasonal affection."

Etiology and Pathogenesis

Pathogenic wind and seasonal pathogens are the predominant etiological factors in this group of illnesses. They invade the upper respiratory tract and the body's surface when the body's resistance is low and when there is a sudden climatic change. The illnesses start from upper respiratory symptoms and clinical manifestations, indicating that the exterior part of the body is invaded and forming an exterior syndrome.

The pathogenic wind combines with cold in the winter, heat in spring, damp-heat in summer, and dryness in autumn, taking advantage of untimely climatic changes to attack the human body. Therefore, different patterns of exterior syndromes may be thus produced in different seasons. The seasonal pathogens also belong to these categories, but usually involve toxic heat, producing an exterior syndrome with a marked fever.

The illnesses are generally self-limited, and in mild cases the pathogens are eliminated when they are in the exterior part of the human body and there is no invasion of the interior. In severe cases, however, the pathogens enter the internal organs, particularly the Lungs, turning the clinical manifestations from an exterior syndrome into an interior one. In some cases, the pathogen may direct invade the interior, such as the gastrointestinal tract.

Syndrome Differentiation

Keys to the traditional diagnosis of syndrome patterns in common cold and influenza:

1. Differentiation of the cold and heat property of the syndrome. Generally speaking, wind-cold affections are characterized by marked chilliness, mild fever and stuffy nose with thin mucous secretion (exterior-cold or wind-cold syndrome), while wind-heat affections are characterized by fever with mild chilliness and sore throat with local redness and swelling (exterior-heat or wind-heat syndrome). A wind-cold syndrome may turn into a wind-heat syndrome at the later stage, marked by sore throat and mucopurulent nasal discharge, though there is no more fever.

2. Recognition of combined pathogenic factors. If pathogenic wind invades the human body in combination with dryness, as occurs in a dry season, the patient usually experiences dryness in the mouth and throat, and dry coughing. If the pathogenic wind is combined with summer-damp, the patient often complains of headache, as though the head were tightly bound, accompanied by nausea or even vomiting.

3. Determination of deficiency or excessiveness. In most cases, the common cold and influenza run an acute and short course, and are of excess type. However, when colds or influenza occur in a patient with a constitution of deficiency, the clinical presentations and the treatment will be changed. The following manifestations indicate a deficiency syndrome: (1) Spontaneous sweating and aversion to wind during chilliness, (2) Prolonged course of the disease, (3) Repeated attacks over a short period of time. In addition, so-called "post-influenzal asthenia" in Western medicine can also be taken as a deficiency syndrome in traditional Chinese medicine.

I. Excess syndromes

1. Wind-cold affection: Chilliness and mild fever with no sweating or thirst, general aching, stuffy and runny nose, sneezing, itching in the throat, coughing with thin expectoration or dry coughing, thin and white coating, and floating, tense pulse.

2. Wind-heat affection: Fever with mild chilliness, sweating, thirst, headache, redness of and pain in the throat, coughing with mucopurulent expectoration, thin and yellowish tongue coating, and floating, rapid pulse.

3. Affection of wind combined with summer-damp: Chilliness with recessive fever which persists in spite of sweating, lassitude, headache as if the head were tightly bound, general aching, nausea or even vomiting, anorexia, fullness in the chest, and yellow greasy tongue coating.

II. Deficiency syndromes

1. Wind affection in *qi* deficiency: Prolonged chilliness and fever, occurring or aggravated when tired, accompanied by headache, stuffy nose, coughing with whitish expectoration, shortness of breath, spontaneous sweating, lassitude, pale tongue with white coating, and floating, weak pulse.

2. Wind affection in *yang* deficiency: Marked chilliness with mild fever, headache, general aching, spontaneous sweating or no sweating, pallid complexion, pale and plump tongue with white coating, and deep and weak pulse.

Herbal Medication

I. Excess Syndromes

1. Wind-cold affection

Principle of treatment: To relieve the exterior syndrome by administering pungent-warm diaphoretics.

Formula of choice: *Jing Fang Baidu San* (Antiphlogistic Powder of Schizonepeta and Saposhnikovia). In case of headache, add *Radix Angelicae Dahuricae* (duhurian angelica root); if the patient complains of occipital pain with stiff neck, add *Radix Puerariae* (kudzuvine root).

2. Wind-heat affection

Principle of treatment: To relieve the exterior syndrome by administering pungent-cool diaphoretics.

Formula of choice: *Yin Qiao San* (Powder of Honeysuckle and Forsythia). For coughing with mucopurulent expectoration, add *Semen Armeniacae Amarum* (bitter apricot seed) and *Fructus Trichosanthis* (snakegourd fruit).

3. Affection of wind combined with summer-damp

Principle of treatment: To dispel wind and remove summer-damp.

Formula of choice: *Huoxiang Zhengqi San* (Powder of Patchouli for Restoring Normal *Qi*).

II. Deficiency syndromes

1. Wind affection in *qi* deficiency

Principle of treatment: To replenish *qi* and relieve the exterior syndrome.

Formula of choice: *Shen Su Yin* (Decoction of Ginseng and Perilla)[1]. For spontaneous sweating, add *Yupingfeng San* (Jade-screen Powder).

2. Wind affection in *yang* deficiency

---

[1]*Shen Su Yin* (Decoction of Ginseng and Perilla): *Radix Ginseng* (ginseng), *Folium Perillae* (perilla leaf), *Radix Puerariae* (kudzuvine root), *Radix Peucedani* (hogfennel root), *Rhizoma Pinelliae* (pinellia tuber), *Poria* (fuling), *Pericarpium Citri Reticulatae* (tangerine peel), *Radix Glycyrrhizae* (licorice root), *Radix Platycodi* (platycodon root), *Fructus Auranti* (bitter orange), and *Radix Aucklandiae* (costus root), to be mixed at the ratio of 3:3:3:3:3:3:2:2:2:2:2 in weight, and pulverized, 12 g each dose after making decoction with three slices of fresh ginger and three pieces of Chinese date. Its ready-to-use preparation is called *Shen Su Wan* (Pill of Ginseng and Perilla).

Principle of treatment: To reinforce *yang* and relieve the exterior syndrome.

Formula of choice: *Mahuang Fuzi Xixin Tang* (Decoction of Ephedra and Wild Ginger)[2].

Patent Medicines

Wind-cold affection: *Ganmao Qingre Chongji* (Antipyretic Granule for Colds)

Wind-heat affection: *Yin Qiao Jie Du Wan* (or *Pian* or *Chongji*) (Detoxicant Pill, Tablets or Granule of Honeysuckle and Forsythia).

Affection of wind combined with summer-damp: *Huoxiang Zhengqi Pian* or *Shui* (Tablet or Liquid of Patchouli for Restoring Normal *Qi*).

Wind affection in qi deficiency: *Shen Su Wan* (Pill of Ginseng and Perilla).

For prevention during an epidemic: *Banlangen Chongji* (Isatis-root Granule); for prevention of repeated colds and influenza in patients with low superficial resistance: *Yupingfeng Wan* (Jade Screen Pill), to be taken for a long period.

Acupuncture

Wind-cold affection: To dispel wind-cold by needling the following points: Dazhui (GV 14), Fengchi (GB 20), Fengmen (BL 12), Hegu (LI 4). Add Taiyang (EX-HN 5) and Yintang (EX-HN 3) for headache, Yingxiang (LU 20) for nasal obstruction, Quchi (LI 11) and Waiguan (TE 5) for fever.

Wind-heat affection: To dispel wind-heat by needling Dazhui (GV 14), Quchi (LI 11), Waiguan (TE 5), Hegu (LI 4). Add Shaoshang (LU 11) for sore throat. Reduction manipulation with retention of the needles for 20-30 minutes.

Prevention of influenza: Needling bilateral Zusanli (ST 36) with reinforcement manipulation and retaining the needles in place for 15 minutes, once during an epidemic. The acupuncture sensation is required to be transmitted to the dorsum of the foot.

BRONCHITIS

Acute bronchitis is likely to be viral in origin, and often follows a common cold or influenza. From the perspective of traditional Chinese medicine, the illness varies in accordance with the weather conditions and the pathogenic factors, as well as the patient's constitution and reaction to the pathogens. Therefore, the illness can be classified into several syndrome patterns and treated differently.

Chronic bronchitis is a condition characterized by persistent or recurrent cough with excessive sputum production over a period of years. Chinese medicine maintains that,

---

[2]*Mahuang Fuzi Xixin Tang* (Decoction of Ephedra and Wild Ginger): *Herba Ephedrae* (ephedra) 5 g, *Radix Aconiti Lateralis Preparata* (prepared aconite lateral root) 3 g, *Herba Asari* (Manchurian wild ginger) 3 g, to be made into a decoction.

besides the Lungs, other organs are involved, and the basic condition is deficiency in property. So, there are a series of tonification methods to improve the condition, which in many instances are more advantageous than modern Western treatment.

Etiology and Pathogenesis

Acute bronchitis is usually due to attack by wind, cold, heat or dryness. These pathogenic factors may impair the normal flow of Lung *qi*, leading to coughing. In addition, colds may give rise to the production of mucoid sputum, and heat to the production of purulent sputum.

In chronic bronchitis, the Lungs, Spleen and Kidneys are involved. From the traditional point of view, coughing is a common symptom of Lung diseases, but the production of sputum is not necessarily confined to disorders of the Lungs. Purulent sputum usually results when exogenous pathogenic factors (particularly heat) attack the Lungs, while production of voluminous nonpurulent phlegm is often attributed to dysfunction of the Spleen. In the latter case, the Lungs merely store the phlegm and cough it up. According to Chinese medical TCM classics, "The Spleen is the source of phlegm, while the Lungs are the place where the phlegm is stored." Shortness of breath with difficulty in exhalation, occurring late in the course of chronic bronchitis indicates that the Kidneys are involved. The Kidneys help the Lungs respire, and impairment of the Kidneys may be manifested by breathlessness with prolonged exhalation.

Syndrome Differentiation

Keys to the traditional diagnosis of syndrome patterns in bronchitis: The crucial point is to differentiate deficiency versus excess. In most cases of acute bronchitis, there are excess syndromes caused by pathogenic wind, cold, heat or dryness, and in most cases of chronic bronchitis there are deficiency syndromes. Since the Lungs, Spleen and Kidneys may be involved, it is important to differentiate which organ is the main one impaired, so that appropriate tonics can be selected.

However, there are complicated cases — excessiveness complicated by deficiency or deficiency complicated by excessiveness. For example, if acute bronchitis occurs in a debilitated person with *qi*, *yin* or *yang* deficiency, the condition is complicated. More frequently, a complicated syndrome occurs in patients suffering from chronic bronchitis with acute exacerbation due to attack of pathogenic factors. In these cases, the excess syndrome should be treated first. In a strictly traditional sense, most patients suffering from chronic bronchitis are considered to be complicated cases, because the phlegm, though it is a product of the Spleen with insufficient function, may in turn become a pathogenic factor that induces coughing. Therefore, expelling the phlegm often plays an important role in the treatment.

I. Acute Bronchitis

1. Hampering of the Lungs by wind-cold: Frequent coughing with white, thin

expectoration, chilliness, fever, headache, general aching, stuffy and runny nose, thin, white tongue coating, and floating pulse.

2. Invasion of the Lungs by wind-heat: Coughing with sticky or yellow phlegm difficult to expectorate, dry mouth and sore throat, fever, mild chilliness; thin yellow tongue coating, and floating, rapid pulse.

3. Impairment of the Lungs by wind-dryness: Dry cough or scanty phlegm difficult to expectorate, itchy throat, dry mouth, chest pain while coughing, reddened tongue tip, yellow, dry tongue coating, and thready, rapid pulse.

II. Chronic Bronchitis

1. *Qi* deficiency of the Spleen and Lungs: Coughing and frothy expectoration with shortness of breath, spontaneous sweating, vulnerability to colds, thin white tongue coating, and weak pulse.

2. *Yin* deficiency of the Lungs and Kidneys: Dry cough with scanty expectoration, dryness of the throat and mouth, heat sensation of the palms and soles, night sweating, reddened tongue with scanty coating, and thready, rapid pulse.

3. *Yang* deficiency of the Spleen and Kidneys: Chronic coughing and dyspnea with prolonged exhalation, aggravated by exertion, accompanied by frothy expectoration, aversion to cold and cool extremities, white and moistened tongue coating, and deep, slippery pulse.

III. Chronic Bronchitis with Acute Exacerbation

1. Accumulation of phlegm-damp in the Lungs: Coughing with expectoration of voluminous thin, whitish phlegm, accompanied by a feeling of oppression in the chest, epigastric distension and anorexia, white greasy tongue coating, and slippery pulse. This is often precipitated by catching a cold, and so there may be symptoms indicating wind-cold affection.

2. Attack of the Lungs by phlegm-heat: Severe coughing with expectoration of sticky, yellow phlegm, feeling of oppression in the chest, bitterness in the mouth and dry throat, sometimes accompanied by fever, yellow, greasy tongue coating, and slippery, rapid pulse.

Herbal Medication

I. Acute Bronchitis

1. Hampering of the Lungs by wind-cold

Principle of treatment: To dispel wind-cold and ventilate the Lungs.

Formula of choice: *Mahuang Tang* (Decoction of Ephedra) minus *Ramulus Cinnamomi* (cinnamon twig) plus *Radix Platycodi* (platycodon root), *Radix Peucedani* (hogfennel root), *Pericarpium Citri Reticulatae* (tangerine peel), and *Folium Perillae* (perilla leaf).

2. Invasion of the Lungs by wind-heat

Principle of treatment: To dispel wind-heat and ventilate the Lungs.

Formula of choice: *Sang Ju Yin* (Decoction of Mulberry Leaf and Chrysanthemum).

3. Impairment of the Lungs by wind-dryness

Principle of treatment: To moisten the Lungs and relieve coughing.

Formula of choice: *Zhisou San* (Cough Powder)[3] plus *Fructus Trichosanthis* (snakegourd fruit), *Bulbus Fritillariae Cirrhosae* (tendrilled fritillary bulb), *Radix Adenophorae* (ladybell root), and *Folium Eriobotryae* (loquat leaf).

II. Chronic Bronchitis

1. *Qi* deficiency of the Spleen and Lungs

Principle of treatment: To replenish *qi,* resolve phlegm and relieve coughing.

Formula of choice: *Sijunzi Tang* (Decoction of Four Noble Ingredients) plus *Yupingfeng San* (Jade-screen Powder), *Radix Asteris* (aster root) and *Flos Farfarae* (coltsfoot flower).

2. *Yin* deficiency of the Lungs and Kidneys

Principle of treatment: To replenish *yin*, moisten the Lungs and relieve coughing.

Formula of choice: *Liuwei Dihuang Tang* (Decoction of Six Ingredients with Rehmannia) plus *Radix Stemonae* (stemona root), *Radix Adenophorae* (ladybell root), *Radix Ophiopogonis* (lilyturf root), *Radix Asteris* (aster root) and *Flos Farfarae* (coltsfoot flower).

3. *Yang* deficiency of the Spleen and Kidneys

Principle of treatment: To warm the Kidneys to receive air, and invigorate the Spleen to resolve phlegm.

Formula of choice: *Gui Fu Bawei Wan* (Pill of Eight Ingredients with Cinnamon and Aconite) plus *Radix Astragali* (milkvetch root), *Rhizoma Atractylodis Macrocephalae* (white atractylodes rhizome), *Fructus Schisandrae* (magnoliavine fruit), and *Herba Asari* (manchurian wild ginger).

III. Chronic Bronchitis with Acute Exacerbation

1. Accumulation of phlegm-damp in the Lungs

Principle of treatment: To remove damp and phlegm.

Formula of choice: *Erchen Tang* (Decoction of Pinellia Tuber and Tangerine Peel) plus *Rhizoma Atractylodis* (atractylodes rhizome), *Cortex Magnoliae Officinalis* (medicinal magnolia bark), *Fructus Aurantii* (bitter orange), and *Radix Asteris* (aster root).

2. Attack of the Lungs by phlegm-heat

Principle of treatment: To clear the Lungs of heat and resolve phlegm.

Formula of choice: *Qingjin Huatan Tang* (Lung-clearing and Phlegm-resolving Decoction)[4].

---

[3]*Zhisou San* (Cough Powder): *Radix Platycodi* (platycodon root), *Herba Schizonepetae* (schizonepeta), *Radix Asteris* (aster root), *Radix Glycyrrhizae* (licorice root), *Radix Stemonae* (stemona root), *Rhizoma Cynanchi Stauntonii* (willowleaf swallowwort rhizome), *Pericarpium Citri Reticulatae* (tangerine peel) to be mixed at the ratio of 4:4:4:4:4:1.5:2 in weight, pulverized and taken 6 g (after mixing with hot water) three times daily or to be made into a decoction with an appropriate dose.

[4]*Qingjin Huatan Tang* (Lung-clearing and Phlegm-resolving Decoction): *Radix Scutellariae* (skullcap root) 9 g, *Fructus Gardeniae* (cape-jasmine fruit) 9 g, *Radix Platycodi* (platycodon root) 9 g, *Bulbus Fritillariae*

Patent Medicines

Wind-cold: *Tongxuan Lifei Wan* (Lung-ventilating Pill)[5].

Wind-heat: *Chuanbei Pipa Tangjiang* (Fritillary and Loquat Syrup).

Phlegm-heat: *Qingqi Huatan Wan* (Qi-clearing and Phlegm-resolving Pill)[6].

Qi deficiency: *Gui Shao Liujun Wan* (Pill of Six Noble Ingredients with Angelica and Peony)[7].

Yin deficiency: *Yangyin Qingfei Gao* (Extract for Nourishing *Yin* and Clearing the Lungs).

Acupuncture

I. Acute Bronchitis

Common points: Dazhui (GV 14), Fengmen (BL 12), Feishu (BL 13), and Zusanli (ST 36).

Additional points according to syndrome differentiation:

Wind-cold: Add Fengchi (GB 20), Chize (LU 5), and Hegu (LI 4).

Wind-heat: Add Yuji (LU 10), Quchi (LI 11), and Fenglong (ST 40).

Wind-dryness: Add Kongzui (LU 6), Yinlingquan (SP 9), and Zhaohai (KI 6).

II. Chronic Bronchitis

Common points: Danzhong (CV 17), Feishu (BL 13), Shenzhu (BL 23), Xuanji (CV 21), and Gaohuangshu (BL 43).

Additional points according to syndrome differentiation:

Phlegm-damp: Zhongfu (LU 1), Fenglong (ST 40), Yinlingquan (SP 9), and Gongsun (SP 4).

Phlegm-heat: Yuji (LU 10), Sanyinjiao (SP 6), and Taixi (KI 3).

Thunbergii (thunberg fritillary bulb) 12 g, *Radix Ophiopogonis* (lilyturf root) 12 g, *Cortex Mori* (mulberry bark) 9 g, *Semen Trichosanthis* (snakegourd seed) 15 g, *Exocarpium Citri Rubrum* (red tangerine peel) 6 g, *Poria* (fuling) 9 g, *Radix Glycyrrhizae* (licorice root) 6 g, to be made into a decoction.

[5]*Tongxuan Lifei Wan* (Lung-ventilating Pill): *Folium Perillae* (perilla leaf), *Radix Peucedani* (hogfennel root), *Radix Platycodi* (platycodon root), *Herba Ephedrae* (ephedra), Radix Scutellariae (skullcap root), *Pericarpium Citri Reticulatae* (tangerine peel), *Poria* (fuling), and *Fructus Aurantii* (bitter orange), *Rhizome Pinelliae* (processed pinellia tuber), *Semen Armeniacae Amarum* (bitter apricot seed), *and Radix Glycyrrhizae* (licorice root), mixed at the ratio of 6:4:4:4:4:4:4:3:3:3 in weight, pulverized and made into honey pills (for each 100 g of the ingredients add 150 g of honey), 12 g of the pills 2-3 times a day.

[6]*Qingqi Huatan Wan* (*Qi*-clearing and Phlegm-resolving Pill): *Rhizoma Pinelliae* (processed pinellia tuber), *Arisema cum bile* (bile-processed arisema), *Radix Scutellariae* (skullcap root), *Semen Trichosanthis* (trichosanthes seed), *Pericarpium Citri Reticulatae* (tangerine peel), *Semen Armeniacae Amarum* (bitter apricot seed), *Fructus Aurantii Immaturus* (immature bitter orange), and *Poria* (fuling) at the ratio of 1.5:1.5:1:1:1:1:1:1 in weight, pulverized, mixed and made into pills, 6-9 g, 2 times a day.

[7]*Gui Shao Liujun Wan* (Pill of Six Noble Ingredients with Angelica and Peony): the ingredients of *Liujunzi Wan* (Pill of Six Noble Ingredients) plus *Radix Angelicae Sinensis* (Chinese angelica root) and *Radix Peoniae Alba* (white peony root), made into pills, 9 g, 2 times a day.

Yang deficiency: Add Dazhui (GV 14), Pishu (BL 20), and Shenshu (BL 23).

BRONCHIAL ASTHMA

Bronchial asthma may be allergic or idiosyncratic. It is often difficult to eliminate the causative agent(s) from the environment of an allergic asthmatic. Drug treatment with Western medicine is effective, e.g., beta-adrenergic agonists, methylxanthines and anticholinergics can cause airway dilatation, and glucocorticoids reduce airway inflammation, but none of them can permanently change the patient's allergic or idiosyncratic state. In addition, all of them have side-effects. Therefore, use of Chinese medicines or acupuncture as a complementary or alternative therapy is advisable for this illness.

Etiology and Pathogenesis

In traditional Chinese medicine, asthma is considered an outcome of the abnormal production of phlegm. This is because the audible wheezing is believed to be due to obstruction of the air passages by phlegm, and remission is commonly preceded by copious expectoration of phlegm.

A constitutional defect that results in abnormal phlegm production is often emphasized. Existence of insidious phlegm in the lungs is taken as the basic mechanism of asthma. A variety of extrinsic factors, such as cold, infections, emotional disturbances, improper diet and physical exertion, may trigger an asthmatic episode by provoking the phlegm to obstruct the air passages.

Although asthma is a respiratory disorder, its pathological changes are not confined to the Lungs. As a rule, the constitutional defect is associated with dysfunction of the Kidneys and the Spleen, since the Kidneys are the foundation of the native constitution, and the Spleen is the source of the acquired constitution.

Syndrome Differentiation

Keys to the traditional diagnosis of syndrome patterns in bronchial asthma: Since the illness is a condition in which cold phlegm or phlegm-heat affects a person with constitutional insufficiency, during an episode the diagnosis should be focused on the differentiation of cold versus heat, while during remission it is important to determine which *zang*-organ is chiefly involved in the functional insufficiency.

I. During an Episode

1. Cold phlegm: Dyspnea with coughing and wheezing preceded by sneezing, watery nasal discharge and itching of the throat, possibly accompanied by chilliness or aversion to cold, and followed by thin, frothy expectoration; whitish, slippery tongue coating, and tense and floating pulse.

2. Phlegm-heat: Asthmatic attack preceded by fever and coughing, accompanied by

thirst, irritability, flushing face, and constipation, and followed by yellow, sticky expectoration; reddened tongue with yellowish, greasy coating, and slippery, rapid pulse.

II. During Remission

1. Deficiency of the Lungs: Spontaneous sweating and susceptibility to catching a cold that induces asthmatic attacks.

2. Deficiency of the Spleen: Frequent expectoration, lassitude, anorexia, abdominal distension after meals and loose bowel movements. The asthmatic attacks are usually precipitated by improper diet.

3. Deficiency of the Kidneys: Shortness of breath, aggravated by exertion, accompanied by aching back and weak legs. Dry throat, reddened tongue and thready pulse indicate Kidney *yin* deficiency. Kidney *yang* deficiency is characterized by cold extremities, aversion to cold, pale tongue and deep, weak pulse.

Herbal Medication

I. During an Episode

1. Cold phlegm

Principle of treatment: To dispel cold, eliminate phlegm and relieve asthma.

Formula of choice: *Xiao Qinglong Tang* (Minor Blue Dragon Decoction).

2. Phlegm-heat

Principle of treatment: To remove heat, eliminate phlegm and relieve asthma.

Formula of choice: *Dingchuan Tang* (Asthma-relieving Decoction).

II. During Remission

1. Lung insufficiency

Principle of treatment: To replenish *qi* and consolidate the body's superficial resistance.

Formula of choice: *Yupingfeng San* (Jade Screen Powder).

2. Spleen insufficiency

Principle of treatment: To invigorate the Spleen and resolve phlegm.

Formula of choice: *Liujunzi Tang* (Decoction of Six Noble Ingredients).

3. Insufficiency of Kidney *yin*

Principle of treatment: To replenish Kidney *yin*.

Formula of choice: *Liuwei Dihuang Tang* (Decoction of Six Ingredients with Rehmannia).

4. Insufficiency of Kidney *yang*

Principle of treatment: To reinforce Kidney *yang*.

Formula of choice: *Shenqi Wan* (Kidney-*qi* Pill).

Patent Medicines

1. During an episode: *Xiao Qinglong Chongji* (Minor Blue Dragon Granule) for

asthma of cold-phlegm type; *Dingchuan Wan* (Asthma-relieving Pill) for asthma of phlegm-heat type.

2. During remission: *Yupingfeng Wan* (Jade-screen Pill) for Lung insufficiency, *Liujunzi Wan* (Pill of Six Noble Ingredients) for Spleen insufficiency, *Liuwei Dihuang Wan* (Pill of Six Ingredients with Rehmannia) for insufficiency of Kidney *yin*, and *Shenqi Wan* (Kidney-*qi* Pill) for insufficiency of Kidney *yang*.

Acupuncture

I. During an episode

Common points: Dingchuan (EX-B 1), Chize (LU 5), Lieque (LU 7), Tiantu (CV 22), and Fenglong (ST 40).

Additional points according to syndrome differentiation:

Cold phlegm: add Dazhui (GV 14), and Fengmen (BL 12).

Phlegm-heat: add Yuji (LU 10), and Hegu (LI 4).

II. During remission

Common points: Dingchuan (EX-B 1), Feishu (BL 13), Gaohuang (BL 43), Guanyuan (CV 4), and Taiyuan (LU 9).

Insufficiency of the Lungs and Spleen: add Pishu (BL 20), and Zusanli (ST 36).

Insufficiency of the Spleen and Kidneys: add Shenshu (BL 23), and Taixi (KI 3).

CHAPTER 17
CARDIOVASCULAR DISEASES

HYPERTENSION

From the traditional Chinese medicine perspective, hypertension is a disorder of the *yin-yang* balance, and the treatment is aimed at restoring the normal balance. Since the balance restoration takes a considerable period of time, the treatment is usually not prompt-acting, but once there is a therapeutic effect, the effect can often last for a long period, even after discontinuance of the treatment. In addition, *yin-yang* imbalance does not equal increased blood pressure, and normal *yin-yang* balance does not necessarily mean normal blood pressure. Therefore, during Chinese medical treatment the patient's general condition improves first, and the blood pressure is lowered afterwards.

Etiology And Pathogenesis

The common etiological factors are emotional disturbances, overstress and improper diet. In different patterns or stages of hypertension, the pathogenic factors may be different.

1. Hyperactivity of Liver *yang*, and up-flaming of Liver fire

The Liver is closely related to psychic and emotional activities. Mental stress or furious anger may cause hyperactivity of Liver *yang*, resulting in irritability, headache and dizziness. Severe hyperactivity of Liver *yang* may turn into Liver fire, which results in irascibility, marked headache or dizziness, flushing face and reddened eyes. This often occurs at the early stage of essential hypertension.

2. *Yin* deficiency of the Liver and Kidneys, and deficiency of *yin* with exuberant *yang*

Stress consumes Kidney *yin*. The Kidneys use their essence to produce marrow, and the brain is the "sea of marrow." In Kidney *yin* deficiency nourishment of the brain is often impaired, and dizziness occurs. There may be other symptoms, such as a hot sensation in the palms and soles, and pain in the heels, indicating Kidney *yin* deficiency. Since the Kidneys and the Liver have the same source in their essential materials, deficiency of Kidney *yin* is usually accompanied by deficiency of Liver *yin* together with exuberant Liver *yang*. In this case, the excessiveness of *yang*, though relative and not absolute, may still lead to irritability and headache, and aggravate dizziness. This is the major mechanism in most chronic cases of essential hypertension.

3. Deficiency of both *yin* and *yang*

Protracted deficiency of *yin* may involve *yang*, and so besides dizziness there may be symptoms indicating *yang* deficiency, such as aversion to cold, nocturia or edema. This is not infrequently encountered in the late stage of essential hypertension, in climacteric hypertension and in renal hypertension.

4. Interior retention of phlegm-damp

Improper diet, overwork and stress or a protracted course of illness may impair the Spleen in transporting and transforming, resulting in the production of damp and phlegm.

Retained phlegm-damp gives rise not only to dizziness, but sometimes also to numbness of the limbs. This may occur in the late stage of hypertension as well as in hypertension with impending apoplectic attack.

Syndrome Differentiation

The crucial point of traditional syndrome diagnosis in hypertension is to determine the different kinds of *yin-yang* imbalance: deficiency or excess of *yin* or *yang*. There may be deficiency of *yin* (Kidney and Liver *yin*) or excess of *yin* (phlegm and damp as pathogenic *yin* factors). There may also be deficiency of *yang* (Kidney *yang*) or excess of *yang* (Liver fire). The duration of illness, precipitating causes, symptoms, tongue pictures and pulse conditions are the main items on which the differential diagnosis is based. Hypertension with hyperactivity of Liver *yang*, deficiency of *yin*, or *yin* deficiency with exuberant *yang* may be asymptomatic. In these cases, examination of the tongue and pulse may give significant clues for differentiating the syndrome patterns.

1. Up-flaming of Liver fire: Headache, dizziness, flushed face and reddened eyes, irritability, bitterness in the mouth, tinnitus, aversion to heat, insomnia, concentrated urine, constipation, reddened tongue with yellow coating, and stringy, rapid and forceful pulse. Hyperactivity of Liver *yang* and up-flaming of Liver fire only differ in degree. In the latter case, there are more marked fire symptoms such as flushed face and reddened eyes, particularly when the symptoms are precipitated by a fit of anger. If the syndrome occurs in an obese person, there may be a sensation of heaviness and distension of the head, and greasy tongue coating, indicating the presence of phlegm-fire.

2. *Yin* deficiency with exuberant *yang*: In *yin* deficiency of the Liver and Kidneys, there is dizziness with blurred vision and a top-heavy feeling, tinnitus, insomnia, aching of the back, pain in the heels, and thready pulse. But *yin* deficiency is often accompanied by relatively exuberant *yang*, manifested by irritability, flushing of the face, reddened tongue with scanty coating, and stringy pulse.

3. Deficiency of both *yin* and *yang*: In addition to the manifestations of *yin* deficiency of the Liver and Kidneys, cool limbs and aversion to cold, palpitations, shortness of breath, edema or nocturia; pale tongue with white coating, and deep, thready pulse weak at the *chi* (cubit) section or irregular pulse.

4. Retention of damp-phlegm: Headache with sensation of pressure in the head, dizziness, sensation of oppression in the chest, nausea and even vomiting, and sometimes numbness of the limbs; corpulent tongue with greasy coating, and stringy, slippery pulse.

Herbal Medication

1. Up-flaming of Liver fire

Principle of treatment: To clear Liver fire.

Formula of choice: *Longdan Xiegan Tang* (Decoction of Gentian to Purge the Liver) plus *Spica Prunellae* (selfheal spike) and *Flos Chrysanthemi* (chrysanthemum flower).

2. *Yin* deficiency with exuberant *yang*

Principle of treatment: To nourish *yin* and subdue *yang*.

Formula of choice: *Qi Ju Dihuang Tang* (Rehmannia Decoction with Wolfberry and Chrysanthemum) plus *Concha Haliotidis* (sea-ear shell) and *Ramulus Uncariae cum Unis* (uncaria stem with hooks).

3. Deficiency of both *yin* and *yang*
Principle of treatment: To reinforce both *yin* and *yang*.
Formula of choice: *Erxian Tang* (Decoction of Two Elixirs).
4. Retention of phlegm-damp
Principle of treatment: To remove phlegm-damp.
Formula of choice: *Erchen Tang* (Decoction of Pinellia Tuber and Tangerine Peel) plus *Rhizoma Gastrodiae* (gastrodia tuber) and *Ramulus Uncariae cum Unis* (uncaria stem with hooks).

Patent Medicines

1. Up-flaming of Liver fire: *Longdan Xiegan Wan* (Pills of Gentian to Purge the Liver) or *Ju Ming Jiangya Wan* (Chrysanthemum-Cinnamon Antihypertensive Pill)[1].
2. *Yin* deficiency with exuberant *yang*: *Qi Ju Dihuang Wan* (Rehmannia Pill with Wolfberry and Chrysanthemum).
3. Deficiency of both *yin* and *yang*: *Gui Lu Erxian Jiao* (Tortoise-Deerhorn Immortals Glue)[2].
4. Retention of phlegm-damp: *Banxia Tianma Wan* (Pinellia and Gastrodia Pill)[3].

Acupuncture

Common points: Baihui (GV 20), Fengchi (GB 20), Zusanli (ST 36), and Quchi (LI 11).
Additional points according to syndrome differentiation:
1. Up-flaming of Liver fire: Xingjian (LR 2), and Taiyang (EX-HN 5).
2. *Yin* deficiency with exuberant *yang*: Sanyinjiao (SP 6), and Taixi (KI 3).
3. Deficiency of both *yin* and *yang*: Qihai (CV 6), and Guanyuan (CV 4).
4. Retention of phlegm-damp: Neiguan (PC 6), and Fenglong (ST 40).
Leave the needles in for 30 minutes.

CORONARY HEART DISEASE (ANGINA PECTORIS)

Traditional Chinese herbal medication is helpful to the relief of angina pectoris in coronary heart disease. It has been shown that some herbal medicines not only reduce the attacks of pectoral pain, but also improve cardiac function and blood circulation, reduce

---

[1]*Ju Ming Jiangya Wan* (Chrysanthemum-Cinnamon Antihypertensive Pills): *Flos Chrysanthemi Indici* (wild chrysanthemum flower) and *Semen Cinnamone* (cinnamon seed) made into pills; 4.5 g, 3 times a day.

[2]*Gui Lu Erxian Jiao* (Tortoise-Deerhorn Immortals Glue): *Carapax et Plastrum Testudinis* (tortoise carapace and plastron), *Cornu Cervi* (deerhorn), *Fructus Lycii* (wolfberry), and *Radix Ginseng* (ginseng) at the ratio of 2:1:0.6:0.3 in weight, made into glue; 6 g to be taken after being mixed with hot water, 2 times a day.

[3]*Banxia Tianma Wan* (Pinellia and Gastrodia Pill): *Rhizoma Pinelliae* (processed pinellia tuber), *Rhizoma Gastrodiae* (gastrodia tuber), *Pericarpium Citri Reticulatae* (tangerine peel), *Rhizoma Atractylodis Macrocephalae* (white atractylodes rhizome), *Massa Fermentata Medicinalis* (medicated leaven), *Radix Codonopsis* (tangshen), *Rhizoma Atractylodis* (atractylodes rhizome), *Radix Astragali* (milkvetch root), *Poria* (fuling), *Semen Sinapis Albae* (white mustard seed), and *Rhizoma Alismatis* (water-plantain tuber), mixed at the ratio of 2:1:3:2:2:1:1:2:2:1:1, and made into honey pills; 10 g, 2 times a day.

myocardial oxygen consumption, and ameliorate the physical and chemical properties of blood. Therefore, herbal medication can be used as an effective therapy alternating with or adjuvant to modern Western treatment.

In myocardial infarction, herbal medication may also help, but it can not be used as an alternative therapy at present. So, this part is not discussed in this book.

Etiology And Pathogenesis

The common feature of angina pectoris is impaired blood flow in the vessels of the heart. The etiological factors that may result in such a pathological change include improper diet, aging, and emotional depression. Excessive rich food may impair the Spleen and Stomach, producing endogenous phlegm-damp or leading to *qi* deficiency. On the one hand, when phlegm-damp invades the Heart, it impedes the flow of the latter's *yang-qi* and the blood, resulting in angina pectoris. On the other hand, *qi* is motive force of blood flow, and *qi* deficiency may be followed by blood stasis. Emotional depression or excessive anxiety often gives rise to depressed Liver with stagnated *qi* and blood. When *qi* stagnation with blood stasis involves the heart vessels, angina pectoris ensues. Kidney insufficiency in the aged often plays an important role in the occurrence of angina pectoris. If Kidney *yin* is insufficient, there is frequently Liver *yin* deficiency and then exuberant Liver *yang,* which disturbs the blood flow. Insufficient Kidney *yang* that fails to promote Heart *yang*, may also lead to *qi* stagnation and blood stasis. In addition, cold causes blood congealing, and so exogenous cold may be a precipitating factor in angina pectoris.

Therefore, in angina pectoris the Heart, Spleen, Kidneys and Liver may be involved, deficiency of *qi*, *yin*, and *yang* are the fundamental pathological changes, and blood stasis, *qi* stagnation, phlegm-damp accumulation, and cold congealing are the precipitating factors.

Syndrome Differentiation

I. Excess syndromes (deficiency in origin)

1. Cold congealing: Severe pectoral pain, precipitated by exposure to cold, pale tongue, and deep, stringy or slow pulse.

2. Blood stasis: Pectoral pain with fixed location, dark or purple tongue or purple spots on the tongue, and stringy, hesitant or irregular pulse.

3. Phlegm turbidity: Pectoral pain accompanied by oppression in the chest, greasy tongue coating, and slippery pulse.

II. Deficiency syndromes

1. Deficiency of *qi* and *yin*: Pectoral pain with feeling of oppression, shortness of breath, spontaneous sweating, dryness in the mouth, reddened tongue with scanty coating, and stringy, thready and weak pulse.

2. *Yin* deficiency with exuberant *yang*: Pectoral pain with feeling of oppression, palpitations, dizziness, headache, tinnitus, lumbar aching, dryness in the mouth, heat sensation in the palms and soles, reddened tongue with scanty coating, and stringy, thready pulse.

3. Deficiency of both *yin* and *yang*: Pectoral pain with a feeling of oppression, shortness of breath, palpitations, soreness and weakness of the back and knees, aversion to cold with cool limbs, heat sensation in the palms and soles, nocturia, dryness of the mouth,

dark red tongue with white coating, and deep, thready and weak or irregular pulse.

Herbal Medication

I. Excess Syndromes

1. Cold congealing

Principle of treatment: To warm and liberate Heart *yang*.

Formula of choice: *Gualou Xiebai Banxia Tang* (Decoction of Trichosanthes, Allium and Pinellia)[4].

2. Blood stasis

Principle of treatment: To promote the flow of *qi* and blood.

Formula of choice: *Tao Hong Siwu Tang* (Decoction of Four Ingredients with Peach Seed and Safflower) plus *Radix Salviae Miltiorrhizae* (red sage root) and *Rhizoma Corydalis* (corydalis tuber).

3. Phlegm turbidity

Principle of treatment: To eliminate phlegm.

Formula of choice: *Erchen Tang* (Decoction of Pinellia Tuber and Tangerine Peel) plus *Fructus Trichosanthis* (snakegourd fruit), *Radix Salviae Miltiorrhizae* (red sage root), *Rhizoma Acori Tatarinowii* (grass-leaved sweetflag rhizome), and *Radix Curcumae* (turmeric root).

II. Deficiency Syndromes

1. Deficiency of *qi* and *yin*

Principle of treatment: To replenish *qi* and *yin* and activate blood.

Formula of choice: *Shengmai Yin* (Pulse-activating Drink) plus *Radix Astragali* (milkvetch root), *Radix Angelicae Sinensis* (Chinese angelica root) and *Radix Salviae Miltiorrhizae* (red sage root).

2. *Yin* deficiency with exuberant *yang*

Principle of treatment: To nourish *yin*, subdue *yang* and activate blood.

Formula of choice: *Qi Ju Dihuang Wan* (Rehmannia Pills with Wolfberry and Chrysanthemum) plus *Concha Haliotidis* (sea-ear shell), *Radix Salviae Miltiorrhizae* (red sage root), and *Fructus Trichosanthis* (snakegourd fruit).

3. Deficiency of both *yin* and *yang*

Principle of treatment: To nourish *yin*, liberate *yang* and activate blood.

Formula of choice: *Shengmai Yin* (Pulse-activating Drink) plus *Ramulus Cinnamomi* (cinnamon twig), *Fructus Trichosanthis* (snakegourd fruit) and *Radix Salviae Miltiorrhizae* (red sage root).

Patent Medicines

During the anginal attack for prompt relief of pain:

Suxiao Jiuxin Wan (Pill for Prompt Relief of Angina Pectoris), 10-15 pills to be taken sublingually.

---

[4]*Gualou Xiebai Banxia Tang* (Decoction of Trichosanthes, Allium and Pinellia): *Fructus Trichosanthis* (snakegourd fruit) 12 g, *Bulbus Allii Macrostemoni* (longstamen onion) 9 g, *Rhizoma Pinelliae* (pinellia tuber) 9 g, *Spiritus* (white spirit) appropriate amount, to be made into decoction.

Guanxin Suhe Wan (Storax Pills for Coronary Heart Disease) 1 pill to be taken orally by chewing.

After the anginal attack for improving myocardial circulation:

Compound *Danshen* (Red Sage Root) Dropping Pills, which contain *Radix Salviae Miltiorrhizae* (red sage root), *Radix Notoginseng* (notoginseng) and *Borneolum Syntheticum* (synthetic borneol), 10 pills to be taken 3 times a day orally or sublingually for 4 weeks.

PULMONARY HEART DISEASE

The following discussion is limited to pulmonary heart disease secondary to chronic bronchitis, chronic asthma and emphysema. Chinese traditional treatment of pulmonary heart disease of other causes is outside the scope of this book.

Etiology and Pathogenesis

Pulmonary heart disease often occurs as a sequela of long-standing repeated attacks of coughing and asthma. Its pathogenesis includes consumption of genuine *qi* and affection of pathogenic factors such as retained fluid, phlegm, and stagnated blood. Among the *zang-fu* organs, the Lungs, heart, Spleen, and Kidneys are involved.

In a chronic respiratory disease, insufficiency of Lung *qi* together with obstruction of the air passages by retained fluid and phlegm causes coughing and asthma. In this case, the Lungs fail to regulate the water passages, and the blood from the vessels of the Lungs cannot all return to the Heart. Therefore, Heart *qi* is impaired. Since the Spleen is in charge of transformation and transportation, when Spleen *yang* is insufficient, essence and *qi* cannot be adequately absorbed and transported to the Lungs, and water-damp as well as phlegm is thus produced, and infused into the Lungs. Insufficiency of Kidney *yang* also leads to retention of water. When the retained water invades the Lungs, it not only aggravates coughing and asthma, but also causes edema; when it interferes with the heart, palpitations and cyanosis ensue.

The above description on the pathogenesis of the clinical picture present in patients with pulmonary heart disease is quite different from the modern Western medical perspective, but it is useful for traditional herbal medication which often helps patients.

Syndrome Differentiation

I. During exacerbation

1. Retained fluid in the Lungs: Coughing with profuse expectoration, dyspnea, oppressive feeling in the chest, abdominal distension, lassitude, lack of strength, anorexia, heavy sensation in the limbs, yellow greasy tongue coating, and stringy, slippery pulse.

2. *Qi* deficiency with blood stasis: Breathlessness, coughing with little expectoration, listlessness, spontaneous sweating, oppressive feeling in the chest, cyanotic lips, dark tongue or purple spots on the tongue, thin tongue coating, and thready and hesitant pulse.

3. *Yin* deficiency of the Lungs and Kidneys: Coughing with difficulty in expectoration, dyspnea with prolonged exhalation, aggravated by exertion, flushed face, heat sensation in the palms and soles, dry throat, reddened tongue with scanty coating, and thready and rapid pulse.

4. *Yang* deficiency of the Spleen and Kidneys: Coughing, dyspnea, profuse foamy expectoration, orthopnea, dark complexion, cool limbs, edema of the legs, pale and plump tongue with slippery, greasy coating, and deep, thready pulse.

II. During remission

1. *Qi* deficiency with phlegm-damp: Coughing with profuse expectoration, oppressive feeling in the chest, spontaneous sweating, vulnerability to colds, lack of strength, pale or plump tongue with slippery and greasy coating, and stringy, thready pulse.

2. *Yin* deficiency of the Lungs and Kidneys: Coughing with scanty expectoration, shortness of breath on exertion, flushed face, dry mouth and throat, reddened tongue with scanty coating, and thready, rapid pulse.

3. Deficiency of *qi* and *yin*: Rapid breathing, spontaneous sweating, lassitude, feeble voice, dry mouth, flushed face, heat sensation in the palms and soles, reddened tongue with thin coating, and deep, thready and rapid pulse.

4. *Yang* deficiency of the Spleen and Kidneys: Rapid breathing with prolonged exhalation, aggravated by exertion, aversion to cold with cool limbs, lack of strength, spontaneous sweating, soreness and weakness of the back and knees, nocturia, edema of legs, pale tongue, and deep, thready pulse.

Herbal Medication

I. During exacerbation

1. Retained fluid in the Lungs

Principle of treatment: To clear the Lungs, remove phlegm and relieve dyspnea.

Formula of choice: *Qingfei Yin* (Lung-clearing Decoction)[5] plus *Rhizoma Pinelliae* (pinellia tuber), *Herba Houttuyniae* (houttuynia) and *Fructus Perillae* (perilla fruit).

2. *Qi* deficiency with blood stasis

Principle of treatment: To clear the Lungs, remove phlegm, replenish *qi* and activate blood.

Formula of choice: *Qingfei Yin* (Lung-clearing Decoction) and *Siwu Tang* (Decoction of Four Ingredients) plus *Radix Astragali* (milkvetch root) and *Semen Persicae* (peach seed).

3. *Yin* deficiency of the Lungs and Kidneys

Principle of treatment: To clear the Lungs, remove phlegm, and replenish *qi* and *yin*.

Formula of choice: *Qingfei Yin* (Lung-clearing Decoction) and *Shengmai Yin* (Pulse-activating Drink).

4. *Yang* deficiency of the Spleen and Kidneys

Principle of treatment: To warm up *yang*, induce diuresis, and resolve phlegm.

Formula of choice: *Xiao Qinglong Tang* (Minor Blue Dragon Decoction) plus *Rhizoma Pinelliae* (pinellia tuber) and *Pericarpium Citri Reticulatae* (tangerine peel).

---

[5]*Qingfei Yin* (Lung-clearing Decoction): *Poria* (fuling) 6 g, *Radix Scutellariae* (skullcap root) 6 g, *Cortex Mori* (mulberry bark) 6 g, *Radix Ophiopogonis* (lilyturf root) 6 g, *Semen Plantaginis* (plantain seed) 6 g, *Fructus Gardeniae* (cape-jasmine fruit) 6 g and *Caulis Clematidis Armandii* (clematis stem) 6 g, to be made into a decoction.

II. During remission

1. *Qi* deficiency with phlegm-damp

Principle of treatment: To replenish *qi* and resolve phlegm.

Formula of choice: *Sijunzi Tang* (Decoction of Four Noble Ingredients) and *Erchen Tang* (Decoction of Pinellia Tuber and Tangerine Peel)

2. *Yin* deficiency of the Lungs and Kidneys

Principle of treatment: To replenish the Lungs and Kidneys.

Formula of choice: *Liuwei Dihuang Wan* (Pills of Six Ingredients with Rehmannia) plus *Shengmai Yin* (Pulse-activating Drink).

3. Deficiency of *qi* and *yin*

Principle of treatment: To replenish *qi* and *yin*.

Formula of choice: *Sijunzi Tang* (Decoction of Four Noble Ingredients) plus *Liuwei Dihuang Wan* (Pills of Six Ingredients with Rehmannia).

4. *Yang* deficiency of the Spleen and Kidneys

Principle of treatment: To warm the Kidneys and invigorate the Spleen.

Formula of choice: *Gui Fu Bawei Wan* (Pills of Eight Ingredients with Cinnamon and Aconite) plus *Sijunzi Tang* (Decoction of Four Noble Ingredients).

Patent Medicines

During acute exacerbation: If there is a wind-cold affection manifested by chills and fever, use *Xiao Qinglong Chongji* (Minor Blue-Dragon Granules). If coughing, dyspnea and profuse expectoration accompany an aching back, dizziness and tinnitus, use *Suzi Jiangqi Wan* (Perilla Pills for Suppressing *Qi*)[6]. If there is aversion to cold with cool extremities, oliguria and edema, use *Jisheng Shenqi Wan* (Revivifying Kidney-*qi* Pills).

During remission

Qi deficiency with phlegm-damp: *Sijunzi Wan* (Pills of Four Noble Ingredients) and *Erchen Wan* (Pills of Pinellia Tuber and Tangerine Peel).

Yin deficiency of the Lungs and Kidneys: *Qiwei Duqi Wan* (Pills of Seven Ingredients for Governing *Qi*)[7].

Deficiency of *qi* and *yin*: *Sijunzi Wan* (Pills of Four Noble Ingredients) plus *Liuwei Dihuang Wan* (Pills of Six Ingredients with Rehmannia).

Yang deficiency of the Spleen and Kidneys: *Gui Fu Bawei Wan* (Pills of Eight Ingredients with Cinnamon and Aconite) plus *Sijunzi Wan* (Pills of Four Noble Ingredients).

VIRAL MYOCARDITIS

Quite a few herbs can inhibit the growth of some kinds of viruses, including

[6]*Suzi Jiangqi Wan* (Perilla Pills for Suppressing *Qi*): *Fructus Perillae* (perilla fruit), *Rhizoma Pinelliae* (processed pinellia tuber), *Cortex Magnoliae Officinalis* (medicinal magnolia bark), *Radix Peucedani* (hogfennel root), Pericarpium Citri Reticulatae (tangerine peel), *Lignum Aquilariae Resinatum* (eagle wood), *Radix Angelicae Sinensis* (Chinese angelica root), *Rhizoma Zingiberis Recens* (fresh ginger), *Fructus Jujubae* (Chinese date), and *Radix Glycyrrhizae* (licorice root), mixed at the ratio of 1:1:1:1:1:0.7:0.7:1:1:1 in weight, made into pills, and taken 3-6 g, 2 times a day.

[7]*Qiwei Duqi Wan* (Pills of Seven Ingredients for Governing *Qi*): Pills made of *Liuwei Dihuang Wan* (Pills of Six Ingredients with Rehmannia) plus *Fructus Schisandrae* (magnoliavine fruit).

coxsachievirus that may cause myocarditis. Since modern Western medicine still lacks safe and effective treatment for acute myocarditis, herbal medication is worthwhile. For chronic viral myocarditis, herbal medication is also helpful if it is administered in accordance with the patient's condition.

Etiology and Pathogenesis

The illness is caused by invasion of evil heat, which consumes *yin*-blood and leads to insufficiency of heart blood or *yin* deficiency with exuberant fire. At the later stage, the Kidneys are also involved.

The main symptom of the illness is palpitations. This may be due to deficiency of heart blood, heart *qi* or heart *yin*, or due to deficiency of Kidney *yin* with exuberant heart fire.

Syndrome Differentiation

I. Acute stage

Retaining of evil heat: Fever with general aching, sore throat, oppressive feeling in the chest, palpitations, reddened tongue with thin dry or yellow coating, and thready, rapid pulse; often occurring in the acute stage.

II. Chronic stage

1. Insufficiency of heart blood: Palpitations, dizziness, pallor, lack of strength, pale tongue, and thready, weak pulse.

2. Deficiency of both *qi* and *yin*: Palpitations, fidgetiness, dizziness, insomnia, lassitude, lack of strength, oppression feeling in the chest, and thready, weak pulse.

3. *Yin* deficiency with exuberant fire: Palpitations, fidgetiness, insomnia, dizziness, tinnitus, lumbar aching, reddened tongue, and thready, rapid pulse.

Herbal Medication

I. Acute stage with retaining of evil heat

Principle of treatment: To clear evil heat and nourish the heart.

Formula of choice: *Yin Qiao San* (Powder of Honeysuckle and Forsythia) plus *Radix* and *Folium Isatidis* (isatis root and leaf), *Radix Salviae Miltiorrhizae* (red sage root) and *Semen Platycladi* (arborvitae seed).

II. Chronic stage

1. Insufficiency of heart blood

Principle of treatment: To replenish *qi* and blood and induce tranquilization.

Formula of choice: *Guipi Tang* (Spleen-invigorating Decoction).

2. Deficiency of both *qi* and *yin*

Principle of treatment: To replenish *qi*, nourish *yin* and induce tranquilization.

Formula of choice: *Sijunzi Tang* (Decoction of Four Noble Ingredients) and *Shengmai Yin* (Pulse-activating Drink) plus *Radix Rehmanniae* (rehmannia root), *Radix Salviae Miltiorrhizae* (red sage root), *Fructus Schisandrae* (magnoliavine fruit) and *Semen Platycladi* (arborvitae seed).

3. *Yin* deficiency with exuberant fire

Principle of treatment: To nourish *yin*, clear away fire and induce tranquilization.

Formula of choice: *Zhi Bai Dihuang Wan* (Rehmannia Pill with Anemarrhena and Phellodendron) plus *Radix Salviae Miltiorrhizae* (red sage root), *Semen Platycladi* (arborvitae seed) and *Fructus Schisandrae* (magnoliavine fruit).

Patent Medicines

I. Acute stage with retaining of evil heat

Patent medicines: *Yinqiao Jiedu Wan* (Detoxicant Pills of Honeysuckle and Forsythia) plus *Banlangen Chongji* (Isatis-root Granules).

II. Chronic stage

1. Insufficiency of heart blood: *Renshen Guipi Wan* (Spleen-invigorating Pills with Ginseng).
2. Deficiency of both *qi* and *yin*: *Sijunzi Wan* (Pills of Four Noble Ingredients) plus *Shenmai Yin* (Pulse-activating Drink).
3. *Yin* deficiency with exuberant fire: *Zhi Bai Dihuang Wan* (Rehmannia Pills with Anemarrhena and Phellodendron).

ARRHYTHMIAS

Arrhythmias are attributed to imbalance of *yin-yang* of the heart, disorders in nourishing the heart, or disturbances of the heart by phlegm-fire or by blood stasis. Therefore, the treatment differs in different conditions. In general, herbal medicines and acupuncture, though not as effective as Western medicines, have no serious side or toxic effects, and so are worth applying to those who complain a lot of palpitations, but have no severe organic lesions of the heart.

Etiology and Pathogenesis

The etiological factors include constitutional weakness, psychic stimulation, excessive anxiety, and exogenous pathogenic factors. All these factors may lead to functional disorders through deficiency of *qi*, *yin*, or blood, or through phlegm-fire, *qi* stagnation, or blood stasis.

Syndrome Differentiation

I. Deficiency syndromes

1. Deficiency of *qi* and blood: Palpitations and shortness of breath, aggravated by exertion, lassitude, insomnia, dizziness, blurred vision, maybe spontaneous sweating, pallid complexion, pale tongue, and irregular pulse.
2. Deficiency of *yin* with exuberant *yang*: Palpitations and restlessness, on and off, accompanied by dizziness, tinnitus, bitterness in the mouth, dreamful sleep or insomnia, malar flush, reddened tongue with yellow coating, and thready, rapid or irregular pulse.

II. Excess syndromes

1. Phlegm-fire: Palpitations, restlessness and oppression feeling in the chest, on and off, accompanied by dizziness, expectoration of sticky sputum, dreamful sleep or insomnia, dryness and bitterness in the mouth, yellow greasy tongue coating, and slippery, rapid pulse.

2. *Qi* stagnation and blood stasis: Palpitations and oppressive feeling in the chest, maybe accompanied by pectoral pain or cyanosis, purplish tongue or purple spots on the tongue, and hesitant or irregular pulse.

Herbal Medication

I. Deficiency syndromes

1. Deficiency of *qi* and blood

Principle of treatment: To nourish *qi* and blood.

Formula of choice: *Guipi Tang* (Spleen-invigorating Decoction) or *Zhigancao Tang* (Honey-fried Licorice Decoction)[8].

2. Deficiency of *yin* with exuberant *yang*

Principle of treatment: To nourish *yin* and induce tranquilization.

Formula of choice: *Tianwang Buxin Dan* (Heavenly King's Heart Tonic).

II. Excess syndromes

1. Phlegm-fire

Principle of treatment: To reduce heat and resolve phlegm.

Formula of choice: *Wendan Tang* (Gallbladder-warming Decoction)[9] plus Rhizoma Coptidis (goldthread rhizome).

2. *Qi* stagnation and blood stasis

Principle of treatment: To remove blood stasis.

Formula of choice: *Xuefu Zhuyu Tang* (Decoction for Removing Blood Stasis in the Chest).

Acupuncture

Common points: Xinshu (BL 15), Jueyinshu (BL 14), Neiguan (PC 6), Shenzhu (GV12), and Shendao (GV 11).

Additional points according to syndrome differentiation:

Deficiency of *qi* and blood: Add Danzhong (CV 17), Guanyuan CV 4), Zusanli (ST 36), Sanyinjiao (SP 6), Pishu (BL 20), and Geshu (BL 17).

Deficiency of *qi* and *yin*: Add Qihai (CV 6), Yinlingquan (SP 9), Zusanli (ST 36), and Taixi (KI 3).

---

[8]*Zhigancao Tang* (Honey-fried Licorice Decoction): *Radix Glycyrrhizae Preparata* (honey-fried licorice root) 12 g, *Rizoma Zingiberis Recens* (fresh ginger) 9 g, *Radix Ginseng* (ginseng) 6 g, *Radix Rehmmaniae* (rehmannia root) 30 g, *Ramulus Cinnamomi* (cinnamon twig) 9 g, *Colla Corii Asini* (donkey-hide gelatin) 6 g, *Radix Ophiopogonis* (lilyturf root) 9 g, *Fructus Cannabis* (hemp seed) 9 g, and *Fructus Jujubae* (Chinese date) 5 pieces, to be made into a decoction.

[9]*Wendan Tang* (Gallbladder-warming Decoction): *Rhizoma Pinelliae* (pinellia tuber) 6 g, *Pericarpium Citri Reticulatae* (tangerine peel) 6 g, *Poria* (fuling) 9 g, *Caulis Bambusae in Taeniam* (bamboo shavings) 3 g, *Fructus Aurantii Immaturus* (immature bitter orange) 6 g, and *Radix Glycyrrhizae* (licorice root) 3 g, to be made into a decoction.

Phlegm-fire: Add Chize (LU 5), Feishu (BL 13), and Fenglong (ST 40).

Qi stagnation and blood stasis: Add Qihai (CV 6), Xuehai (SP 10), Danzhong (CV 17), and Ximen (PC 4).

In all syndrome patterns, uniform reinforcement-reduction with 30 minutes retention of needles is used.

CHAPTER 18
DIGESTIVE DISEASES

CHRONIC GASTRITIS

Chronic gastritis may be asymptomatic, but many patients complain of chronic anorexia, dyspepsia and persistent epigastric pain. Traditional Chinese therapeutic experience in relieving these symptoms by the unique method of syndrome diagnosis is useful for the treatment of chronic gastritis. According to modern research, the successful treatment of these syndromes also brings about histological improvement of the stomach.

Etiology and Pathogenesis

In traditional Chinese medicine, the clinical manifestations of chronic gastritis are usually considered an outcome of the following factors.

1. Improper diet

Irregular food intake, overeating or hunger, indulgence in cold and raw food, and consumption of too much greasy food or alcoholic drinks can impair the *qi* of the Spleen and Stomach. These pathogenic factors may disturb Stomach *qi*, which fails to descend, resulting in its stagnation, and hence chronic anorexia, dyspepsia and epigastric pain.

2. Emotional disturbances

Emotional disturbances often impair the normal function of *qi*. For example, anxiety makes the *qi* depressed, rage causes the *qi* to flow adversely upward, and worry makes the *qi* stagnate. All these disorders may further lead to anorexia, dyspepsia and epigastric pain, as occurring in chronic gastritis.

3. Weak constitution

The functions of the Spleen and Stomach are often weakened in the aged, during a chronic illness, or due to taking excessive drugs cool or cold in property. These individuals are apt to develop chronic gastritis with dyspepsia and anorexia. When the above factors impair the Spleen and Stomach, various mechanisms and pathological changes may take place in the occurrence of chronic gastritis. First of all, these factors can directly cause stagnation or deficiency of Spleen and Stomach *qi*. Secondly, stagnated Liver *qi* may be transformed into heat, resulting in retained heat in the Stomach. In addition, deficiency of Spleen *qi* may develop into deficiency of *yang* with cold manifestations, or produce damp, and then phlegm, and as a result, retention of phlegm-damp in the Spleen and Stomach. Protracted stagnation of Stomach *qi* may lead to impairment of Stomach *yin*, and hence *yin* deficiency of the Stomach, which is sometimes accompanied by heat symptoms.

Syndrome Differentiation

Keys to the traditional diagnosis of syndrome patterns in chronic gastritis: Just like syndrome differentiation in many other diseases, the crucial point for the diagnosis of chronic gastritis is to differentiate excess versus deficiency, and heat versus cold. Generally speaking, most chronic gastritis patients are in a state of deficiency (deficiency of *qi*, *yin* or *yang*), but in many of them the condition is complicated by excessiveness (stagnated *qi*, phlegm-damp or undigested food). The differentiation is important because a deficiency state should be treated with tonics, while the presence of excessive pathogenic factors should be eliminated with corresponding therapies.

It is equally important to differentiate cold and heat. The differentiation mainly depends upon symptoms such as aversion to cold or heat, and the color of the tongue and its coating. Drugs hot or warm in property are suitable for cold syndromes, and drugs cold or cool in property for heat syndromes.

I. Excess Syndromes

1. Stagnation of *qi* in the Liver and Stomach: Epigastric distension and oppressive feeling in the chest, alleviated by belching, anorexia, difficulty in defecation; thin but greasy tongue coating, and stringy pulse.

2. Retained heat in the Liver and Stomach: Epigastric distension and burning pain, irritability, acid regurgitation, dryness and bitterness in the mouth, constipation; reddened tongue, yellow coating, and stringy, rapid pulse.

3. Interior retention of phlegm-damp: Epigastric distension and fullness, dizziness, nausea, feeling of heaviness; turbid greasy tongue coating, and slippery pulse.

4. Retention of undigested food: Epigastric distension and pain, foul belching, acid regurgitation, nausea or even vomiting; thick greasy tongue coating, and stringy, slippery pulse.

II. Deficiency Syndromes

1. Deficiency of Spleen and Stomach *qi*: Epigastric fullness, anorexia, listlessness, lack of strength; sallow or pale complexion, pale tongue with white coating, and weak pulse.

2. Deficiency of Stomach *yin*: Dull epigastric pain with burning feeling, decreased food intake in spite of feeling hungry, preference for cold beverages; reddened tongue with scanty coating, and stringy, thready and rapid pulse.

3. Deficiency of Spleen and Stomach *yang* (deficiency-cold of the Spleen and Stomach): Epigastric distension and pain, alleviated by warmth, preference for hot drinks and food, vomiting of watery fluid, loss of appetite, lassitude, cool limbs; pale and flabby tongue with white coating, and weak, thready pulse.

Herbal Medication

I. Excess Syndromes

1. Stagnation of *qi* in the Liver and Stomach

Principle of treatment: To soothe the Liver, regulate *qi*, and harmonize the Stomach.

Formula of choice: *Chaihu Shugan San* (Bupleurum Powder for Soothing the Liver).

2. Retained heat in the Liver and Stomach

Principle of treatment: To remove heat from the Liver and harmonize the Stomach.

Formula of choice: *Zuojin Wan* (Goldthread-Evodia Pill) plus *Radix Peoniae Alba* (white peony root) and *Radix Glycyrrhizae* (licorice root).

3. Interior retention of phlegm-damp

Principle of treatment: To eliminate phlegm-damp and regulate the Spleen and Stomach.

Formula of choice: *Pingwei San* (Stomach-pacifying Powder) plus *Radix Scutellariae* (skullcap root) and *Caulis Bambusae in Taeniam* (bamboo shavings).

4. Retention of undigested food

Principle of treatment: To promote digestion, and harmonize the Stomach.

Formula of choice: *Baohe Wan* (Lenitive Pill) plus *Rhizoma Atractylodis Macrocephalae* (white atractylodes rhizome), *Fructus Aurantii Immaturus* (immature bitter orange) and *Cortex Magnoliae Officinalis* (medicated magnolia bark).

II. Deficiency Syndromes

1. Deficiency of Spleen and Stomach *qi*

Principle of treatment: To replenish Spleen *qi* and harmonize the Stomach.

Formula of choice: *Xiang Sha Liujunzi Tang* (Decoction of Six Noble Ingredients with Costus and Amomum).

2. Deficiency of Stomach *yin*

Principle of treatment: To nourish *yin* and regulate the Stomach.

Formula of choice: *Yiguan Jian* (Ever-effective Decoction).

3. Deficiency of Spleen and Stomach *yang* (Deficiency-cold of the Spleen and Stomach)

Principle of treatment: To tonify the Spleen and Stomach and expel cold.

Formula of choice: *Huangqi Jianzhong Tang* (Astragalus Decoction for Strengthening the Middle Energizer).

Patent Medicines

Chaihu Shugan Wan (Bupleurum Pill for Soothing the Liver) or *Sini San* (Powder for Relieving Stagnation with Cold Limbs), 6-9 g, 3 times a day for stagnation of *qi* in the Liver and Stomach.

Zuojin Wan (Goldthread-Evodia Pill), 3-6 g, 3 times a day, for retained heat in the Liver and Stomach with acid regurgitation.

Xiang Sha Liujunzi Wan (Pill of Six Noble Ingredients with Costus and Amomum), 9 g, 2 times a day, for deficiency of Spleen and Stomach *qi*.

Jiawei Baohe Wan (Supplemented Lenitive Pill)[1], 6-12 g, 3 times a day, for retention of undigested food.

Huangqi Jianzhong Wan (Astragalus Pill for Strengthening the Middle Energizer), 9 g, 3 times a day, for deficiency of Spleen and Stomach *yang*.

Acupuncture

Selection of points: Pishu (BL 20), Weishu (BL 21), Zhongwan (CV 12), Zhangmen (LR 13), Qihai (CV 6), and Zusanli (ST 36).

[1] *Jiawei Baohe Wan* (Supplemented Lenitive Pill): Pill made of *Baohe Wan* (Lenitive Pill) plus *Rhizoma Atractylodis Macrocephalae* (white atractylodes rhizome), *Fructus Aurantii Immaturus* (immature bitter orange) and *Cortex Magnoliae Officinalis* (medicated magnolia bark).

Use two or three of the above points each time. Reinforcement manipulation with warming needling is preferred. Treat the patient once daily or every other day. A course of treatment consists of 30 sessions.

PEPTIC ULCER

Because of the characteristic symptoms of this ailment, particularly chronic and recurrent food-related epigastric pain, numerous patients with peptic ulcers, though the diagnosis was not made with the aid of modern techniques, were treated by traditional Chinese medicine in the past and rich experience has been thus accumulated. The introduction of H_2-antagonists and H^+-K^+-ATPase inhibitors into the modern Western treatment of peptic ulcers has greatly improved the therapeutic effects, but the classical experience achieved by Chinese medicine is still of use, especially for those who worry about the side effects of chemical agents.

Etiology and Pathogenesis

Since peptic ulcers have similar clinical manifestations to chronic gastritis, the etiology and pathogenesis of the two diseases are considered similar. The etiological factors include improper diet, emotional disturbances, and constitutional weakness, and the common pathophysiological changes are stagnation of Liver *qi* which involves the Spleen and Stomach, deficiency of Spleen and Stomach *qi*, deficiency of Spleen and Stomach *yin*, and deficiency of Spleen and Stomach *yang*. In peptic ulcer cases, deficiency of Spleen and Stomach *yang* (deficiency-cold of the Spleen and Stomach) is most frequently encountered.

Syndrome Differentiation

Keys to the traditional diagnosis of syndrome patterns in peptic ulcer cases: The crucial points for the pattern diagnosis of peptic ulcers are the differentiation of excess versus deficiency, cold versus heat, and involvement of *qi* versus involvement of blood. Attack on the Stomach by stagnated Liver *qi*, and retention of stagnated blood are of excess pattern or excess as an incidental, and deficiency as the fundamental. Deficiency of Stomach *yin*, and deficiency of Stomach *yang* (deficiency-cold of the Stomach) are of deficiency pattern.

1. Disharmony of the Liver and Stomach: Epigastric distension and pain, referring to the hypochondriac regions, accompanied by frequent belching, and often aggravated by anger; thin white tongue coating, and stringy taut pulse.

2. Deficiency-cold of the Spleen and Stomach: Dull epigastric pain alleviated by pressure and warmth or relieved after eating, and precipitated by cold or fatigue, vomiting of watery fluid, lassitude, cool limbs, cool extremities, loose stools; pale tongue with white coating, and weak and fine pulse.

3. Deficiency of Stomach *yin*: Dull or burning epigastric pain, aggravated in the afternoon, accompanied by dryness in the mouth and throat, impaired appetite, diminished food intake, constipation; dry reddened tongue with scanty or exfoliative coating, and thready and rapid pulse.

4. Retention of stagnated blood: Stabbing pain in the epigastrium with tenderness, aggravated after meals, maybe accompanied by tarry stools; purple or dark tongue, and hesitant or deep and stringy pulse.

Herbal Medication

1. Disharmony of the Liver and Stomach
Principle of treatment: To relieve stagnated Liver *qi* and harmonize the Stomach.
Formula of choice: *Chaihu Shugan San* (Bupleurum Powder for Soothing the Liver).
2. Deficiency-cold of the Spleen and Stomach
Principle of treatment: To strengthen the Middle Energizer and warm the Stomach.
Formula of choice: *Huangqi Jiangzhong Tang* (Astragalus Decoction for Strengthening the Middle Energizer) plus *Liang Fu Wan* (Pill of Galangal and Aconite)[2].
3. Deficiency of Stomach *yin*
Principle of treatment: To replenish Stomach *yin*.
Formula of choice: *Yiguan Jian* (Ever-effective Decoction).
4. Retention of stagnated blood
Principle of treatment: To remove blood stasis and relieve pain.
Formula of choice: *Shixiao San* (Shixiao Powder)[3].

Patent Medicines

Xiaoyao Wan (Ease Pill), 5 g, 2 times a day, for disharmony between the Liver and Stomach.

Huangqi Jianzhong Wan (Astragalus Pill for Strengthening the Middle Energizer), 9 g, 3 times a day, for deficiency-cold of the Spleen and Stomach.

Liang Fu Wan (Pill of Galangal and Aconite), 5 g, 3 times a day, for epigastric pain due to deficiency-cold.

Fuzi Lizhong Wan (Aconite Pill for Regulating the Middle Energizer), 5 g, 3 times a day, for epigastric pain due to deficiency-cold.

Zuojin Wan (Goldthread-Evodia Pill), 3-6 g, 3 times a day, for acid regurgitation.

Yuanhu Zhitong Pian (Corydalis Analgesic Tablet)[4], 4-6 tablets, 3 times a day, for epigastric pain due to *qi* stagnation and blood stasis.

Xiang Sha Yangwei Wan (Costus and Amomum Stomach-nourishing Pill)[5], 6 g, 3

---

[2]*Liang Fu Wan* (Pill of Galangal and Aconite): *Rhizoma Galangae* (Galangal rhizome) and *Rhizoma Cyperi* (Cyperus tuber), pulverized and mixed in equal weight, and made into pills.

[3]*Shixiao San* (Shixiao Powder): *Pollen Typhae* (cat-tail pollen) and *Feces Trogopteronri* (trogopterus dung) pulverized and mixed in equal weight. *Shixiao* means "cannot help smiling," describing the marked effect of the powder that can stop the severe pain for which the patient is sobbing.

[4]*Yuanhu Zhitong Pian* (Corydalis Analgesic Tablets): *Rhizoma Corydalis* (corydalis tuber) 445 g and *Radix Angelicae Dahuricae* (dahurian angelica root) 223 g, made into 1,000 tablets, 4-6 tablets 2-3 times a day.

[5]*Xiang Sha Yangwei Wan* (Costus and Amomum Stomach-nourishing Pill): *Radix Codonopsis* (tangshen) 60 g, *Rhizoma Atractylodis Macrocephalae* (white atractylodes rhizome) 60 g, *Rhizoma Atractylodis* (atractylodes rhizome) 40 g, *Poria* (fuling) 40 g, *Herba Pogostemonis* (cablin patchouli) 40 g, *Cortex Magnoliae Officinalis* (medicated magnolia bark) 24 g, *Fructus Amomi Rotundus* (round cardamom) 24 g, *Rhizoma Pinelliae* (pinellia tuber) 20 g, *Fructus Amomi* (spiny amomum fruit) 16 g, *Rhizoma Cyperi*

times a day, for weakness of the Stomach with *qi* stagnation.

Acupuncture

Common points: Pishu (BL 20), Weishu (BL 21), Zhongwan (CV 12), Zhangmen (LR 13), Zusanli (ST 36), and Neiguan (PC 6).

Additional points according to syndrome differentiation:

Disharmony between the Liver and Stomach: Add Yanglingquan (GB 34), and Taichong (LR 3). Uniform reinforcement-reduction manipulation is used.

Deficiency-cold of the Spleen and Stomach: Add Guanyuan (CV 4), and Qihai (CV 6). Reinforcement manipulation with warming needling is indicated.

Retention of stagnated blood: Add Geshu (BL 17), Sanyinjiao (SP 6), and Gongsun (SP 4). Reduction manipulation is preferred.

COLITIS

Colitis is a general term for a group of inflammatory disorders of the colon. Their common clinical feature is diarrhea. Acute colitis may be caused by a variety of infectious agents, and most of them can be satisfactorily treated with Western medicine, but colitis may also be associated with antibiotics. Chronic inflammatory bowel diseases, such as ulcerative colitis and Crohn's disease, often present problems of complexity. In the Western medical management of these diseases, continuous corticosteroid administration may be helpful, but the patients are at the risk of developing the complications of chronic steroid therapy. A considerable number of patients are believed to require surgical intervention. However, even after colectomy, recurrence is not unusual, particularly in cases of Crohn's disease. Traditional Chinese medicine has abundant experience in the treatment of various kinds of diarrhea, including diarrhea in these complicated conditions. It seems reasonable to give the patients the alternative conservative therapy before their colons are resected. Since Chinese therapeutic experience of diarrhea is not limited to chronic colitis, and the above-mentioned chronic inflammatory bowel diseases may also reveal acute symptoms, the discussion in this section will cover various aspects of colitis.

Etiology and Pathogenesis

Acute colitis is an illness due to exogenous affection of the Spleen and Stomach, particularly damp affection. The damp pathogen is often combined with pathogenic heat or cold, causing colitis of damp-heat pattern or cold-damp pattern. Acute diarrhea due to overeating, and indigestion can also be discussed under the heading of acute colitis.

In chronic colitis, insufficiency of the Spleen usually plays the primary role. Damp also exists, but it is endogenous, due to the diminished function of the Spleen. The causal factors of Spleen insufficiency include improper diet, emotional disturbances, and a chronic disease that impairs the Spleen function. In the majority of cases, however, chronic

---

(cyperus tuber) 40 g, *Pericarpium Citri Reticulatae* (tangerine peel) 40 g, *Radix Aucklandiae* (costus root) 16 g, *Massa Fermentata Medicinalis* (medicated leaven) 24 g, *Fructus Hordei Germinatus* (germinated barley) 24 g, and *Radix Glycyrrhizae* (licorice root) 10 g, to be pulverized, mixed, and made into pills; 6-9 g, 2 times a day.

colitis comes from acute diarrhea without proper treatment, since long-term diarrhea may injure the Spleen.

Syndrome Differentiation

I. Acute Colitis

1. Cold-damp affection: Watery diarrhea accompanied by abdominal pain and borborygmi, loss of appetite, sometimes chilliness, fever and headache; thirst but with no desire to drink, diminished amount of urine, white greasy tongue coating, and relaxed pulse.

2. Damp-heat affection: Diarrhea accompanied by abdominal pain and tenesmus, burning sensation in the anus, concentrated urine, reddened tongue with greasy yellow coating, and slippery and rapid pulse.

3. Food stagnation: Diarrhea with stools containing undigested food and offensive smell, foul belching, epigastric distension and abdominal pain alleviated after bowel movement, loss of appetite, thick greasy tongue coating, and slippery and rapid pulse.

II. Chronic Colitis

1. Weakness of the Spleen and Stomach: Recurrent episodes of diarrhea aggravated by a rich diet and accompanied by anorexia, sallow complexion, listlessness, lassitude, pale tongue with white coating, and weak, thready pulse.

2. Impairment of the Spleen by stagnated Liver *qi*: Diarrhea preceded by abdominal pain and borborygmi, accompanied by distension in the chest and flanks, belching and loss of appetite, thin coating of the tongue, and stringy pulse. Episodes of diarrhea are often precipitated by psychic stress or emotional tension.

3. *Yang* deficiency of the Spleen and kidney: Diarrhea before dawn accompanied by borborygmi and pain around the umbilicus which is alleviated after bowel movement, preference for warmth applied to the abdomen, aversion to cold with cool limbs, aching and weakness of the loins and knees, pale tongue with white coating, and deep, thready and weak pulse.

Herbal Medication

I. Acute Colitis

1. Cold-damp affection

Principle of treatment: To dispel cold-damp and invigorate the Spleen.

Formula of choice: *Huoxiang Zhengqi San* (Powder of Patchouli for Restoring Normal *Qi*).

2. Damp-heat affection

Principle of treatment: To eliminate damp-heat.

Formula of choice: *Gegen Qin Lian Tang* (Decoction of Kudzuvine, Skullcap and Goldthread).

3. Food stagnation

Principle of treatment: To promote digestion and remove the stagnated food.

Formula of choice: *Baohe Wan* (Lenitive Pill) plus *Rhizoma Coptidis* (goldthread rhizome).

II. Chronic Colitis

1. Weakness of the Spleen and Stomach

Principle of treatment: To invigorate the Spleen and remove damp.

Formula of choice: *Shen Ling Baizhu Wan* (Pill of Ginseng, Poria and White Atractylodes)

2. Impairment of the Spleen by stagnated Liver *qi*

Principle of treatment: To soothe the Liver and invigorate the Spleen.

Formula of choice: *Tongxie Yaofang* (Essential Formula for Diarrhea with Abdominal Pain).

3. *Yang* deficiency of the Spleen and kidney

Principle of treatment: To warm up the kidneys, invigorate the Spleen and relieve diarrhea.

Formula of choice: *Sishen Wan* (Pill of Four Miraculous Ingredients).

Patent Medicines

Huoxiang Zhengqi Shui (Liquid of Patchouli for Restoring Normal *Qi*), 10 ml, 3 times a day, for acute colitis due to mild cold-damp affection.

Xiang Sha Liujunzi Wan (Pill of Six Noble Ingredients with Costus and Amomum), 6 g, 2 times a day, for chronic diarrhea due to weakness of the Spleen and Stomach.

Shen Ling Baizhu Wan (Pill of Ginseng, Poria and White Atractylodes), 6 g, 2 times a day, for chronic diarrhea due to weakness of the Spleen and Stomach.

Fuzi Lizhong Wan (Aconite Pill for Regulating the Middle Energizer), 6 g, 2 times a day, for chronic diarrhea due to deficiency-cold of the Spleen and Stomach.

Sishen Wan (Pill of Four Miraculous Ingredients), 6 g, 2 times a day, for *yang* deficiency of the Spleen and kidneys.

Acupuncture

I. Acute Colitis

Selection of points: Shangjuxu (ST 37), Xiajuxu (ST 39), Liangqiu (ST 34), Tianshu (ST 25), and Yinlingquan (SP 9).

Additional points according to syndrome differentiation: For cold-damp affection, add Shenque (CV 8, moxibustion), Liangmen (ST 21), and Guanmen ((ST 22); for damp-heat affection, add Quchi (LI 11), Dazhui (GV 14), and Neiting (ST 44); for food stagnation, add Shanglian (LI 9), Xialian (LI 8), and Zhongwan (CV 12).

II. Chronic Colitis

Selection of points: Zhongwan (CV 12), Tianshu (ST 25), Guanyuan (CV 4), and Zusanli (ST 36).

Additional points according to syndrome differentiation: For weakness of the Spleen and Stomach, add Pishu (BL 20), Weishu (BL 21), and Gongsun (SP 4); for stagnated Liver *qi*, add Ganshu (BL 18), Xingjian (LR 2), and Yanglingquan (GB 34); for *yang* deficiency of the Spleen and kidney, add Pishu (BL 20), Zhangmen (LR 13), Mingmen (GV 4, moxibustion), and Guanyuan (CV 4, moxibustion).

Appendix

Herbal enema therapy for ulcerative colitis: Herbal retention enema may be applied to patients with ulcerative colitis after evacuation of the colon and a cleansing enema with 500 ml of 5% infusion of tea-leaves. All kinds of enemata should be kept at body temperature, and three hours of retention is preferred.

1. Enema for general use: *Radix Angelicae Sinensis* (Chinese angelica root), *Calamina* (calamine), *Radix Angelicae Dahuricae* (dahurian angelica root), *Talcum* (talc), *Succinum* (amber), *Sanguis Draconis* (dragon's blood), *Radix Glycyrrhizae* (licorice root), and *Borneolum* (borneol).

2. Enema for damp-heat pattern: *Radix Scutellariae* (skullcap root), *Rhizoma Coptidis* (goldthread rhizome), *Radix Angelicae Dahuricae* (dahurian angelica root), *Flos Sophorae* (pagodatree flower), *Os Sepiae* (cuttlefish bone), *Herba Patriniae* (patrinia), and *Radix Glycyrrhizae* (licorice root).

3. Enema for conditions involving stagnated Liver *qi* and impaired Spleen: *Radix Saposhnikoviae* (saposhnikovia root), *Rhizoma Atractylodis Macrocephalae* (white atractylodes rhizome), *Radix Peoniae Alba* (white peony root), *Radix Bupleuri* (thorowax root), *Pericarpium Citri Reticulatae* (tangerine peel), *Radix Linderae* (spicebush root), and *Radix Curcumae* (turmeric root).

4. Enema for weakness of the Spleen and Stomach: *Radix Astragali* (milkvetch root), *Radix Glycyrrhizae* (licorice root), *Rhizoma Atractylodis Macrocephalae* (white atractylodes rhizome), *Radix Angelicae Sinensis* (Chinese angelica root), *Radix Codonopsis* (tangshen), *Radix Bupleuri* (thorowax root), *Rhizoma Cimicifugae* (bugbane rhizome), *Pericarpium Citri Reticulatae* (tangerine peel), *Resina Olibani* (frankincense), and *Myrrha* (myrrh).

5. Enema for deficiency of kidney *yang*: *Sulfur*, *Radix Aconiti Lateralis Preparata* (prepared aconite lateral root), *Fructus Psoraleae* (scurfpea fruit), *Herba Epimedii* (epimedium), *Radix Angelicae Dahuricae* (dahurian angelica root), *Radix Glycyrrhizae* (licorice root), and *Pericarpium Granati* (pomegranate rind).

VIRAL HEPATITIS

Although different types of hepatitis viruses such as HAV, HBV, HCV, HEV and HBV-associated delta agent have been recognized, all of them produce clinically similar illnesses. The early symptoms of acute hepatitis include malaise, fatigue, anorexia, nausea, vomiting, jaundice and pain in the liver area. There may be mild fever. The typical morphologic lesions of all kinds of hepatitis are often similar, and consist of panlobular inflammation, hepatic cell necrosis, and various degrees of cholestasis. If the hepatocyte necrosis and inflammation persist for more than 6 months, chronic hepatitis is considered.

Chronic hepatitis refers to chronic persistent hepatitis, and chronic active hepatitis. Most patients with chronic persistent hepatitis are asymptomatic, although some may complain of anorexia, fatigue, and occasionally of nausea and vomiting. There is usually a slightly enlarged liver with elevation of serum aminotransferase. Chronic active hepatitis is characterized by continuing necrosis, active inflammation, and fibrosis which may lead to liver failure, cirrhosis and death.

Based on the symptoms, therapeutic experience with hepatitis in traditional Chinese medicine has been achieved in association with the treatment of "jaundice," "hypochondriac pain" and "stagnation syndromes."

Etiology and Pathogenesis

Epidemic pathogens or pathogenic damp-heat is considered to be the major cause of hepatitis, particularly in its acute stage, whether there is jaundice or not.

1. Epidemic pathogens infect the Liver and Gallbladder, resulting in damp-heat which affects the smooth flow of Liver *qi* and secretion of bile, and leads to jaundice, anorexia and malaise.

2. Improper diet or abnormal weather causes dysfunction of the Spleen in transportation and transformation, resulting in retention of damp-heat in the Spleen and Stomach, which further injures the Liver and Gallbladder.

3. Exuberant pathogenic damp-heat accumulated in the interior of the body for a long time impairs vital essence; as a result, deficiency of *yin*, *yang*, *qi* or blood syndromes may occur.

4. Prolonged stagnation of Liver *qi* may lead to blood stasis, manifested by stabbing pain, firm and enlarged liver and spleen, and other related signs.

Syndrome Differentiation

Keys to the traditional diagnosis of syndrome patterns in viral hepatitis:

1. Diagnosis of *yang*-jaundice versus *yin*-jaundice: Acute affection due to damp-heat often results in *yang*-jaundice, characterized by a lustrous yellow discoloration of the skin and sclera. In chronic cases, especially when *yang-qi* of the body is impaired, the jaundice leads to dark yellow discoloration of sclera and smoky-colored skin. It is believed that damp-heat has turned into cold-damp, and the jaundice is of the *yin* type.

2. Determination of preponderance of heat over damp or vice versa: The pathogens of viral hepatitis are usually considered as damp-heat in Chinese medicine. Because of different types of viruses and different routes of infection, in some patients the pathogenic damp may be preponderant, in some patients the pathogenic heat may be preponderant, and in others both damp and heat are prominent. If heat is preponderant, there are marked heat manifestations such as fever, thirst, constipation, reddened tongue with yellow coating and rapid pulse. If damp is preponderant, there are marked damp manifestations such as a sensation of heaviness in the body, anorexia, stuffy feeling in the chest, abdominal distension, greasy tongue coating and slippery pulse.

3. Differentiation of deficiency and excess: Most acute hepatitis cases are of the excess type, while the majority of chronic hepatitis patients are in a condition of deficiency or deficiency complicated with excess.

4. Recognition of *qi* stagnation versus blood stasis: *Qi* stagnation and blood stasis are two common pathological changes in hepatitis, particularly in chronic hepatitis. *Qi* stagnation is characterized by pain over the liver area with no definitely fixed location and accompanied by a sensation of distention but with no marked tenderness. Blood stasis usually develops later, and is characterized by stabbing or pricking hypochondriac pain, fixed in location and accompanied by hepatosplenomegaly with tenderness as well as dark complexion, presence of spider nevus,

purple tongue or purple spots on the tongue.

I. Acute hepatitis

1. Acute hepatitis with jaundice

Acute hepatitis with jaundice is usually considered as a damp-heat affection. The pathogenic heat may be preponderant over the damp, and the pathogenic damp may be preponderant over the heat, but in severe cases, both the pathogenic damp and heat may be prominent.

(1) Preponderance of heat over damp: Fever, jaundice, anorexia, dark urine, constipation, dryness and bitterness of the mouth, fatigue, reddened tongue, yellow tongue coating, and rapid or stringy and rapid pulse.

(2) Preponderance of damp over heat: Fever, jaundice, lassitude, distension in the stomach, anorexia, nausea, vomiting, loose stools, white and greasy tongue coating, and soft, slippery pulse.

(3) Prominence of both damp and heat: Fever, deep and persistent jaundice, anorexia, nausea, vomiting, lassitude, constipation, thick, yellow and greasy tongue coating, and stringy, rapid or slippery and rapid pulse. In severe cases, there may be coma, hemorrhage and ascites, as in fulminating hepatitis.

2. Acute hepatitis without jaundice

Acute hepatitis without jaundice is usually considered a mild damp-heat infection in which only the normal flow of Liver *qi* is impaired while the bile secretion is still intact. The syndrome diagnosis pertains to stagnation of Liver *qi*, manifested by mild impairment of appetite, fatigability, pain in the liver area, and stringy pulse.

II. Chronic hepatitis

1. Stagnation of Liver *qi* with Spleen insufficiency: Pain in the liver area and distension in the epigastrium, impaired appetite, stools sometimes loose and sometimes bound, fatigability, lack of strength, and plump tongue with thin whitish coating.

2. Deficiency of both *qi* and *yin*: Dull pain in the liver area, hot sensation in the palms and soles, night sweating, dizziness, lack of strength, reddened tongue with thin coating, and thready, stringy or thready, stringy and rapid pulse.

3. Interior accumulation of cold-damp: Chronic jaundice with dim-colored discoloration, epigastric distension, anorexia, cool limbs averse to cold, fatigability and lack of strength, loose stools, white greasy tongue coating, and deep, relaxed pulse.

4: *Qi* stagnation and blood stasis: Dull complexion, hypochondriac pain, hepatosplenomegaly, emaciation, lassitude, anorexia, abdominal distension, sometimes spider nevus; dark and purplish tongue with white coating, and stringy, thready pulse.

Herbal Medication

I. Acute Hepatitis

1. Acute hepatitis with jaundice

Principle of treatment: To clear damp-heat.

Formula of choice: *Yinchenhao Tang* (Oriental Wormwood Decoction) plus *Radix Isatidis* (isatis root).

Modifications of the formula according to syndrome differentiation: For preponderance of heat over damp, add *Cortex Phellodendri* (phellodendron bark) and *Radix Glycyrrhizae* (licorice root). For preponderance of damp over heat, subtract *Radix et Rhizoma Rhei* (rhubarb) and add *Wuling San* (Powder of Five Drugs with Poria). For prominence of both damp and heat, add *Radix Scutellariae* (skullcap root), *Rhizoma Coptidis* (goldthread rhizome), *Cortex Moutan* (moutan bark) and *Pulvis Cornus Bubali Concentratus* (concentrated buffalo horn powder).

2. Acute hepatitis without jaundice

Principle of Treatment: To restore the normal flow of Liver *qi*.

Formula of choice: *Xiao Chaihu Tang* (Minor Bupleurum Decoction).

II. Chronic Hepatitis

1. Stagnation of Liver *qi* with Spleen insufficiency

Principle of treatment: To soothe the Liver and invigorate the Spleen.

Formula of choice: *Chaihu Shugan San* (Bupleurum Powder for Soothing the Liver).

2. Deficiency of both *qi* and *yin*

Principle of treatment: To replenish *qi* and nourish *yin*.

Formula of choice: *Yiguan Jian* (Ever Effective Decoction) plus *Sijunzi Tang* (Decoction of Four Noble Ingredients).

3. Interior accumulation of cold-damp

Principle of treatment: To remove damp with warming drugs.

Formula of choice: *Pingwei San* (Stomach-pacifying Powder) plus *Yinchenhao Tang* (Oriental Wormwood Decoction) and *Radix Aconiti Lateralis Preparata* (prepared aconite lateral root).

4. *Qi* stagnation and blood stasis

Principle of treatment: To regulate *qi* and remove blood stasis.

Formula of choice: *Xiaoyao San* (Ease Powder) plus *Tao Hong Siwu Tang* (Decoction of Four Ingredients with Peach Seed and Safflower).

Patent Medicines

Chuipencao Chongji (Stringy Stonecrop Granule)[6], 10 g, 3 times a day, or *Chuipencao Tangjiang* (Stringy Stonecrop Syrup), 10-30 ml, 3 times a day, for acute and chronic hepatitis.

Jigucao Wan (Prayer-bead Pill) for chronic hepatitis.

Chaihu Shugan Wan (Bupleurum Pill for Soothing the Liver), 6-9 g, 3 times a day, for chronic hepatitis with stagnation of Liver *qi*.

Diphenyldiester, a substance extracted from *Fructus Schisandrae* (magnoliavine fruit), is effective for reducing serum transaminase in hepatitis, but a relapse may occur after stopping the treatment.

Radix Sophorae Tonkinensis (tongking sophora root) Injection. Inject 10 ml (containing 50 mg total alkaloids of tongking sophora root) intramuscularly daily for 2 months may turn blood HBV-DNA and HBeAg negative in active chronic cases.

---

[6] *Chuipencao Chongji* (Stringy Stonecrop Granule) or *Chuipencao Tangjiang* (Stringy Stonecrop Syrup) is composed of *Herba Sedi* (stringy stonecrop), *Folium Ardisiae Japonicae* (Japanese ardisia leaf) and sugar.

LIVER CIRRHOSIS

In Western medicine, cirrhosis is considered an irreversible pathological change, and the management is chiefly supportive or limited to treatment of the complications of portal hypertension. In traditional Chinese medicine, the enlargement and firmness of the liver and spleen is taken as a kind of stagnation, and it is believed that some herbs to eliminate blood stasis are able to soften the hard masses.

Etiology and Pathogenesis

The common causal factors are improper diet and infection.

1. Improper diet, particularly excessive intake of alcohol, impairs the function of the Spleen in transporting and transforming water-damp, so that the retained damp is condensed into phlegm, which impedes the normal flow of *qi* and blood in the Liver. Long-term blood stasis produces the pathological changes in the Liver.

2. A chronic infection of viral hepatitis or schistosomiasis also causes long-term stagnation of *qi* and blood in the Liver and Spleen.

The *zang-fu* organs mainly involved in this disease are the Liver, Spleen and Kidneys. Stagnation of Liver *qi* leads to blood stasis, and insufficiency of the Spleen produces damp. A long-standing accumulation of damp produces ascites. Protracted disorders of the Liver and Spleen often involve the Kidneys. If Kidney *yang* is impaired, excretion of water with urine is diminished, and ascites is aggravated. If Kidney *yin* is impaired, there will be *yin* deficiency in both the Liver and Kidneys, with exuberant fire, which causes hemorrhages. At the last stage, failure of the Liver, Spleen and Kidneys disturbs the Heart (mental activities), resulting in coma.

Syndrome Differentiation

Keys to the traditional diagnosis of syndrome patterns in liver cirrhosis: In the early stage of the disease, Liver depression with Spleen insufficiency, *qi* stagnation and blood stasis are the main patterns. When ascites is formed, there is accumulation of water-damp. In the late stage of the disease, the Kidneys are usually involved, and either *yang* deficiency of the Spleen and Kidneys, or *yin* deficiency of the Liver and Kidneys, or both, may occur. In most cases, the syndrome is deficiency (deficiency of the Liver, Spleen and Kidneys) complicated with excess (*qi* stagnation, blood stasis, and water accumulation).

1. Liver depression with Spleen insufficiency: Dull pain of distension in the hypochondriac region, epigastric stuffiness, sometimes nausea, diarrhea, and fatigue, particularly after ingestion of improper food, pale tongue with thin white coating, and stringy pulse.

2. *Qi* stagnation with blood stasis: Distended feeling in the hypochondriac region, with hepatosplenomegaly and fixed pain, dark complexion, purplish tongue with thin coating, and stringy pulse.

3. Retention of stagnated blood in the Liver: Abdominal distension with tense ascites, distended abdominal veins, spider nevi on the face, neck and chest, liver palms, dark lips, purple tongue or purple spots on the tongue with thin coating, and deep, stringy pulse, or stringy, hesitant pulse.

4. Accumulation of water-damp: Distended abdomen with shifting dullness or fluid

sensation, edema of the lower extremities, epigastric distress, anorexia, oliguria, difficult bowel movements; dark-red tongue or purple spots on the tongue, and stringy, thready pulse.

5. *Yang* deficiency of the Spleen and Kidneys: Abdominal distension with ascites, edema in the loins and legs, anorexia, cold limbs, aversion to cold, scanty dilute urine; sallow complexion, pale and purplish tongue, and deep, thready pulse.

6. *Yin* deficiency of the Liver and Kidneys: Distended abdomen with thin limbs, dark complexion, purple lips, dryness in the mouth, heat sensation in the palms and soles, epistaxis, scanty urine, reddened or dark purple tongue with scanty or no coating, and stringy, thready pulse.

Herbal Medication

1. Liver depression with Spleen insufficiency

Principle of treatment: To soothe the Liver, invigorate the Spleen and replenish *qi*.

Formula of choice: *Xiaoyao San* (Ease Powder) plus *Liujunzi Tang* (Decoction of Six Noble Ingredients).

2. *Qi* stagnation with blood stasis

Principle of treatment: To promote the flow of *qi* and eliminate stagnated blood.

Formula of choice: *Gexia Zhuyu Tang* (Decoction for Removing Blood Stasis below the Diaphragm)[7].

3. Retention of stagnated blood in the Liver

Principle of treatment: To promote *qi* and blood flow, remove blood stasis, and induce diuresis.

Formula of choice: *Xuefu Zhuyu Tang* (Decoction for Removing Blood Stasis in Chest) plus *Wuling San* (Powder of Five Drugs with Poria).

4. Accumulation of water-damp

Principle of treatment: To reduce ascites for symptomatic relief, and then treat as retention of stagnated blood in the Liver.

Formula of choice: *Semen Pharbitis* (pharbitis seed), 3 g, ground into powder, to be taken in the morning before breakfast daily for 2-3 days. (It can be administered only when the patient is intolerant of gross ascites, but his genuine *qi* is not in an extremely deficient state.)

5. *Yang* deficiency of the Spleen and Kidneys

Principle of treatment: To warm and tonify the Spleen and Kidneys, and induce diuresis.

Formula of choice: *Fuzi Lizhong Wan* (Aconite Pill for Regulating the Middle Energizer) plus *Wuling San* (Powder of Five Drugs with Poria).

6. *Yin* deficiency of the Liver and Kidneys

Principle of treatment: To nourish Liver and Kidney *yin* and induce diuresis.

Formula of choice: *Yiguan Jian* (Ever-effective Decoction) plus *Zhuling Tang*

---

[7]*Gexia Zhuyu Tang* (Decoction for Removing Blood Stasis below the Diaphragm): *Feces Trogopterorum* (trogopterus dung) 9 g, *Radix Angelicae Sinensis* (Chinese angelica root) 9 g, *Rhizoma Chuanxiong* (chuanxiong) 6 g, *Semen Persicae* (peach seed) 9 g, *Cortex Moutan* (moutan bark) 6 g, *Radix Peoniae Rubra* (red peony root) 6 g, *Radix Linderae* (spicebush root) 6 g, *Rhizoma Corydalis* (corydalis tuber) 3 g, *Radix Glycyrrhizae* (liquorice root) 9 g, *Rhizoma Cyperi* (cyperus tuber) 3 g, *Flos Carthami* (safflower) 9 g, to be made into a decoction.

(Decoction of Polyporus)[8].

CHOLECYSTITIS AND CHOLELITHIASIS

In most instances, cholecystitis is associated with gallstones. Antibiotic and supportive therapy may lead to a temporary remission in cholecystitis without severe complications such as empyema, but cholecystectomy is often the treatment of choice for cholecystitis and common bile duct stones. After cholecystectomy, however, some patients continue to complain of symptoms similar to those which occur in chronic cholecystitis. Extracorporeal lithotripsy is now an effective treatment in selected patients with gallbladder calculi, but there remain several problems, e.g., how to expel all the stone fragments, and how to prevent recurrence. Therefore, despite the achievements of modern Western medicine, plenty of room for complementary or alternative therapy is still left.

Etiology And Pathogenesis

From the viewpoint of traditional Chinese medicine, cholecystitis is a disease mainly related to dysfunction of the Liver, Gallbladder, Spleen and Stomach caused by improper diet and emotional disturbances. Since the Liver is responsible for smoothing and regulating the flow of *qi*, including the *qi* to promote bile flow, stagnated Liver *qi* may interfere with the normal bile discharge from the Gallbladder. Retained bile in the Gallbladder will turn into damp-heat, and lead to jaundice and pain in the right upper abdomen.

Impaired function of the Spleen and Stomach may result in accumulation of damp-heat in the middle energizer. When damp-heat invades the Liver and Gallbladder, it often causes pain and jaundice. Therefore, the common pathophysiological changes in cholecystitis are considered to be stagnation of Liver and Gallbladder *qi*, and damp-heat in the Liver and Gallbladder.

When stagnated bile is condensed by damp-heat, gallstones are formed. The existence of gallstones further aggravates the morbid condition of the Liver and Gallbladder, with frequent recurrence.

Syndrome Differentiation

In cholecystitis, the crucial point in traditional diagnosis is to differentiate *qi* stagnation from damp-heat. The former corresponds to chronic cholecystitis, and the latter to acute pyogenic inflammation of the gallbladder.

1. *Qi* stagnation of the Liver and Gallbladder: Mild and transient dull pain in the right upper abdomen, accompanied by bitterness in the mouth, nausea, anorexia or epigastric distress after meals; thin white tongue coating and stringy pulse. There is no fever, chill, jaundice or pain during remission, but the symptoms often recur repeatedly.

2. Damp-heat in the Liver and Gallbladder: Acute onset of severe pain in the right

---

[8] *Zhuling Tang* (Decoction of Polyporus): *Polyporus* (chuling), *Poria* (fuling), *Rhizoma Alismatis* (water-plantain tuber), *Colla Cori Asini* (donkey-hide gelatin) and *Talcum* (talc) each 9 g, to be made into a decoction.

upper abdomen, accompanied by chills and fever, jaundice, nausea, anorexia, thirst, constipation and reddened tongue with greasy coating. The gallbladder may be palpable, with tenderness.

Herbal Medication

1. *Qi* stagnation of the Liver and Gallbladder
Principle of treatment: To soothe the Liver and relieve pain.
Formula of choice: *Chaihu Shugan San* (Bupleurum Powder for Soothing the Liver).
2. Damp-heat in the Liver and Gallbladder
Principle of treatment: To purge the Liver and Gallbladder of damp-heat.
Formula of choice: *Da Chaihu Tang* (Major Bupleurum Decoction).

For expelling gallstones, some effective formulas have been designed. The following can be taken as an example: *Herba Lysimachiae* (loosestrife) 30 g, *Herba Artemisiae Scopariae* (oriental wormwood) 15 g, *Radix Curcumae* (turmeric root) 15 g, *Fructus Aurantii* (bitter orange) 10 g, *Radix Aucklandiae* (costus root) 10 g, and *Radix et Rhizoma Rhei* (unprocessed rhubarb) 10 g, to be made into a decoction.

Patent Medicines

Dan Zhi Xiaoyao Wan (Ease Pill with Moutan and Gardenia), 6 g, 2 times a day, for chronic cholecystitis with frequent attacks of right upper abdominal pain.

Longdan Xiegan Wan (Gentian Pill to Purge the Liver), 6 g, 2 times a day, for cholecystitis with damp-heat affection.

Acupuncture

Acupuncture can be used as a complementary measure for symptomatic relief of cholecystitis.

Selection of points: Ganshu (BL 18), Danshu (BL 19), Riyue (GB 24), *Qi*men (LR 14) and Dannang (EX-LE 6).

Additional points according to syndrome differentiation: For damp-heat, add Dazhui (GV 14), Quchi (LI 11) and Waiguan (TE 5); for *qi* stagnation, add Neiguan (PC 6) and Gongsun (SP 4).

Repeated manipulation of the needles or application of electro-acupuncture is preferred.

PANCREATITIS

Besides the use of analgesics, prohibition of oral alimentation and application of nasogastric suction are two of the Western conventional measures to treat acute pancreatitis. Both measures are aimed at reducing pancreatic secretion. Chinese medicine holds a different view: Abdominal pain in pancreatitis is usually due to obstruction, and the effective way to treat this condition is to remove the obstruction and promote the pancreatic juice flow. The commonest herb used for this purpose is *Radix et Rhizoma Rhei* (rhubarb). Recent research has revealed that rhubarb can increase the discharge of pancreatic juice, but its major action is the marked inhibition of the activities of various pancreatic enzymes, including pancreatic amylase, trypsin, chymotrypsin, elastase, lipase and kallikrein.

Etiology And Pathogenesis

The most common causal factors of pancreatitis are emotional upset (particularly anger), and improper diet (eating too much at one meal, and excessive intake of alcohol). The pathogenesis is quite complicated from the perspective of traditional Chinese medicine. The pathogenetic links include depression of the *qi* function, accumulation of pathogenic factors, exuberance of heat or damp-heat, stasis of blood, and adverse flow of *qi* and blood. In modern Western medicine, they correspond to functional disorders, obstruction, inflammation, circulatory disturbances and toxic shock, respectively.

The course of pancreatitis can be divided into three stages. In the early stage, genuine *qi* is strong and the pathological changes are mild, manifested chiefly by depressed *qi* function and accumulated pathogenic factors. In the intermediate stage, genuine *qi* is still adequate, but the pathological changes become severer, usually manifested by accumulated pathogenic factors, exuberant heat or damp-heat and blood stasis. In the late stage, genuine *qi* is inadequate. If the pathogenic factors penetrate deeply, shock and other complications may occur; and if the pathogenic factors linger, the disease becomes chronic, with repeated recurrence.

Syndrome Differentiation

Pancreatitis is a diagnosis of Western medicine. After the diagnosis is established, the crucial point is to determine whether the case is acute or chronic, severe or mild. Mild or moderate cases (usually called "edematous pancreatitis" in Western medicine) can be treated with Chinese medicine alone, but in severe cases ("necrotizing pancreatitis" in Western medicine) herbal medication should not be used to replace surgical intervention. Acute pancreatitis of mild or moderate severity and chronic pancreatitis can be classified as follows:

1. Stagnation of Liver *qi*: Epigastric and hypochondriac pain and distension, accompanied by belching, retching and constipation, or by alternate chills and fever; thin yellow coating of the tongue, stringy or stringy and tense pulse. This pattern often occurs in mild cases of acute pancreatitis or chronic pancreatitis.

2. Excessive heat in the Spleen and Stomach: Stabbing abdominal pain with tenderness, accompanied by nausea, vomiting, chills and high fever, thirst, concentrated urine, constipation, reddened tongue with thick, dry, yellow coating, and full, rapid pulse, as seen in acute pancreatitis of moderate severity.

3. Damp-heat in the Liver and Gallbladder: Severe pain in the upper abdomen with alternate chills and fever, jaundice, nausea, vomiting, reddened tongue with yellow, greasy coating, and stringy, slippery and rapid pulse. This pattern corresponds to acute pancreatitis complicated with biliary infection.

4. Weakness of the Spleen and Stomach: Repeated attacks of abdominal pain accompanied by lassitude, belching, abdominal distension, loose stools, emaciation, plump tongue with white, greasy coating, and soft, weak pulse. The syndrome is often

encountered in chronic pancreatitis or the convalescence stage of acute pancreatitis.

Herbal Medication

1. Stagnation of Liver *qi*
Principle of treatment: To relieve *qi* stagnation.
Formula of choice: *Da Chaihu Tang* (Major Bupleurum Decoction).
2. Excessive heat in the Spleen and Stomach
Principle of treatment: To purge toxic heat.
Formula of choice: *Da Chengqi Tang* (Drastic Purgative Decoction) plus *Radix Scutellariae* (skullcap root), *Rhizoma Coptidis* (goldthread rhizome) and *Caulis Bambusae in Taeniam* (bamboo shavings).
3. Damp-heat in the Liver and Gallbladder
Principle of treatment: To eliminate damp-heat.
Formula of choice: *Longdan Xiegan Tang* (Decoction of Gentian to Purge the Liver) plus *Da Chaihu Tang* (Major Bupleurum Decoction).
In all the above three patterns the formulas contain *Radix et Rhizoma Rhei* (rhubarb).
4. Weakness of the Spleen and Stomach
Principle of treatment: To invigorate the Spleen, replenish *qi* and arrest diarrhea.
Formula of choice: *Shen Ling Baizhu San* (Powder of Ginseng, Poria and White Atractylodes).

Acupuncture

Selection of points: Zusanli (ST 36), Xiajuxu (ST 39), Zhongwan (CV 12), Sanyinjiao (SP 6).

Additional points according to symptoms: For vomiting, add Neiguan (PC 6) and Yanglingquan (GB 34); for fever, add Quchi (LI 11) and Hegu (LI 4).

Apply strong stimulation to all the points, and retain the needles.

CHAPTER 19

BLOOD DISORDERS

ANEMIA

Among various kinds of anemias, the management of aplastic anemia is one of most challenging aspects of modern Western medicine. Testosterone is only effective in mild cases. Combined use of Chinese herbal medicine can improve the effect of testosterone. Since various kinds of anemias may show similar syndromes, the following discussion is not limited to aplastic anemia.

Etiology and Pathogenesis

The formation of blood is related to the function of the Heart, Spleen and Kidneys. Weakness of the Spleen depletes the source of *qi* and blood formation. Failure of the Spleen to control blood causes persistent loss of blood, aggravating anemia. The Kidneys govern the bones and the production of bone marrow. Insufficiency of Kidney essence impairs the formation of marrow and the regeneration of blood. The Heart governs blood. Insufficiency of the Heart also leads to anemia.

Syndrome Differentiation

1. Deficiency of both *qi* and blood: Pallor or sallow complexion, dizziness, blurred vision, palpitations, shortness of breath, anorexia, delayed menstrual with pale discharge in women; pale tongue with white coating, and thready, weak pulse.

2. Insufficiency of both Heart and Spleen: Pallor, lassitude, lack of strength, abdominal distension, loose bowel movements, palpitations, insomnia, anorexia, pale tongue, and thready, rapid pulse.

3. Insufficiency of both Spleen and Kidneys: Dizziness, tinnitus, palpitations, shortness of breath, aversion to cold with cool extremities, soreness and weakness of back and knees, abdominal distension, loose bowel movements, pale tongue, and deep, thready pulse.

4. Deficiency of Liver and Kidney *yin*: Pallor, low fever in the afternoon, dizziness, blurred vision, tinnitus, insomnia, soreness and weakness of the back and knees, dryness of the throat and mouth, night sweating, heat sensation in the palms and soles, menorrhagia or incessant menstrual discharge in women, pale tongue with scanty coating, and stringy, thready pulse.

5. Deficiency of both *yin* and *yang*: Pallor, dizziness, tinnitus, soreness and weakness of the back and knees, aversion to cold with cool extremities, spontaneous and night sweating, pale tongue, and deep, thready and weak pulse or deep, thready and rapid pulse.

Herbal Medication

1. Deficiency of both *qi* and blood

Principle of treatment: To replenish *qi* and blood.

Formula of choice: *Bazhen Tang* (Decoction of Eight Precious Ingredients) plus *Radix Astragali* (milkvetch root).

2. Insufficiency of both Heart and Spleen

Principle of treatment: To invigorate the Spleen, replenish *qi* and nourish Heart blood.

Formula of choice: *Guipi Tang* (Spleen-invigorating Decoction).

3. Insufficiency of both Spleen and Kidneys

Principle of treatment: To invigorate the Spleen and reinforce the Kidneys.

Formula of choice: *Sijunzi Tang* (Decoction of four Noble Ingredients) and *Zuogui Yin* (Yin-directing Decoction) plus *Rhizoma Curculiginis* (curculigo rhizome) and *Herba Epimedii* (epimedium).

4. Deficiency of Liver and Kidney *yin*

Principle of treatment: To nourish Liver and Kidney *yin*.

Formula of choice: *Da Buyuan Jian* (Major Origin-tonic Decoction)[1].

5. Deficiency of both *yin* and *yang*

Principle of treatment: To tonify both *yin* and *yang*.

Formula of choice: *Shiquan Dabu Wan* (Pill of Ten Powerful Tonics) plus *Radix Polygoni Multiflori* (fleeceflower root) and *Radix Morindae Officinalis* (morinda root).

Patent Medicines

Deficiency of both *qi* and blood: *Bazhen Wan* (Pill of Eight Precious Ingredients).

Insufficiency of both the Heart and the Spleen: *Renshen Guipi Wan* (Spleen-invigorating Pill with Ginseng).

Insufficiency of both the Spleen and the Kidneys: *Sijunzi Wan* (Pill of Four Noble Ingredients) plus *Zuogui Wan* (Yin-directing Pill).

Deficiency of Liver and Kidney *yin*: *Da Buyuan Jian Wan* (Pill of Major Origin-tonic Decoction).

Deficiency of both *yin* and *yang*: *Shiquan Dabu Wan* (Pill of Ten Powerful Tonics).

---

[1] *Da Buyuan Jian* (Major Origin-tonic Decoction): *Fructus Corni* (dogwood fruit) 9 g, *Rhizoma Dioscoreae* (Chinese yam) 9 g, *Cortex Eucommiae* (eucommia bark) 9 g, *Radix Angelicae Sinensis* (Chinese angelica root) 9 g, *Fructus Lycii* (wolfberry) 9 g, *Radix Codonopsis* (tangshen) 15 g, *Radix Rehmanniae Preparata* (prepared rehmannia root) 15 g, and *Radix Glycyrrhizae* (licorice root) 6 g, to be made into a decoction. It is also made into ready-to-use honey pills, called *Da Buyuan Jian Wan* (Pill of Major Origin-tonifying Decoction).

Acupuncture

Acupuncture may be helpful in mild cases of anemia. The following points are often used: Zusanli (ST 36), Hegu (LI 4), Gaohuangshu (BL 43), Geshu (BL 17), and Xuanzhong (GB 39), with moderate stimulation and 30-60 minutes retention of needles.

LEUKOPENIA

In traditional Chinese medicine there is no such a diagnosis as leukopenia. The decreased blood white cell count can only be recognized by means of modern laboratory techniques, but patients with leucopenia can be effectively treated with traditional therapies.

Etiology and Pathogenesis

According to Chinese medical concepts, the production of white blood cells is believed to be closely related to the Spleen and Kidneys. Congenital insufficiency, excessive strain, and sexual overindulgence may impair the Kidney function, resulting in diminished production of *qi* and blood. An improper diet often gives rise to dysfunction of the Spleen and Stomach. In the long run, blood disorders develop. In exogenous affections, when the pathogens invade the blood system or the bone marrow, leukopenia occurs. The use of toxic drugs may also impair the Spleen and Kidneys, leading to inhibition of blood production. Recent studies have revealed that Spleen and Kidney tonics are useful for the prevention and treatment of leukopenia caused by chemotherapy and radiotherapy in cancer patients.

Syndrome Differentiation

1. Insufficiency of both the Heart and the Spleen: Lassitude, lack of strength, dizziness, blurred vision, insomnia, palpitations, anorexia, abdominal distension, loose stools, pale tongue with thin white coating, and thready, weak pulse.

2. Deficiency of both *qi* and blood: Pallor, palpitations, insomnia, hot sensation in the palms and soles, dizziness, blurred vision, lack of strength, spontaneous or night sweating, pale tongue, and thready, weak pulse.

3. Deficiency of Spleen and Kidney *yang*: Lassitude, lack of strength, dizziness, tinnitus, abdominal distension, loose stools, aching and weakness of the lower back and knees, aversion to cold with cold limbs, pale and plump tongue with tooth prints, and deep, thready pulse.

Herbal Medication

1. Insufficiency of both the Heart and the Spleen

Principle of treatment: To tonify the Heart and the Spleen.

Formula of choice: *Guipi Tang* (Spleen-Invigorating Decoction) plus *Caulis*

Spatholobe (spatholobus stem).

2. Deficiency of both *qi* and blood

Principle of treatment: To replenish *qi* and blood.

Formula of choice: *Bazhen Tang* (Decoction of Eight Precious Ingredients) plus *Radix Astragali* (milkvetch root) and *Caulis Spatholobe* (spatholobus stem).

3. Deficiency of Spleen and Kidney *yang*

Principle of treatment: To warm and tonify the Spleen and Kidneys.

Formula of choice: *Yougui Yin* (*Yang*-directing Decoction).

Leukopenia itself may not produce symptoms. In asymptomatic cases, it is often treated with Spleen or *qi* tonics. Leukopenia is most frequently found in cancer patients who receive chemotherapy and/or radiotherapy. Since chemotherapeutic agents and irradiation usually cause adverse gastrointestinal reactions and general weakness, Spleen and *qi* tonics together with Stomach-pacifying herbs are indicated. Patients with leukopenia are vulnerable to complication of infections. If there is such a complication, the treatment should be first directed to control the infection.

Patent Medicines

Lingzhi Pian (Lucid Ganoderma Tablet), 1 g, 3 times a day, or *Lingzhi Jiaonang* (Lucid Ganoderma Capsule), 2 g, 3 times a day.

Ciwujia Jingao (*Extractum Acanthopanacis Senticosi*, Thorny Acanthopanax Extract), 0.3 g, 3 times a day.

Acupuncture

Principle of treatment: To invigorate the Spleen and replenish *qi*.

Selection of points: Zusanli (ST 36), Sanyinjiao (SP 6), Dazhui (GV 14), Xuehai (SP 10), Pishu (BL 20), Shenshu (BL 23), and Geshu (BL 17).

Manipulation: Reinforcement needling or moxibustion.

CHAPTER 20

RENAL DISEASES

ACUTE GLOMERULONEPHRITIS

The prognosis of acute glomerulonephritis is often good, but in some patients heavy proteinuria leading to nephrotic syndrome may develop. Neither steroids nor cytotoxic drugs are appropriately indicated. Herbal medication in Chinese medicine is useful, and seldom causes side effects.

Etiology and Pathogenesis

In most cases acute glomerulonephritis follows an infection, particularly a pharyngeal or cutaneous infection. From the traditional Chinese medical perspective, the infection is considered an invasion of wind, cold, damp, or toxic heat. Ordinarily, they are common pathogenic factors that cause exogenous affections of the Lungs. Since the Lungs are responsible for regulating the water passages, exogenous pathogens may interfere with the downward flow of water to the Kidneys and Bladder, and hence edema develops, marked in the upper portion of the body. Pathogenic damp that causes cutaneous infection may also impair the Kidney function and induce edema. In both cases, the edema is due to excessiveness of pathogenic factors, and is called "*yang*-edema" in order to differentiate it from "*yin*-edema" occurring in chronic glomerulonephritis and in other conditions characterized by a deficiency state.

Syndrome Differentiation

As an illness of excessiveness, the crucial point of diagnosis is to differentiate the property of the pathogenic factor(s). The common pathogenic factors include wind-cold, wind-heat, wind-damp, and damp-heat.

1. Wind-cold: Chilliness, fever and coughing at the onset, and then oliguria and generalized edema, more marked at the head and face, thin and white tongue coating, and floating and tense pulse (but deep pulse if the wrist is edematous).

2. Wind-heat: Oliguria and puffiness of the eyelids after an attack of sore throat with fever; thin yellow tongue coating, and slippery and rapid pulse.

3. Cold-damp: Pitting edema over the limbs, oliguria, lassitude, abdominal distention and loose stools, often occurring after drenching, white greasy tongue coating, and deep, soft pulse.

4. Damp-heat: Anasarca, oliguria, dryness and bitterness in the mouth, distress in the chest, abdominal distention, often occurring after a pyogenic skin infection or after upper respiratory infection when the exterior syndromes have disappeared, yellow greasy tongue coating, and slippery, rapid pulse.

Herbal Medication

1. Wind-cold

Principle of treatment: To dispel wind-cold and induce diuresis.

Formula of choice: *Yuebi Tang* (Decoction for Relieving Edema)[1] with substraction of gypsum and addition of *Rhizoma seu Radix Notopterygii* (notopterygium rhizome or root) and *Radix Saposhnikoviae* (saposhnikovia root).

2. Wind-heat

Principle of treatment: To dispel wind-heat and induce diuresis.

Formula of choice: *Yuebi Tang* (Decoction for Relieving Edema) plus *Flos Lonicerae* (honeysuckle flower) and *Fructus Forsythiae* (forsythia fruit).

3. Cold-damp

Principle of treatment: To remove cold-damp and induce diuresis.

Formula of choice: *Wuling San* (Powder of Five Drugs with Poria).

4. Damp-heat

Principle of treatment: To remove damp-heat.

Formula of choice: *Xiaoji Yinzi* (Decoction of Field Thistle)[2].

CHRONIC GLOMERULONEPHRITIS

Chronic glomerulonephritis is a major cause of death from kidney disease, accounting for at least one-third of patients with terminal renal failure requiring dialysis or transplantation. The treatment of chronic glomerulonephritis in Western medicine is only supportive and symptomatic. Although trials with steroids, cytotoxic agents, non-steroidal anti-inflammatory agents and anticoagulants have been performed for many years, unequivocal evidence of a favorable effect has yet to be provided. Chinese herbal therapy is worth recommending in the treatment of this chronic kidney disease, not only for its independent use, but also for its combined use with steroids to minimize the latters' adverse side effects.

---

[1]*Yuebi Tang* (Decoction for Relieving Edema): *Herba Ephedrae* (ephedra) 9 g, *Gypsum Fibrosum* (gypsum) 180 g, *Rhizoma Zingerberis Recens* (fresh ginger) 9 g, *Radix Glyccyrhizae* (licorice root) 5 g, and *Fructus Jujubae* (Chinese date) 6 g, to be made into a decoction.

[2]*Xiaoji Yinzi* (Decoction of Field Thistle): *Radix Rehmanniae* (rehmannia root) 30 g, *Herba Cirsii* (field thistle) 15 g, *Talcum* (talc) 15 g, *Caulis Aristolochiae Manshuriensis* (manshurian dutchmanspipe stem) 9 g, *Pollen Typhae* (cat-tail pollen) 9 g, *Nodus Nelumbinis Rhizomatis* (lotus node) 9 g, *Herba Lophatheri* (lophatherum) 9 g, *Radix Angelicae Sinensis* (Chinese angelica root) 6 g, *Fructus Gardeniae* (cape-jasmine fruit) 9 g, and *Radix Glycyrrhizae* (licorice root) 6 g, to be made into a decoction.

Etiology and Pathogenesis

From the traditional Chinese medical perspective, chronic glomerulonephritis is due to overstrain or fatigue in most cases, and a deficiency condition of the Kidneys and/or the Spleen is the key link in its pathogenesis.

The formation of edema in chronic glomerulonephritis is attributed to deficiency of Kidney *yang* or Spleen *yang*, but not to dysfunction of the Lungs. Only during exacerbation following an upper respiratory infection, the involvement of Lung in the formation of edema is considered.

Protein present in the urine is considered to be a loss of essence which should be normally stored in the Kidneys. Therefore, proteinuria is attributed to insufficiency of the Kidneys. However, the Spleen has the function to send the essence upward. Insufficiency of the Spleen also leads to downward pouring of the essence.

Hypertension is also often encountered in chronic glomerulonephritis. In most cases, hypertension is due to deficiency of *yin* with exuberant *yang*.

Hematuria is often considered to be a manifestation resulting from internally retained damp-heat which injures small renal vessels.

Although the fundamental pathogenesis of chronic glomerulonephritis is deficiency of the Spleen and Kidneys, the presence of exogenous pathogenic factors should not be neglected, particularly if the patient is treated with a large dose of steroids.

Syndrome Differentiation

1. Deficiency of Spleen *qi* with edema: Chronic edema, oliguria, sallow complexion, lassitude, lack of strength, anorexia, loose stools, pale tongue with thin white coating, and deep, relaxed pulse.

2. *Yang* deficiency of the Spleen and Kidneys with anasarca: Generalized edema with ascites, oliguria, pale and puffy complexion, lassitude, lack of strength, aversion to cold with cool limbs, pale and plump tongue with teeth prints, and deep, thready pulse.

3. Deficiency of *qi* and *yin*: No edema or mild edema, pallid complexion, lack of strength, soreness in the back and knees, dizziness, tinnitus, heat sensation in the palms and soles, thin tongue coating, and thready, rapid pulse.

4. *Yin* deficiency of the Liver and Kidneys with exuberant *yang*: Malar flush, dizziness, tinnitus, soreness and weakness of the back and legs, heat sensation in the palms and soles, dryness of the mouth, and stringy, thready pulse.

5. Accumulation of damp-heat: Flushed face, obesity, bitterness in the mouth and dryness of the throat, yellow greasy tongue coating, and slippery, rapid pulse, usually occurring in nephritic patients treated with steroids for long periods.

Herbal Medication

1. Deficiency of Spleen *qi* with edema

Principle of treatment: To invigorate Spleen *qi* and induce diuresis.

Formula of choice: *Fangji Huangqi Tang* (Decoction of Tetrandra and Astragalus)[3].

2. *Yang* deficiency of the Spleen and Kidneys with anasarca: To warm Kidney *yang* and induce diuresis.

Formula of choice: *Zhenwu Tang* (the Water God's Decoction)[4]. Add *Radix Astragali* (milkvetch root) for heavy albuminuria.

3. Deficiency of *qi* and *yin*: To replenish Spleen *qi* and Kidney *yin*.

Formula of choice: *Da Buyuan Jian* (Major Origin-tonic Decoction)[5]. Add *Radix Astragali* (milkvetch root) for heavy albuminuria.

4. *Yin* deficiency of the Liver and Kidneys with exuberant *yang*: To replenish *yin* and subdue the exuberant *yang*.

Formula of choice: *Qi Ju Dihuang Tang* (Rehmannia Decoction with Wolfberry and Chrysanthemum) plus *Ramulus Uncariae cum Uncis* (uncaria stem with hooks) and *Spika Prunellae* (selfheal spike).

5. Accumulation of damp-heat: To remove damp-heat.

Formula of choice: *Zhibai Dihuang Tang* (Rehmannia Decoction with Anemarrhena and Phellodendron) and *Longdan Xiegan Tang* (Decoction of Gentian to Purge the Liver).

In all the above patterns, *Herba seu Radix Cirsii Japonici* (Japanese thistle), *Herba Cirsii* (field thistle) and *Rhizoma Imperatae* (cogongrass rhizome) are added for hematuria.

Patent Medicines

Liuwei Dihuang Wan (Pill of Six Ingredients with Rehmannia) for chronic glomerulonephritis with *yin* deficiency.

Qi Ju Dihuang Wan (Rehmannia Pill with Wolfberry and Chrysanthemum) for chronic glomerulonephritis with renal hypertension.

Jingui Shenqi Wan (Kidney-*qi* Pill of Golden Chamber) for chronic glomerulonephritis with *yang* deficiency.

Shenyan Siwei Pian (Anti-nephritic Tablet of Four Ingredients)[6] for chronic glomerulonephritis with edema and proteinuria.

---

[3]*Fangji Huangqi Tang* (Decoction of Tetrandra and Astragalus): *Radix Stephaniae Tetrandrae* (tetrandra root) 12 g, *Radix Astragali* (milkvetch root) 15 g, *Radix Glycyrrhizae* (licorice root) 6 g, and *Rhizoma Atractylodis Macrocephalae* (white atractylodes rhizome) 9 g, to be made into a decoction.

[4]*Zhenwu Tang* (the Water God's Decoction): *Poria* (fuling) 9 g, *Rhizoma Atractylodis Macrocephalae* (white atractylodes rhizome) 9 g, *Radix Peoniae Alba* (white peony root) 6 g, *Rhizoma Zingiberis Recens* (fresh ginger) 9 g, and *Radix Aconiti Lateralis Preparata* (prepared aconite lateral root) 9 g, to be made into a decoction.

[5]See Footnote 1 of Anemia in Chapter 19.

[6]*Shenyan Siwei Pian* (Anti-nephritic Tablets of Four Ingredients): *Fructus Gardeniae* (cape-jasmine fruit), *Folium Pyrrosiae* (pyrrosia leaf), *Radix Astragali* (milkvetch root), *Radix Scutellariae* (skullcap root)

Appendix:
Use of Herbal Medication in Steroid Therapy

Adverse side effects and complications are inevitable when steroids are used continuously at large doses. The side effects and complications can be divided into two major categories—those arising from prolonged use of large doses and those that, on stopping treatment, occur as a result of suppression of the hypothalamo-pituitary-adrenal axis.

Those in the first category chiefly involve the endocrinological system (weight gain with Cushingoid distribution, moon face, hirsutism, and diabetes mellitus), skeletal system (osteoporosis), neuro-psychiatric changes (insomnia, restlessness, and depression), sodium retention with hypertension, and liability to opportunistic infection. From the Chinese medical perspective, most of these side effects can be considered to be Kidney *yin* deficiency with exuberant *yang* or fire. Herbs to nourish *yin* and purge fire, e.g., *Zhibai Dihuang Tang* (Rehmannia Decoction with Anemarrhena and Phellodendron), are effective for minimizing the side effects. In the course of steroid therapy, it is better to start the herbal decoction in the second week.

During the withdrawal of steroids, the above-mentioned fire manifestations spontaneously disappear, and *yin* deficiency turns to *yang* deficiency. *Qi* tonics, e.g., *Radix Astragali* (milkvetch root) and *Radix Codonopsis* (tangshen), *yang* tonics, e.g., *Herba Epimedii* (epimedium) and *Fructus Psoraleae* (scurfpea fruit), and cold-dispelling herbs, e.g., *Radix Aconiti Lateralis Preparata* (prepared aconite lateral root) and *Cortex Cinnamomi* (cinnamon bark) are then indicated. Combined use of these herbs not only facilitates the withdrawal of steroids, but also greatly prevents the suppression of the hypothalamo-pituitary-adrenal axis.

Subsequent administration of Kidney and Spleen tonics may prevent recurrence after discontinuance of steroids. The common herbal formula used for this purpose is *Da Buyuan Jian* (Major Origin-tonic Brew)[7] plus *Sijunzi Tang* (Decoction of Four Noble Ingredients).

INFECTIONS OF THE URINARY TRACT

Urinary tract infections are a common source of morbidity, and although the introduction of antibiotics and antibacterial chemical agents has greatly reduced their morbidity, the mortality from these infections has remained high. Many patients with end-stage kidney failure have been suffering from chronic pyelonephritis. Lowered human defensive mechanisms may play an important role in rendering the infections intractable and persistent. Chinese medicine emphasizes reinforcing genuine *qi* in chronic infections, and so either herbal medication or acupuncture or both may be used as a complementary therapy in the treatment of urinary tract infections, particularly when they become chronic.

---

[7]See Footnote 1 of Anemia in Chapter 19.

Etiology and Pathogenesis

The pathogens that infect the urinary tract are usually taken as damp-heat because fever, dysuria and turbid urine are the common clinical features. The conditions that often precipitate the infection include lack of cleanness of the external genitalia, sexual activities, pregnancy and delivery.

At the onset, the pathogens invade the Bladder, leading to dysfunction of the Bladder, manifested by frequency and urgency of urination and urodynia. Damp-heat often gives rise to fever and pyuria. If the pathogenic damp-heat is transformed into fire which injures the blood vessels, hematuria ensues. Long-standing infection usually involves the Kidneys, resulting in insufficiency of the Kidneys. When the infection is not properly treated in the acute stage, it turns chronic. Lingering of damp-heat impairs genuine *qi*, and the condition becomes a mixture of excess and deficiency. There may be deficiency of Kidney *yin*, deficiency of *qi* and blood, and deficiency of Spleen and Kidney *yang*. In chronic cases, exacerbation repeatedly occurs, being particularly due to fatigue.

Syndrome Differentiation

The disease chiefly involves the Kidneys and Bladder, and the main pathogenesis is damp-heat in the Bladder with or without Kidney insufficiency. During the acute stage, the condition is usually an excess case, due to accumulation of damp-heat. In chronic cases the pathogens are still present, but on a deficiency basis.

1. Downward pouring of damp heat: Fever with dysuria, frequency and urgency, burning pain in the urethra, suprapubic or lumbar pain, reddened tongue with yellow coating, and slippery, rapid pulse.

2. Deficiency of Kidney *yin* with lingering damp-heat: Dysuria with frequent urination, lumbar aching, dizziness, tinnitus, dryness of the mouth and throat, sometimes accompanied by low fever, slightly reddened tongue with thin yellow coating, and stringy, thready pulse.

3. Deficiency of both *qi* and *yin* with remnant damp-heat: Lumbar aching, lower abdominal distension, lassitude, lack of strength, sometimes accompanied by low fever, dysuria and frequent urination, insomnia, dryness of the mouth, reddened tongue tip, and deep, thready pulse.

4. Deficiency of Spleen and Kidney *yang* with remnant damp-heat: Dysuria with dripping of urine, nocturia, coldness and pain in the loins and knees, puffy face and ankle edema, lassitude, lack of strength, anorexia, abdominal distension, loose stools, pale tongue with thin white coating, and deep, thready and weak pulse.

Herbal Medication

1. Downward pouring of damp heat

Principle of treatment: To clear up toxic heat and relieve strangury.

Formula of choice: *Bazheng San* (Overall Correction Powder) plus *Cortex*

Phellodendri (phellodendron bark).

2. Deficiency of Kidney *yin* with lingering damp-heat

Principle of treatment: To replenish Kidney *yin*, clear up heat, and induce diuresis.

Formula of choice: *Zhi Bai Dihuang Wan* (Rehmannia Pill with Anemarrhena and Phellodendron) plus *Rhizoma Imperata* (cogongrass rhizome) and *Semen Plantaginis* (plantain seed).

3. Deficiency of both *qi* and *yin* with remnant damp-heat

Principle of treatment: To replenish *qi* and *yin*, and clear up heat.

Formula of choice: *Buzhong Yiqi Tang* (Decoction for Reinforcing the Middle Energizer and Replenishing *Qi*) plus *Zhi Bai Dihuang Wan* (Rehmannia Pill with Anemarrhena and Phellodendron).

4. Deficiency of Spleen and Kidney *yang* with remnant damp-heat

Principle of treatment: To warm and tonify the Kidneys and the Spleen, and relieve dysuria.

Formula of choice: *Jisheng Shenqi Wan* (Revivifying Kidney-*qi* Pill) plus *Radix Astragali* (milkvetch root) and *Rhizoma Atractylodis Macrocephalae* (white atractylodes rhizome).

Patent Medicines

Ganlu Xiaodu Dan (Sweet-dew Antiphlogistic Pill)[8] for acute infection of urinary tract with damp-heat syndromes.

Zhi Bai Dihuang Wan (Rehmannia Pill with Anemarrhena and Phellodendron) used during the remission period with *yin* deficiency and remnant damp-heat.

Acupuncture

1. Acute stage

Selection of points: Weizhong (BL 40), Xialiao (BL 34), Yinlingquan (SP 9), and Shugu (BL 65).

Additional points according to symptoms: For fever, add Quchi (LU 11); for hematuria, add Xuehai (SP 10) and Sanyinjiao (SP 6); for dribbling of urine, add Guanyuan (CV 4) and Qihai (CV 6); for lower abdomen distension and pain, add Ququan (LR 8).

2. Chronic stage.

Selection of points: Weizhong (BL 40), Yingu (KI 10), Fuliu (KI 7), Zhaohai (KI 6),

[8]*Ganlu Xiaodu Dan* (Sweet-dew Antiphlogistic Pills): *Talcum* (talc), *Herba Artemisiae Scopariae* (oriental wormwood), *Radix Scutellariae* (skullcap root), *Rhizoma Acori Tatarinowii* (grass-leaved sweetflag), *Bulbus Fritillariae Cirrhosae* (tendrilled fritillary bulb), *Caulis Aristolochiae Manshuriensis* (manchurian dutch-manspipe stem), *Rhizoma Belamcandae* (belamcanda rhizome), *Fructus Forsythiae* (forsythia fruit), *Herba Menthae* (peppermint), *Fructus Amomi Rotundus* (round cardamom), and *Herba Agastachis* (giant-hyssop) mixed at the ratio of 3:2.2:2:1.2:1:1:0.8:0.8:0.8:0.8:0.8 in weight, and made into pills, 9 g, 2 times a day.

and Taixi (KI 3).

Additional points according to symptoms: For backache, add Guanyuan (CV 4) and Shenshu (BL 23); for night sweating, add Fuliu (KI 7, reinforcement) and Hegu (LI 4, reduction); for frequent and painful urination, add Zhongji (CV 3) and Yinlingquan (SP 9).

Adjuvant points according to syndrome differentiation: For deficiency of both *qi* and *yin* with remnant damp-heat, add Qihai (CV 6) and Zhongwan (CV 12); for deficiency of Spleen and Kidney *yang* with remnant damp-heat, add Guanyuan (CV 4) and Shenshu (BL 23) for moxibustion.

URINARY STONE AND RENAL COLIC

In the past, a urinary stone could be removed only by a surgical operation if it did not pass spontaneously. In Western medicine, the spontaneous passage of stones is chiefly aided by maintaining a high fluid intake and a short burst of vigorous diuretic therapy. Now, extracorporeal lithotripsy can cause in situ fragmentation of stones in the kidneys or proximal ureter. This greatly improves the non-surgical treatment of urolithiasis. Even then, Chinese medical treatment is still of use. Acupuncture usually gives immediate relief of renal colic caused by urinary stones; herbal medicines promote the passage of small stones or stone fragments after lithotripsy, dissolve urinary stones of certain patterns, and prevent stone recurrence.

Etiology and Pathogenesis

Damp-heat accumulated in the lower energizer evaporates fluid, making the impure substances of the urine precipitate and forming calculi. When the calculus obstructs the urinary tract, impairing the related *qi* function, stagnation of *qi* causes colicky pain. *Qi* stagnation may lead to blood stasis, which aggravates the pain. In addition, heat injures the vessels, leading to frenetic movement of the blood, and hence hematuria. In a lengthy course of the illness, the Spleen and Kidneys are impaired, manifested by dull pain in the loins, listlessness and thready pulse.

Syndrome Differentiation

1. Downward pouring of damp-heat: Sudden onset of severe or colicky pain in the loins or flank, radiating downwards, accompanied by frequency and urgency of painful urination, hematuria, bitterness in the mouth, and fever, yellow greasy tongue coating, and slippery, rapid pulse.

2. *Qi* stagnation and blood stasis: Distending pain in the loins or flank, dull, prickly or colicky, and fixed in location, accompanied by hematuria, dark complexion, purple dark tongue or purple spots on the tongue, and thready, hesitant pulse.

3. Kidney insufficiency: Dull or colicky pain in the loins or flank, aggravated by fatigue, accompanied by dripping of urine after micturition, soreness and weakness of the

back and knees or irregular menstruation, listless complexion, and deep, thready pulse.

Herbal Medication

1. Downward pouring of Damp-heat: To clear damp-heat and expel stones.

Formula of choice: *Niaodao Paishi Tang* (Decoction for Expelling Urinary Stones)[9].

2. *Qi* stagnation and blood stasis: To regulate *qi*, activate blood and expel stones.

Formula of choice: *Shaofu Zhuyu Tang* (Decoction for Removing Blood Stasis in the Lower Abdomen) plus *Herba Lysimachiae* (loosestrife).

3. Insufficiency of the Spleen and Kidneys: To tonify the Spleen and Kidneys, and expel stones.

Formula of choice: *Buzhong Yiqi Tang* (Decoction for Reinforcing the Middle Energizer and Replenishing *Qi*) and/or *Liuwei Dihuang Tang* (Decoction of Six Ingredients with Rehmannia) plus *Herba Lysimachiae* (loosestrife) and *Spora Lygodii* (climbing-fern spores).

4. Deficiency of Kidney *yang*: To warm the Kidneys and expel stones.

Formula of choice: *Yougui Yin* (*Yang*-directing Decoction) plus *Herba Lysimachiae* (loosestrife) and *Spora Lygodii* (climbing-fern spores).

Patent Medicines

Jinqiancao Chongji (Loosestrife Granule)[10] chiefly for prevention of stone recurrence.

Herba Lysimachiae (loosestrife), 30 g daily to be taken as tea. Its action of dissolving phosphate and oxalate stones has been demonstrated.

Acupuncture

Common points: Shenshu (BL 23), Jingmen (GB 25), Pangguangshu (BL 28), and Zhongji (CV 3).

Adjuvant points according to syndrome diagnosis:

Downward pouring of damp-heat: Yinlingquan (SP 9), Sanyinjiao (SP 6), Weiyang (BL 39), and Taichong (LR 3).

Qi stagnation and blood stasis: Qihai (CV 6), Xuehai (SP 10), and Zusanli (ST 36).

Insufficiency of the Spleen and Kidneys: Pishu (BL 20), and Guanyuan (CV 4).

Additional points according to the location of the stone:

---

[9]Niaodao Paishi Tang (Decoction for Expelling Urinary Stones): Herba Lysimachiae (loosestrife) 30 g, Spora Lygodii (climbing-fern spores) 18 g, Folium Pyrrosiae (pyrrosia leaf) 15 g, Rhizoma Sparganii (burreed tuber) 9 g, Otolithum Pseudosciaenae (otolith) 15 g, Semen Persicae (peach seed) 9 g, Radix Cyathulae (cyathula root) 9 g, Talcum (talc) 18 g, Semen Vaccariae (cow-herb seed) 9 g, to be made into decoction.

[10]*Jinqiancao Chongji* (Loosestrife Granule): *Herba Lysimachiae* (loosestrife), *Folium Pyrrosiae* (pyrrosia leaf), and *Herba Plantaginis* (plantain).

The kidney or upper portion of the ureter: add Sanjiaoshu (SP 6), Tianshu (ST 25), and Qihai (CV 6).

The middle or lower portion of the ureter: add Shuidao (ST 28), and Ciliao (BL 32).

Reducing manipulation with repeated strong stimulation is recommended. It is advisable to retain the needles at least for 30 minutes after the colicky condition is ameliorated.

RETENTION OF URINE

Non-obstructive retention of urine, such as occurs in postoperative and postpartum conditions is often immediately relieved by acupuncture, but in retention of urine due to obstruction by organic lesions acupuncture is not indicated.

Acupuncture

Selection of points: Ciliao (BL 32), Zhongliao (BL 33), Baihuanshu (BL 30), Shenshu (BL 23), Sanjiaoshu (BL 22), Zhongji (CV 3), Qugu (CV 2), Sanyinjiao (SP 6), and Yinlingquan (SP 9).

When needling the points of the lower abdomen and back, it is preferable to direct the acupuncture sensation downwards to the urethra or perineum.

INCONTINENCE OF URINE

Incontinence of urine is often due to insufficient function of the Kidneys or sinking of Spleen *qi*, which makes the Bladder unable to restrain a natural urine discharge. In addition, incontinence of urine also occurs in paraplegia.

Acupuncture

The treatment principle is to invigorate the Spleen and reinforce the Kidneys for improving the Bladder function.

Selection of points: Zhongji (CV 3), Guanyuan (CV 4), Qihai (CV 6), Dahe (KI 12), Sanyinjiao (SP 6), Taixi (KI 3), Fuliu (KI 7), Mingmen (GV 4), Shenshu (BL 23), and Qihaishu (BL 24). Uniform reinforcement-reduction manipulation with 20-30 minutes retention of needles is advisable. Select three or four of above points in one session of treatment every other day. A course of treatment consists of ten sessions.

MALE INFERTILITY

The causes of male infertility are multifarious, ranging from various abnormalities of the generative organs to abnormalities of intercourse. Unfortunately, in modern Western medicine it is unusual to find a remediable cause of infertility in the male, and the treatment of the cause can be achieved in only a minority of instances. Chinese medicine views the problem from a different angle, and it does help some of the subjects who have not been benefited by Western medicine.

Etiology and Pathogenesis

Abnormalities of spermatogenesis (such as oligospermia, azoospermia, and cacospermia) and most abnormalities of intercourse (such as impotence, and retrograde ejaculation) are attributed to insufficiency of the Kidneys, either Kidney *yin* or Kidney *yang*. Since Kidney essence (including sperm) and blood are of the same source, abnormalities of spermatogenesis may also be related to deficiency of *qi* and blood. In addition, infection of genital organs, and varicocele that cause seminal abnormalities are considered as damp-heat affection and stasis of Liver vessels respectively.

Syndrome Differentiation

1. Deficiency of Kidney *yin*: Soreness of the back and weakness of the legs, dryness of the mouth, heat sensation in the palms and soles, constipation, reddened tongue with scanty coating, and thready, rapid pulse; abnormalities of sperm, including decreased volume of the ejaculate, absence of liquefaction, aspermia or oligospermia.

2. Deficiency of Kidney *yang*: Soreness of the back and weakness of the legs, aversion to cold with cool limbs, desire for hot drinks, impotence or inability to maintain an erection to achieve ejaculation, loose stools, frequent diluted urination, plump tongue with thin white and moistened coating, and deep, weak pulse; thin seminal fluid with decreased number and reduced motility of sperms.

3. Deficiency of *qi* and blood: Lassitude and lack of strength, pale tongue with scanty coating, and deep, thready pulse, or abnormalities of sperm with no subjective symptoms.

4. Downward pouring of damp-heat: Dull pain in the lower abdomen, heavy sensation in the legs, lassitude, lack of strength, dryness of the mouth, frequent and turbid urination, wetness of the scrotum, reddened tongue with yellow greasy coating, and slippery, rapid pulse; leukocytes in the seminal fluid with decreased number and reduced motility of sperm.

5. Stasis of Liver vessels: Varicocele, often on the left side, accompanied by dull pain in the lower abdomen, oligospermia and low motility of sperms.

Herbal Medication

1. Deficiency of Kidney *yin*
Principle of treatment: To replenish Kidney *yin*.
Formula of choice: *Zuogui Yin* (*Yin*-directing Decoction).
2. Deficiency of Kidney *yang*
Principle of treatment: To invigorate Kidney *yang*.

Formula of choice: *Yougui Yin* (*Yang*-directing Decoction).

3. Deficiency of *qi* and blood

Principle of treatment: To replenish *qi* and blood, and tonify the Kidneys.

Formula of choice: *Gui Lu Erxian Jiao* (Tortoise-Deerhorn Immortals Glue)[11] plus *Wuzi Yanzong Wan* (Pill of Five Kinds of Seeds for Offspring).

4. Downward pouring of damp-heat

Principle of treatment: To remove damp-heat from the Lower Energizer.

Formula of choice: *Longdan Xiegan Tang* (Decoction of Gentian to Purge the Liver) plus *Semen Cuscutae* (dodder seed), *Radix Dipsaci* (teasel root) and *Radix Morindae Officinalis* (morinda root).

5. Stasis of Liver vessels

Principle of treatment: To warm the Liver and promote the patency of its vessels.

Formula of choice: *Nuangan Jian* (Liver-warming Decoction)[12].

Patent Medicines

1. Deficiency of Kidney *yin*: *Zuogui Wan* (*Yin*-directing Pill) or *Zhi Bai Dihuang Wan* (Rehmannia Pill with Anemarrhena and Phellodendron), 6-9 g, 2 times a day.

2. Deficiency of Kidney *yang*: *Yougui Wan* (*Yang*-directing Pill) or *Jinsuo Gujing Wan* (Golden Lock Pill of Semen Discharge), 6-9 g, 2 times a day.

3. Deficiency of *qi* and blood: *Gui Lu Erxian Jiao* (Tortoise-Deerhorn Immortals Glue), 3 g, taken in the morning after mixing with wine and boiling water. *Wuzi Yanzong Wan* (Pill of Five Kinds of Seeds for Offspring), 6 g, 2 times a day.

4. Downward pouring of damp-heat: *Longdan Xiegan Wan* (Gentian Pill to Purge the Liver), 5 g, 3 times a day, until damp-heat syndrome disappears, and then treat according to one of the other syndromes.

5. Stasis of Liver vessels: *Juhe Wan* (Tangerine Seed Pill)[13], 6-9 g, 2 times a day.

Acupuncture

Selection of points: (1) Taixi (KI 3), Sanyinjiao (SP 6), Zusanli (ST 36), Qihai (CV

---

[11]*Gui Lu Erxian Jiao* (Tortoise-Deerhorn Immortals Glue): *Glutinum Plastri Testudinis* (tortoise plastron glue) 12 g, *Gelatinum Cornu Cervi* (deerhorn glue) 9 g, *Fructus Lycii* (wolfberry) 15 g, *Radix Ginseng* (ginseng) 9 g, to be made into a decoction.

[12]*Nuangan Jian* (Liver-warming Decoction): *Radix Angelicae Sinensis* (Chinese angelica root) 9 g, *Fructus Lycii* (wolfberry) 9 g, *Poria* (fuling) 6 g, *Fructus Foeniculi* (fennel) 6 g, *Cortex Cinnamomi* (cinnamon bark) 6 g, *Radix Linderae* (spicebush root) 6 g, and *Lignum Aquilariae Resinatum* (eagle wood) 3 g, to be made into a decoction.

[13]*Juhe Wan* (Tangerine Seed Pill): *Semen Citri Reticulatae* (tangerine seed), *Sargassum* (seaweed), *Thallus Laminariae* (sea tangle), *Fructus Toosendan* (Sichuan chinaberry), *Semen Persicae* (peach seed), *Cortex Magnoliae Officinalis* (medicinal magnolia bark), *Caulis Aristolochiae Manshuriensis* (manchurian dutchmanspipe stem), *Fructus Aurantii Immaturus* (immature bitter orange), *Rhizoma Corydalis* (corydalis tuber), *Cortex Cinnamomi* (cinnamon bark), and *Radix Aucklandiae* (costus root), pulverized, mixed at equal amount in weight, and made into pills; 5 g, 3 times a day.

6), and Shenshu (BL 23); (2) Fuliu (KI 7), Gongsun (SP 4), Lieque (LU 7), Guanyuan (CV 4), and Mingmen (GV 4).

Manipulation: Alternatively use the above two groups of points. Puncturing Taixi (KI 3), Sanyinjiao (SP 6), Zusanli (ST 36), Fuliu (KI 7), Gongsun (SP 4), and Lieque (LU 7), apply uniform reinforcement-reduction with moderate stimulation and retention of needle for 20 minutes. Puncturing Qihai (CV 6) or Guanyuan (CV 4), direct the needle tip downward to cause a transmission of acupuncture sensation down to the external genitalia, and then withdraw the needle immediately. Apply moxibustion to Shenshu (BL 23) and Mingmen (GV 4), and also to Qihai (CV 6) and Guanyuan (CV 4) after needling.

CHAPTER 21

ENDOCRINE AND METABOLIC DISORDERS

HYPERTHYROIDISM

Hyperthyroidism can be well treated with antithyroid therapy (e.g., propylthiouracil) in modern Western medicine. However, leukopenia is a common undesirable side effect of antithyroid drugs, and on rare occasions agranulocytosis occurs. Allergic reactions such as skin rashes, drug fever, and arthralgias are not infrequently encountered. In addition, Western antithyroid therapy usually has no effect on ophthalmopathy; on the contrary, it may sometimes cause enhancement of ophthalmopathy. Chinese herbal medication and acupuncture, though not so effective as propylthiouracil, have no undesirable side effects, and so can be used as complementary treatment. Their effect on ophthalmopathy is worth special investigation.

Etiology and Pathogenesis

Hyperthyroidism is usually related to the emotions. In most cases, it occurs after emotional trauma or stress. The Liver is the first to be affected. Depressed Liver *qi* turns into fire. Fire accumulated in the Liver Meridian impairs Liver *yin,* and subsequently Kidney *yin*, and "kindles" Heart fire, leading to the damage of Heart *yin*. *Yin* deficiency further gives rise to exuberant fire, thus making the illness persistent, even though the emotional trauma or stress is over. Therefore, the main pathogenesis at the initial stage is *yin* deficiency with exuberant fire, with the Liver, Kidneys and Heart involved.

However, impairment of *yin* affects *yang*, and Spleen *yang* is often impaired in this case. Impaired Spleen *yang* leads to production of damp, which turns into phlegm after long-standing retention. Damp-phlegm accumulated in the neck forms a goiter or enlarged thyroid gland. Damp-phlegm can further go upward to the eyes, causing protrusion of the eyeballs (exophthalmos). Fire affecting the Heart causes palpitations. If it affects the Liver, it makes the patient irascible, and if it affects the Stomach, it leads to hyperorexia with emaciation.

Syndrome Differentiation

In most cases, the illness is jumbled with deficiency and excess. The deficiency conditions involve the Liver, Kidneys and Spleen; the excess conditions are related with stagnated *qi*, exuberant fire, and accumulated phlegm.

1. *Yin* deficiency with exuberant fire: Flushing face with abnormally protruded eyeballs, tremors of hands, palpitations, excessive sweating, irascibility, bitterness in the mouth and dryness of the throat, abnormal increase of appetite and food intake but with loss of weight, congested eyes with photophobia, insomnia and dreamful sleep, enlarged thyroid gland, reddened tongue with thin yellow coating, and stringy, rapid or slippery, rapid pulse.

2. Deficiency of both *qi* and *yin*: Oppression feeling in the chest and shortness of breath, palpitations, aversion to heat, excessive sweating, fidgetiness, insomnia, lassitude, lack of strength, emaciation, enlarged thyroid gland, slightly reddened tongue with thin white coating, and thready, rapid pulse.

3. Depressed Liver with insufficiency of the Spleen: Distented feeling in the chest and abdomen, tastelessness in the mouth, anorexia, lassitude, lack of strength, loose stools, abnormally protruding eyes, tremors of the tongue and hands, irregular menstruation in women, enlarged thyroid gland, pale tongue with thin white coating, and stringy, thready pulse.

4. Accumulation of phlegm with stagnated *qi*: Irritability and irascibility, aversion to heat, excessive sweating, abdominal distension, anorexia, hypochondriac pain and distension, enlarged thyroid gland, pale and plump tongue with white, greasy coating, and slippery, rapid pulse.

Herbal Medication

1. *Yin* deficiency with exuberant fire

Principle of treatment: To nourish *yin* and purge fire.

Formula of choice: *Zhi Bai Dihuang Tang* (Rehmannia Pill with Anemarrhena and Phellodendron).

2. Deficiency of both *qi* and *yin*

Principle of treatment: To replenish *qi*, nourish *yin*, and subdue Liver *yang*.

Formula of choice: *Shengmai Yin* (Pulse-activating Drink) plus *Qi Ju Dihuang Wan* (Rehmannia Pill with Wolfberry and Chrysanthemum).

3. Depressed Liver with insufficiency of the Spleen

Principle of treatment: To soothe the Liver, invigorate the Spleen, and resolve phlegm.

Formula of choice: *Xiaoyao San* (Ease Powder) plus *Liujunzi Tang* or *Liujunzi Wan* (Decoction or Pill of Six Noble Ingredients).

4. Accumulation of phlegm with stagnated *qi*

Principle of treatment: To soothe the Liver, regulate the flow of *qi*, and resolve phlegm.

Formula of choice: *Chaihu Shugan San* (Bupleurum Powder for Soothing the Liver).

Patent Medicines

Xiakucao Gao (*Extractum Prunellae Inspissatum*, common selfheal extract), 9 g, 2 times a day.

Acupuncture

Selection of points: Neiguan (PC 6), Jianshi (PC 5), Shenmen (HT 7), Zusanli (ST 36), Sanyinjiao (SP 6), Taixi (KI 3), Fuliu (KI 7), Taichong (LR 3), Zhaohai (KI 6), and Guanyuan (CV 4). Use 4-5 points each time, and puncture with reduction manipulation.

Auxiliary points selected according to symptoms: Add Tianzhu (BL 10), and Fengchi (GB 20) for exophthalmos (preferably direct the acupuncture sensation to the eyes); add Zhongwan (CV 12) for polyphagia.

DIABETES MELLITUS

In traditional Chinese medicine, diabetes is called *xiaoke*, which means emaciation and thirst. As early as in the 2nd century A.D., a formula for treating this illness was initiated, which is still used in the treatment of certain patterns of diabetes mellitus. In 752 A.D., the sweetness of urine was recorded. So, over a long period of time, a mass of therapeutic experience on diabetes mellitus has been collected.

Etiology and Pathogenesis

The causal factors of the illness are either inborn (hereditary) or acquired. The acquired factors include improper diet, particularly excessive intake of sweet food, emotional trauma, overstrain, and exogenous affections. Any of the factors may lead to the production of heat which consumes *yin*, so that dryness-heat impairs the functioning of the Lungs, Stomach and Kidneys, resulting in diabetes mellitus. Therefore, the major pathological changes are *yin* deficiency and dryness-heat.

Syndrome Differentiation

1. Dryness-heat in the Lungs: Dire thirst with strong desire for drinks, polyuria, increased intake of food, loss of body weight, reddened tongue with dry and yellow coating, and slippery, rapid pulse.

2. Dryness-heat in the Stomach: Increased appetite and food intake, thirst, constipation; dry reddened tongue, and forceful pulse.

3. *Yin* deficiency of the Lungs and Kidneys: Polyuria with increased appetite and emaciation, sometimes accompanied by dizziness and blurred vision, reddened tongue with little coating, and thready and rapid pulse.

4. Deficiency of both *yin* and *yang*: Polyuria with turbid creamy urine, dark complexion, dryness of the mouth and throat, aching and weakness of the back and knees, aversion to cold, pale tongue with dry, white coating, and deep, thready and weak pulse.

5. *Qi* deficiency with blood stasis: Thirst but no desire for drinks, numbness of limbs with abnormal sensation, lassitude, lack of strength, dark tongue with purple spots or congested sublingual veins, and deep and hesitant pulse.

Herbal Medication

1. Dryness-heat in the Lungs
Principle of treatment: To purge heat from the Lungs and relieve dryness.
Formula of choice: *Baihu Jia Renshen Tang* (White Tiger Decoction Plus Ginseng).
2. Dryness-heat in the Stomach
Principle of treatment: To purge heat from the Stomach and replenish fluid.
Formula of choice: *Yunü Jian* (Gypsum Decoction)[1] plus Rhizoma Coptidis (goldthread rhizome).
3. *Yin* deficiency of the Lungs and Kidneys
Principle of treatment: To nourish Kidney *yin*.
Formula of choice: *Liuwei Dihuang Wan* (Pill of Six Ingredients with Rehmannia).
4. Deficiency of both *yin* and *yang*
Principle of treatment: To tonify both *yin* and *yang*.
Formula of choice: *Jingui Shenqi Wan* (Kidney-*Qi* Pill of the Golden Chamber).
5. *Qi* deficiency with blood stasis
Principle of treatment: To replenish *qi* and remove blood stasis.
Formula of choice: *Buyang Huanwu Tang* (*Yang*-reinforcing Decoction for Treating Hemiplegia).

Patent Medicines

Dryness in the Lungs and Stomach: *Yuquan Wan* (Jade Spring Pill)[2].
Yin deficiency of the Kidneys: *Liuwei Dihuang Wan* (Pill of Six Ingredients with Rehmannia).
Yang deficiency of the Kidneys: *Jingui Shenai Wan* (Kidney-*Qi* Pill of the Golden Chamber).

Acupuncture

Common points: Feishu (BL 13), Pishu (BL 20), Shenshu (BL 23), Zusanli (ST 36), and Taxi (KI 3).

Adjuvant points according to syndrome differentiation: For dryness-heat in the Lungs, add Shaoshang (LU 11), Yuji (LU 10), Geshu (BL 17), and Xinshu (BL 15); for

---

[1] *Yunü Jian* (Gypsum Decoction): *Gypsum Fibrosum* (gypsum) 15-30 g, *Rhizoma Anemarrhenae* (anemarrhena rhizome) 4.5 g, *Radix Rehmanniae* Preparata (prepared rehmannia root) 9-30 g, *Radix Ophiopogonis* (lilyturf root) 6 g, and *Radix Achyranthis Bidentatae* (twoteethed achyranthes) 4.5 g, to be made into a decoction.

[2] *Yuquan Wan* (Jade Spring Pills): *Radix Trichosanthis* (snakegourd root), *Radix Pueraricae* (kudzuvine root), *Radix Ophiopogonis* (lilyturf root), *Radix Ginseng* (ginseng), *Poria* (fuling), *Fructus Mume* (black plum), *Radix Glycyrrhizae* (licorice root), *Radix Astragali* (milkvetch root), and *Radix Astragali Preparata* (processed milkvetch root) mixed at the ratio of 3:3:2:2:2:2:2:1:1 in weight and made into pills, to be taken 6 g, 2-3 times a day.

dryness-heat in the Stomach, add Zhongwan (CV 12), Weishu (BL 21), Neiting (ST 44), and Sanyinjiao (SP 6); for *yin*-deficiency of the Kidneys, add Guanyuan (CV 4), Fuliu (KI 7), Shuiquan (KI 5), and Mingmen (GV 4).

OBESITY

Limitation of calories below caloric expenditure is often made difficult by the metabolic changes that occur in response to caloric restriction. Anorexiants are frequently used in the Western treatment of obesity. However, problems of habituation, addiction, and drug abuse limit their usefulness. Use of thyroid hormone supplements also produces side effects, particularly in those with cardiovascular complications. Therefore, herbal medication and acupuncture may serve as an alternative or complementary therapy whenever dietary restriction is needed.

Etiology and Pathogenesis

Obesity can be classified as excess and deficient. In excess conditions, improper diet with rich food acts on the Spleen, producing phlegm-damp, which accumulating in the body, leads to obesity. Improper diet may impair the function of the Spleen, giving rise to *qi* deficiency. In the latter case, though obese, the patient is in a deficiency condition.

Syndrome Differentiation

1. Interior accumulation of phlegm-damp: Obesity accompanied by good appetite, dizziness, somnolence, salivation, oppression feeling in the chest, shortness of breath, slow in movement, greasy tongue coating, and slippery pulse.

2. Weakness of the Spleen and Stomach (*qi* deficiency): Obesity accompanied by indolence, lassitude, abdominal distension, loss of appetite, mild edema- of the legs, thin and white tongue coating, and thready pulse.

Herbal Medication

1. Interior accumulation of phlegm-damp

Principle of treatment: To remove phlegm and damp.

Formula of choice: *Daotan Tang* (Phlegm-abducting Decoction)[3].

2. *Qi* deficiency

Principle of treatment: To invigorate the Spleen and replenish *qi*.

[3]*Daotan Tang* (Phlegm-abducting Decoction): *Poria* (fuling) 9 g, *Rhizoma Pinnelliae* (pinellia tuber) 12 g, *Pericarpium Citri Reticulatae* (tangerine peel) 6 g, *Radix Glycyrrhizae* (licorice root) 3 g, *Rhizoma Arisaematis* (Jack-in-the-pulpit tuber) 5 g, *Fructus Aurantii* Immaturus (immature bitter orange) 6 g, and *Rhizoma Zingiberis Recens* (fresh ginger) 3 slices, to be made into a decoction.

Formula of choice: *Liujunzi Tang* (Decoction of Six Noble Ingredients).

Patent Medicines

Phlegm-damp: *Fangfeng Tongsheng Wan* (Miraculous Saposhnikovia Pill).
Qi deficiency: *Jiangzhi Jianfei Chongji* (Lipid-reducing Slimming Granule)[4].

Acupuncture

For obesity of the phlegm-damp pattern, the principle of treatment is to dispel damp and dissolve phlegm. The points used are chiefly Zhongwan (CV 12), Weishu (BL 21), Zusanli (ST 36), Fenglong (ST 40), and Neiguan (PC 6), and application of strong stimulation with reduction manipulation is preferred. For obesity of the *qi*-deficiency type, the treatment is aimed at invigorating the Spleen and replenishing *qi.* The points used are: Pishu (BL 20), Zusanli (ST 36), Qihai (CV 6), Liangqiu (ST 34), and Lieque (LU 7), and application of weak stimulation with reinforcement manipulation is indicated.

---

[4] *Jiangzhi Jianfei Chongji* (Lipid-reducing Slimming Granule): *Radix Salviae Miltiorrhizae* (red sage root), *Rhizoma Alismatis* (water-plantain tuber), *Radix Polygoni Multiflori* (fleeceflower root), *Fructus Crataegi* (hawthorn fruit), *Radix Astragali* (milkvetch root), *Radix Ophiopogonis* (lilyturf root), *Rhizoma Dioscoreae* (Chinese yam), and *Folium Theae* (tea leaf).

CHAPTER 22

GYNECOLOGICAL DISEASES

TRADITIONAL CHINESE FEMALE PHYSIOLOGY

The uterus is an important female organ, from which menstruation originates, and in which the offspring develops before birth. It is considered an "extraordinary organ" because it functions as a *fu*-organ when it discharges the menstrual flow and removes the fetus and placenta during deLivery, but it also acts like a *zang*-organ as it stores the fetus, essence, and blood during pregnancy and the intermenstrual period.

Menstruation is the monthly sanguineous discharge peculiar to women. It begins at the age of puberty (13-15 years) and extends to the menopause (around 49 years of age). Normally, the menstrual cycle is about 28 days, and the menstrual period lasts 3-7 days. The menstrual blood does not coagulate, and there is only mild abdominal soreness during menstrual discharge.

Leukorrhea is a whitish, viscid and odorless secretion, discharged from the vagina. From the traditional Chinese medical perspective, leukorrhea is a kind of *yin*-fluid stored in the Kidneys, governed by Conception Vessel, and restrained by Belt Vessel. The secretion moistens the vagina, and increases in amount around the menstrual period, during the ovulation period and pregnancy.

Pregnancy is the condition being with child, marked by cessation of the menses, nausea in the morning, and progressive enlargement of the abdomen. The duration of pregnancy is about 280 days. After deLivery, the breasts secrete milk to feed the infant.

Menstruation, leukorrhea secretion, pregnancy and lactation are all related with the function of the *zang-fu* organs, meridians, *qi* and blood, "tiankui" (sex-stimulating essence) and the uterus.

***Qi* and blood** are the material basis from which menstruation, pregnancy and lactation originate. The main constituent of menses is blood. During pregnancy essence and blood are needed for nourishing the fetus. Milk is produced from blood. However, the production, circulation, and regulation of blood all depend on the function of *qi*. So, it is said in traditional Chinese medicine that female physiology is based on *qi* and blood.

The Liver, Spleen and Kidneys are the *zang*-organs closely related to the female physiology. The Kidneys store essence and are responsible for reproduction. Only when the Kidney *qi* is exuberant and enough *tiankui* is produced at the due time, the Thoroughfare and Conception Vessels will be full, and menstruation, vaginal secretion and pregnancy will be normal.

The Spleen has the function of digestion and transportation, and the Stomach receives the food taken. The two organs are the source of *qi* and blood, and hence are also closely related to menstruation, pregnancy and lactation.

The Liver, a reservoir of blood, has the function of smoothing and regulating the flow of *qi* and blood, and so adjusts the menstrual cycle and the amount of menstrual discharge.

The Thoroughfare, Conception, Governor and Belt Vessels are the meridians directly related to the female physiology. The Thoroughfare Vessel, also called the "sea of blood," originates in the uterus in women. The blood from all *zang-fu* organs converges in the Thoroughfare Vessel. When the Thoroughfare Vessel fills at regular intervals, a normal menstrual cycle is formed. During pregnancy, menstruation ceases and the blood in the Thoroughfare Vessel is used for nourishing the fetus.

The Conception Vessel, the "sea of *yin* meridians," also originates in the uterus in women, governs all the essence, blood and fluid, and provides the major source for nourishing the fetus.

The Governor Vessel, the "sea of *yang* meridians," rules *yang qi* in the human body. The Governor and Conception Vessels, communicating with each other, regulate *qi* and blood, and maintain the normal female physiology.

The Belt Vessel runs around the waist, meeting the Thoroughfare, Conception and Governor Vessels, and restraining the function of the latter three vessels, so that *qi* and blood flowing to the uterus can be kept when a normal range.

Tiankui is the Chinese name for sex-stimulating essence in both men and women. It is an essence produced and stored in the Kidneys, and has the action of promoting development, regulating menstruation and facilitating reproduction.

TRADITIONAL CHINESE FEMALE PATHOLOGY

The Etiology and pathogenesis of gynecological diseases are the same as those of internal diseases, but the following points are often emphasized:

1. Exogenous pathogenic factors, especially cold, heat and damp are apt to involve blood in women, leading to blood stasis.

2. Emotional factors often easily cause disturbances of *zang-fu* organs in women.

3. Dysfunction of *zang-fu* organs, particularly dysfunction of the Liver, Spleen and Kidneys, is the rudimentary pathogenesis of gynecological diseases. The Kidneys govern the Conception Vessel, the Liver rules the Thoroughfare Vessel, and the Spleen is in charge of the Belt Vessel. Insufficiency of the Kidneys often gives rise to irregular menstruation, threatened abortion, infertility, or amenorrhea; depression of the Liver causes dysmenorrhea, epimenorrhea, or amenorrhea; insufficiency of the Spleen leads to prolapse of the uterus, metrorrhagia or metrostaxis.

4. Disorders of *qi* and blood are the main pathogenetic link in gynecological diseases. Most of the above etiological factors acting on *qi* and blood, lead to *qi* stagnation, *qi* deficiency, blood deficiency, blood stasis, cold or heat in blood, and hence various illnesses marked by abnormal menstruation, morbid leukorrhea, infertility or untimely

delivery.

5. Impairment of the Thoroughfare, Conception, Governor and Belt Vessels directly causes gynecological diseases, as the three vessels originate in the uterus, and the last one regulates all of them.

DYSMENORRHEA

Dysmenorrhea is a common complaint in women of childbearing age. Although organic diseases may be found in a considerable proportion of the patients, dysmenorrhea due only to functional disorders is not infrequently encountered. In the latter cases, Chinese medicine, including acupuncture, can often give much help.

Etiology and Pathogenesis

Dysmenorrhea is chiefly due to impeded flow of *qi* and blood, which may be caused by the following factors:

Emotional disturbances. Stagnation of *qi* and blood in the uterus produces pain during menstruation.

Living in a cold, damp place or exposure to cold while wading across a river, or excessive intake of cold and raw food may lead to lingering of cold in the uterus. Congealing of blood by cold impedes the blood flow and causes pain.

In individuals with chronic diseases or weak constitutions, *qi* and blood are usually inadequate. When the blood supply to the uterine vessels is insufficient, the blood flow will also be impeded, causing pain.

Syndrome Differentiation

1. *Qi* stagnation: Lower abdominal pain preceding or during the menstrual period, referring to the flanks and chest, decreased amount of menstrual flow mixed with blood clots, irritability, thin and white tongue coating, and stringy pulse.

2. Blood stasis: Lower abdominal cramps preceding or during the menstrual period, stabbing in character and aggravated by pressure, decreased amount of dark menstrual blood mixed with clots, and alleviation of pain after discharge of clots, purple tongue or purple spots on the tongue, and deep and hesitant pulse.

3. Congealed cold: Lower abdominal pain accompanied by a cold sensation and tenderness preceding or during the menstrual period, alleviated by warmth, delayed and scanty menstruation, and presence of blood clots, dark tongue with white greasy coating, and deep and tense pulse.

4. Deficiency of *qi* and blood: Continuous dull pain during and following the menstrual period, alleviated by warmth and pressure, scanty pale-colored menstrual flow, pallor, lassitude, lack of strength, palpitations, shortness of breath, pale tongue with thin coating, and thready and weak pulse.

Herbal Medication

1. *Qi* stagnation

Principle of treatment: To smooth the flow of *qi* and relieve pain.

Formula of choice: *Xiaoyao San* (Ease Powder) plus *Rhizoma Corydalis* (corydalis tuber).

2. Blood stasis

Principle of treatment: To remove blood stasis and relieve pain.

Formula of choice: *Shaofu Zhuyu Tang* (Decoction for Removing Blood Stasis in the Lower Abdomen) plus *Rhizoma Corydalis* (corydalis tuber).

3. Congealed cold

Principle of treatment: To dispel cold-damp, regulate the flow of *qi* and remove blood stasis.

Formula of choice: *Wenjing Tang* (Menses-warming Decoction)[1] plus *Rhizoma Corydalis* (corydalis tuber).

4. Deficiency of *qi* and blood

Principle of treatment: To reinforce *qi* and blood.

Formula of choice: *Shiquan Dabu Wan* (Pill of Ten Powerful Tonics).

Patent Medicines

Qi stagnation and blood stasis: *Yimu Wan* (Motherwort Pill)[2].

Congealed cold with blood deficiency: *Aifu Nuangong Wan* (Uterus-warming Pill of Argyi and Cyperus).

Deficiency of *qi* and blood: *Bazhen Yimu Wan* (Pill of Eight Precious Ingredients with Motherwort)[3].

Acupuncture

Common points: Guanyuan (CV 4), Zhongji (CV 3), Ciliao (BL 32), Diji (SP 8), and Xuehai (SP 10).

Additional points according to syndrome differentiation: For *qi* stagnation and blood

---

[1] *Wenjing Tang* (Menses-warming Decoction): *Fructus Evodiae* (evodia fruit) 9 g, *Radix Angelicae Sinensis* (Chinese angelica root) 9 g, *Radix Peoniae Rubra* (red peony root) 6 g, *Rhizoma Chuanxiong* (chuanxiong) 6 g, *Radix Ginseng* (ginseng) 6 g, *Ramulus Cinnamomi* (cinnamon twig) 6 g, *Colla Corii Asini* (donkey-hide gelatin) 9 g, *Cortex Moutan* (moutan bark) 6 g, *Rhizoma Zingiberis Recens* (fresh ginger) 6 g, *Radix Glycyrrhizae* (licorice root) 6 g, *Rhizoma Pinelliae* (pinellia tuber) 6 g, and *Radix Ophiopogonis* (lilyturf root) 9 g, to be made into a decoction.

[2] *Yimu Wan* (Motherwort Pill): *Herba Leonuri* (motherwort), *Radix Angelicae Sinensis* (Chinese angelic root), *Rhizome Chuanxiong* (chuanxiong), and *Radix Aucklandiae* (costus root), mixed at the ratio of 8:4:2:0.75 in weight, and made into honey pills to be taken 9 g, 3 times a day.

[3] *Bazhen Yimu Wan* (Pill of Eight Precious Ingredients with Motherwort): honey pills made of *Bazhen Wan* (Pill of Eight Ingredients) plus *Herba Leonuri* (motherwort), to be taken 9 g, 2 times daily, starting one week before the menstrual period.

stasis, add Taichong (LR 3) and *Qi*chong (ST 30); for congealed cold, add Shuidao (ST 28) and Dahe (KI 12); for deficiency of *qi* and blood, add Pishu (BL 20) and Sanyinjiao (SP 6).

Start acupuncture one week before the menstrual period, once daily.

DYSFUNCTIONAL UTERINE BLEEDING

Dysfunctional uterine bleeding is abnormal bleeding from the uterus not related to threatened or incomplete abortion or to generalized bleeding diathesis. The causes of dysfunctional uterine bleeding can be divided into those associated with ovulatory cycles and those associated with anovulatory cycles. In Chinese medicine, however, the causal factors of this illness are viewed in a different way.

Etiology and Pathogenesis

The illness is often attributed to the following four factors:

1. Blood heat. Heat invading the Thoroughfare and Conception Vessels causes frenetic movement of the blood, and hence bleeding. In excess conditions, the heat often originates from an exuberant *yang* constitution, spicy hot food, fire transformed from a depressed Liver, or affection by evil heat. In deficiency conditions, the heat may derive from a deficient *yin* constitution, chronic illness, or impairment of *yin* after massive bleeding.

2. Kidney insufficiency. Deficiency of Kidney *qi* may lead to dysfunction of the Thoroughfare and Conception Vessels, manifested by uterine bleeding. Deficiency of Kidney *yin* may give rise to endogenous heat or fire which causes uterine bleeding. In these cases, constitutional insufficiency, climacteric changes and chronic illnesses that involve the Kidneys are the common etiological factors.

3. *Qi* deficiency. Improper diet, overstrain or excessive worry and anxiety impair Spleen *qi*, so that blood cannot be kept flowing within the vessels, resulting in bleeding.

4. Blood stasis. Depressed Liver *qi* due to emotional or psychic trauma often leads to blood stasis. If the stagnated blood is retained in the Thoroughfare and Conception Vessels or during menstruation, it prevents the circulating blood from flowing in the vessels, and hence causes bleeding.

Syndrome Differentiation

1. Bleeding due to excessive heat in blood: Irregular menstruation with advanced period and profuse deep red and thick discharge, flushed face, headache, irritability, dryness of the throat and bitterness in the mouth, constipation, reddened tongue with dry yellow coating, and slippery and forceful pulse.

2. Bleeding due to *yin* deficiency with heat in blood: Prolonged, incessant bleeding with bright red discharge, malar flush, fidgetiness, insomnia, dry and red lips, soreness and weakness of the back and legs, heat sensation in the palms and soles, reddened tongue with little or no coating, and deep, thready pulse.

3. Bleeding due to insufficient Kidney *qi*: Profuse or incessant bleeding with pale-colored discharge, soreness and weakness of the back and knees, aversion to cold with cool limbs, pale tongue with thin coating, and thready pulse, particularly weak at the *chi* section.

4. Bleeding due to *qi* deficiency: Profuse or incessant bleeding with pale-colored and thin discharge, pale and puffy complexion, lassitude, lack of strength, palpitations, spontaneous sweating, loss of appetite, abdominal distension, loose stools, pale tongue with thin coating, and thready and weak pulse.

5. Bleeding due to blood stagnation: Profuse or incessant bleeding with dark red discharge mixed with clots, accompanied by lower abdominal pain which is alleviated after the clots are discharged, dark tongue or purple spots on the tongue, and thready and hesitant pulse.

Herbal Medication

1. Bleeding due to excessive heat in blood
Principle of treatment: To remove heat from blood.
Formula of choice: *Qingjing Tang* (Menses-clearing Decoction)[4].
2. Bleeding due to *yin* deficiency with heat in blood
Principle of treatment: To nourish *yin*, clear heat, and arrest bleeding.
Formula of choice: *Gujing Wan* (Menses-securing Pill)[5].
3. Bleeding due to insufficient Kidney *qi*
Principle of treatment: To tonify Kidney *qi*.
Formula of choice: *Yougui Yin* (*Yang*-directing Decoction).
4. Bleeding due to *qi* deficiency
Principle of treatment: To replenish *qi*.
Formula of choice: *Guipi Tang* (Spleen-invigorating Decoction).
5. Bleeding due to blood stagnation
Principle of treatment: To remove stagnated blood and arrest bleeding.
Formula of choice: *Siwu Tang* (Decoction of Four Ingredients) plus *Shixiao San* (Wonderful Powder for Relieving Pain of Blood Stasis) and *Radix Notoginseng* (notoginseng).

Patent Medicines

Patent medicines can only be used as a maintenance treatment after the bleeding has

---

[4]*Qingjing Tang* (Menses-clearing Decoction): *Cortex Moutan* (Moutan bark) 6 g, *Radix Peoniae Alba* (white peony root) 6 g, *Radix Rehmanniae Preparata* (prepared rehmannia root) 6 g, *Cortex Lycii* (wolfberry bark) 15 g, *Herba Artemisiae Annuae* (sweet wormwood) 6 g, *Poria* (fuling) 3 g, *Cortex Phellodendri* (phellodendron bark) 1.5 g, to be made into a decoction.

[5]*Gujing Wan* (Menses-securing Pill): *Radix Scutellariae* (skullcap root) 30 g, *Radix Peoniae Alba* (white peony root) 30 g, *Plastrum Testudinis* (tortoise plastron) 30 g, *Cortex Ailanthi* (tree-of-heaven bark) 21 g, *Cortex Phellodendri* (phellodendron bark) 9 g, *Rhizoma Cyperi* (flatsedge tuber) 7.5 g, to be made into pills, 9 g, 1-2 times a day.

already been arrested.

Bleeding due to excessive heat in blood: *Gujing Wan* (Menses-securing Pill).

Yin deficiency with heat in blood: *Erzhi Wan* (Pill of Two Solstices)[6].

Bleeding due to *qi* deficiency: *Guipi Wan* (Spleen-invigorating Pill) or *Buzhong Yiqi Wan* (Pill for Reinforcing the Middle Energizer and Replenishing *Qi*)

Acupuncture

Common points: Qihai (CV 6), Sanyinjiao (SP 6), Pishu (BL 20), Ganshu (BL 18), Yinbai (SP 1), and Jiaoxin (KI 8).

Additional points according to syndrome differentiation: For *qi* deficiency, add Yinjiao (CV 7), Zusanli (ST 36), and Gaohuang (BL 43); for blood heat, add Xuehai (SP 10), Dadun (LR 1), and Shuiquan (KI 5); for blood stasis, add Qichong (ST 30), Taichong (LR 3), and Diji (SP 8); and for *yin* deficiency, add Taixi (KI 3) and Yingu (KI 10).

AMENORRHEA

Physiological amenorrhea occurs during pregnancy and lactation, and after menopause. Pathological amenorrhea is defined as failure of menarche by age 16 (primary amenorrhea) or the absence of menstruation for 6 months in a woman with previous periodic menses (secondary amenorrhea). The major underlying physiological derangements include: (1) anatomic defects, (2) ovarian failure, and (3) chronic anovulation with or without estrogen present. Except for anatomic defects, other derangements may be treated with herbal medication and/or acupuncture.

Etiology and Pathogenesis

In traditional Chinese medicine, amenorrhea is classified into two categories: deficiency and excess. The former is usually attributed to deficiency of *qi*, blood, the Liver, and the Kidneys, while the latter to *qi* stagnation, blood stasis and accumulation of phlegm. The common causal factors in the former are abortion, postpartum hemorrhage, and chronic diseases, and those in the latter are usually exogenous affection of wind-cold or cold-damp, and internal injury due to emotional stress.

Syndrome Differentiation

I. Deficiency Syndromes

1. Deficiency of both *qi* and blood: Amenorrhea with dizziness, tinnitus, palpitations, shortness of breath, lassitude, pale tongue, and deep, thready pulse.

---

[6]*Erzhi Wan* (Pill of Two Solstices): *Fructus Ligustri Lucidi* (glossy privet fruit), and *Folium Camptothecae* (camptotheca leaf) mixed and made into honey pills, 15 g, 2 times a day. Glossy privet fruit should be collected at the winter solstice, and camptotheca leaf at the summer solstice, hence the name.

2. Deficiency of Kidney *yang*: Amenorrhea with an old-looking complexion, atrophy of breasts, soreness of the back, aversion to cold, cool limbs, pale tongue with white coating, and deep, relaxed pulse.

3. Deficiency of Kidney *yin*: Amenorrhea with an old-looking complexion, atrophy of breasts, emaciation, heat sensation in the palms and soles, night sweating, peeled tongue coating, and thready, rapid pulse.

II. Excess Syndromes

1. *Qi* stagnation and blood stasis: Amenorrhea with depression, irritability, oppression feeling in the chest, pain in the flank, distension in the lower abdomen, purple tongue edges or purple spots on the tongue, and stringy or hesitant pulse.

2. Obstruction by phlegm: Amenorrhea with obesity, oppression feeling in the chest, abdominal distention, nausea, expectoration, tastelessness in the mouth, white greasy tongue coating, and thready, slippery pulse.

Herbal Medication

I. Deficiency Syndromes

1. Deficiency of both *qi* and blood

Principle of treatment: To replenish *qi* and blood.

Formula of choice: *Bazhen Yimu Wan* (Pill of Eight Precious Ingredients with Motherwort)[7].

2. Deficiency of Kidney *yang*

Principle of treatment: To warm and reinforce the Kidneys.

Formula of choice: *Yougui Yin* (*Yang*-directing Decoction).

3. Deficiency of Kidney *yin*

Principle of treatment: To replenish Kidney *yin*.

Formula of choice: *Liuwei Dihuang Tang* (Decoction of Six Ingredients with Rehmannia).

II. Excess Syndromes

1. *Qi* stagnation and blood stasis

Principle of treatment: To regulate *qi* and remove blood stasis.

Formula of choice: *Shaofu Zhuyu Tang* (Decoction for Removing Blood Stasis in the Lower Abdomen).

2. Obstruction by phlegm

Principle of treatment: To resolve phlegm.

Formula of choice: *Cang Fu Daotan Tang* (Phlegm-abducting Decoction with Atractylodes and Cyperus)[8].

---

[7]*Bazhen Yimu Wan* (Pill of Eight Precious Ingredients with Motherwort): Honey pills consisting of *Bazhen Wan* (Pill of Eight Precious Ingredients) and *Herba Leonuri* (motherwort), 6 g, 2 times a day.

[8]*Cang Fu Daotan Tang* (Phlegm-abducting Decoction with Atractylodes and Cyperus): *Poria* (fuling) 9 g, *Rhizoma Pinelliae* (pinellia tuber) 9 g, *Pericarpium Citri Reticulatae* (tangerine peel) 5 g, *Radix*

Patent Medicines

The following ready-to-use preparations are used for treating amenorrhea of deficiency pattern: *Bazhen Yimu Wan* (Pill of Eight Precious Ingredients with Motherwort), *Danggui Wan* (Chinese Angelica Pill), and *Jixueteng Gao* (Concentrated Decoction of Spatholobus Stem).

The following ready-to-use preparations are used for treating amenorrhea of the excess type: *Xiaoyao Wan* (Ease Pill) for relieving *qi* stagnation, *Yueju Wan* (Pill for Removing Stagnation) for resolving phlegm, and *Yimucao Gao* (*Extractum Leonuri,* Motherwort Extract) for removing blood stasis.

Acupuncture

I. Deficiency Syndromes

Selection of points: Pishu (BL 20), Shenshu (BL 23), Qihai (CV 6), and Zusanli (ST 36).

Manipulation: Reinforcement with moxibustion.

II. Excess Syndromes

Selection of points: Zhongji (CV 3), Hegu (LI 4), Sanyinjiao (SP 6), Xuehai (SP 10), and Fenglong (ST 40).

Manipulation: Reduction. Moxibustion is not indicated.

PREMENSTRUAL SYNDROME

Premenstrual syndrome is a symptom complex of cyclic irritability and depression accompanied by edema, breast engorgement and abdominal bloating, occurring during the few days prior to menses. In Western medicine, since the cause of premenstrual syndrome is not yet clearly known, there is no consensus about therapy. In Chinese medicine, however, much experience in treating this illness has been accumulated, although there is no such diagnostic term as premenstrual syndrome.

Etiology and Pathogenesis

The illness is chiefly related to emotional disturbances and dysfunction of the Liver and the Spleen. Stagnated Liver *qi*, which is transformed into fire, deficiency of blood, which leads to exuberant Liver fire, and deficiency of Spleen and Kidney *yang*, which leads to edema, are the major pathogenic factors.

Glycyrrhizae (licorice root) 3 g, *Rhizoma Arisaematis* (Jack-in-the-pulpit tuber) 9 g, *Rhizoma Atractylodis* (atractylodes rhizome) 9 g, *Rhizoma Cyperi* (cyperus tuber) 12 g, *Fructus Aurantii* (bitter orange) 9 g, *Rhizoma Zingiberis Recens* (fresh ginger) 3 slices, and *Massa Fermentata Medicinalis* (medicated leaven) 9g, to be made into a decoction.

Syndrome Differentiation

1. Stagnation of Liver *qi*: Irregular menstruation with breast engorgement, oppressed feeling in the chest, irritability and insomnia preceding the menstrual period, normal tongue and stringy pulse.

2. Deficiency of Liver blood with exuberant fire: Advanced menstrual period with profuse discharge, preceded by dizziness, headache, irritability, and insomnia, emaciation, reddened tongue, and stringy, rapid pulse.

3. *Yang* deficiency of the Spleen and Kidneys: Delayed menstrual period with scanty, pale discharge, preceded by edema of the face and limbs, or diarrhea, abdominal bloating or discomfort, lassitude; white and slippery tongue coating, and deep or thready, weak pulse.

Herbal Treatment

1. Stagnation of Liver *qi*

Principle of treatment: To soothe the Liver.

Formula of choice: *Xiaoyao San* (Ease Powder) plus *Rhizoma Cyperi* (cyperus tuber), *Radix Curcumae* (turmeric root), and *Radix Salviae Miltiorrhizae* (red sage root).

2. Deficiency of Liver blood with exuberant fire

Principle of treatment: To nourish the Liver and clear fire.

Formula of choice: *Qi Ju Dihuang Wan* (Rehmannia Pill with Wolfberry and Chrysanthemum) plus *Ramulus Uncariae cum Uncis* (uncaria stem with hooks), and *Fructus Tribuli* (puncture-vine fruit).

3. *Yang* deficiency of the Spleen and Kidneys

Principle of treatment: To warm the Kidneys and invigorate the Spleen.

Formula of choice: *Jiangu Tang* (Fortifying Decoction)[9] plus *Rhizoma Zingiberis* (stir-baked ginger), and *Radix Aucklandiae* (costus root).

Patent Medicines

1. Stagnation of Liver *qi*: *Xiaoyao Wan* (Ease Pill), 6 g, 2 times a day, starting from one week before the period up to the end of the period.

2. Deficiency of Liver blood with exuberant fire: *Qi Ju Dihuang Wan* (Rehmannia Pill with Wolfberry and Chrysanthemum), starting one week before the period and up to the end of the period.

3. *Yang* deficiency of the Spleen and Kidneys: *Fuzi Lizhong Wan* (Aconite Pill for Regulating the Middle Energizer), 6 g, 2 times a day, starting one week before the period and up to the end of the period.

---

[9] *Jiangu Tang* (Fortifying Decoction): *Radix Codonopsis* (tangshen) 10 g, *Rhizoma Atractylodis Macrocephalae* (white atractylodes rhizome) 10 g, *Poria* (fuling) 10 g, *Semen Coicis* (coix seed) 10 g, and *Radix Morindae Officinalis* (morinda root) 10 g, to be made into a decoction.

Acupuncture

Selection of points: Hegu (LI 4), Sanyinjiao (SP 6), Shenmen (HT 7), Qihai (CV 6), and Yintang (EX-HN 3)

Uniform reinforcement-reduction manipulation 3-5 days before the menstrual period once a day.

MENOPAUSAL SYNDROME

A considerable number of women in their climacteric periods develop symptoms serious enough to seek medical assistance. The symptoms include hot flushes, irritability, anxiety and nervousness. Since these symptoms are chiefly related to estrogen deficiency, the treatment in Western medicine is appropriate administration of estrogen. However, this therapy has its restraints, for protracted estrogen treatment might induce neoplastic changes in estrogen-sensitive tissues. Therefore, Chinese medicines are useful as an alternative therapy in the treatment of this syndrome.

Etiology and Pathogenesis

The *yin-yang* imbalance in menopausal syndrome is chiefly related to the decline of Kidney *qi* and deficiency of *tiankui* along with the physiological changes. In addition, psychic factors such as overstress and emotional strain may also be blamed for the occurrence of this syndrome.

Syndrome Diagnosis and Treatment

1. Deficiency of Kidney *yin*: flushed face, sweating, fidgetiness, irritability, anxiety, headache, dizziness, tinnitus, soreness of the back, heat sensation in the palms and soles, irregular menstruation with bright red discharge, reddened tongue with scanty coating, and thready and rapid pulse.

2. Deficiency of Kidney *yang*: Dark complexion, listlessness, aversion to cold with cool limbs, soreness and cold feeling in the back and knees, anorexia, abdominal distension, loose stools, maybe accompanied by profuse uterine bleeding or excessive thin leukorrhea; pale or plump tongue with thin white coating and teeth prints, and deep, thready and weak pulse.

3. Deficiency of both Kidney *yin* and *yang*: Sometimes flushed face with a hot sensation and sweating, and sometimes aversion to cold with cool limbs, accompanied by dizziness, tinnitus and soreness of the back, thin tongue coating, and deep and thready pulse.

Herbal Medication

1. Deficiency of Kidney *yin*

Principle of treatment: To nourish Kidney *yin*.

Formula of choice: *Zuogui Yin* (*Yin*-directing Decoction).

2. Deficiency of Kidney *yang*

Principle of treatment: To warm the Kidneys and the Spleen.

Formula of choice: *Yougui Yin* (*Yang*-directing Decoction) plus *Lizhong Wan* (Pill for Regulating the Middle Energizer).

3. Deficiency of both Kidney *yin* and *yang*

Principle of treatment: To tonify both *yin* and *yang*.

Formula of choice: *Erxian Tang* (Decoction of Two Elixirs).

Patent Medicines

Qi Ju Dihuang Wan (Rehmannia Pill with Wolfberry and Chrysanthemum) for deficiency of Kidney *yin*.

Gengnian'an Tablet (Menopause-quieting Tablet)[10] for deficiency of Kidney *yin* or deficiency of both Kidney *yin* and *yang*.

Gengniankang Tablet (Health Tablet for Menopause)[11] for deficiency of Kidney *yang*.

Acupuncture

Selection of points: Baihui (GV 20), Neiguan (PC 6), Shenmen (HT 7), Zusanli (ST 36), Sanyinjiao (SP 6), and Taichong (LR 3).

Uniform reinforcement-reduction manipulation with 20 minutes retention of needles.

INFERTILITY

Infertility, the failure to become pregnant after 2 years of unprotected intercourse, is one of the common complaints for which women seek medical assistance. Here, the male factors that account for infertility are excluded. Among the female factors, failure of ovulation and luteal phase dysfunction cause infertility in a considerable number of women. In these cases, Chinese medicine may have beneficial results. Even in infertility due to pelvic factors, Chinese medical therapy is still worthwhile trying.

Etiology and Pathogenesis

Infertility in women with no congenital defects is mostly due to Kidney insufficiency,

---

[10] *Gengnian'an Tablet* (Menopause-quieting Tablet): *Radix Rehmanniae* (steamed rehmannia root), *Radix Polygoni Multiflori* (fleeceflower root), *Rhizoma Alismatis* (water-plantain tuber), *Poria* (fuling), *Fructus Schisandrae* (magnoliavine fruit), *Radix Scrophulariae* (figwort root), *Concha Margaritifera Usta* (mother-of-pearl), *Fructus Tritici Levis* (light wheat), etc. pulverized, mixed and made into tablets.

[11] *Gengniankang Tablet* (Health Tablet for Menopause): composed of Extractum Schisandrae Liquidum (magnoliavine extract), Extractum Acanthopanacis Liquidum (acanthopanax extract), and Extractum Cornis Cervi Pantitrichi (antler extract); 0.9 g, 2-3 times a day.

as the Kidneys are responsible for reproduction, but some other factors such as Liver depression, phlegm-damp and blood stasis may also have an impact on fertility.

If Kidney *yang* is insufficient, it fails to warm up the uterus, and so fertility is impossible. In Kidney *yin* deficiency, the Thoroughfare and Conception Vessels cannot be filled with adequate essence and blood, and the uterus is thus poorly nourished, so that fertility is impaired. Kidney *yin* deficiency often produces exuberant fire, which may also interfere with fertility.

Liver depression due to emotional disturbances may lead to disharmony between *qi* and blood, uncoordination between Thoroughfare and Conception Vessels, and consequently infertility.

In obese individuals and in those who take excessive amounts of rich food, the Spleen function is often impaired and phlegm-damp produced. Phlegm-damp may obstruct the uterine vessels, making fertility impossible.

Attack of pathogenic cold during menstruation may result in blood stasis in the uterine vessels, interfering with the fusion of the ovum with a sperm.

Syndrome Differentiation

According to the pathogenesis, infertility can be classified into the following syndrome patterns:

1. Kidney *yang* deficiency: Infertility with delayed menstruation, scanty pale menstrual discharge or even amenorrhea, dark complexion, soreness and weakness of the back and legs, sexual hypesthesia, pale tongue with white coating, and deep, thready or slow pulse.

2. Kidney *yin* deficiency: Infertility in short-tempered women with advanced menstruation, scanty red menstrual discharge or normal menstrual flow, emaciation, soreness and weakness of the back and legs, dizziness, blurred vision, palpitations, insomnia, dryness in the mouth, heat sensation in the palms and soles, reddened tongue with little coating, and thready and rapid pulse.

3. Liver depression: Infertility in irritable and depressed women with irregular menstruation and dysmenorrhea, breast distension preceding the menstrual period, normal or slightly dark tongue, and stringy pulse.

4. Phlegm-damp: Infertility in obese women with delayed menstruation or even amenorrhea, profuse leukorrhea, pale and puffy complexion, dizziness, palpitations, white and greasy tongue coating, and slippery pulse.

5. Blood stasis: Infertility in women with delayed menstruation, scanty dark menstrual discharge containing blood clots and accompanied by lower abdominal pain and tenderness, purple tongue or purple spots on the edges of the tongue, and thready, stringy pulse.

Herbal Medication

1. Kidney *yang* deficiency

Principle of treatment: To warm up the Kidneys, replenish *qi* and blood, and regulate Thoroughfare and Conception Vessels.

Formula of choice: *Bazhen Tang* (Decoction of Eight Precious Ingredients) plus *Semen Cuscutae* (dodder seed), *Cortex Eucommiae* (eucommia bark), and *Cornu Cervi Degelatinatum* (deglued antler).

2. Kidney *yin* deficiency

Principle of treatment: To nourish *yin* essence and blood.

Formula of choice: *Yangjing Zhongyu Tang* (Essence-nourishing Decoction for Fertility)[12].

3. Liver depression

Principle of treatment: To relieve depression and nourish blood.

Formula of choice: *Kaiyu Zhongyu Tang* (Antidepressant Decoction for Fertility)[13]

4. Phlegm-damp

Principle of treatment: To resolve phlegm-damp and regulate menstruation.

Formula of choice: *Qigong Wan* (Uterus-arousing Pill)[14].

5. Blood stasis

Principle of treatment: To remove blood stasis.

Formula of choice: *Shaofu Zhuyu Tang* (Decoction for Removing Blood Stasis in the Lower Abdomen).

Patent Medicines

Infertility due to Kidney insufficiency: *Shen Gui Lurong Wan* (Ginseng, Cinnamon and Antler Pill)[15], 9 g, 2 times daily, discontinued during the menstrual period.

Infertility due to Liver depression: *Xiaoyao Wan* (Ease Pill), 4 g, 2 times daily.

Infertility due to blood stasis: *Guizhi Fuling Wan* (Cinnamon and Poria Pill)[16], 3 g,

---

[12] *Yangjing Zhongyu Tang* (Essence-nourishing Decoction for Fertility): *Radix Peoniae Alba* (white peony root) 12 g, *Radix Angelicae Sinensis* (Chinese angelica root) 12 g, *Radix Rehmanniae Preparata* (prepared rehmannia root) 15 g, and *Fructus Corni* (dogwood fruit) 9 g, to be made into a decoction.

[13] *Kaiyu Zhongyu Tang* (Antidepressant Decoction for Fertility): *Rhizoma Atractylodis Macrocephalae* (white atractylodes rhizome) 9 g, *Radix Angelicae Sinensis* (Chinese angelica root) 12 g, *Radix Peoniae Alba* (white peony root) 9 g, *Poria* (fuling) 9 g, *Cortex Moutan* (moutan bark) 9 g, *Rhizoma Cyperi* (cyperus tuber) 9 g, and *Radix Trichosanthis* (snakegourd root) 9 g, to be made into a decoction.

[14] *Qigong Wan* (Uterus-arousing Pill): *Rhizoma Pinelliae* (pinellia tuber) 12 g, *Rhizoma Atractylodis* (atractylodes rhizome) 9 g, *Rhizoma Cyperi* (cyperus tuber) 9 g, *Pericarpium Citri Reticulatae* (tangerine peels) 6 g, *Massa Fermentata Medicinalis* (medicated leaven) 9 g, *Poria* (fuling) 9 g, and *Rhizoma Chuanxiong* (chuanxiong) 6 g, to be made into pills.

[15] *Shen Gui Lurong Wan* (Ginseng, Cinnamon and Antler Pill): *Radix Ginseng* (ginseng), *Cornu Cervi Pantotrichum* (pilose antler), *Radix Glycyrrhizae* (licorice), *Radix Dipsaci* (teasel root), *Cortex Cinnamomi* (cinnamon bark), *Radix Astragali* (milkvetch root), *Radix Codonopsis* (tangshen), *Rhizoma Atractylodis Macrocephalae* (white atractylodes rhizome), *Radix Peoniae Alba* (white peony root), *Radix Angelicae Sinensis* (Chinese angelica root), *Radix Polygalae* (milkwort root), *Fructus Lycii* (wolfberry), *Herba Cistanchis* (cistanche), *Pericarpium Citri Reticulatae* (tangerine peel), *Poria* (fuling), and *Radix Rehmanniae Preparata* (prepared rehmannia root) mixed at the ratio of 1:1:1:1:1:2:2:2:2:2:2:2:2:1.6:1.6:2.4 in weight, pulverized and made into honey pills, 9 g, 2 times daily.

[16] *Guizhi Fuling Wan* (Cinnamon and Poria Pill): *Ramulus Cinnamomi* (cinnamon twig), *Poria* (fuling), *Cortex Moutan* (moutan bark), *Radix Peoniae Rubra* (red peony root), and *Semen Persiae* (peach

2 times daily.

Acupuncture

Infertility due to Kidney *yin* deficiency: Shenshu (BL 23), Hegu (LI 4) and Qihai (CV6).

Infertility due to Kidney *yang* deficiency: Sanyinjiao (SP 6), Mingmen (GV 4) and Qihai (CV 6).

Infertility due to Liver depression: Guanyuan (CV 4), Yanglingquan (GB 34) and Zusanli (ST 36).

Infertility due to phlegm-damp: Zhongji (CV 3), Sanyinjiao (SP 6) and Taichong (LR 3).

Retain the needles for 10-20 minutes, and apply moxibustion to the points on the abdomen after needling.

OLIGOGALACTIA

In traditional Chinese medicine, deficient lactation is considered as a result either of insufficient milk production or of obstructed milk flow. In either case, acupuncture may be helpful.

Etiology and Pathogenesis

Deficient lactation secretion can be classified into two patterns according to the pathogenesis:

1. Deficiency of *qi* and blood. Milk is derived from blood, and its secretion needs the action of *qi*. Thus, if *qi* and blood are insufficient, secretion of milk is impaired.

2. Stagnation of Liver *qi*. The flow of milk in the lactiferous ducts also needs the action of *qi*. If emotional or psychic influences make the Liver depressed and *qi* stagnates, the milk flow will be impeded, resulting in deficient lactation with galactostasis.

Syndrome Differentiation

It is of crucial significance to differentiate excess from deficiency. Oligogalactia due to inadequate production of milk is a deficiency condition, while that due to stagnation of Liver *qi* is an excess condition. The treatment of the two conditions should be different in principle.

1. Deficiency of *qi* and blood: No secretion or insufficient secretion of thin milk after deLivery, soft breast with no distention, pallor complexion, lassitude, anorexia, pale tongue with scanty coating, and thready and thin pulse.

2. Stagnation of Liver *qi*: Insufficient or no secretion of milk after deLivery, accompanied by distension in the chest and flank, or emotional depression, anorexia, thin

---

kernel) mixed at equal amount, pulverized and made into pills; 3-5 g, 2 times daily.

yellow tongue coating, and stringy, thready or rapid pulse.

Acupuncture

Common points: Danzhong (CV 17), Shaoze (SI 1), and Rugen (ST 18)

Additional points according to syndrome differentiation:

Deficiency of *qi* and blood: Pishu (BL 20), and Zusanli (ST 36)

Stagnation of Liver *qi*: Ganshu (BL 18), and Taichong (LR 3)

When needling at Danzhong (CV 17), the needle is directed to the breast transversely.

ABNORMAL FETAL POSITION

Abnormal fetal position refers to occipitoposterior, breech, transverse and oblique positions after the 28th week of pregnancy. It may cause difficult labor if not corrected before deLivery. Knee-chest position can give some help to the correction, but moxibustion is more effective.

Moxibustion

Selection of point: Zhiyin (BL 67).

Manipulation: Ask the subject to void urine, loosen her belt, and lie on her back with the legs bent. The feet are exposed to moxibustion. Either direct moxibustion (3-5 units) or moxibustion with a moxa stick (15-30 minutes) is applied once daily until the fetal position is corrected. Laser moxibustion can also be used instead.

CHAPTER 23

SKIN DISEASES

Skin diseases, though located on the superficial portion of the body, are mostly not diagnosed as exterior syndromes; they are often considered as derangements of internal *zang-fu* organs with pathological changes of the skin. The causes of skin diseases are the same as those of internal diseases, namely, exogenous pathogens and internal injuries.

The common symptoms of skin diseases include swelling, pain, itching and suppuration. Swelling is usually attributed to obstruction of meridians with accumulation of *qi* and blood.

Pain is frequently due to stagnated flow of *qi* and blood. Pain accompanied by tenderness is of excess type, while pain alleviated by pressure is of deficiency type. Pain which is not accompanied by reddening of the local skin and can be alleviated by warmth is of the cold type, while pain which is accompanied by reddening of the local skin and can be alleviated by a cold compress is of the heat type. Pain wandering in location is caused by wind, while pain fix in location is due to blood stasis.

Itching is a symptom indicating wind, damp, heat, parasites or blood deficiency. Generalized itching is often due to wind; itching accompanied by exudation signifies damp; itching with dry and desquamative skin frequently results from blood deficiency.

Suppuration is either due to internal heat that makes the tissue putrid or due to stagnation of *qi* and blood that deprives the tissue of nutrition.

URTICARIA

Urticaria is one of the diseases related to immediate-type hypersensitivity. Identification of the etiological factors and their elimination provide the most satisfactory therapeutic results. However, this may not be feasible in many cases. Antihistamines and sympathomimetic agents often give symptomatic relief, but persistent existence or repeated recurrence of this vexatious skin trouble is not infrequently encountered. Some alternative therapy is therefore necessary.

Etiology and Pathogenesis

Urticaria characterized by sudden appearance and disappearance of wheals accompanied by severe itching is considered as an affection by wind, either exogenous or endogenous. In acute cases, exogenous wind is the major causal factor, which attacks constitutionally weak individuals. Wind that invades the human body is usually combined with cold or heat. In chronic cases, wind that causes repeated recurrence of urticaria is mostly endogenous, originating from blood deficiency.

Syndrome Differentiation

1. Wind-heat: Erythematous wheals accompanied by a severe itching and burning sensation, aggravated by warmth and alleviated by cold; reddened tongue, and floating and rapid pulse (often seen in acute urticaria).

2. Wind-cold: Blanched wheals accompanied by severe itching, occurring after exposure to cold or wind, and relieved by warmth, thin white tongue coating, and floating, tense pulse (often seen in cold urticaria).

3. Wind-dryness: Recurrent attacks of urticaria, persisting for months or years, aggravated at night or during fatigue, accompanied by disturbed sleep and dizziness, thin white tongue coating, and thready pulse (often seen in chronic urticaria).

Herbal Medication

1. Wind-heat

Principle of treatment: To dispel wind-heat.

Formula of choice: *Jing Fang Tang* (Decoction of Schizonepeta and Saposhnikovia)[1].

2. Wind-cold

Principle of treatment: To dispel wind-cold.

Formula of choice: *Mahuang Tang* (Decoction of Ephedra).

3. Wind-dryness

Principle of treatment: To nourish blood and dispel wind.

Formula of choice: *Danggui Yinzi* (Chinese Angelica Decoction)[2].

Patent Medicines

Fangfeng Tongshen Wan (Miraculous Pill of Saposhnikovia) for urticaria due to wind-heat.

---

[1] *Jing Fang Tang* (Decoction of Schizonepeta and Saposhnikovia): *Herba Schizonepetae* (schizonepeta) 9 g, *Radix Saposhnikoviae* (saposhnikovia root) 9 g, *Periostracum Cicadae* (cicada slough) 6 g, *Cortex Phellodendri* (phellodendron bark) 9 g, *Fructus Forsythiae* (forsythia fruit) 12 g, *Gypsum Fibrosum* (gypsum) 30 g, *Radix Sophorae Flavescentis* (flavescent sophora root) 9 g, *Cortex Dictamni* (dittany bark) 9 g, *Rhizoma Cimicifugae* (bugbane rhizome) 3 g, *Radix Glycyrrhizae* (licorice root) 6 g, and *Radix Scutellariae* (skullcap root) 9 g, to be made into a decoction.

[2] *Danggui Yinzi* (Chinese Angelica Decoction): *Radix Angelicae Sinensis* (Chinese angelica root) 6 g, *Radix Rehmanniae* (rehmannia root) 6 g, *Radix Peoniae Alba* (white peony root) 6 g, *Rhizoma Chuanxiong* (chuanxiong) 6 g, *Radix Polygoni Multiflori* (fleeceflower root) 6 g, *Herba Schizonepetae* (schizonepeta) 6 g, *Radix Saposhnikoviae* (saposhnikovia root) 6 g, *Fructus Tribuli* (puncture-vine fruit) 6 g, *Radix Astragali* (milkvetch root) 3 g, and *Radix Glycyrrhizae* (licorice root) 3 g, to be made into a decoction.

Acupuncture

Selection of Points: Quchi (LI 11), Hegu (LI 4), Xuehai (SP 10), and Sanyinjiao (SP 6).

Manipulation: Reducing method.

ECZEMA

Eczema usually refers to endogenous or constitutional dermatitis. It is a multifactorial disease, and to avoid all factors that cause irritation of the skin is a difficult task. In some patients, long-term corticosteroid therapy is required in Western medical treatment. Chinese medicine as an alternative therapy is therefore of great value.

Etiology and Pathogenesis

Eczema is a skin disease caused by pathogenic wind, damp and heat. Wind induces itching, damp-heat affecting the skin gives rise to vesiculation and then watery discharge. In chronic eczema, the condition is usually complicated by blood deficiency.

Syndrome Differentiation

I. Acute Eczema

1. Wind-damp-heat: Acute onset of erythema, infiltration, and vesiculation accompanied by severe itching, erosion and exudate discharge after scratching, yellow greasy tongue coating, and stringy, rapid pulse.

2. Wind-dryness: Localized skin lesion with infiltration, scales and crusts, accompanied by local burning and itching.

II. Chronic Eczema

Localized skin lesion characterized by thickening and roughness of the skin with lichenoid changes, marks of scratching, adherent scales of shed epithelium, blood crusts, pigmentation, and maybe accompanied by various degrees of redness, erosion and exudation. If wind is preponderant, there is severe itching, if damp is preponderant, there is weeping exudation, and if heat (fire) is preponderant, there is marked local redness.

Herbal Medication

I. Acute eczema

1. Wind-damp-heat

Principle of treatment: To dispel wind, remove damp and clear up heat.

Formula of choice: *Bixie Shenshi Tang* (Hypoglaucous Yam Decoction for

Removing Damp)[3].

2. Wind-dryness

Principle of treatment: To dispel wind, remove heat and arrest itching.

Formula of choice: *Xiaofeng San* (Wind-dispelling Powder)[4].

II. Chronic eczema

Principle of treatment: To nourish blood and dispel wind.

Formula of choice: *Siwu Tang* (Decoction of Four Ingredients) plus *Radix Saposhnikoviae* (saposhnikovia root), *Cortex Dictamni* (dittany bark), *Fructus Tribuli* (puncture-vine fruit), and *Periostracum Cicadae* (cicada slough).

Additional ingredients: For preponderant wind, add *Fructus Xanthii* (cocklebur fruit); for preponderant damp, add *Cortex Dictamni* (dittany bark); for preponderant fire, add *Radix Scutellariae* (skullcap root).

Patent Medicines

I. Acute eczema

Xiaofeng Zhiyang Chongji (Wind-dispelling Pruritus-relieving Granule), 1 pack, 3-4 times a day. (The composition of *Xiaofeng Zhiyang Chongji* is the same as that of *Xiaofeng San*).

Fangfeng Tongshen Wan (Miraculous Pill of Saposhnikovia), 5 g, 3 times a day.

II. Chronic eczema

Longdan Xiegan Wan (Gentian Pill to Purge the Liver), 5 g, 3 times a day.

Acupuncture

Common points: Dazhui (GV 14), Quchi (LI 11), Zusanli (ST 36), Sanyinjiao (SP 6), and Shenmen (HT 7).

Additional points according to syndrome differentiation: For damp-heat, add Yinlingquan (SP 9), and Feishu (BL 13); for blood deficiency, add Ximen (PC 4), and Xuehai (SP 10).

---

[3]*Bixie Shenshi Tang* (Hypoglaucous Yam Decoction): *Rhizoma Dioscoreae Hypoglaucae* (hypoglaucous yam) 15 g, *Semen Coicis* (coix seed) 15 g, *Poria* (fuling) 9 g, *Cortex Moutan* (moutan bark) 9 g, *Rhizoma Alismatis* (water-plantain tuber) 6 g, *Talcum* (talc) 12 g, and *Medulla Tetrapanacis* (ricepaper-plant pith) 3 g, to be made into a decoction.

[4]*Xiaofeng San* (Wind-dispelling Powder): *Radix Angelicae Sinensis* (Chinese angelica root) 3 g, *Radix Saposhnikoviae* (saposhnikovia root) 3 g, *Radix Rehmanniae* (rehmannia root) 3 g, *Periostracum Cicadae* (cicada slough) 3 g, *Rhizoma Anemarrhenae* (anemarrhena rhizome) 3 g, *Radix Sophorae Flavescentis* (flavescent sophora root) 3 g, *Semen Sesami Nigrum* (black sesame) 3 g, *Herba Schizonepetae* (schizonepeta) 3 g, *Rhizoma Atractylodis* (atractylodes rhizome) 3 g, *Fructus Arctii* (burdock fruit) 3 g, *Gypsum Fibrosum* (gypsum) 3 g, *Radix Glycyrrhizae* (licorice root) 1.5 g, and *Caulis Aristolochiae Manshuriensis* (manchurian dutchmanspipe stem) 1.5 g, to be made into a decoction.

Manipulation: Reducing method applied to 3-5 points each time every other day for 6 days as a course of treatment. When needling at Xuehai (SP 10), direct the tip of the needle obliquely upward to induce acupuncture sensation up to the abdomen.

HERPES ZOSTER

Herpes zoster, or "shingles," is an acute inflammatory virus disease, characterized by groups of small vesicles on inflammatory bases occurring in the cutaneous areas supplied by certain nerve trunks, and often associated with severe neuralgic pain. Although antiviral chemotherapy such as parental administration of acyclovir or vidarabine is effective for herpes zoster, it has been associated with side effects. Therefore, Chinese medical treatment is still of use.

Etiology and Pathogenesis

Herpes zoster is often caused by invasion of the Liver and Gallbladder Meridians by pathogenic wind-fire or accumulation of damp-heat in the Spleen and stomach. In the former case, the wind-fire runs along the Liver and Gallbladder Meridians, and causes vesicles on the skin. In the latter case, the retained damp-heat in combination with the virulent pathogen, invades the skin and leads to the formation of vesicles. In both cases, there is obstruction of *qi* and blood flow, and hence severe pain.

Syndrome Differentiation

1. Liver fire: Skin lesions usually located in the flank with local inflammation and clusters of vesicles, associated with burning sensation and stabbing pain, but with no rupture, reddened tongue, and stringy, rapid pulse.

2. Spleen damp: Skin lesions often located on the chest or face with scattered vesicles as big as soybeans, which often burst and are associated with severe pain, yellow and greasy tongue coating, and slippery, rapid pulse.

Herbal Medication

1. Liver fire

Principle of treatment: To purge Liver fire.

Formula of choice: *Longdan Xiegan Tang* or *Longdan Xiegan Wan* (Decoction or Pill of Gentian to Purge the Liver) plus *Radix Isatidis* (isatis root).

2. Spleen damp

Principle of treatment: To eliminate damp from the Spleen.

Formula of choice: *Chushi Weiling Tang* (Poria and Polypore Decoction for

Eliminating Damp)[5] plus *Radix Isatidis* (isatis root).

Patent Medicines

For both patterns *Banlangen Chongji* (Isatis Granules) can be used.

Acupuncture

Distant points: Neiguan (PC 6), Hegu (LI 4), Zusanli (ST 36), Yanglingquan (GB 34), and Xuehai (SP 10), to be punctured with reduction manipulation.

Local points: points around the skin lesion, to be transversely punctured centripetally.

NEURODERMATITIS

Neurodermatitis, a chronic itching lichenoid eruption due to nervous disorder, often occurring on the axillary and pubic regions, is a common clinical problem. Local steroids are helpful, but acupuncture may promote healing.

Etiology and Pathogenesis

At the early stage, itching is caused by pathogenic wind-heat retention in the cutaneous tissue. Later, when wind leads to dryness in blood, impairing the nutrition of the skin, lichenoid eruptions appear, and the skin becomes thick and rough.

Syndrome Differentiation

1. Wind-heat: At the early stage of neurodermatitis with a few eruptions and slight reddening of the local skin, accompanied by itching.

2. Blood-dryness: Dry skin lesions with local thickening, desquamation, and extreme itch which leads to persistent scratching with oozing.

Acupuncture

Common points: Fengchi (GB 20), Dazhui (GV 14), Xuehai (SP 10), Quchi (LI 11),

---

[5] *Chushi Weiling Tang* (Poria and Polypore Decoction for Eliminating Damp): *Rhizoma Atractylodis* (atractylodes rhizome), 12 g, *Cortex Magnoliae Officinalis* (medicinal magnolia bark) 12 g, *Pericarpium Citri Reticulatae* (tangerine peel) 12 g, *Poria* (fuling) 9 g, *Polyporus* (zhuling) 9 g, *Rhizoma Alismatis* (water-plantain tuber) 12 g, *Talcum* (talc) 12 g, *Radix Saposhnikoviae* (saposhnikovia root) 9 g, *Fructus Gardeniae* (cape-jasmine fruit) 9 g, *Caulis Aristolochiae Manshuriensis* (manchurian dutchmanspipe stem) 5 g, *Cortex Cinnamomi* (cinnamon bark) 6 g, and *Radix Glycyrrhizae* (licorice root) 5 g, to be made into a decoction.

Neiguan (PC 6), Weizhong (BL 40), Zhaohai (KI 6), and Ashi.

Additional points according to syndrome differentiation: For wind-heat, add Yinlingquan (SP 9), Taibai (SP 3), and Taiyuan (LU 9); for blood-dryness, add Sanyinjiao (SP 6), Zusanli (ST 36), and Geshu (BL 17).

Manipulation: Needle at 4-5 of the above-mentioned points each time with strong stimulation. Ashi points are selected around the skin lesion, and the puncturing needles are directed toward the center of the lesion.

PRURITUS

Pruritus is the term used when itching is the primary complaint unaccompanied by visible skin lesions or systemic diseases predisposing to itch. It is usually due to dryness and desiccation of the stratum corneum. Use of antihistamines is often limited because of their sedative effect. Acupuncture may provide satisfactory relief.

Etiology and Pathogenesis

Pruritus often occurs before sleeping, precipitated by stress, weather changes, alcoholic drinks or spicy hot food. According to Chinese medicine, this is due to constitutional anomaly with heat in blood and further attack by wind-heat which halts in the skin, or due to blood deficiency with exuberant Liver *qi* which turns to wind and causes dryness, impairing the cutaneous nutrition.

Syndrome Differentiation

1. Wind-dryness and blood-heat: Pruritus of short duration, often occurring in young adults, dry skin with desquamation.

2. Blood deficiency with Liver exuberance: Pruritus of long duration, often occurring in the elderly, precipitated by emotional stress or weather changes, reddened skin with rhagades.

Patent Medicines

Xiaofeng Zhiyang Chongji (Wind-dispelling Pruritus-relieving Granules), 1 pack, 3 times a day. (The composition of *Xiaofeng Zhiyang Chongji* is the same as *Xiaofeng San,* cf. Eczema)

Acupuncture

Main points: (1) Quchi (LI 11), Hegu (LI 4), and Fengmen (BL 12); (2) Xuehai (SP 10), Geshu (BL 17), and Zusanli (ST 36).

Additional points according to syndrome differentiation: For wind-dryness and blood-heat, add Fengchi (GB 20), Taixi (KI 3), and Sanyinjiao (SP 6); for blood deficiency with Liver exuberance, add Ganshu (BL 18), and Taichong (LR 3).

Manipulation: Use the main points group (1) and (2) alternatively and apply reduction manipulation with retention of needles for 15 minutes.

CHAPTER 24

NEUROLOGICAL AND PSYCHIATRIC DISORDERS

HEADACHE

Headache is one of the commonest symptoms for which patients seek medical help. In most cases, the pain is not related to the brain and meninges. Many of the extracranial organs are prone to give rise to pain, but the muscles and arteries of the scalp are the commonest source of headache. In the latter case, acupuncture seems to be the most satisfactory therapy, though drugs, either chemical in Western medicine or herbal in Chinese medicine, are also frequently used.

Syndrome Differentiation

I. Headache due to Exogenous Affections

1. Wind-cold

Headache precipitated or aggravated by exposure to wind and cold, referring to the nape, and alleviated by warmth, no thirst, maybe accompanied by stuffy and runny nose, thin white tongue coating, and floating and tense pulse.

2. Wind-heat

Headache accompanied by distension feeling, aggravated by warmth, flushing face, thirst, maybe accompanied by fever and constipation, thin yellow tongue coating, and floating, rapid pulse.

3. Wind-damp

Headache as if the head were tightly bound, heaviness feeling all over the body, oppression feeling in the chest, impaired appetite, loose stools, white greasy tongue coating, and soft pulse.

II. Headache due to Endogenous Injury

1. Exuberance of Liver *yang*

Headache, marked at the temporal region, aggravated by anger, accompanied by dizziness, irritability, irascibility, insomnia, or hypochondriac pain and bitterness in the mouth; thin yellow tongue coating, and stringy, rapid pulse.

2. *Qi* deficiency

Dull pain in the head, aggravated by fatigue, accompanied by lassitude, lack of strength, anorexia, palpitations, shortness of breath, sometimes aversion to cold with cool limbs; thin white tongue coating, and thready, weak pulse.

3. Blood deficiency

Headache, dizziness, palpitations, insomnia, dreamful sleep, blurred vision, numbness of the limbs, pale tongue, and thready pulse.

4. Kidney insufficiency

Headache with a feeling of emptiness, accompanied by dizziness, tinnitus, aching and weakness of the lower back and legs; reddened tongue, and deep, thready and weak pulse.

5. Phlegm-damp

Headache with feeling of haziness, oppression in the chest, nausea and even vomiting, white greasy tongue coating, and stringy, slippery pulse.

6. Blood stasis

Persistent pricking or stabbing headache with fixed location, purple tongue or purple spots on the tongue, and stringy, hesitant pulse.

Herbal Medication

I. Headache due to Exogenous Affections

1. Wind-cold

Principle of treatment: To dispel wind-cold.

Formula of choice: *Chuanxiong Chatiao San* (Tea-blended Chuanxiong Powder)[1].

2. Wind-heat

Principle of treatment: To dispel wind-heat.

Formula of choice: *Sang Ju Yin* (Decoction of Mulberry Leaf and Chrysanthemum).

II. Headache due to Endogenous Injuries

1. Exuberance of Liver *yang*

Principle of treatment: To soothe the Liver and subdue the exuberant *yang*.

Formula of choice: *Tianma Gouteng Yin* (Decoction of Gastrodia and Uncaria Stem).

2. *Qi* deficiency

Principle of treatment: To replenish *qi*.

Formula of choice: *Buzhong Yiqi Tang* (Decoction for Reinforcing the Middle Energizer and Replenishing *Qi*); add *Rumulus Cinnamomi* (cinnamon twig) 9 g and *Herba Asari* (manchurian wildginger) 1.5 g to the decoction if there is aversion to cold with cool limbs.

3. Blood deficiency

Principle of treatment: To nourish blood.

Formula of choice: *Siwu Tang* (Decoction of Four Ingredients) plus *Flos Chrysanthemi* (chrysanthemum flower) 9 g and *Fructus Viticis* (chastetree fruit) 9 g.

4. Kidney insufficiency

Principle of treatment: To replenish Kidney *yin*.

Formula of choice: *Qi Ju Dihuang Tang* (Rehmannia Decoction with Wolfberry and Chrysanthemum).

---

[1]*Chuanxiong Chatiao San* (Tea-blended Chuanxiong Powder): *Rhizoma Chuanxiong* (chuanxiong) 12 g, *Herba Schizonepetae* (schizonepeta) 12 g, *Radix Angelicae Dahuricae* (dahurian angelica root) 6 g, *Rhizoma Notopterygii* (notopterygium rhizome) 6 g, *Radix Glycyrrhizae* (licorice root) 6 g, *Herba Asari* (manchurian wildginger) 3 g, *Radix Saposhnikoviae* (saposhnikovia root) 4.5 g, and *Herba Menthae* (peppermint) 24 g, mixed and ground into powder, 6 g of the powder blended with green tea to be taken twice a day.

5. Phlegm-damp

Principle of treatment: To remove damp and resolve phlegm.

Formula of choice: *Erchen Tang* (Decoction of Pinellia Tuber and Tangerine Peel) plus *Radix Angelicae Dahuricae* (dahurian angelica root).

6. Blood stasis

Principle of treatment: To remove blood stasis.

Formula of choice: *Tao Hong Siwu Tang* (Decoction of Four Ingredients with Peach Seed and Safflower) plus *Radix Angelicae Dahuricae* (dahurian angelica root).

Patent Medicines

Wind-cold headache: *Chuanxiong Chatiao San* (Tea-blended Chuanxiong Powder), 6 g, 2 times a day.

Wind-heat headache: *Xiong Ju Shangqing Wan* (Chuanxiong-Chrysanthemum Pill for Clearing the Head)[2], 6 g, 2 times a day.

Phlegm-damp heaeache: *Banxia Tianma Wan* (Pinellia-Gastrodia Pill)[3], 6 g, 2 times a day.

Liver-*yang* headache: *Longdan Xiegan Wan* (Pill of Gentian to Purge the Liver), 6 g, 2 times a day.

Headache due to depressed Liver *qi*: *Dan Zhi Xiaoyao Wan* (Ease Pill with Moutan and Gardenia), 6 g, 2 times a day.

Headache due to Kidney *yin* deficiency: *Qi Ju Dihuang Tang* (Rehmannia Pill with Wolfberry and Chrysanthemum), 6 g, 2 times a day.

Headache due to *qi* and blood deficiency: *Renshen Guipi Wan* (Spleen-invigorating Pill with Ginseng), 6 g, 2 time a day.

Acupuncture

I. Treatment according to syndrome differentiation

Wind-cold: Fengfu (GV 16), Fengchi (GB 20), Waiguan (TE 5), and Dazhui (GV 14), with reducing manipulation.

Wind-heat: Fengmen (BL 12), Taiyang (EX-HN 5), Quchi (LI 11), Shaoshang (LU 11), Dazhui (GV 14), and Hegu (LI 4), with reducing manipulation.

---

[2]*Xiong Ju Shangqing Wan* (Chuanxiong-Chrysanthemum Pills for Clearing the Head): *Flos Chrysanthemi* (chrysanthemum flower), *Radix Scutellariae* (skullcap root), *Radix Platycodi* (platycodon root), *Fructus Gardeniae* (cape-jasmine fruit), *Fructus Forsythiae* (forsythia fruit), *Radix Saposhnikoviae* (saposhnikovia root), *Fructus Viticis* (chestetree fruit), *Herba Schizonepetae* (schizonepeta), *Radix Glycyrrhizae* (licorice root), *Rhizoma Coptidis* (goldthread rhizome), *Rhizoma seu Radix Notopterygii* (notopterygium), *Rhizoma Chuanxiong* (chuanxiong), *Herba Menthae* (peppermint), *Rhizoma et Radix Ligustici* (ligusticum root), and *Radix Angelicae Dahuricae* (dahurian angelica root), pulverized, mixed at the ratio of 12:6:1.5:1.5:1.5:1.5:1.5:1.5:1:1:1:1:1:2:4 in weight, and made into pills; 6 g, 2-3 times a day.

[3]*Banxia Tianma Wan* (Pinellia-Gastrodia Pill): *Rhizoma Pinelliae* (pinellia tuber), *Rhizoma Gastrodiae* (gastrodia tuber), *Radix Astragali* (milkvetch root), *Radix Ginseng* (ginseng), *Rhizoma Atractylodis Macrocephalae* (white atractylodes rhizome), *Rhizoma Atractylodis* (atractylodes rhizome), *Poria* (fuling), *Rhizoma Alismatis* (water-plantain tuber), *Massa Fermentata Medicinalis* (medicated leaven), *Fructus Hordei Germinatus* (germinated barley), *Pericarpium Citri Reticulatae* (tangerine peel), and *Cortex Phellodendri* (phellodendron bark)

Exuberance of Liver *yang*: Taichong (LR 3), Taiyang (EX-HN 5), Xingjian (LR 2), Fengchi (GB 20), Ganshu (BL 18), and Taixi (KI 3), with reducing manipulation.

Deficiency of *qi* and blood: Baihui (GV 20), Pishu (BL 20), Qihai (CV 6), Guanyuan (CV 4), and Zusanli (ST 36), with reinforcing manipulation.

Kidney insufficiency: Shenshu (BL 23), Mingmen (GV 4), Taixi (KI 3), and Guanyuan (CV 4), with reinforcing manipulation.

Phlegm-damp: Fengchi (GB 20), Zhongwan (CV 12), Fenglong (ST 40), Lieque (LU 7), and Weishu (BL 21), with reducing manipulation.

Blood stasis: Xuehai (SP 10), Geshu (BL 17), local tender points and distant points selected according to the affected meridian, with reducing manipulation.

II. Treatment according to the affected meridian

Occipital headache (Foot-Taiyang Meridian): Fengfu (GV 16), Tianzhu (BL 10), Fengchi (GB 20), Houding (GV 19), and Kunlun (BL 60).

Temporal headache (Foot-Shaoyang Meridian): Shuaigu (GB 8), Taiyang (EX-HN 5), Xuanzhong (GB 39), Zulinqi (GB 41), and Touwei (ST 8).

Frontal headache (Foot-Yangming Meridian): Yintang (EX-HN 3), Shangxing (GV 23), Hegu (LI 4), and Neiting (ST 44).

Vertical headache (Foot-Jueyin Meridian): Baihui (GV 20), Taichong (LR 3), Xingjian (LR 2), and Fengfu (GV 16).

MIGRAINE

Migraine is a complex syndrome characterized by episodic headache, usually limited on one side, and preceded by visual disturbances, nausea and vomiting as prodromal symptoms. Vascular instability is the probable cause of migraine. Ergotamine has long been regarded as a specific agent for constricting the dilated arteries, but it is far less effective than might be supposed. Particularly if migraine is frequent, chronic administration of ergotamine is undesirable, as ergotism with gangrene of the limbs may result. Other drugs such as anti-serotonin agents and beta-blocking agents may be effective, but they all have some restraints or side effects when used continuously. Acupuncture is recommended for chronic migraine.

Etiology and Pathogenesis

The commonest pattern of migraine is that due to exuberant Liver *yang*. Emotional depression with stagnated Liver *qi* which turns into Liver fire (exuberant Liver *yang*) or insufficiency of Liver and Kidney *yin* with relatively exuberant Liver *yang* may lead to disorders of the head, manifested by migraine. In some other cases, migraine is caused by retention of cold-fluid or blood stasis. Retained fluid due to insufficiency of Spleen *yang* or stagnated blood in a long-term depression of *qi* flow may interfere with the free flow of the clear *yang* in the meridians and collaterals of the head, resulting in migraine.

Syndrome Differentiation

1. Migraine of the Liver-*yang* pattern: One-sided periodic headache with distending

pain, dizziness, irritability, insomnia, dryness of the mouth, congested eyes, reddened tongue with scanty coating, and stringy, rapid pulse.

2. Migraine of the retained-fluid pattern: One-sided periodic headache with heavy sensation in the head, fullness in the chest, nausea, vomiting, cool limbs, white greasy tongue coating, and stringy, slippery pulse.

3. Migraine of stagnated-blood pattern: One-sided periodic headache with a chronic course and fix in location, accompanied by a purple tongue, and stringy or deep, hesitant pulse.

Acupuncture

Principle of treatment: To regulate *qi* flow in the local meridians. In addition, to pacify the Liver *yang* if it is exuberant, to invigorate the Spleen and Stomach if there is retained fluid, and to normalize the blood flow if it is in stagnation.

Common points: Local painful points, Sizhukong (TE 23), Shuaigu (GB 8), Hanyan (GB 4), Xuanlu (GB 5), Hegu (LI 4), Lieque (LU 7), and Zulinqi (GB 41).

Additional points according to syndrome differentiation: For Liver *yang*, add Sishencong (EX-HN 1), Yifeng (TE 17), and Fengchi (GB 20); for retained fluid, add Zhongwan (CV 12).

Manipulation: Horizontal insertion of the needles with strong stimulation is applied to the points on the head. Joined puncture is used for Sizhukong (TE 23) and Shuaigu (GB 8) and for Hanyan (GB 4) and Xuanlu (GB 5), i.e., puncturing two adjoining points with one insertion of the needle. Electro-acupuncture often provides a satisfactory effect. The best result is achieved if the patient is treated at the prodromal stage of the episode.

TRIGEMINAL NEURALGIA

Trigeminal neuralgia is characterized by brief but frequent paroxysms of intense pain strictly confined to the distribution of the trigeminal nerve. The pain is excruciating, and often described as piercing or knife-like. The paroxysms may be spontaneous or provoked by touching certain areas on the face, lips, or tongue (so-called trigger zones) or by movement of these parts. Eating and speaking may become extremely difficult. Analgesics and sedatives are usually necessary. Carbamazepine is the drug of choice, but unfortunately a considerable number of patients cannot tolerate the drug in the dosage required to alleviate pain. If drug treatment fails, surgical therapy may be offered. Since acupuncture can provide relief to neuralgic patients, application of this simple and safe therapy is recommended before surgical therapy or even before administration of drugs.

Etiology and Pathogenesis

In Chinese medicine, this illness was traditionally called "facial pain." Since the pain usually occurs in transient paroxysms, evil wind in combination with cold, invading and obstructing the related meridians, is considered to be the major causal factor. However, upward invasion of excessive Liver- and Stomach-fire or fire secondary to *yin* deficiency may also interfere with the clarity of the head, resulting in paroxysmal facial pain.

Syndrome Differentiation

According to the pathogenesis, trigeminal neuralgia can be classified into three syndrome patterns: wind-cold, excessive Liver- and Stomach-fire, and *yin* deficiency with exuberant fire. In wind-cold pattern, the paroxysm is precipitated or aggravated by exposure to cold, the pain may be accompanied by a cooling sensation, and the tongue coating is usually thin and white. In the pattern of excessive Liver- and Stomach-fire, the pain is accompanied by irritability, thirst, constipation, reddened tongue with yellow coating, and rapid pulse. In the pattern of *yin* deficiency with exuberant fire, the patient is usually emaciated with malar flush, and thready, rapid and weak pulse.

Acupuncture

Reducing manipulations with continuous twisting and long retention of needles is necessary. Selection of points may follow either of the two programs listed below.

I. Treatment according to syndrome differentiation

Common points for trigeminal neuralgia: Xiaguan (ST 7), Fengchi (GB 20), Zulinqi (GB 41), and Zhiyin (BL 67).

Additional points: For wind-cold affection, add Fengchi (GB 20), Fengmen (BL 12), and Waiguan (TE 5); for Liver-fire, add Ganshu (BL 18), Shenshu (BL 23), and Taichong (LR 3); for *yin* deficiency, add Sanyinjiao (SP 6), Taixi (KI 3), and Xuehai (SP 10).

II. Treatment according to the affected nerve branch

Common distant points: Hegu (LI 4), Zulinqi (GB 41), and Neiting (ST 44).

Local points:

Affection of the ophthalmic branch: Cuanzhu (BL 2), Yangbai (GB 14), and Yuyao (EX-HN 4)

Affection of the maxillary branch: Sibai (ST 2), Juliao (ST 3), and Quanliao (SI 18).

Affection of the mandibular branch: Xiaguan (ST 7), Jiache (ST 6), and Chengjiang (CV 24).

For relieving pain, reduction manipulation is required.

INTERCOSTAL NEURALGIA

Intercostal pain due to primary neuritis is rare. In most cases, intercostal neuralgia is secondary, particularly postherpetic. When organic lesions such as pleurisy and cancer are excluded, acupuncture may be the major treatment of intercostal neuralgia.

Etiology and Pathogenesis

According to Chinese medicine, intercostal neuralgia may be due to attack of the collateral meridians by wind-heat or caused by traumatic injury with stagnated blood. In some cases, emotional upset may lead to *qi* stagnation and then blood stasis in the Liver Meridian, which will also cause intercostal pain.

Syndrome Differentiation

1. Wind-heat: Intercostal pain accompanied by chilliness and fever, and floating, rapid pulse.

2. *Qi* stagnation: Intercostal pain accompanied by distented feeling in the flank, occurring after emotional upset, and stringy pulse.

3. Blood stasis: Intercostal pain, stabbing or pricking in character, occurring after a traumatic injury.

Acupuncture

The principle of acupuncture treatment is to regulate *qi* and activate blood.

Common points: Zhigou (TE 6), Taichong (LR 3), Xingjian (LR 2), and Yanglingquan (GB 34).

Additional points according to syndrome:

Wind-heat: Fengchi (GB 20), Quchi (LI 11), and Waiguan (TE 5).

Qi stagnation: Guangming (GB 37), Ligou (LR 5), and Qiuxu (GB 40).

Blood stasis: Ganshu (BL 18), Qimen (LR 14), and Geshu (BL 17).

SCIATICA

Sciatica may be attributed to inflammatory neuritis of the sciatic nerve, but in most cases the cause is pressure on the root or trunk of the sciatic nerve. Acupuncture treatment is often recommended if no urgent surgical intervention is required.

Etiology And Pathogenesis

Primary sciatica (sciatic neuritis) is attributed to invasion of the related meridian by pathogenic wind-cold-damp. Secondary sciatica (pressure on the sciatic nerve) is often due to trauma or overstrain.

Acupuncture

Primary sciatica: Huantiao (GB 30), Weizhong (BL 40), Chengshan (BL 57), Kunlun (BL 60), Fengshi (GB 31), Zhibian (BL 54), and Yanglingquan (GB 34).

Secondary sciatica: Dachangshu (BL 25), Qihaishu (BL 24), Zhibian (BL 54), Huantiao (GB 30), Weizhong (BL 40), Yanglingquan (GB 34), and Kunlun (BL 60).

When needling the points in the lumbar and gluteal regions, it is preferable to direct the acupuncture sensation downwards. However, the manipulation should not be repeated in the same session of treatment, in order to avoid injury to the nerve.

POSTAPOPLECTIC HEMIPLEGIA

Rehabilitation after a stroke presents great complexity. Acupuncture is one of various measures. The earlier this simple therapy is applied, the better the outcome.

Etiology and Pathogenesis

Apoplexy is called "wind-stroke" in Chinese medicine. This means that the apoplectic seizure is caused by wind, endogenous and not exogenous. Once the endogenous wind in combination with phlegm invades the brain and collateral meridians, there is transient loss of consciousness followed by hemiplegia. After the acute onset, *qi* and blood flow in the collaterals is obstructed, and the motory and sensory disturbances of the involved side persist.

Acupuncture

Principle of treatment: To dispel wind, activate blood and remove obstruction from the collateral meridians.

Major points:

Aphasia: Yamen (GV 15), and Lianquan (CV 23).

Facial paralysis: Xiaguan (ST 7), Dicang (ST 4), Jiache (ST 6), Yifeng (TE 17), Sibai (ST 2), Hegu (LI 4), Yingxiang (LI 20), Cuanzhu (BL 2), Yangbai (GB 14), Quanliao (SI 18), and Chengjiang (CV 24).

Paralysis of the upper limb: Tianding (LI 17), Quchi (LI 11), Xiaoluo (TE 12), Sidu (TE 9), Jianyu (LI 15), Shousanli (LI 10), Hegu (LI 4), Quze (PC 3), Neiguan (PC 6), and Sanjian (LI 3).

Paralysis of the lower limb: Huantiao (GB 30), Fengshi (GB 31), Weiyang (BL 39), Chongmen (SP 12), Biguan (ST 31), Zusanli (ST 36), Yanglingquan (GB 34), Futu (ST 32), Xuanzhong (GB 39), and Jiexi (ST 41).

Additional points according to syndrome pattern or other symptoms: Add Tiantu (CV 22), Neiguan (PC 6), Fenglong (ST 40) and Gongsun (SP 4) for obese patients with phlegm; add Taichong (LR 3), Ganshu (BL 18) for exuberant Liver fire; add Taixi (KI 3), Zhaohai (KI 6) for *yin* deficiency with reddened tongue and dryness in the mouth; add Sishencong (EX-HN 1), Qiangjian (GV 18), and Naohu (GV 17) for slowness in mental activities.

In most cases, reduction manipulation is indicated.

BELL'S PALSY

From the traditional Chinese medical perspective, Bell's palsy is a paralytic condition due to wind-cold attack of the meridians on the face. Acupuncture is often effective when it is used at the early stage.

Acupuncture

Principle of treatment: To dispel wind-cold from the meridians. Combined use of local and distant points is preferable.

Major points: Fengchi (GB 20), Dicang (ST 4), Jieche (ST 6), Sibai (ST 2), Hegu (LI 4), Zusanli (ST 36), and Neiting (ST 44).

Additional points: Add Shuigou (GV 26), and Heliao (LI 19) for salivation, add Yifeng (TE 17) for pain in the mastoid region; add Chengjiang (CV 24) for deviation of nasolabial sulcus.

At the beginning of acupuncture treatment, only superficial punctures with light stimulation at fewer points is preferable. The number of punctured points and the stimulation can be gradually increased in the course of treatment.

INSOMNIA

Insomnia is a common complaint. Physical causes of insomnia are comparatively few. In most cases, insomnia is a psychophysiological disorder, resulting mainly from the self-stimulation engendered by anxiety, worry, or depression. Sleeping pills are routinely used for treating this disorder, but their continuous use in chronic cases may cause adverse side or toxic effects. Herbal medicines and acupuncture can be effectively used as alternative measures.

Etiology and Pathogenesis

Insomnia is often caused by emotional or psychic disturbances. Anxiety and anger make the Liver depressed, and the depressed Liver *qi* may be transformed into fire, which interferes with the normal functions of the Heart. Excessive anxiety may also impair the Heart (mind) and the Spleen, and insomnia occurs due to inadequate supply of nutrients and blood to the Heart.

In the aged and the patients suffering from chronic diseases, *qi* and blood are insufficient to nourish the Heart, thus leading to palpitations and insomnia. *Qi* deficiency may also involve the Heart and the Gallbladder, impairing one's sleep and making one vulnerable to fright. Consumption of Kidney essence may break down the normal balance between the Heart and the Kidneys, and incoordination between the Heart and the Kidneys may also be manifested as insomnia.

Syndrome Differentiation

According to the pathogenesis, insomnia can be classified into the following syndrome patterns:

1. Depressed Liver with exuberant fire: Insomnia accompanied by irritability, irascibility, thirst, yellow coating, and stringy, rapid pulse.

2. Incoordination of the Heart and the Kidneys: Insomnia accompanied by dizziness, tinnitus, dryness in the mouth, heat sensation in the palms and soles, palpitations, forgetfulness, lumbar aching, reddened tongue, and thready, rapid pulse.

3. Deficiency of both the Heart and the Spleen: Dreamful sleep with early waking, palpitations, forgetfulness, dizziness, lassitude, lack of strength, anorexia, pallid complexion, and thready, weak pulse.

4. Deficiency of the Heart and the Gallbladder: Dreamful sleep with wakefulness, susceptibility to fright, and stringy, thready pulse.

Herbal Medication

1. Depressed Liver with exuberant fire

Principle of treatment: To purge the Liver of fire.

Formula of choice: *Longdan Xiegan Tang* (Decoction of Gentian to Purge the Liver).

2. Incoordination of the Heart and the Kidneys

Principle of treatment: To coordinate the Heart and the Kidneys.

Formula of choice: *Liuwei Dihuang Wan* (Pill of Six Ingredients with Rehmannia) plus *Rhizoma Coptidis* (goldthread rhizome) and *Cortex Cinnamomi* (cinnamon bark).

3. Deficiency of both the Heart and the Spleen

Principle of treatment: To nourish the Heart and the Spleen.

Formula of choice: *Guipi Tang* (Spleen-invigorating Decoction).

4. Deficiency of the Heart and the Gallbladder

Principle of treatment: To replenish *qi* and induce tranquilization

Formula of choice: *Anshen Wan* (Tranquilizing Pill)[4].

Patent Medicines

1. Depressed Liver with exuberant fire: *Longdan Xiegan Wan* (Gentian Pill to Purge the Liver).
2. Incoordination of the Heart and the Kidneys: *Tianwang Buxin Dan* (Heavenly King's Heart Tonic).
3. Deficiency of both the Heart and the Spleen: *Renshen Guipi Wan* (Spleen-invigorating Pill with Ginseng).
4. Deficiency of the Heart and the Gallbladder: *Anshen Wan* (Tranquilizing Pill).

Acupuncture

Common points: Shenmen (HT 7), and Sanyinjiao (SP 6) to induce tranquilization.

Adjuvant points according to syndrome differentiation:

1. Depressed Liver with exuberant fire: Ganshu (BL 18), and Jianshi (PC 5), Taichong (LR 3).
2. Incoordination of the Heart and the Kidneys: Xinshu (BL 15), Shenshu (BL 23), and Taixi (KI 3).
3. Deficiency of both the Heart and the Spleen: Xinshu (BL 15), and Jueyinshu (BL 14).
4. Deficiency of the Heart and the Gallbladder: Xinshu (BL 15), Danshu (BL 19), and Daling (PC 7).

Manipulation: Uniform reinforcement-reduction or reinforcement.

NARCOLEPSY

Narcolepsy is a chronic disorder characterized by involuntary daytime sleep episodes. The symptoms range from mild drowsiness intruding upon lecture hours or social events, to severe sleepiness in which subjects spend nearly the entire day, unable to work.

---

[4]*Anshen Wan* (Tranquilizing Pill): *Radix Ginseng* (ginseng), *Radix Angelicae Sinensis* (Chinese angelica root), *Poria* (fuling), *Semen Ziziphi Spinosae* (spiny jujube seed), *Semen Armeniacae Amarum* (bitter apricot seed), *Radix Peoniae Rubra* (red peony root), *Exocarpium Citri Rubrum* (red tangerine peel), *Fructus Schisandrae* (magnoliavine fruit), *Rhizoma Pinelliae* (pinellia tuber), *Radix Glycyrrhizae* (licorice root), *and Rhizoma Zingiberis* (ginger).

The onset is usually insidious in the second decade. Once the predisposition to excessive sleepiness starts, it is likely to last a lifetime if not treated. In Western medicine, the treatment is symptomatic with stimulants such as amphetamine, methylphenidate, and pemoline. Their continuous use is limited, due to side effects. The therapeutic experience of traditional Chinese medicine may be helpful to those with narcolepsy.

Etiology And Pathogenesis

Wakefulness is attributed to *yang*, and sleepiness to *yin*. Narcolepsy is a condition characterized by excessive *yin* with insufficient *yang*. This is usually closely related to disorders of the Spleen. Insufficiency of the Spleen may give rise to retained phlegm-damp, which inhibits clear *yang*. In addition, deficiency of Spleen *qi* or *yang* itself may directly lead to sleepiness.

Syndrome Differentiation

Narcolepsy can be divided into three patterns: Retention of phlegm-damp, weakness of Spleen *qi*, and insufficiency of Spleen *yang*.

1. Retention of phlegm-damp: Excessive daytime sleepiness accompanied by heavy sensation in the body, fullness in the chest, and impaired appetite, white greasy tongue coating, and soft, relaxed pulse.

2. Weakness of Spleen *qi*: Excessive daytime sleepiness accompanied by indolence, particularly after meals.

3. Insufficiency of Spleen *yang*: Excessive daytime sleepiness accompanied by lassitude, aversion to cold, cool limbs, spontaneous sweating, and weak pulse.

Herbal Medication

1. Retention of phlegm-damp

Principle of treatment: To eliminate phlegm-damp and invigorate the Spleen.

Formula of choice: *Pingwei San* (Stomach-pacifying Powder) plus *Herba Pogostemonis* (cablin patchouli), *Herba Eupatorii* (eupatorium), and *Semen Coicis* (coix seed).

2. Weakness of Spleen *qi*

Principle of treatment: To replenish *qi* and invigorate the Spleen.

Formula of choice: *Liujunzi Tang* (Decoction of Six Noble Ingredients).

3. Insufficiency of Spleen *yang*

Principle of treatment: To warm and tonify *yang-qi*.

Formula of choice: *Lizhong Tang* (Decoction for Regulating the Middle Energizer).

Patent Medicines

1. Retention of phlegm-damp: *Erchen Wan* (Pill of Tangerine Peel and Pinellia Tuber)

2. Weakness of Spleen *qi*: *Buzhong Yiqi Wan* (Pill for Reinforcing the Middle Energizer and Replenishing *Qi*).

3. Insufficiency of Spleen *yang*: *Fuzi Lizhong Wan* (Aconite Pill for Regulating the

Middle Energizer).

Acupuncture

Selection of points: Xinshu (BL 15), Pishu (BL 20), Shenmen (HT 7), Neiguan (PC 6), and Zusanli (ST 36).

Manipulation: When puncturing the back-*shu* points, direct the tip of the needle toward the spine, and twirl it to make the transmission of acupuncture sensation to the chest. When puncturing points on the limbs, twirl the needle to make proximal transmission of the acupuncture sensation.

EPILEPSY

Epilepsy is a group of disorders characterized by chronic, recurrent seizures, either convulsive when they are accompanied by motor manifestations, or manifest by sensory, cognitive, emotional changes. In this section, however, only epilepsy with tonic-clonic seizures is discussed.

Etiology and Pathogenesis

Epilepsy is a group of disorders caused by multiple factors. Emotional, dietary, and constitutional factors that lead to dysfunction of *zang-fu* organs (particularly the Liver) with turbid phlegm retention and *qi* derangement may result in obstruction of the "mental orifices" by Liver wind combined with phlegm, and hence epileptic seizures.

Syndrome Differentiation

I. During the Seizures

1. Liver wind with phlegm turbidity: The seizure is often preceded by dizziness, an oppressive feeling in the chest and lack of strength.

2. Liver fire with phlegm-heat: Similar seizure as described above, but in the interseizure periods irascible temperament, insomnia, bitterness and dryness in the mouth, constipation, reddened tongue with yellow coating, and stringy, rapid pulse.

II. The Interseizure State

1. *Yin* deficiency of the Liver and Kidneys: Hot temper, disturbed sleep, impaired memory, backache, dizziness, difficult emptying of the bowels, reddened tongue, and thready, rapid pulse.

2. Weakness of the Spleen and Stomach: Lassitude and listlessness, poor appetite, sallow complexion, emaciation, loose stools, pale tongue, and soft, thready pulse.

Herbal Medication

I. During the Seizures

1. Liver wind with phlegm-turbidity

Principle of treatment: To extinguish wind, eliminate phlegm and induce tranquilization.

Formula of choice: *Dingxian Wan* (Epilepsy-relieving Pill)[5].

2. Liver fire with phlegm-heat

Principle of treatment: To purge the Liver of fire and eliminate phlegm.

Formula of choice: *Longdan Xiegan Tang* (Decoction of Gentian to Purge the Liver) plus *Ditan Tang* (Decoction for Cleansing the Heart of Phlegm).

II. The Interseizure State

1. *Yin* deficiency of the Liver and Kidneys

Principle of treatment: To nourish the Liver and Kidneys and induce tranquilization.

Formula of choice: *Zuogui Wan* (*Yin*-directing Pill) plus *Semen Platycladi* (arborvitae seed) and *Magnetitum* (magnetite).

2. Weakness of the Spleen and Stomach

Principle of treatment: To invigorate the Spleen, replenish *qi* and harmonize the Stomach.

Formula of choice: *Liujunzi Tang* (Decoction of Six Noble Ingredients).

Patent Medicines

Yixian Wan (Anti-epilepsy Pill)[6] for various patterns of epilepsy.

Dingxian Wan (Epilepsy-relieving Pill) for epilepsy of the phlegm-heat pattern.

Mengshi Guntan Wan (Mica Pill for Eliminating Phlegm)[7] for epilepsy due to fire and phlegm.

Heche Wan or *Heche Dazao Wan* (Placenta Pill)[8] for interseizure state with *yin* deficiency.

Liujunzi Wan (Pill of Six Noble Ingredients) for interseizure state with weakened Spleen.

---

[5]*Dingxian Wan* (Epilepsy-relieving Pill): *Rhizoma Gastrodiae* (gastrodia tuber) 30 g, *Bulbus Fritillariae Cirrhosae* (tendrilled fritillary bulb) 30 g, *Rhizoma Pinelliae* (pinellia tuber) 30 g, *Poria* (fuling) 30 g, *Poria cum Radice Pino* (fushen) 30 g, *Rhizoma Arisematis cum Felle Bovis* (bile-processed jack-in-the-pulpit tuber) 15 g, *Rhizoma Acori Tatarinowii* (grass-leaved sweetflag rhizome) 15 g, *Scorpio* (scorpion) 15 g, *Radix Glycyrrhizae* (licorice root) 15 g, *Bombyx Batryticatus* (white-stiff silkworm) 15 g, *Succinum* (amber) 15 g, *Medulla Junci* (rush pith) 15 g, *Pericarpium Citri Reticulatae* (tangerine peel) 20 g, *Radix Polygalae* (milkwort root) 20 g, *Radix Salviae Miltiorrhizae* (red sage root) 60 g, *Radix Asparagi* (asparagus root) 60 g, and *Cinnabaris* (cinnabar) 9 g, to be pulverized, mixed and made into pills, 6 g twice a day.

[6]*Yixian Wan* (Anti-epilepsy Pill): *Rhizoma Typhonii* (typhonium tuber) 40 g, *Rhizoma Arisematis* (Jack-in-the-pulpit tuber) 80 g, *Rhizoma Pinelliae* (pinellia tuber) 80 g, *Fructus Gleditsiae Abnormalis* (small gleditsia) 400 g, *Bombyx Batryticatus* (white-stiff silkworm) 80 g, *Zaocys* (black-tailed snake) 80 g, *Scolopendra* (centipede) 2 g, *Scorpio* (scorpion) 16 g, *Alumen* (alum) 120 g, *Realgar* (realgar) 12 g, and *Cinnabaris* (cinnabar) 16 g, to be pulverized, mixed, and made into pills, 3 g, 2-3 times a day.

[7]*Mengshi Guntan Wan* (Mica Pill for Eliminating Phlegm): *Radix et Rhizoma Rhei* (rhubarb), *Radix Scutellariae* (skullcap root), *Lapis Micae Aureae* (mica), and *Lignum Aquilariae Resinatum* (eagle wood) to be mixed at the ratio of 16:16:2:1 in weight, and made into pills, 6 g, 2 times a day.

[8]*Heche Wan* or *Heche Dazao Wan* (Placenta Pill): *Placenta Hominis* (human placenta), *Radix Asparagi* (asparagus root), *Radix Ophiopogonis* (lilyturf root), *Radix Achyanthis Bidentatae* (twoteethed achyranthes root), *Cortex Eucommiae* (eucommia bark), *Cortex Phellodendri* (phellodendron bark), *Radix Rehmanniae* (rehmannia root), *Carapax et Plastrum Testudinis* (tortoise carapace and plastron), pulverized, mixed at the ratio of 1:1:1:1:1.5:1.5:2:2, and made into pills; 6 g, 2 times a day.

Acupuncture

Principle of treatment: To extinguish wind and eliminate phlegm.

Points used during seizures: Baihui (GV 20), Shuigou (GV 26), Houxi (SI 3), and Yongquan (KI 1).

Points used in interseizure periods: Jiuwei (CV 15), Dazhui (GV 14), Yaoqi (EX-B 9), Jianshi (PC 5), and Fenglong (ST 40).

DEPRESSION

"Depression" in traditional Chinese medicine is defined as a disease caused by emotional constraint with stagnation of *qi*, manifested by lowering of the spirits, uneasiness, irritability, irascibility or inclination to sob or cry, distension and pain in the hypochondriac region, insomnia, or the feeling of a foreign body in the throat. It is not the equivalent of depression in Western medicine, but they share some common features, and so the discussion of the former may be applied to the latter.

Etiology and Pathogenesis

1. Anger impedes the smooth flow of Liver *qi*, resulting in stagnation. Long-standing stagnant *qi* may be transformed into fire or impairment of the Spleen with production of phlegm, giving rise to irritability, hypochondriac distension and pain, and the feeling of a foreign body in the throat.

2. Emotional disturbance and anxiety affecting the Liver and Spleen may further impair *qi* and blood of the Heart (mind), leading to a lowering of the spirits, uneasiness and insomnia.

Syndrome Differentiation

1. Stagnation of Liver *qi*: Low-spiritedness, uneasiness, hypochondriac distension and pain, epigastric fullness, belching, anorexia, abnormal bowel movements, thin and greasy tongue coating, and stringy pulse.

2. Transformation of stagnated *qi* into fire: Irritability and irascibility, hypochondriac distension and fullness, bitterness and dryness of the mouth, accompanied by headache, congested eyes and tinnitus, or by acid regurgitation and constipation, reddened tongue and yellow coating, and stringy, rapid pulse.

3. Accumulation of phlegm with stagnated *qi*: Depressed mood, suffocating sensation in the chest, distension and pain in the flanks, feeling of a foreign body in the throat which is neither able to be spat out nor swallowed, white slippery tongue coating and stringy, slippery pulse.

4. Deficiency of Heart *yin*: Palpitations, forgetfulness, insomnia, dream-disturbed sleep, heat sensation in the palms and soles, night sweating, dryness of the throat and mouth, reddened and dry tongue, and thready, rapid pulse.

5. Insufficiency of both Heart and Spleen: Anxiety with suspicions, dizziness, lack of energy, palpitations, insomnia, forgetfulness, anorexia, sallow complexion, pale tongue with thin white coating, and thready pulse.

Herbal Medication

1. Stagnation of Liver *qi*

Principle of treatment: To soothe the Liver and regulate the flow of *qi,* and relieve emotional depression.

Formula of choice: *Chaihu Shugan San* (Bupleurum Powder for Soothing the Liver).

2. Transformation of stagnated *qi* into fire

Principle of treatment: To soothe the Liver, clear the Liver of fire and relieve emotional depression.

Formula of choice: *Dan Zhi Xiaoyao San* (Ease Powder with Moutan and Gardenia).

3. Accumulation of phlegm with stagnated *qi*

Principle of treatment: To remove the stagnated *qi*, resolve phlegm and relieve emotional depression.

Formula of choice: *Banxia Houpo Tang* (Decoction of Pinellia and Magnolia).

4. Deficiency of Heart *yin*

Principle of treatment: To replenish *yin*-blood of the Heart and calm the mind.

Formula of choice: *Tianwang Buxin Dan* (Heavenly King's Tonic for the Heart).

5. Insufficiency of both Heart and Spleen

Principle of treatment: To invigorate the Spleen, nourish the Heart, and replenish *qi* and blood.

Formula of choice: *Guipi Tang* (Spleen-invigorating Decoction).

Patent Medicines

Yueju Wan (Pill for Removing Stagnation) used for depression due to stagnation of Liver *qi*.

Xiaoyao Wan (Ease Pill) used for depression due to stagnation of Liver *qi* with insufficiency of the Spleen.

Danzhi Xiaoyao Wan (Ease Pill with Moutan and Gardenia) used for depression due to stagnation of *qi* with fire.

Tianwang Buxin Dan (Heavenly King's Tonic for the Heart) used for depression with deficiency of Heart *yin*.

Renshen Guipi Wan (Spleen-invigorating Pill with Ginseng) used for depression with insufficiency of both Heart and Spleen.

Acupuncture

1. Stagnation of Liver *qi*

Selection of points: Ganshu (BL 18), Danzhong (CV 17), Zhongwan (CV 12), Zusanli (ST 36), Gongsun (SP 4), and Taichong (LR 3).

Manipulation: Uniform reinforcement-reduction is applied.

2. Transformation of stagnated *qi* into fire

Selection of points: Shangwan (CV 13), Zhigou (TE 6), Yanglingquan (GB 34), Xingjian (LR 2), and Xiaxi (GB 43).

Manipulation: Reduction is applied to dispel the fire.

3. Accumulation of phlegm with stagnated *qi*

Selection of points: Tiantu (CV 22), Danzhong (CV 17), Neiguan (PC 6), Fenglong

(ST 40), and Taichong (LR 3).

Manipulation: Uniform reinforcement-reduction is applied.

4. Deficiency of Heart *yin*

Selection of points: Xinshu (BL 15), Juque (CV 14), Shenmen (HT 7), Sanyinjiao (SP 6), and Taichong (LR 3).

Manipulation: Uniform reinforcement-reduction is applied.

5. Insufficiency of both Heart and Spleen

Selection of points: Xinshu (BL 15), Geshu (BL 17), Pishu (BL 20), Juque (CV 14), Shenmen (HT 7), and Zusanli (ST 36).

Manipulation: Reinforcement or uniform reinforcement-reduction is applied.

CHAPTER 25

LOCOMOTIVE DISORDERS

SPRAIN

In sprains, there is injury of the tendons and meridians, which causes impairment of *qi* flow in the meridians and local stagnation of *qi* and blood. Acupuncture, regulating the flow of *qi* and blood, not only relieves pain, but also helps to cure sprains.

Acupuncture

Shoulder: Jianyu (LI 15), Jianliao (TE 14), and Jianzhen (SI 9).

Elbow: Quchi (LI 11), Xiaohai (SI 8), and Tianjin (TE 10).

Wrist: Yangchi (TE 4), Yangxi (LI 5), Yanggu (SI 5), and Yaotongdian (EX-UE 7).

Waist: Shenshu (BL 23), Yaoyangguan (GV 3), and Weizhong (BL 40).

Hip: Huantiao (GB 30), Zhibian (BL 54), and Chengfu (BL 36).

Knee: Liangqiu (ST 34), Xiyan (EX-LE 5), Yinlingquan (SP 9), and Yanglingquan (GB 34).

Ankle: Jiexi (ST 41), Kunlun (BL 60), Qiuxu (GB 40), and Sanyinjiao (SP 6).

In all the above conditions, local tender points may be added.

In acute sprain reduction, manipulation is indicated, while in chronic cases it is preferable to add moxibustion to acupuncture, or apply warming needling.

CRICK IN THE NECK

Improper position during sleep, turning of the neck with a heavy burden, or attack on the nape by wind-cold may cause a crick in the neck. Acupuncture may quickly relieve the pain and muscle stiffness.

Acupuncture

Major points: Tender point, Laozhen (an extra point located on the dorsum of the hand between the second and third metacarpal bones, 0.5 *cun* proximal to the metacarpo-phalangeal articulation).

Additional points: Add Houxi (SI 3) if the muscle stiffness and pain is on the posterolateral side of the neck; add Zhongzhu (TE 3) and Xuanzhong (GB 39) if the lateral side of the neck is affected; and add Hegu (LI 4) and Lieque (LU 7) if the anterior aspect of the neck is involved.

Reduction manipulation is indicated. While applying manipulation to the distant points, ask the patient to try to turn the neck.

HEEL PAIN

Heel pain may be due to hyperosteogeny or due to kidney insufficiency. The former is a kind of degenerative change, while the latter is often accompanied by soreness and weakness of the back and legs. In both cases, acupuncture-moxibustion is useful, but the principle of treatment and the punctured points are different.

Acupuncture

Heel pain due to hyperosteogeny: Moxibustion applied to the tender points, Kunlun (BL 60) and Taixi (KI 3).

Heel pain due to kidney insufficiency: Acupuncture or moxibustion applied to Zhaohai (KI 6), Taixi (KI 3), Shenshu (BL 23), and Fuliu (KI 7).

FROZEN SHOULDER

Frozen shoulder is caused by trauma, overstrain, or attack of wind-cold-damp which impairs the function of the tendons and the flow of *qi* and blood in the meridians and collaterals over the shoulder.

Acupuncture

Principle of treatment: To soothe the tendons and smooth the flow of *qi* and blood in the meridian and collaterals.

Points: Jianyu (LI 15), Jianliao (TE 14), Hegu (LI 4), Tianding (LI 17), Jugu (LI 16), Jianzhen (SI 9), Binao (LI 14), Tianzong (SI 11), and Quyuan (SI 13).

Manipulation: Warming needling is preferable.

LUMBAGO

Lumbago or back pain is experienced by most people. It has many possible causes, mechanical, inflammatory, neurological, etc. If there is no need for specific treatment (e.g., antibiotics for infections or urgent surgical intervention for structural anomalies), acupuncture is an effective therapy. This was even recorded in Western medical textbooks decades ago.

Etiology and Pathogenesis

Among the various categories of lumbago, only the following three are discussed in this section: cold-damp lumbago, lumbar muscle sprain, and lumbago due to kidney insufficiency.

Cold-damp lumbago is usually attributed to wind-cold affections or staying in a wet place where the pathogenic wind-cold-damp lodges in the related meridians, impairing the normal flow of *qi*.

Lumbar muscle sprain results from trauma which injures the related muscles and meridians. In chronic cases, blood stasis often plays an important role in the origination of pain.

Lumbago due to kidney insufficiency is the outcome of overstrain, sexual indulgence or chronic illnesses.

Syndrome Differentiation

1. Cold-damp lumbago: Backache with sensation of heaviness and inability of movement, sometimes chronic with intermittent pain, and aggravated by exposure to cold or sudden weather changes.

2. Lumbar muscle sprain: Chronic backache, fixed in location, precipitated by exertion or fatigue, aggravated by turning over, and accompanied by local stiffness.

3. Lumbago due to kidney insufficiency: Gradual onset of dull backache, persistent and continuous, accompanied by weakness of the legs and lack of strength.

Acupuncture

Common points: Shenshu (BL 23), Weizhong (BL 40), and Jiaji (EX-B 2).

Adjuvant points according to syndrome differentiation: For cold-damp, add Fengfu (GV 16); for sprain, add Geshu (BL 17) and Ciliao (BL 32); for kidney insufficiency, add Zhishi (BL 52) and Taixi (KI 3).

Manipulations: Reduction for cold-damp lumbago; uniform reinforcement-reduction for sprain, and reinforcement for kidney insufficiency.

ARTHRITIDES AND RHEUMATOID ARTHRITIS

Diseases characterized by joint pain with inflammatory process and accompanied by ankylosis, deformities, numbness or muscular atrophy are called "*bi* syndrome" in Chinese medicine. *Bi* means obstruction of the collateral meridians of the limbs by pathogenic factors resulting in arthralgia, numbness and impaired motility. *Bi* syndrome includes a variety of articular and musculoskeletal disorders such as rheumatoid arthritis, osteoarthropathy and peripheral neuritis. In order to avoid confusion in terminology, the term "arthritides" will be used instead of "*bi* syndromes."

Etiology and Pathogenesis

1. Weak constitution vulnerable to exogenous affections. A person with a weak constitution is apt to be invaded by wind, damp, cold or heat from outside. Owing to lack of adequate body's resistance, the pathogens further enter the muscles, tendons and bones, resulting in arthritides. If the patient used to be deficient in *yang*, the result is usually obstruction of *qi* and blood circulation in the collaterals by wind, cold and damp (wind-cold-damp arthritides). If the patient used to be deficient in *yin*, his *yang* is relatively exuberant, and the result may be obstruction of the collaterals by wind, heat and damp (wind-heat-damp arthritides).

2. Invasion of the exogenous pathogens. The common exogenous pathogens are wind, cold, damp and heat. Although the pathogens tend to attack people with weak constitutions, they also affect healthy individuals who have been exposed to cold and damp for a long period of time (e.g., staying in a cold place without adequate measures to keep warm, underwater operations, sleeping in the open, or exposure to draught, rain or snow). The result will be affection by wind, cold and damp, but the pathogens may be transformed into heat, giving rise to arthritides of the wind-heat-damp type.

3. Retention of phlegm and stagnation of blood. In chronic cases, long-term impairment of *qi* and blood circulation will lead to blood stasis and condensation of damp into phlegm. Stagnated blood and phlegm, combined with each other or with exogenous pathogens, further obstruct the collaterals deep in the bones, rendering the disease stubborn. Joint swelling with deformities occurring in the late stage of the disease is usually attributed to retention of phlegm and stagnated blood.

In addition, although the disease chiefly involves the collaterals of the limbs, the pathogens may also be transmitted interiorly, bringing about disorders in the *zang-fu* organs. For example, the heart may be involved, manifested by cardiac palpitations and shortness of breath.

Syndrome Differentiation

Key points to the traditional syndrome diagnosis:

1. Differentiation of excess and deficiency

Similar to other diseases, arthritides should first be classified as excess and deficiency syndromes. Generally speaking, most arthritides in the early stages are excessive in pathogens. After repeated attacks, long-termed obstruction of the collaterals by pathogens impairs the nutritive supply and defensive energy on the one hand, and formation of phlegm and stagnated blood on the other. Therefore, the arthritides are usually characterized by deficiency of genuine *qi,* together with excess of pathogenic factors. In the late stage, when there is consumption of *qi* and blood with lack of nourishment to the tendons and bones, the arthritides usually enter the deficiency state. However, the duration of the disease is not the only criterion for the differentiation of excess and deficiency. In some cases, an acute disease may occur in a patient with deficiency of *qi* and blood, and there is a deficiency state at the very beginning. On the other hand, if cold-damp or damp-heat persists or phlegm with stagnated blood retains in a chronic case, the syndrome will still be excessive in character.

2. Differentiation of the patient's constitution

Differentiation of the patient's constitution is also of great significance. A constitution deficiency in *yang* is usually characterized by obesity, puffy and pale or yellowish complexion, aversion to wind, lack of strength, loose stools, plump and pale tongue and feeble pulse. Arthritides in patients with *yang* deficiency is often of the wind-cold-damp type.

A constitution deficiency in *yin* is usually characterized by emaciation, dark complexion, malar flush, night sweating, insomnia, constipation, thin and reddened tongue, and thready, rapid pulse. Arthritides in patients with *yin* deficiency is often of the wind-heat-damp type.

3. Recognition of the pathogenic factors

The common pathogenic factors of arthritides are wind, cold, damp and heat. Each of them has its own characteristic features. Wind is characterized by migratory pain, moving from one site to another without fixed location, together with thin white tongue coating and a floating pulse. Cold has a congealing action, which causes severe pain fixed in location and accompanied by muscular contracture. The pain may be aggravated by exposure to cold and alleviated by warmth. The tongue coating is white and the pulse tense. Damp is characterized by the lingering course of disease. It often affects the joints of the lower part of the body accompanied by a feeling of heaviness and marked swelling. The tongue coating is white and greasy, and the pulse soft. Heat causes severe joint pain with redness, swelling, hotness and tenderness. There may be general symptoms such as high fever and thirst. The tongue is reddened, coating yellow and dry, and the pulse slippery and rapid.

In chronic cases, the presence of phlegm and stagnated blood should be carefully considered, especially when ordinary treatment for wind, cold and damp or wind, heat and damp fails. Joint swelling due to damp is usually diffuse and soft, without severe pain, while joint swelling due to phlegm and stagnated blood in combination is hard, accompanied by severe pain and numbness of the limb. In stagnation of blood, the pulse is thready and hesitant, the tongue purplish with purple spots. In retention of phlegm, the pulse is soft and relaxed, and the tongue coating white and greasy.

I. Arthritides of the Excess Type

1. Arthritis due to wind, cold and damp

This type of arthritis is often encountered in early rheumatoid arthritis and osteoarthropathy without acute inflammatory manifestations. It may be further divided into three patterns.

(1) Wind arthritis (migratory arthralgia): Joint and muscle pain, moving from one to another, usually involving multiple joints, particularly the fingers, wrists, elbows, knees and ankles. The pain may be accompanied by an exterior syndrome characterized by aversion to wind and mild fever. The tongue coating is thin and white, and the pulse slow.

(2) Cold arthritis (agonizing arthralgia): Severe muscle and joint pain, fixed in location, alleviated by warmth and aggravated by exposure to cold, with impairment of articular motility and without local redness and heat. The tongue coating is white, and the pulse stringy and tense.

(3) Damp arthritis (weighty arthralgia): Muscle and joint soreness, fixed in location, accompanied by impairment of joint motion, swelling and numbness. The tongue coating is white and greasy, and the pulse soft and slow.

2. Arthritis due to wind, damp and heat (heat arthritis): This type of arthritis is often encountered in acute rheumatic arthritis or acute exacerbation of rheumatoid arthritis, manifested by acute onset of point pain with local redness, heat and swelling, alleviated by cold and aggravated by exposure to heat, accompanied by loss of joint motion. There may be fever, sweating, and thirst, erythema or subcutaneous nodules. The tongue coating is yellow, and the pulse rapid.

3. Stubborn arthritis: Chronic arthritis with repeated recurrences, manifested by ankylosis and deformities of the joints, severe pain fixed in location, dark discoloration of the surrounding skin, loss of joint motion or presence of numbness. The affected joint(s) may be reddened and swollen, associated with general symptoms such as fever and thirst, or may be felt cold with aggravated pain during weather changes and alleviation by warmth. The pulse is often thready and hesitant, and there may be purple spots on the tongue.

II. Arthritides of the Deficiency Type

1. Arthritis with deficiency of *qi* and blood: Chronic arthritis with joint pain varying in severity, aggravated by flexion and extension, and maybe accompanied by muscle twitching or contracture; sallow complexion, cardiac palpitation, lack of strength, shortness of breath, spontaneous sweating, emaciation, anorexia, loose stools, pale tongue with white coating or no coating, soft and weak pulse or thready and feeble pulse.

2. Arthritis with deficiency of *yang*: Chronic arthritis with joint pain, stiffness and deformities, accompanied by cold feeling and muscle atrophy, pale complexion, aversion to cold, cold limbs, loose stools, pale tongue, and deep, weak pulse.

3. Arthritis with deficiency of *yin*: Chronic arthritis with joint pain and muscular contracture, aggravated on motion; lassitude, lack of strength, night sweating, dizziness, tinnitus, constipation, or persistent low fever, reddened tongue with scanty coating, and thready pulse.

Herbal Medication

I. Arthritides of Excess Type

1. Arthritis due to wind, cold and damp

(1) Wind arthritis

Principle of treatment: To remove wind from the collaterals, and dispel cold and damp.

Formula of choice: *Juanbi Tang* (Decoction for Treating *Bi* Syndromes)[1] plus *Radix Saposhnikoviae* (saposhnikovia root).

(2) Cold arthritis

Principle of treatment: To warm up the meridian by dispelling cold, and to eliminate wind and damp.

Formula of choice: *Juanbi Tang* (Decoction for Treating *Bi* Syndromes) plus *Radix Aconiti Lateralis* (aconite lateral root).

(3) Damp arthritis

Principle of treatment: To eliminate damp by invigorating the spleen, and dispel wind and cold.

Formula of choice: *Juanbi Tang* (Decoction for Treating *Bi* Syndromes) plus *Radix Stephaniae Tetrandrae* (tetrandra root) and *Semen Coicis* (coix seed).

2. Arthritis due to wind, damp and heat (Heat arthritis)

Principle of treatment: To clear heat, wind and damp from the collaterals.

Formula of choice: *Baihu Jia Guizhi Tang* (White Tiger Decoction with Cinnamon Twig).

3. Stubborn arthritis

Principle of treatment: To eliminate stagnated blood and retained phlegm from the collaterals.

Formula of choice: *Xiao Huoluo Wan* (Pill for Activating Circulation in Collateral Meridians—Mild Recipe).

II. Arthritides of Deficiency Type

1. Arthritis with deficiency of *qi* and blood

Principle of treatment: To replenish *qi* and blood, warm the meridians and relieve arthralgia.

Formula of choice: *Huangqi Guizhi Wuwu Tang* (Decoction of Five Ingredients with Astragalus and Cinnamon)[2] plus *Radix Angelicae Sinensis* (Chinese angelica root).

2. Arthritis with deficiency of *yang*

Principle of treatment: To reinforce *yang*.

Formula of choice: *Zhenwu Tang* (the Water God's Decoction)[3].

3. Arthritis with deficiency of *yin*

Principle of treatment: To replenish liver and kidney *yin*.

Formula of choice: *Liuwei Dihuang Tang* (Decoction of Six Ingredients with

---

[1]*Juanbi Tang* (Decoction for Treating *Bi* Syndromes): *Rhizoma Notopterygii* (notopterygium rhizome) 3 g, *Radix Angelicae Pubescentis* (pubescent angelica root) 3 g, *Cortex Cinnamomi* (cinnamon bark) 1.5 g, *Radix Gentianae Macrophyllae* (large-leaf gentian root) 3 g, *Radix Angelicae Sinensis* (Chinese angelica root) 9 g, *Rhizoma Chuanxiong* (chuanxiong) 2 g, *Radix Glycyrrhizae* (licorice) 1.5 g, *Caulis Piperis Kadsurae* (kadsura pepper stem) 6 g, *Ramulus Mori* (mulberry twig) 9 g, *Resina Olibani* (frankincense) 1.5 g, and *Radix Aucklandiae* (costus root) 1.5 g, to be made into a decoction.

[2]*Huangqi Guizhi Wuwu Tang* (Decoction of Five Ingredients with Astragalus and Cinnamon): *Radix Astragali* (astragalus root) 12 g, *Radix Peoniae Alba* (white peony root) 9 g, *Ramulus Cinnamomi* (cinnamon twig) 9 g, *Rhizoma Zingiberis Recens* (fresh ginger) 12 g, *Fructus Jujubae* (Chinese date) 4 pieces, to be made into a decoction.

[3]See Footnote 4 of Chronic Glomerulonephritis in Chapter 20.

Rehmannia) plus *Radix Angelicae Sinensis* (Chinese Angelica root) and *Radix Peoniae Alba* (white peony root).

Arthritis with deficiency of *qi* and blood together with deficiency of liver and kidney *yin* is common among the chronic cases of the deficiency type. *Duhuo Jisheng Tang (Wan)* (Decoction or Pill of Pubescent Angelica and Mulberry Mistletoe) is the popular formula for the treatment.

Patent Medicines

Xiaohuoluo Wan (Pill for Activating Circulation in Collateral Meridians—Minor Recipe) for cold arthritis.

Duohuo Jisheng Wan (Pill of Pubescent Angelica and Mulberry Mistletoe) for arthritis with deficiency of *qi* and blood together with deficiency of liver and kidney *yin*.

Mugua Wan (Chaenomeles Fruit Pill) for chronic arthritis with joint pain.

Wangbi Chongji (Granule for Arthritis with Deformity)[4] for chronic rheumatoid arthritis with deformities.

Leigongteng Pian (Tripterygium Wilfordii Tablets)[5] for rheumatoid arthritis.

Acupuncture

Selection of points according to the affected joints.

Shoulder: Jianyu (LI 15), Jianliao (TE 14), Jianzhen (SI 9), and Naoshu (SI 10).

Scapula: Tianzong (SI 11), Bingfeng (SI 12), Jianwaishu (SI 14), and Gaohuangshu (BL 43).

Elbow: Quchi (LI 11), Chize (LU 5), Tianjing (TE 10), Waiguan (TE 5), and Hegu (LI 4).

Wrist: Yangchi (TE 4), Yangxi (LI 5), Yanggu (SI 5), and Waiguan (TE 5).

Fingers: Houxi (SI 3), Sanjian (LI 3), and Baxie (EX-UE 9).

Hip: Huantiao (GB 30), Yinmen (BL 37), and Juliao (GB 29).

Knee: Liangqiu (ST 34), Dubi (ST 35), Neixiyan (EX-LE 4), Yanglingquan (GB 34), Xiyangguan (GB 33), and Yinlingquan (SP 9).

Leg: Chengshan (BL 57), and Feiyang (BL 58).

Ankle: Jiexi (ST 41), Shangqiu (SP 5), Qiuxu (GB 40), Kunlun (BL 60), and Taixi

---

[4]*Wangbi Chongji* (Granules for Arthritis with Deformity): *Radix Rehmanniae* (rehmannia root), *Radix Aconiti Lateralis* (aconite lateral root), *Rhizoma Drynariae* (drynaria rhizome), *Herba Epimedii* (epimedium), *Radix Angelicae Pubescentis* (pubescent angelica root), *Ramulus Cinnamomi* (cinnamon twig), *Radix Saposhnikoviae* (saposhnikovia root), *Scolopendra* (centipede), *Rhizoma Anemarrhenae* (anemarrhena rhizome), *Spina Gleditsiae* (gleditsia thorn), *Radix Peoniae alba* (white peony root), *Flos Carthami* (safflower), *Radix Clematidis* (clematis root), *Herba Lycopodii* (club-moss), and *Fructus Psoraleae* (scurfpea fruit), to be pulverized and made into granules, 10-20 g taken after being mixed with boiling water.

[5]*Tripterygium wilfordii Hook f.* was found effective in the treatment of rheumatoid arthritis in 1969. Its clinical use was limited, owing to the adverse side effects, particularly on the digestive and reproductive systems, caused by its diterpene and alkaloid contents. Later, its multi-glucosides were found to be as effective as the entire herb, but with much less side effects. Now, Leigongteng Pian (Tripterygium Wilfordii Tablet) is prepared only from the multi-glucosides. The recommended dosage is 30 mg daily.

(KI 3).

Toes: Gongsun (SP 4), Shugu (BL 65), and Bafeng (EX-LE 10).

Back: Shuigou (GV 26), Shenzhu (GV 12), and Yaoyangguan (GV 3).

General aching: Houxi (SI 3), Shenmai (BL 62), Dabao (SP 21), and Geshu (BL 17).

Additional points according to syndrome differentiation.

Wind arthritis: Fengmen (BL 12), and Geshu (BL 17).

Cold-damp arthritis: Zusanli (ST 36), and Shangqiu (SP 5).

Heat arthritis: Dazhui (GV 14), and Quchi (LI 11).

Stubborn arthritis: Yanglingquan (GB 34), Xuanzhong (GB 39), and Dazhu (BL 11).

Deficiency of *qi* and blood: Pishu (BL 20), Geshu (BL 17), Guanyuan (CV 4), and Zusanli (ST 36).

Deficiency of liver and kidney *yin*: Shenshu (BL 23), Taixi (KI 3).

Defciiency of kidney *yang*: Shenshu (BL 23), and Guanyuan (CV 4).

Manipulations:

Wind arthritis is treated with needling, and cold arthritis with moxibustion or warming needling. For heat arthritis, reducing manipulation is indicated; for damp arthritis, shallow insertion with reinforcing manipulation is advisable.

APPENDIX 1

MAJOR REFERENCES

Part One

(1) 季钟朴主编（Ji Zhongpu, chief-editor）：现代中医生理学基础 （*Physiological Basis of Modernized TCM*）(in Chinese), Beijing, Xueyuan Press, 1991.

(2) 彭瑞骢主编（Peng Ruicong, chief-editor）：医学辨证法 (*Medical Dialectics*) (in Chinese), Beijing, People's Medical Publishing House, 1992.

(3) 沈自尹主编(Shen Ziyin, chief-editor): 中医学 (*Traditional Chinese Medicine*) (in Chinese), Shanghai, Shanghai Science and Technology Press, 1995.

(4) 印会河主编（Yin Huihe, chief-editor）：中医基础理论 (*Basic Theories of Traditional Chinese Medicine*) (in Chinese), Shanghai, Shanghai Science and Technology Press, 1984.

(5) 李德新 (Li Dexin): 实用中医基础学 (*Basic Studies in Practical Traditional Chinese Medicine*) (in Chinese), Shenyang, Liaoning Science and Technology Press, 1985.

(6) 邓铁涛主编（Deng Tietao, chief-editor）: 实用中医诊断学（*Practical Traditional Chinese Diagnosis*）(in Chinese), Shanghai, Shanghai Science and Technology Press, 1988.

(7) 梁运通 (Liang Yuntong): 黄帝内经类析 (*Classified Analysis of Huangdi's Internal Classic*) (in Chinese), Huhhot, Inner Mongolia People's Publishing House, 1986.

(8) Xie Zhufan, Lou Zhicen and Huang Xiaokai: *Classified Dictionary of Traditional Chinese Medicine*, Beijing, New World Press, 1994.

Part Two

(1) 凌一揆主编 (Ling Yikui, chief-editor): 中药学 (*Traditional Chinese Pharmaceutics*) (in Chinese), Shanghai Science and Technology Press, 1984.

(2) 沈映君主编 (Shen Yingjun, chief-editor): 中药药理学 (*Pharmacology of Traditional Chinese Medicines*) (in Chinese), Shanghai, Shanghai Science and Technology Press, 1997.

(3) 王筠默主编 (Wang Junmo, chief-editor): 中药药理学 (*Pharmacology of Traditional Chinese Medicines*) (in Chinese), Shanghai, Shanghai Science and Technology Press, 1985.

(4) 许济群主编 (Xu Jiqun, chief-editor): 方剂学 (*Traditional Chinese Formulary*) (in Chinese), Shanghai, Shanghai Science and Technology Press, 1985.

(5) 傅衍魁、尤荣辑主编 (Fu Yankui and You Rongji, chief-editors): 医方发挥 (*Elaborations on Traditional Chinese Formulas*) (in Chinese), Shenyang, Liaoning Science and Technology Press, 1984.

(6) *Pharmacopoeia of the People's Republic of China* (English Edition, 1992).

Part Three

(1) Cheng Xinnong (chief-editor): *Chinese Acupuncture and Moxibustion*, Beijing, Foreign Languages Press, 1987.

(2) 裘沛然、陈汉平主编 (Qiu Peiran and Chen Hanping, chief-editors): 新编中国针灸学 (*Newly Compiled Chinese Acupuncture and Moxibustion*), Shanghai, Shanghai Science and Technology Press, 1992.

(3) *State Standard of the People's Republic of China: The Location of Acupoints*, Beijing, Foreign Languages Press, 1990.

(4) 张香桐、季钟朴、黄家驷主编 (Zhang Xiangtong, Ji Zhongpu and Huang Jiasi, chief-editors): 针灸针麻研究 (*Researches on Acupuncture-Moxibustion and Acupuncture-Anesthesia*) (in Chinese), Beijing, Science Press, 1986.

(5) 府强主编（Fu Qiang, chief-editor）: 实用针灸疗法临床大全 (*A Complete Book of Practical Acupuncture-Moxibustion*) (in Chinese), Beijing, Press of Traditional Chinese Medicine, 1991.

(6) 孙国杰主编 (Sun Guojie, chief-editor): 针灸学 (*Acupuncture and Moxibustion*), Shanghai, Shanghai Science and Technology Press, 1997.

Part Four

(1) Xie Zhufan and Liao Jiazhen: *Traditional Chinese Internal Medicine*, Beijing, Foreign Languages Press, 1993.

(2) 王永炎主编 (Wang Yongyan, chief-editor): 中医内科学 (*Traditional Chinese Internal Medicine*) (in Chinese), Shanghai, Shanghai Science and Technology Press, 1997.

(3) 罗元凯主编 (Luo Yuankai, chief-editor): 中医妇科学 （*Traditional Chinese Gynecology*）, Shanghai, Shanghai Science and Technology Press, 1994.

(4) 沈自尹主编 (Shen Ziyin, chief-editor): 中医学 (*Traditional Chinese Medicine*) (in Chinese), Shanghai, Shanghai Science and Technology Press, 1995.

(5) 王显明 (Wang Xianming): 中医内科辨证学 (*Traditional Differential Diagnosis of Internal Diseases*) (in Chinese), People's Medical Publishing House, 1984.

(6) 孙国杰、涂晋文主编 (Sun Guojie and Tu Jinwen, chief-editors): 中医治疗学 (*Therapeutics of Traditional Chinese Medicine*) (in Chinese), Beijing, Press of Chinese Medical Sciences, 1992.

APPENDIX 2

CLASSICAL CHINESE MEDICAL LITERATURE QUOTED

Ben Cao Gang Mu (本草纲目) (*Compendium of Materia Medica*) compiled by Li Shizhen, a gigantic and most comprehensive work published with detailed description of the appearance, properties, method of collection, preparation and use of each substance.

Bin Hu Mai Xue (濒湖脉学) (*Binhu's Pulse Studies*), a monograph on pulse diagnosis written by Li Shizhen (also called Li Binhu) in 1564.

Gu Shi Yi Jing (顾氏医镜) (*Gu's Mirror of Medicine*), a comprehensive book of theoretical and clinical medicine compiled by Gu Jing and published in 1718.

Huang Di Nei Jing (黄帝内经) (*Huangdi's Canon of Medicine*) or Nei Jing (内经) (*The Canon of Medicine*) for short, also known as *The Yellow Emperor's Internal Classic*, the oldest and greatest medical classic extant in China, a product of unknown authors in the Warring States Period (475-221 B.C.). The book consists of two parts: Su Wen (素问) (*Plain Questions*) and Ling Shu (灵枢) (*Miraculous Pivot*). The former includes various subjects of medicine, such as anatomy and physiology, cause of disease, pathology, symptomology, diagnosis, treatment and prevention of disease, health protection, integrity of human and nature, application of the theories of *qi, yin-yang* and the Five Elements in medicine. The latter is also known as Zhen Jing (针经) (*Canon of Acupuncture*). It also covers various aspects of medicine, but has a more detailed discussion on meridians and needling.

Jing Yue Quan Shu (景岳全书) (*Jingyue's Complete Works*), a book written by Zhang Jiebin, also called Zhang Jingyue, and published in 1624. He extracted the essence of various schools and made a systematical analysis of the traditional Chinese diagnosis and treatment.

Lei Jing (类经) (*Classified Canon*), a rearrangement of Nei Jing (*The Canon of Medicine*) compiled by Zhang Jiebin and published in 1624.

Mai Jing (脉经) (*The Pulse Classic*), written by Wang Shuhe in the third century, the earliest comprehensive and standard work dealing with sphygmology.

Mai Jue (脉决) (*Key to Pulse-Taking*), written in rhymes by Wang Shuhe in the third century.

Nan Jing (难经) (*Classic of Difficulties*), a book appeared in the first or second century B.C.. It deals with fundamental medical theories and expounds the main points of Nei Jing (The Canon of Medicine) in the form of questions and answers.

Nan Jing Ji Zhu (难经集注) (*Collection of Annotations on Classics of Difficulties*), compiled by Wang Jiusi, Wang Weiyi et al. in the 11th century.

Nei Jing (内经) (*The Canon of Medicine*), same as Huang Di Nei Jing (黄帝内经).

Shang Han Za Bing Lun (伤寒杂病论) (*Treatise on Febrile and Miscellaneous Diseases*), written by Zhang Zhongjing at the beginning of the third century. The book was rearranged by Wang Shuhe and was later divided into two books: Shang Han Lun (*Treatise on Febrile Diseases*) and Jin Gui Yao Lue Fang Lun (*Synopsis of Prescriptions of the Golden Chamber*). Both books lay the foundation of Chinese clinical medicine, particularly syndrome differentiation and treatment.

Shi Si Jing Fa Hui (十四经发挥) (*Exposition of the Fourteen Meridians*), written in 1341 by Hua Shou, who made a marked development of the meridian theory.

Yi Lin Gai Cuo (医林改错) (*Errors in Medicine Corrected*), a book written in 1830 by Wang Qingren, who insisted on making anatomical observations on internal organs of the human body. In the book the author corrected certain mistakes in the previous conceptions and suggested new methods of treating blood stasis.

Yi Guan (医贯) (*Key Link of Medicine*), a book on medical theories, written by Zhao Xianke in 1687.

YI Xue Ru Men (医学入门) (*The ABC of Medicine*) , an influential elementary book of medicine written in rhythmical prose by Li Yan in 1575.

Zhen Jing (针经) (*The Canon of Acupuncture*), another name of the book Ling Shu (*Miraculous Pivot*), one of the two parts of Nei Jing (*The Canon of Medicine*).

Zhen Jiu Jia Yi Jing (针灸甲乙经) (*ABC Classic of Acupuncture and Moxibustion*), the earliest exclusive and systemized book on acupuncture and moxibustion, written by Huangfu Mi in about 259

Zhen Jiu Feng Yuan (针灸逢源) (*Source of Acupuncture and Moxibustion*), a monograph compiled by Li Xuechuan in 1815. In the book, 361 points of the fourteen meridians and 96 extra points are listed.

INDICES

GENERAL INDEX

(Page numbers in **boldface** indicate major discussions.)

INDEX OF PINYIN NAMES OF MEDICINAL SUBSTANCES, HERBAL FORMULAS, PATENT MEDICINES AND ACUPOINTS

HERBAL FORMULAS (INCLUDING PATENT MEDICINES)

(Page numbers in **boldface** indicate major discussions.)

MEDICINAL SUBSTANCES

PINYIN NAMES OF ACUPOINTS

INDEX OF LATIN NAMES OF MEDICINAL SUBSTANCES

ACKNOWLEGEMENT

The author is indebted to Ms Li Ning, Dr Zhang Xuezhi and other colleagues of the Institute of Integration of Chinese and Western Medicine, the First Clinical Medical College of Peking University, for their kind help in preparing the relevant materials.

图书在版编目（CIP）数据
实用中医学 / 谢竹藩著. —北京：外文出版社，2000.1
ISBN 7-119-02375-6

I. 实...II. 谢... III. 中医学 IV. R2

中国版本图书馆 CIP 数据核字（2000）第 60383 号

责任编辑　徐明强　李振国
执行编辑　胡开敏
封面设计　陈　军
彩图制作　唐　宇
插图绘制　李　宁

Home Page:
http://www.flp.com.cn
Email Address:
Info@flp.com.cn
Sales@flp.com.cn

实 用 中 医 学
谢竹藩 著

*

外文出版社出版
（中国北京百万庄大街 24 号）
邮政编码 100037
中国国际图书贸易总公司发行
（中国北京车公庄西路 35 号）
北京邮政信箱第 399 号　邮政编码 100044
2000 年（16 开）第 1 版
2000 年第 1 版第 1 次印刷
（英）
ISBN 7-119-02375-6 / R・177 (外)
15000 (精)
14-E-3326S